HEALTHY DECISIONS

HEALTHY DECISIONS

Clint E. Bruess
University of Alabama at Birmingham

Glenn E. Richardson
University of Utah

Chapters 3 and 5 written by:

Susan J. Laing
Department of Veterans Affairs Medical Center
Birmingham, Alabama

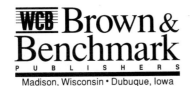
WCB Brown & Benchmark
PUBLISHERS

Madison, Wisconsin • Dubuque, Iowa

Book Team

Executive Editor *Scott Spoolman*
Developmental Editor *Susan J. Butler*
Production Editor *Debra DeBord*
Designer *Elise A. Lansdon*
Art Editor/Processor *Carla Goldhammer*
Photo Editor *Robin Storm*
Visuals/Design Developmental Consultant *Marilyn A. Phelps*
Visuals/Design Freelance Specialist *Mary I. Christianson*
Publishing Services Specialist *Sherry Padden*
Marketing Manager *Pamela S. Cooper*
Advertising Manager *Jodi Rymer*

WCB Brown & Benchmark

A Division of Wm. C. Brown Communications, Inc.

Executive Vice President/General Manager *Thomas E. Doran*
Vice President/Editor in Chief *Edgar J. Laube*
Vice President/Sales and Marketing *Eric Ziegler*
Director of Production *Vickie Putman Caughron*
Director of Custom and Electronic Publishing *Chris Rogers*

Wm. C. Brown Communications, Inc.

President and Chief Executive Officer *G. Franklin Lewis*
Corporate Senior Vice President and Chief Financial Officer *Robert Chesterman*
Corporate Senior Vice President and President of Manufacturing *Roger Meyer*

The credits section for this book begins on page 405 and is
considered an extension of the copyright page.

Copyedited by Laura Beaudoin.

Cover photo: © Lori Adamski Peek/Tony Stone Images

A Times Mirror Company

Library of Congress Catalog Card Number: 92–82966

ISBN 0–697–17043–8
        0–697–21449–4 (B/W version)

Printed in the United States of America by Wm. C. Brown Communications, Inc.,
2460 Kerper Boulevard, Dubuque, IA 52001

10 9 8 7 6 5 4 3 2 1

To Susan J. Laing, with thanks for her creative writing,
her constant support, and her role in a beautiful
relationship.

C. B.

To Kathleen, my best friend, my soul mate, for her
strength, comfort, support, and joy for living. To my
children, Brannon, Tavan, Jordan, and Lauren, my
source for playfulness, tenderness, hugs, hope for the
future, and cherished Kodak moments.

G. R.

Brief Contents

Contents

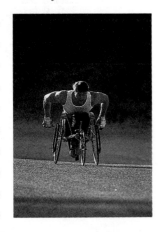

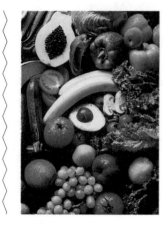
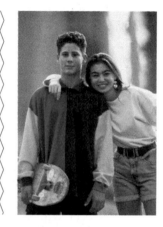

PART IV

Chemical Choices 196

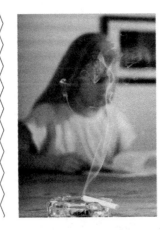

CHAPTER 9

Psychoactive Drugs 198

CHAPTER 10

Alcohol 217

CHAPTER 11

Tobacco 236

PART **V**

Choices and Disease 256

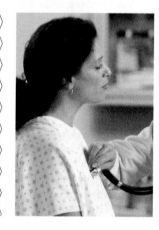

CHAPTER **12**

Communicable Diseases 258

CHAPTER **13**

**Cardiovascular, Cancer, and
Other Chronic Disease 277**

PART **VI**

*Choices and the Aging
Process 308*

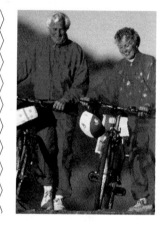

CHAPTER **14**

Aging, Death, and Dying 310

PART **VII**

*Choices and the World
Around You 334*

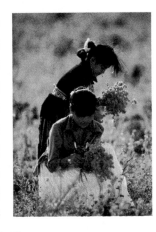

CHAPTER **15**

Environmental Health 336

CHAPTER **16**

Consumer Choices 352

Preface

Having jointly taught personal health courses at seven different colleges, we have found constant challenges. With so much ongoing research and the constant development and advocacy of new health products and services, we are challenged to provide up-to-date information about a great variety of health topics. With the many personal health students outside the typical college-age range, we are further challenged to present material on health needs and issues that arise throughout life. Finally, with the vast amount of health information, products, and services available—much of which is complex, confusing, often controversial, and even contradictory—we are challenged to provide health information within a context that leads to healthy decision making.

In *Healthy Decisions,* we have responded to these challenges just as we did in three editions of *Decisions for Health.* Although *Healthy Decisions* is shorter than *Decisions for Health,* we have still produced a text that instructors and students can use to make personal health a valuable learning experience. By providing up-to-date information, by involving the students in activities related to various health issues, and by providing a framework on which students can build sound decision-making skills, this text enables students to become informed health consumers who are also skilled decision makers.

Why Is *Healthy Decisions* Needed?

While *Decisions for Health* has been successful through three editions, in some colleges and universities there is a need for a briefer text. Perhaps a course is offered for only one or two credits, or perhaps an instructor desires to have a book that has less detail. At the same time, however, both students and instructors want to maintain an emphasis on accurate and up-to-date health knowledge, which provides the foundation for sound health decision making. In *Healthy Decisions,* we continue our tradition of accurate and up-to-date health information and maintain our unique approach to health decision making. Careful attention has been given to reducing the size and cost of the text while further enriching its key ingredients.

Organization and Emphasis

Healthy Decisions is unique in its thorough emphasis on decision making. The first chapter lays the groundwork for the development of decision-making skills, with its emphasis on total health, health behavior, and health decision making. The second chapter stresses the importance of the interdependent aspects of health. The remaining chapters build upon these themes while dealing with nutrition, physical activity, and weight-control choices; sexual choices; chemical choices; choices and disease; choices and the aging process; and choices and the world around you. The text helps the student integrate health information into an overall decision-making model. Health is primarily a product of life-styles, and students will find that they can use this text to help improve their life-styles and, hence, improve their health.

Features of *Healthy Decisions*

Students are assisted in the decision-making process by the following text features:

1. Key questions
2. Chapter outlines
3. Health assessments
4. Issue boxes
5. Information boxes
6. Health actions boxes
7. Chapter summaries

8. Commitment activities
9. Additional readings
10. Life-style contracts
11. Glossary

Key questions help students focus on the direction the chapter is going.

Chapter outlines give students an up-front overview of chapter content.

Health assessments, found at the beginning of each chapter, give the student an opportunity to assess present health status or their feelings related to health topics contained within the chapter. These were developed especially for *Healthy Decisions* and *Decisions for Health* and help the reader become personally involved in the content to follow.

Issue boxes throughout *Healthy Decisions* present opposing sides of many contemporary controversies. Consideration of these issues helps students become more involved while learning about health and health decisions.

Information boxes provide fresh information that supplements the usual material found in a personal health text and enlivens particular topics.

Health actions boxes relate to the topics within each chapter and help students consider how they can take related mental, physical, spiritual, and interdependent actions as steps to healthier living.

Chapter summaries help students recall where the chapter text has taken them.

Commitment activities are found at the end of every chapter and are designed to prompt readers to act on health problems they have studied within the chapter. It is well known that long-lasting health behavior changes are more likely to occur if learners are immediately and actively involved in appropriate positive health activities.

Additional readings provide motivated learners with sources of new information.

Life-style contracts are found at the end of each part of the text. The process of assessing health behavior, providing instruction, and then contracting for behavior changes is an appropriate formula for helping students make commitments to improve their health status. Students and instructors should pay particular attention to chapter 1, where the use of life-style contracts is described in detail.

Most researchers believe that students should effectively modify only one or two behaviors at a time. An attempt to modify numerous behaviors will likely result in frustration and failure in several areas. The purpose of the life-style contract is to allow students the chance to consider the behavioral changes that can occur with each topic area. After consideration of the assessments, and their own degrees of readiness and motivation, students may then select the areas that fit their needs and complete the life-style contracts that correspond with those areas. It is assumed that some of the contracts will be left blank and reserved for another time.

The **glossary** facilitates understanding of necessary health terminology. Terms are boldfaced within the text to alert students to their importance.

Unique Approaches to Health

Healthy Decisions is designed to provide accurate health information and promote sound health decision making. In addition, the decision-making theme is enhanced with a model for action based upon resiliency skills. As explained in the first two chapters, the model describes the process of acquiring protective skills and adjustment skills to promote cutting edge thinking in health education.

Each of the major parts of the text also contains a brief **PNI** (Psychoneuroimmunology) discussion. This relatively new and exciting area of health education research examines the way we think (*psycho*), which then affects the central nervous system (*neuro*), and in turn affects our immune system (*immunology*). These boxes invite students to better understand the relationship between the mind and the body as it relates to the topics in each part.

Supplements

A number of aids are available to help both the instructor and the student experience the best learning situation possible while using *Healthy Decisions.*

The **Instructor's Manual** promotes an optimal learning experience for students while providing an invaluable and easy-to-use resource for instructors.

The **Test Item File** to accompany *Healthy Decisions* was written exclusively for this text and consists of over one thousand objective test questions, including multiple choice, true–false, and matching questions.

The printed Test Item File is also available in Windows, Macintosh, and two DOS Graphics formats of MicroTest, a user-friendly test-generating software program produced by Chariot Software Group.

A free subscription to *The University of California–Berkeley Wellness Newsletter* is yours with adoption of this text to ensure you continue to receive the most current health information possible for your course.

The **Brown & Benchmark Personal Health Transparency Set** (revised in 1993) is available for your use with this text. *The AIDS Booklet,* Second Edition, by Frank Cox, updated semiannually, is also available with *Healthy Decisions* at your request. The **Brown & Benchmark Video Library** is another resource available to qualified adopters of *Healthy Decisions.*

If you have further questions about supplements available to you through Brown & Benchmark, feel free to contact your local sales representative or call the customer service department at 1–800–338–5371.

Acknowledgments

A number of people have contributed to the development of this book, and we would like to thank the most obvious ones. Again, we are thankful to Susan J. Laing for her overall suggestions, her writing of the chapters on nutrition and weight control, and for her creation of an outstanding Instructor's Manual.

Although Chris Rogers has gone on to higher responsibilities within the Brown & Benchmark organization, *Healthy Decisions* is a direct result of his editorial creativity and encouragement. We miss our regular interactions with him but appreciate all he did to help make our books as good as they are. Our developmental editor, Susie Butler, deserves special recognition. She inherited us and has learned to work well with us. Her thorough analysis of our work, her flexibility, and her support for what we want to do are particularly appreciated.

Our appreciation also goes to the following individuals for their review and suggestions, which helped in the development of *Healthy Decisions:*

- Norm Hoffman
  Bakersfield College
- Gaye Osborne
  Morehead State University
- Jan Mittleider
  College of Southern Idaho
- Carolyn M. Allred
  Central Piedmont Community College
- David D. Delmer
  Montgomery College
- Patricia Kenney
  Penn State University
- Silvea E. Thomas
  Kingsborough Community College of Brooklyn
- Rick Barnes
  East Carolina University
- Anita Scandurra
  Ferris State University

HEALTHY DECISIONS

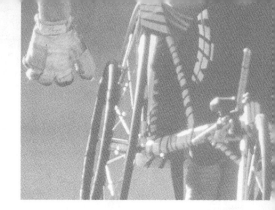

PART I

Making Healthy Choices

THE FOUNDATION FOR HEALTHY DECISIONS IS ESTABLISHED IN CHAPTER 1. A MODEL FOR ACTION IS DESCRIBED, EMPHASIZING HEALTH SKILLS, RESILIENCY, AND STRENGTH INTERVENTION. THE FIRST CHANCE TO APPLY THE MODEL IS FOUND IN CHAPTER 2. ITS FOCUS IS ON SKILLS THAT CAN HELP YOU BE MENTALLY HEALTHY, THE POINTS OF INTERVENTION FOR STRESS MANAGEMENT, AND WAYS YOU CAN EFFECTIVELY MANAGE STRESS.

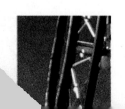

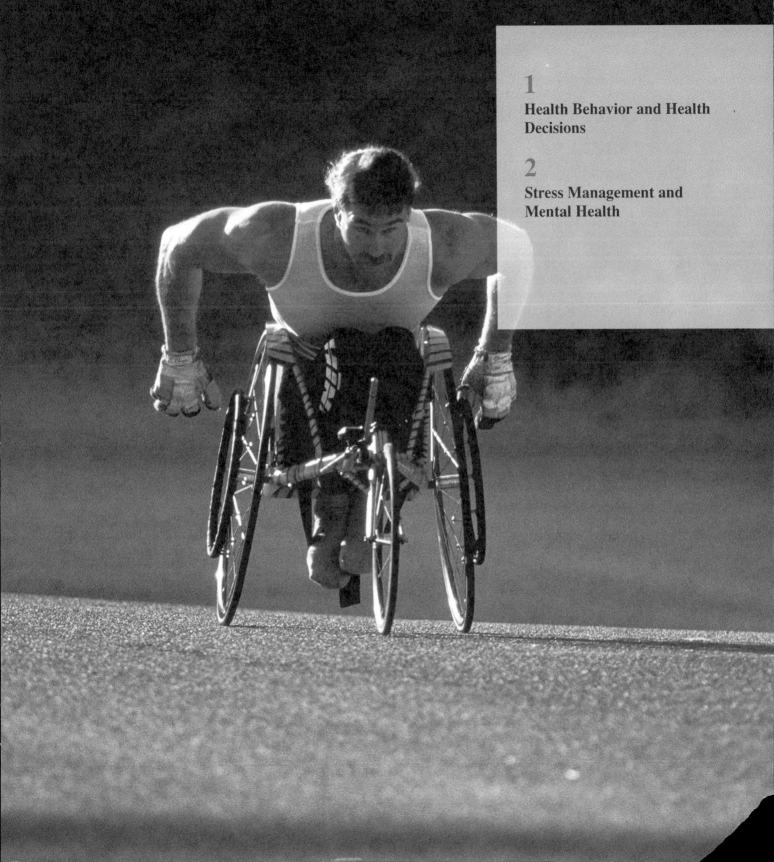

CHAPTER 1

Health Behavior and Health Decisions

Key Questions

- What is health?
- What factors influence health?
- How consistent is your health behavior?
- What motivates health behavior?
- How can you change your health behavior?
- How does one health decision affect another?
- What are the steps in health decision making?
- What factors influence health decisions?
- How can you plan to avoid poor health and strive for optimal health?
- How do strength intervention and life-style contracting work?

Chapter Outline

Each day you make decisions that affect your well-being in the days and even years to come. How can you know which choices are best? A steady stream of health information flows from many sources, and many of these sources are unreliable.

There is a national interest in health. Fitness programs for all ages and body types abound. In addition, national health promotion and disease prevention objectives have been developed by the U.S. government. The most recent edition of these objectives, *Promoting Health/Preventing Disease: Year 2000 Objectives for the Nation* (1990), contains major goals related to infant mortality, life expectancy, chronic disability, years of healthy life, and disparity in life expectancy among individuals. The government's goal of increasing years of healthy life to at least sixty-five years for all individuals is a clear indicator of our improved quality of life as well as quantity.

Despite abundant information and interest in health, surveys show that we actually know little about health. Furthermore, we have few guidelines to evaluate all the advice offered. This text provides basic information and the necessary

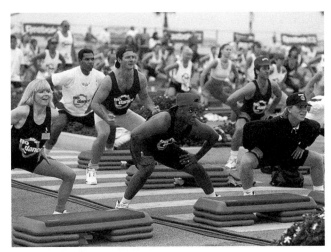

Health is a national preoccupation.

decision-making techniques to make intelligent choices about health. This first chapter explores what health means, what influences your health behavior, and health decision making.

Views of Health

Historically, various cultures have viewed health in different ways. Most views have clustered around two definitions of health: health as absence of illness and infirmity or health as a positive state of being.

Health as Absence of Illness and Infirmity

Many individuals view health as the absence of illness and infirmity (lack of vitality). According to this view, if you aren't sick, you must be healthy. At various times in history, health problems have been attributed to the gods or to unsanitary conditions. Modern medicine, however, emphasizes scientifically proven treatment with drugs and surgery and prevention of disease through vaccinations, cleanliness, and good nutrition.

Health as a Positive State of Being

Many individuals view health as not just freedom from illness but as an overall positive condition. Health consists of several different components, including mental, emotional, social, physical, occupational, and spiritual health.

Mental health is the capacity to cope with life's circumstances, to grow emotionally, to develop to our fullest potential, and to expand in awareness and consciousness. **Emotional health,** while related to mental health, is the ability to express emotions comfortably and appropriately. This might include choosing *not* to express emotions in certain situations.

Social health includes good relations with others, the presence of a supportive culture, and successful adaptation to the environment. **Physical health,** what

---

many individuals think of first when considering overall health, obviously includes efficient bodily functioning, resistance to disease, and the physical capacity to respond appropriately to varied events.

Occupational health is a more recently added component of health (Eberst 1985). It includes feelings of comfort and accomplishment related to one's daily tasks. For those employed outside the home, the aspects of a job make up occupational health. For those who work at home or remain at home for other reasons, occupational health is still a function of daily tasks. For example, you might assess this component of health by answering such questions as, Do I feel a sense of accomplishment from my daily tasks? and Am I basically happy with the way I spend most of my "occupational" time?

Spiritual health is also an important component of overall health (Bensley 1991). While spiritual health has not always been viewed as a component of health in our culture, there is increased recognition that it is significant in health-related decision making (Goodloe and Arreola 1992). Optimal spiritual health includes the ability to discover and express your purpose in life; to experience love, joy, peace, and fulfillment; and to help yourself and others achieve full potential (Chapman 1987). For some, spiritual health includes the belief in a Supreme Being, but for others this is not necessary. Spiritual health might include answers to the questions Who am I? Why am I here? and Where am I going? Complete the accompanying Health Assessment, and you will have a clearer picture of this important health component.

A continuum can be constructed for each component of health, with poor health and optimal health described for each component. While various descriptions might be used, sample continuums are found in figure 1.1.

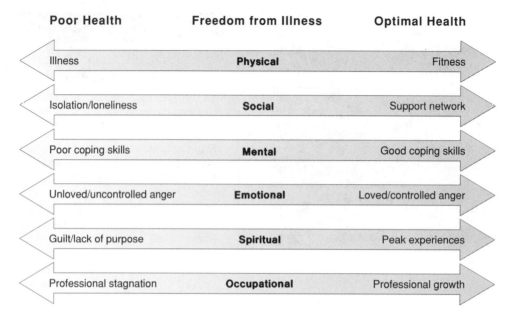

Poor Health	Freedom from Illness	Optimal Health
Illness	**Physical**	Fitness
Isolation/loneliness	**Social**	Support network
Poor coping skills	**Mental**	Good coping skills
Unloved/uncontrolled anger	**Emotional**	Loved/controlled anger
Guilt/lack of purpose	**Spiritual**	Peak experiences
Professional stagnation	**Occupational**	Professional growth

Figure 1.1

The components of health.

Though it is easier to speak separately about the components of health, they actually form a whole. The word **health,** in fact, comes from an Old English root meaning "wholeness." A change in any one of the components affects the others. For example, if your social environment subjects you to racial prejudice and discrimination, anxiety and a lowered sense of self-worth can result. This in turn can lower resistance to disease. Another example is that if your level of social health is not what you want it to be, your self-concept (part of mental health) might be influenced, and your eating and exercise patterns (part of physical health) might be altered. On the other hand, if you are pleased with your progress in a fitness program, your good feelings can have a positive impact on your self-concept and even your relationships with others. Well-being in all components is necessary for comprehensive health. The interaction of all components of health is shown in figure 1.2 on page 8.

Health is dynamic rather than static. It is constantly changing, and your choices can directly influence your level of health. Also, your health and health maintenance may differ from someone else. You and another individual may vary considerably in blood pressure, weight, and the amount of sleep you each get although you have similar diet and exercise habits. What health means, too, is likely to be different for you than for someone else. You may be content with a small circle of friends, for example, while another individual needs a variety of social interactions to consider himself or herself socially healthy.

There is increasing scientific evidence that mind-body interactions are at the root of both health and disease. Psychological factors have a role in causing the onset and course of many chronic disorders. Psychological factors

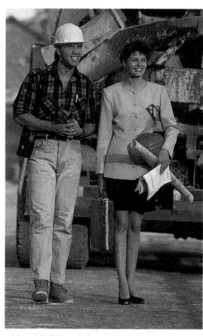

Occupational health is an important component of our overall health.

can also promote a positive state of health. In addition, psychological, emotional, psychosocial, and behavioral interventions are at least as effective as many purely medical treatments (Pelletier 1992).

There is no question that the complex interactions of the mind, body, and soul work together to influence our health. You will see many examples of such interactions in this text and throughout life.

1. Are you happy with your

   social health status? _____ yes _____ no

   physical health status? _____ yes _____ no

   emotional health status? _____ yes _____ no

   occupational health status? _____ yes _____ no

   spiritual health status? _____ yes _____ no

   mental health status? _____ yes _____ no

2. Are you motivated to enhance your health in reference to

   social health status? _____ yes _____ no

   physical health status? _____ yes _____ no

   emotional health status? _____ yes _____ no

   occupational health status? _____ yes _____ no

   spiritual health status? _____ yes _____ no

   mental health status? _____ yes _____ no

3. Are you actively doing something to improve your

   social health status? _____ yes _____ no

   physical health status? _____ yes _____ no

   emotional health status? _____ yes _____ no

   occupational health status? _____ yes _____ no

   spiritual health status? _____ yes _____ no

   mental health status? _____ yes _____ no

For the following items, mark what you would probably do in each case.

4. You are at a party, and some of your friends offer you a drug. You really don't want to try it, but they are persistent. What would you do?
   a. definitely go along with them
   b. probably go along with them
   c. probably not go along with them
   d. definitely not go along with them

5. Some of your friends are pressuring you to go to a movie that you really don't want to see or feel it is wrong to see. What would you do?
   a. definitely go along with them
   b. probably go along with them
   c. probably not go along with them
   d. definitely not go along with them

6. Some other students found an exact copy of a test you are going to take tomorrow. They want you to study the test with them, but you think it is wrong. What would you do?
   a. definitely go along with them
   b. probably go along with them
   c. probably not go along with them
   d. definitely not go along with them

7. I do those things that are consistent with what I believe.
   ____ agree   ____ disagree

8. I rarely do things that I think are morally wrong.
   ____ agree   ____ disagree

9. I behave in accordance with my value system.
   ____ yes   ____ no

10. I seem to have plenty of energy to do what I have to do.
    ____ yes   ____ no

11. I am rarely too tired to do something I want to do.
    ____ yes   ____ no

12. I have a zest for living.
    ____ yes   ____ no

Scoring/Interpretation

Questions 1–3 help you assess your motivation and pursuit of health. If you answered no to any of these questions, evaluate whether you should do something about that component of your health. One component can drag down other components, and conversely, efforts to enhance a component of health can positively affect another.

Questions 4–6 are an assessment of your peer resistance skills. Score your responses as follows:

For each *a* give yourself 1 point.
For each *b* give yourself 2 points.
For each *c* give yourself 3 points.
For each *d* give yourself 4 points.

A score of 10 or more points indicates good peer resistance skills. A score of 7–9 points indicates moderate peer resistance skills. A score of 6 or less points indicates poor peer resistance skills.

Questions 7–9 assess whether your behaviors are consistent with your value system. An answer of no to any of these questions might suggest conflict between what you believe is right and what you are doing, resulting in guilt. Congruence between these two important dimensions of health is important for happiness.

Questions 10–12 assess your energy level and quality of life. Positive responses indicate a zest for living and the energy to live life to the fullest. Negative responses indicate that you should do something to find that zest. The chapters in this text will give you some suggestions to find increased energy.

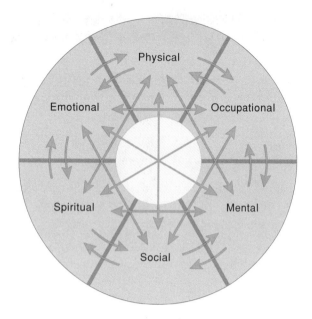

Figure 1.2
Interaction of all health components.

Health for What?

Good health is essential to a good quality of life. To enjoy life more, to be more productive in life's activities, and to live at a higher level of existence are the primary reasons for pursuing good health.

Health and Life-Style

Not long ago, the greatest strides in improving human health were made by individuals doing something for others, such as digging city sewer systems and developing vaccines for diseases. There is still much to be done, but in the industrialized world at least, the greatest future improvements in individual health will come from actions people take for themselves.

Many current Western health problems are actually self-inflicted. Lung cancer and various circulatory ailments often result from an individual's choice to smoke cigarettes. Degeneration of circulatory and respiratory systems is often traced to a lifetime of relative physical inactivity.

Life-style, that is, your customary pattern of behavior, dramatically affects your health. Your decisions concerning personal care, drugs, sexual relations, and other health-related matters may help or hinder you throughout your life.

Control and Responsibility

Clearly, some factors that influence the length or quality of life, such as gender at birth and the health history of your ancestors, are completely out of your control. Other factors, such as where you live, the quality of drinking water, and the kind of work you do now or in the future, *may* be within your control to change, depending on your age, the

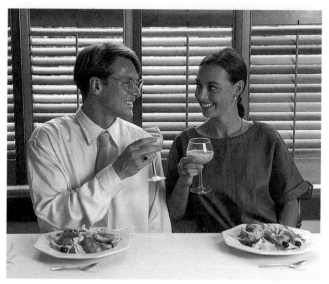

Your decisions probably influence your health more than anything else.

amount of money you have, and other circumstances. Many health-related factors clearly *are* within control—such as what you eat and whether you smoke, take sleeping pills nightly, exercise regularly, practice stress management, or drink heavily. It may also be possible to reduce the risk from factors that cannot be changed, such as heredity, if you understand how these factors affect well-being. For example, if early death due to stroke runs in your family, your life-style can be altered to reduce the likelihood of stroke, thereby increasing life expectancy.

Many experts believe the next major health revolution in the United States will be a direct result of improved life-styles. To develop a healthier life-style, you need (1) an awareness of present patterns of behavior and their health consequences, (2) adequate health knowledge, and (3) the capacity to make intelligent decisions about health issues based on this knowledge and self-awareness. One example of the direct effects of these three factors is the reduction in cardiovascular disease in the United States in the past twenty years. Many individuals have learned how their behavior patterns influence the development of this disease. They have acquired sound knowledge about the disease and made more intelligent decisions to reduce the likelihood of developing it.

Consistent Health Behavior

Most people are inconsistent in their health behaviors. They may exercise regularly but go years without a physical examination. Others are critical of marijuana smokers but regularly overindulge in alcohol. Still others take pride in shopping wisely for health products but fail to use the same consumer skills when making other health decisions.

Do such inconsistencies mean that we really don't value our health? Sometimes. But to conclude that someone doesn't value health because health behavior is inconsistent ignores the fact that good health is not always an individual's priority. For example, a woman who runs into a burning building is more concerned with saving the life of a family member than with risking her own health.

We often do things that affect health positively or negatively, though the motivation may not be health related. For example, a man may follow good dental practices just to look more attractive or eat certain foods for taste and appearance rather than nutritional value.

Sometimes motivation conflicts with the desire for health and well-being. For example, a woman may want to have sexual intercourse but also fear an unwanted pregnancy. While not all activities need be health oriented, understanding the motivation and the health-related consequences of behavior can help you plan more effectively for future well-being.

Motivations for Health Behavior

Motivation is the psychological force that prods you to act. Actions are influenced by many factors. For example, you may delay seeking medical attention because you suspect your symptoms are a sign of something quite serious. Fear about health can prevent individuals from acquiring information needed to make sound decisions and from facing health problems in a rational and constructive way (Price, Galli, and Slenker 1985). As complicated as motivation for health behavior can be, four main motivations underlie most health behavior: social pressure, health habits, attitudes and values, and knowledge.

Social Pressure

Actions taken to look more masculine or feminine, to gain praise or avoid embarrassment, or to appear more mature are all motivated by **social pressure**—that is, by the desire or belief that you need to go along with or rebel against others' actions or expectations. Because we are social animals, thoughts and actions are heavily influenced by the opinions and actions of others, particularly those of peers (social equals).

Our actions, then, are strongly influenced by our perceptions of how often family, friends, and associates engage in a particular type of health behavior (i.e., its social acceptability). Peer and family influence can be an important tool in promoting health (Norman 1987). One good example of how social pressure has changed attitudes and behavior is drinking and driving. Alcohol-related fatalities used to be considered accidents. Today, there is a tendency to view them as a result of criminal or immoral behavior.

Health Habits

When an action is performed routinely and without thought, it becomes a **habit.** Actions that affect health often result from habits developed as a result of social or parental pressure. Most children, for example, began to brush their teeth nightly because their parents insisted. Many began to smoke because they desired acceptance from an admired family member or friend who smoked.

The more an act is repeated, the easier it becomes, and the more comfortable and self-assured you feel. As habits become increasingly ingrained, you may forget both the original reasons for doing them and their potential health effects.

Attitudes and Values

Attitudes and **values** influence health behavior in many ways. Attitudes are feelings about facts and behaviors. Values are ideas we believe in and cherish. You might engage in some practices, such as running, reading, or eating sweets, purely for pleasure. These activities may have beneficial, harmful, or no real consequences for health. You might engage in or avoid other behaviors because of personal or religious values. Your values may dictate whether or not you choose to become a vegetarian or to smoke, drink, or have premarital sexual activity. It is clear that the values we place on health do influence specific health behaviors (Abood and Conway 1992).

Health-related behavior may also reflect specific attitudes toward health. Have you ever been in excellent physical condition and run, swam, or done some other physical activity relatively easily for long periods of time? If so, you probably also know that it feels great to be in good shape. This feeling can influence your attitude toward a physically active life-style. Not knowing this sensation can have the opposite effect.

If we fail to recognize the influence of health behaviors on our present and future health, we are again viewing health in a very limited fashion—simply the absence of disease. If, on the other hand, our attitudes and values cause us to prevent health problems and promote positive health by making wise health decisions today, we are consciously considering the consequences of our health behaviors.

Knowledge

Though we may not always act as reasonably as we could, we are not simply the victims of emotions, habits, and environmental influences. We take action or avoid action mainly because we are aware of the health benefits or risks. For instance, you might take certain vitamins, refuse to ride with a drunk driver, and get periodic physical checkups.

Because individuals seem most at ease when what they know is consistent with their attitudes and values, we often seek information to support personal attitudes while ignoring information that does not. This tendency takes effort to overcome. We find many reasons to ignore information we receive. Instead, we tend to respond to knowledge only when it becomes important to us. For example, some individuals pay no attention to salt intake until they develop high blood pressure. This discrepancy between personal health behavior and general health knowledge is one of the most publicized dilemmas in the field of health education (Hamrick, Anspaugh, and Smith 1980).

Motivations for health behavior can be complex. When an individual wants to change behavior, social pressures, health habits, attitudes and values, and knowledge about the health behavior need to be considered. For example, if you want to quit smoking, you must consider role models and possible sources of support; when, where, and why you have the habit of lighting a cigarette; personal values and reasons for quitting; and what is known about the benefits of being a nonsmoker. The chances of successfully changing a health behavior increase dramatically when you adopt an approach that considers your motivations.

It all boils down to making decisions that improve health and enhance well-being. Your view of what health means, your reasons for valuing a healthy life-style, and your motivations in choosing health behaviors are all components of the health choices you make. Let's look more closely at how we can make better health-related decisions and put them into practice.

Decision Making: A Systematic Approach

No one can make you do anything about the quality of your life-style—except you. Each day you make decisions that affect your health. When a decision is made, it often affects other decisions. There might even be a series of needed decisions—each decision might influence the next one. Even our friends in the comics are faced with this dilemma, as shown vividly by Calvin and Hobbes.

A **decision tree** diagrams the possible choices and steps in decision making. Figure 1.3 illustrates the choices and steps that might be used when deciding whether to drink alcohol. Even this simple example shows that health decisions are often quite complex.

You can have greater control over personal health if you understand how decisions are made and what influences

them. To facilitate this, we now look at how to make decisions and then at what is needed to put these decisions into practice.

Taking an active role in immediate and long-term personal well-being is a four-stage process of thought and action. These stages are (1) *recognition* of a health-related problem; (2) *evaluation* of alternative courses of action; (3) *implementation* of the course decided on; and (4) *review* of the decision.

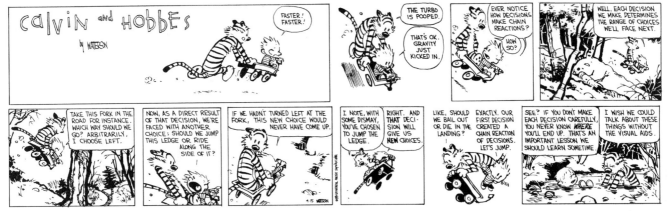

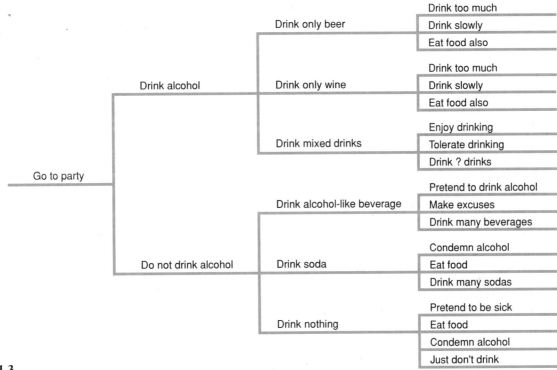

Figure 1.3

A decision tree: deciding whether to use alcohol at a party.

Recognition

Only when we recognize that there is a problem to be solved or a goal to be reached can a conscious decision be made. If you drink alcohol or smoke cigarettes, for example, you may decide whether or not to quit when friends quit, when you read an article on the physical dangers of smoking or drinking, or when you feel negative physical effects. Or, perhaps you feel a need to begin an exercise program because of changes in your physical appearance or your ability to run around with young children. To make the best decision, the issue to be resolved or the goal to be reached should be defined as precisely as possible. For example, does "drinking" include beer and caffeinated drinks? Does "smoking" mean marijuana as well as tobacco? What would be the purpose of the fitness program?

Evaluation

Having recognized the need to make a decision, it is time to gather relevant information, analyze the possible choices, and decide on the best alternative. For example, the decision could be to drink wine only with dinner guests or not to drink before a long commute. The decision might be to stop smoking altogether or to set aside time each day for a fitness program.

1. **Recognition**—Perhaps a physically inactive person becomes concerned about his or her lack of exercise. This could result from increased knowledge about the health benefits of physical activity, the influence of a friend, or numerous other factors. For whatever reason, the need to develop a personal activity program is recognized.

2. **Evaluation**—Then the person needs information, such as the effects of different types of exercise on the body, possible exercise programs available, facilities close to home, cautions to keep in mind, etc. The available choices need to be evaluated so the best alternative can be selected.

3. **Implementation**—Once the best alternative is chosen, it is put into action. Many factors needing consideration are mentioned later in this chapter. Steps that need to be taken and personal, social, and other characteristics that influence the implementation of an exercise program also need attention.

4. **Review**—After giving the exercise program a fair chance, it is appropriate to analyze it to be sure it is working as desired. Are results being achieved? Is the program satisfactory? Should other factors or alternatives be considered? If things are going well, then the exercise program should be continued. If not, perhaps steps 2 and 3 need to be used again to look at other possible alternatives.

Implementation

Once a decision is reached based on analysis and learning, it is time to put it into practice. In the case of alcohol consumption or cigarette addiction, the decision might be to quit outright or to cut down gradually. If fitness is the goal, changes in daily habits may be needed. In these cases, only personal behavior is being altered. In other health matters, however, it may be concluded that the environment also must be changed to have a healthier life. Suppose, for example, you live near a chemical plant whose waste is polluting streams and seeping into the water supply. If you decide not to move, talking to neighbors and petitioning officials to halt the pollution are two possible courses of action.

Review

After putting your decision into practice, a periodic review is needed. Are desired results being achieved, or should another alternative be tried? You may decide to quit alcohol or cigarettes completely instead of just cutting down. Or, perhaps you decide to try different exercises as part of a fitness program.

Perhaps after making your decision, you learn something new that raises questions about your choice. If so, start the decision-making process again. In fact, according to different circumstances, many of your choices will require you to rethink your decision. Personal and group values will also strongly influence your decisions.

The major influences on decision making are the same ones that affect health behavior in general: social pressure, health habits, attitudes and values, and knowledge. For example, a man might reluctantly decide to sniff cocaine at a party because of friends' urging (social pressure) and because their acceptance is desired. Or, a woman might decide to eat junk food, for instance, simply because that is what she usually has for dinner (habit).

Attitudes about disobeying the law can influence whether an individual drinks when underage. Also, a woman who knows little about prenatal care (knowledge) may make an uninformed and potentially disastrous decision to take certain drugs.

Research is lacking on exactly why some individuals are more likely to behave in ways that promote their health. It does seem, however, that those with more positive behaviors feel better about themselves, their bodies, their appearance, and their feelings of moral and personal worth (Bergmann & Greenberg 1991).

A Model for Action

To better understand health decision making, a model that describes the process of preventing poor health and striving for optimal health may help (Richardson et al. 1990). To simplify the model, we will view life like a game of golf. The golfer often practices hard to become skillful. There are obstacles (sand traps, water hazards, etc.) and problems (wind, leaves, hills, etc.), however, and the golfer must contend with these during the game. The golfer's skills, and the way in which problems are handled, directly influence the quality of the golf game. So it is with health decisions and life.

The mind and body strive to remain balanced. Examples of balance can be found related to all health components. For example, when biological functioning varies from normal, the body's mechanisms try to regain balance. When psychological functioning is out of balance (e.g., uncontrolled anger), you can initiate ways to return to a balanced state. The mechanism may be socially appropriate (vigorous exercise, relaxation techniques) or inappropriate (violence, property destruction), but over time you can usually revert to a balanced (unangered) state.

How can you tell a good decision from a bad one? Unfortunately, there is no simple standard. You cannot judge by the chosen behavior alone, because a practice that is good for one person or group may not be good for another. Should you have an affair outside of marriage? You might answer this question very differently if you lived in the Muslim world, where the consequences of an affair are often much more severe than in the United States. Similarly, we might judge the decision by a seventy-year-old person to continue smoking as reasonable but the same decision by a pregnant woman as thoughtless.

The best preliminary way to judge the quality of a decision is to assess carefully the process used in arriving at it. Here is a helpful checklist:

1. Have I fairly examined all the alternatives?

2. Have I examined all the relevant information, not just the information I wanted to hear?

3. Have I considered all the probable consequences of my decision, including non–health-related consequences?

4. Am I being realistic about my chances of success with this choice?

5. Can I feel comfortable with this decision in the future? Does my chosen course of action fit with my values and goals in life, or am I simply responding to social pressure or habit?

6. Am I willing to put the effort into making this decision work?

Once you have implemented your decision, as suggested earlier, you should review whether your course is still appropriate and working successfully.

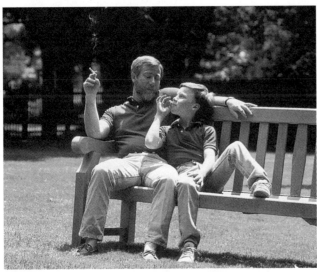
Observing others can influence health behavior.

Spiritual balance can best be viewed as a blending of values and behavior. It exists when you choose a value or belief system that provides guidelines for living and then abide by that system. If blending does not occur between values and behavior, imbalance of the spiritual component of health results. This can cause guilt, for example, which subsides when values and behavior are again aligned.

Life Event Reactions and Skills

As we mentioned, as golfers follow a course, challenges and stressors appear in many forms, such as sand traps, lakes, hills, and even noise. This happens in life, also, as we encounter various experiences, stressors, challenges, and risks. These are referred to as **life events.** They are the many positive and negative influences that may cause disruption or changes. Life events may result in pressure to engage in addictive behaviors (such as excessive television watching, use of chemical substances to try to maintain balance, food misuse, or inappropriate sexual behavior).

How well you handle life events, just as how well golfers handle problems on the course, determines how healthy you are. The more skilled golfer usually has a better score (in golf a better score is a lower score), and the more skilled individual has better health and handles problems in a more positive way. Understanding protective skills, negotiation, disruption, disorganization, and adjustment skills is basic to health promotion.

Protective Skills

Well-developed golf skills assist golfers in obtaining a better score. Golfers can protect themselves from potential problems by learning how to deal with these problems before they occur. Certain **protective skills** also prepare individuals to deal with life's problems while promoting higher levels of health. For example, certain protective skills can be learned to enhance such biological factors as overall medical condition, tolerance for pain, healing capabilities, fitness level, and state of fatigue. Protective skills might be enhanced by exercise, rest, meditation, proper nutrition, and avoidance of harmful substances.

Additional skills to help protect individuals are explained throughout this text. Examples are stress management skills, decision-making skills, and value/behavioral congruence. Not all skills are necessary at all times, but some must be functional to provide at least minimal protection.

Negotiation

Golfers use their skills to negotiate (deal with) problems as they develop. Skill with different clubs or in difficult situations (e.g., next to a tree) is often needed. We must also develop skills to negotiate life events. Which negotiating mechanism or stress-management technique is best depends on the nature of the life event and its effect. For example, you might find that ignoring an individual with a negative attitude might be the best tactic; however, another person might choose to use a different method, such as talking with the individual and finding a way to deal with his or her problem. You may negotiate easily or have difficulty dealing with problems. If there is much difficulty, it is probable that disruption will be experienced.

Disruption

Golfers who lose concentration, become angry, or perhaps experience fatigue have problems shooting a good score. They are disrupted and actually out of balance with what it takes to play good golf. The long-term effect of the **disruption** could be positive or negative. For example, perhaps next time a golfer will know how to better deal with anger so it does not cause disruption. On the other hand, a negative result could be that the golfer stops trying because her anger ruins her golf game.

Flach (1989) suggests that experiencing disruption in life can be beneficial. Although the pain of being out of balance is unpleasant, disruption can be part of a process that enhances **resiliency.** The person can become better skilled, better able to bounce back from problems, and stronger next time. For example, if you fear certain social situations, you might become more resilient by participating in such situations and finding ways to be successful in them. Disruption forces the resilient individual to look inward, adapt to life events, and possibly develop new skills.

Disruption can be an opportunity to grow and learn. While the mechanism is certainly different, an analogy can be drawn to muscle development. After strenuous exercise, muscles are fatigued and "torn down." Although the individual is initially weaker and exhausted, the body responds. Through a rebuilding process, muscles become a little stronger than before the exercise experience. The results of enhancing psychological and/or spiritual resiliency are not as predictable as muscle development from a time perspective, but recovery and growth are inevitable for the resilient person.

Many individuals take on challenges because they know they are growth opportunities. Golfers often like to play new and difficult courses just for the challenge. A disruption is not necessarily negative. It may be an exciting opportunity to accomplish something. Sometimes disorganization occurs, however, and this can also help individuals effectively face the challenge.

Disorganization

Disorganization is a temporary state when one or more of the components of health become disrupted. Perhaps a new challenge requires you to formulate a plan without the benefit of previous related experiences. This can cause a state of disorganization. Or there may be complete collapse of your view of the world, such as with the death of someone close. This might necessitate building a new support system, establishing a new social life, or making other major adjustments. The part of life that is most affected by the life event must become disorganized in order to create a place for the new.

Golfers who undergo a slump may, for a time, lose their skills and become disorganized or be unable to pull their games together. To remedy this problem, they may need to rethink the way they play the game and adopt a whole new approach to golf.

Individuals do not usually stay in a state of disorganization for long. A new state of balance must be established in order to function. To do this, you might think about what you experienced and how you might avoid the problem next time. Attempts to return to balance ideally result in positive adjustment.

Adjustment Skills

Adjustment is the process of returning to balance. It can involve creatively putting your life back together or recovering through systematic problem solving. Golfers in a difficult position behind a tree must solve the problem quickly and take action based on skills and past experiences. The process of adjustment in life may take a few minutes or several years, depending on the severity of the life event and the adjustment capacity of the individual.

Adjustments to Promote Health and Prevent Problems

Whether you are trying to improve your level of health or prevent potential health problems, there are four basic ways to adjust to life events. Continuing with the golf analogy, a comparison of golf scores is appropriate. For those nongolfers, a score of par on a hole is generally considered good. One stroke below par is called a birdie, one stroke above par is called a bogey, and two strokes above par is called a double bogey. Obviously, birdies and pars help the golf score more than bogeys and double bogeys. Here is a comparison between golf scores and ways to deal with disorganization:

1. resilient adjustment = birdie
2. balanced adjustment = par
3. faulty adjustment = bogey
4. problematic adjustment = double bogey

Resilient Adjustment

Resilient adjustment (a birdie—a fine golf score) is the optimal type of adaptation. Golfers may have a badly misplaced shot. But because they stay calm, keep a good mental outlook, and wisely apply their skills, they are able to recover and make up for the bad shot. They return to their normally high level of play and *learn something in the process.*

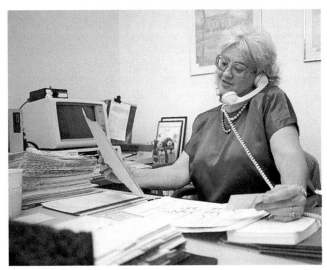
The resilient person manages life events and learns from them.

The key is to benefit from all that a life event offers. While adjusting, we learn new skills, gain more self-understanding, and better comprehend personal, social, and environmental influences. Through the experience, resilient individuals put life back together in a way that results in more protective skills to adjust to future life events. For example, perhaps the next time you experience problems with personal relationships, you will know new ways to work them out.

Balanced Adjustment

Balanced adjustment (a par—good golf score, but not one that benefits future adjustment as much as a birdie) means returning to the same level of functioning that existed prior to the life event. A golfer might get into trouble with a bad stroke, such as hitting into a sand trap. She might be able to deal with it and return to her previous level of play. But, she may make the same mistake again because she has not added to her understanding or variety of skills.

Those who return to the same level do not learn from their experiences and will likely have similar problems until they learn from the life event. For example, an individual who has difficulty controlling body weight might lose weight in a weight-control program but not learn how to prevent the problem from occurring again. The same reasons for failure are likely to come up repeatedly.

Faulty Adjustment

Faulty adjustment (a bogey—not a score that makes a good golfer happy) results when the impact of the life event is so great that the individual has fewer protective skills than before the event. A golfer might make a mistake and take several strokes to make up for it. The game suffers for the next several holes, because the golfer loses concentration and confidence.

In the face of failure, there may be a loss of self-esteem, of a sense of adventure, or of high expectations. Generally, the person makes a minimal attempt at balanced adjustment but ultimately becomes resigned to a lower level of functioning. It is as if the person thinks it is not possible to get pars and birdies and must settle for bogeys.

Many health topics discussed throughout this text relate to faulty adjustment. For example, some experience problems with alcohol, tobacco, life-style diseases, obesity, or sexuality. If the problems are life threatening or cause dysfunctions, there may be problematic adjustment.

Problematic Adjustment

Problematic adjustment (a double bogey—a score that tends to ruin the total golf score for good golfers) reflects the need for psychotherapy. A golfer might encounter a problem and be unable to cope successfully with it. Not only is the score ruined for the day, but the golfer goes into a slump: he has problem after problem with all his golf game. He develops bad habits that actually prevent him from playing golf successfully. He stalks off the course in disgust—whacking the ball into a tree on purpose because of frustration. His only hope might be getting professional help to straighten out his game.

Individuals demonstrate problematic adjustment to life events by abusing chemical substances, exhibiting violent behaviors, threatening or even attempting suicide, showing difficulty controlling behaviors, and becoming antisocial. For example, trying to escape reality with excessive use of alcohol or other drugs or losing your temper for no reason are signs of problematic adjustment.

The model for the prevention of health problems is illustrated in figure 1.4. Individuals are represented in the circles as negotiating with life events, going through disruption and disorganization, and then adjusting in one of four ways. The promotion of optimal health and the prevention of health problems involve the same steps. Wise health decisions, influenced by many factors, result in an increase in the ability to deal with life events.

Strength Intervention and Life-Style Contracting

The focus of this text is on achieving a high level of health rather than on health problems. Emphasizing strengths is a powerful way to help make health decisions that promote optimal health and, at the same time, makes it easier to continue implementing these decisions. This emphasis on strengths is basic to an understanding of how to make better health decisions (Richardson and Berry 1987).

Strength intervention means influencing health behavior by building on existing strengths. It is the basis for the remainder of this chapter, which focuses on **life-style contracting** (making a personal plan for improving health behaviors) as an important way to improve health.

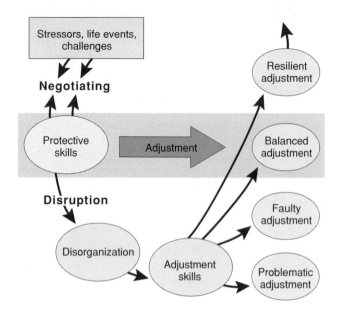

Figure 1.4

A model for preventing health problems.

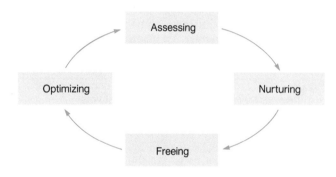

Figure 1.5

Stages of strength intervention.

To use this method it is first necessary to understand the four stages of strength intervention: assessing, nurturing, freeing, and optimizing (fig. 1.5).

Assessing means determining personal strengths, motivations, existing support systems, barriers to life-style change, and factors determining comfort and happiness. **Nurturing** means giving care and attention to the factors that produce strength in life. Remember the concept of total health and the interaction of all components of health (see fig.1.1), and note that building strengths in one health area (such as physical) can positively affect another health area (such as mental). Focusing on strengths provides a boost in other areas of life.

Freeing means achieving freedom from disabling habits. At the negative end of the continuum for each component of health, a burden is implied. Although subject to individual interpretation, the disability end of the spiritual component could be defined as guilt. One might

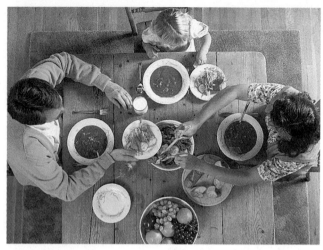

Everyone has areas of strength on which to build healthy behaviors.

believe a set of values is right, for example, but behave differently than those values dictate. Freedom can be conceptualized with any health risk factor. It might include liberation from the effects of such factors as distress, hate, excess weight, or tobacco.

Optimizing means striving to reach high-level health in one health component at a time. This means incorporating positive health behaviors. For example, you might focus on joy in the workplace to improve occupational health.

Assessing personal strengths is a logical start when considering health behavior change. Complete the Health Assessment before continuing.

Life-style contracting is used throughout this text to help you consider health decisions that might alter behaviors and improve your health. Life-style contracting is a systematic approach to making a commitment to life-style change. Strength intervention seems to be the most pleasant and effective approach to life-style contracting.

A life-style contract is shown in figure 1.6. Refer to this figure as we discuss the various parts of the contract. You will choose the areas in which your health most needs improvement and do life-style contracts in those areas. For example, you might want to stop smoking, lose weight, and manage stress better. Another person might prefer to improve communication skills and nutritional practices.

Select a behavior you want to change. You will combine the concept of strength intervention with the results of your health assessments. The first factor to consider (part I.A of the life-style contract) is whether the strength area needs *nurturing*. If you feel the necessary strength, comfort, and support are being provided, go on to *freeing* and *optimizing*. Those areas that represent either freeing or optimizing factors should be identified, with consideration given to those that appear to be beneficial to your health.

The most vital decision-making assessment is the identification of individual **motivation.** It is better to work on something you want to work on and build on the success for future behaviors. Building on the success of

Personal Strengths

1. List those now living who consistently make you the happiest and give you the most support, strength, or comfort.

   a. _____

   b. _____

   c. _____

   d. _____

2. List, in order, the specific activities (types of exercising, recreating, reading, visiting, and so on) that make you the happiest or make you feel good.

   a. _____

   b. _____

   c. _____

   d. _____

3. When you were younger, what activities gave you strength, comfort, happiness, or support? Reflect on one of several ages. Select those things from the list that you do not do now (e.g., listening to music with friends, going to movies, dancing, camping, going on trips by yourself).

   a. _____

   b. _____

   c. _____

   d. _____

4. Describe some elements of an ideal or fantasy day that you could have if you had no responsibilities or commitments but yet are within moral and financial limitations.

   a. _____

   b. _____

   c. _____

   d. _____

Apperception (Building on Earlier Success)

5. Reflect for a moment over the past several years and write down any habit you broke, any habit you intentionally started, or any behavior you modified and were able to continue to the present. Check any of the following items or write some that are not listed.

   ____ stopped smoking

   ____ lost weight

   ____ began an exercise program

   ____ improved a relationship with someone

   ____ improved my diet

   ____ stopped eating so many sweets

   ____ started using time management or organized my day better

   ____ stopped drinking (or excessive drinking)

   ____ began to give more time to loved ones or friends

   ____ became less moody

   ____ others (list) _____

   _____

6. If you were able to answer item 5, identify which of the following approaches you used (mark as many as apply).

   ____ family support

   ____ friend(s) support

   ____ read some material on it and did it myself

   ____ just made up my mind to do it

   ____ got professional help

   ____ made it part of the enjoyable things I do

   ____ my physician (health professional) told me to do it

   ____ I felt the time had come to make the change

   ____ others (list) _____

   _____

7. The reason I changed a habit in the past was

   ____ I just felt ready to change.

   ____ I was motivated to change.

   ____ there was an incentive for me to change.

   ____ the idea of a change seemed fun.

   ____ I was challenged by the idea of changing.

   ____ I was encouraged by significant people in my life.

   ____ I had a positive attitude about the change.

   ____ others (list) _____

   _____

8. The reason I chose the habit I chose was because (please check all appropriate responses)

   ____ I knew I would feel better if I changed this habit.

   ____ an important person in my life helped me select this behavior.

   ____ it was something I always wanted to change.

   ____ I kept hearing about it from the media or other sources.

   ____ others (list) _____

   _____

Locus of Control (Control Over Your Health)

9. My health status is determined mostly by how I live.

    ____ agree   ____ not sure   ____ disagree

10. How I feel is determined mostly by how my doctor and other health professionals care for me.

    ____ agree   ____ not sure   ____ disagree

11. Whether I get sick or not is a matter of good or bad luck.

    ____ agree   ____ not sure   ____ disagree

12. I am in control of my health.

    ____ agree   ____ not sure   ____ disagree

13. If I actively do things to improve my health, I will undoubtedly feel better.

    ____ agree   ____ not sure   ____ disagree

14. Whether I am sick or well has little to do with how I live.

    ____ agree   ____ not sure   ____ disagree

Scoring/Interpretation

Most of the Health Assessments in this text are to help you complete a life-style contract, which is explained in this chapter. Questions 1–4 help you reflect on areas of personal strength. Questions 5–8 help you consider past successes in changing a health behavior. Using the same principles and methods you used to change past behavior helps you plan your current health challenge.

Questions 9–14 help determine your perspective of control over your health or health locus of control. Score as follows:

Questions 9, 12, and 13	*Questions 10, 11, and 14*
agree = 3 points	agree = 1 point
not sure = 2 points	not sure = 2 points
disagree = 1 point	disagree = 3 points

Total your points. The following is an interpretation of your score.

14–16 points: You perceive yourself as in control of your health status.

11–13 points: You perceive yourself as in moderate control of your health and some control by those around you or chance.

below 11 points: You perceive yourself as a product of your environment or your health is controlled by chance or other people.

The life-style analysis form is to help you plan your behavior change project. You can look at this tool to determine where you can incorporate positive behaviors into your life-style.

Life-Style Analysis

Directions: Take a day that could be labeled typical for you. A generally stressful day should be the typical day you reflect on. As best you can, note the activities you do during different times of the day. Indicate the periods when you eat, sleep, drive, work, recreate, watch television, take breaks during work, socialize, and so on until another activity is listed. For example, if you generally go to sleep at 11:00 P.M. and wake up at 6:30 A.M., you need only write sleep once at 11:00 P.M. and then write your next activity at 6:30 A.M.

12:00 (noon) _____

:15 _____

:30 _____

:45 _____

1:00 P.M. _____

:15 _____

:30 _____

:45 _____

2:00 P.M. _____

:15 _____

:30 _____

:45 _____

3:00 P.M. _____

:15 _____

:30 _____

:45 _____

4:00 P.M. _____

:15 _____

:30 _____

:45 _____

5:00 P.M. _____

:15 _____

:30 _____

:45 _____

6:00 P.M. _____

:15 _____

:30 _____

:45 _____

7:00 P.M.	_____	:30	_____
:15	_____	:45	_____
:30	_____	4:00 A.M.	_____
:45	_____	:15	_____
8:00 P.M.	_____	:30	_____
:15	_____	:45	_____
:30	_____	5:00 A.M.	_____
:45	_____	:15	_____
9:00 P.M.	_____	:30	_____
:15	_____	:45	_____
:30	_____	6:00 A.M.	_____
:45	_____	:15	_____
10:00 P.M.	_____	:30	_____
:15	_____	:45	_____
:30	_____	7:00 A.M.	_____
:45	_____	:15	_____
11:00 P.M.	_____	:30	_____
:15	_____	:45	_____
:30	_____	8:00 A.M.	_____
:45	_____	:15	_____
12:00 (midnight)	_____	:30	_____
:15	_____	:45	_____
:30	_____	9:00 A.M.	_____
:45	_____	:15	_____
1:00 A.M.	_____	:30	_____
:15	_____	:45	_____
:30	_____	10:00 A.M.	_____
:45	_____	:15	_____
2:00 A.M.	_____	:30	_____
:15	_____	:45	_____
:30	_____	11:00 A.M.	_____
:45	_____	:15	_____
3:00 A.M.	_____	:30	_____
:15	_____	:45	_____

```
┌─────────────────────────────────────────────────────────────────────────────────────┐
│                    ◆  Life-Style Contracting Using Strength Intervention  ◆            │
│                                                                                       │
│  I. Behavioral selection                          III. Support groups                 │
│     A. Factors to consider before making               A. Who _____│
│        a behavioral selection                             _____│
│        1. Nurturing _____               _____│
│        2. Freeing _____            B. Role _____│
│        3. Optimizing _____               _____│
│        4. Motivation/readiness _____            C. Organized support _____│
│        5. Apperception _____               _____│
│        6. Barriers to change_____                _____│
│     B. Behaviors I will change (no more than two) IV. Trigger responses _____│
│        _____           _____│
│        _____           _____│
│                                                    V. Starting date _____│
│  II. The plan                                     VI. Date/sequence the contract       │
│     A. General plan _____           will be reevaluated _____│
│        _____           _____│
│     B. Substitution _____      VII. Evidences of reaching goal _____│
│        _____           _____│
│     C. Confluence _____     VIII. Rewards when contract is          │
│        _____           completed _____│
│     D. Systematic enhancement _____           _____│
│        _____      IX. Signature of client _____│
│     E. When _____       X. Signature of facilitator _____│
│     F. Where _____       XI. Additional conditions/comments: _│
│     G. Intensity _____           _____│
│     H. Preparation _____           _____│
│        _____                                           │
│     I. With whom _____                                           │
└─────────────────────────────────────────────────────────────────────────────────────┘
```

Figure 1.6

Life-style contract.

earlier experience is referred to as **apperception.** Perhaps you have been successful in solving health-related problems. From these successes you can derive methods and procedures that might apply to the current behavior changes desired. In addition, successes with simpler problems can help build the confidence needed when dealing with more difficult problems. (It might be helpful to again look at items 5–8 in the Health Assessment on page 17, since those items deal with apperception.)

Barriers to change (part I.A.6 in fig. 1.6) should also be considered. Finances, working hours, social support (or lack of it), or other reasons may dictate that a different behavior be selected or modified based on feasibility.

Most behavior change specialists recommend contracting for no more than one or two behaviors at a time. Attempting to change several behaviors at one time generally builds failure into the life-style contract. It might be possible to contract for more than two behaviors if they are closely related, such as weight control, fitness, stress control, and nutritional practices; however, this should be done only with extreme caution.

While formulating a general plan (part II.A), it is important to be detailed to avoid unexpected pitfalls. Questions that need to be resolved include how, when, where, and with whom. Substitution, confluence, apperception (already discussed in part I of the contract), and systematic enhancement are several methods in strength intervention that resolve the questions of how and when.

The most obvious intervention strategy is **substitution** (part II.B)—substituting positive behaviors for negative behaviors or for nonproductive time. For example, you might eliminate one television show and replace it by cooking a nutritious meal, exercising, or devoting time to spiritual reading. There is also substitution in cases where an unhealthy activity is deleted from a life-style. To take away smoking, late night snacking, or other behaviors though without replacing them generally results in failure. For example, one man pet his dog every time he had a

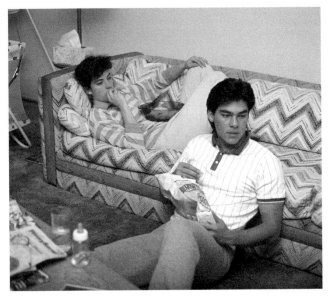

(a)

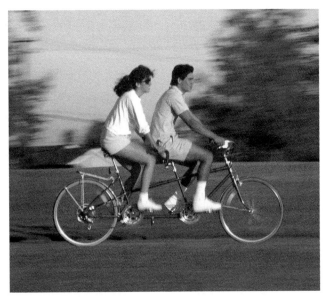

(b)

Substituting one behavior for another might help promote health. For example, substituting the behavior in *(b)* for the behavior in *(a)* would be helpful.

craving for a cigarette, another chewed sugarless gum, and another jumped on his minitramp.

Confluence (part II.C) is the combining or linking of activities or behaviors for time efficiency. The possibilities are limited only by your creativity. Examples include listening to spiritual music while jogging, working on communication skills with a spouse/partner while cooking a nutritious meal, or studying while riding a stationary bicycle.

An important psychological principle is evident when you combine a strength and a weakness. If the two are somewhat matched, the strength usually wins out. **Systematic enhancement** (part II.D) is an approach to using strength with weakness. The strength dimension provides a supportive environment and promotes success. For example, one man who wanted to stop smoking determined that his primary strength dimension was social and his primary support person was his wife. Using systematic enhancement, he was most likely to be successful in his effort to stop smoking if initially he abstained from smoking in the presence of his wife. He might then progress to not smoking in any social situation and then move to not smoking in all situations.

The question of *when* (part II.E) is a personal one that is also influenced by outside factors. For example, starting an exercise program means finding the right time of day to fit it into your schedule. Controlling body weight has different "when" implications, and stopping smoking has still others. It is important to consider the timing of events, which has an impact on attempts to improve health behaviors.

The issue of *where* (part II.F) may or may not be a critical one, but it should be considered. One glaring example of a "where" problem arises with jogging or walking. In seasonal climates, many individuals find themselves inactive in winter. The plan needs to build in a bad-weather alternative, such as cross-country skiing, snowshoeing, exercise bikes, or other acceptable alternatives. Another consideration of "where" is a place to do the activity. At the beginning of a program, when great motivation is felt, you might be willing to get in your car and drive to an exercise facility. When motivation is not so high, however, convenience may be more of a factor.

Intensity (part II.G) may or may not be applicable to a specific contract. For example, it would relate to an exercise program but probably not to contracts designed to improve time-management skills. Even though most parts of the contract apply to all strength-improvement programs, there may be a few parts that do not.

Preparation (part II.H) usually becomes obvious once the plan is designed. It could involve getting equipment, learning new information, making arrangements to meet people at a certain time, or other acts to be successful.

With whom (part II.I) is another consideration that might not always be necessary, but it can be very helpful. While some goals can be accomplished alone, others might be enhanced by the presence and even the assistance of another person.

One or more **support groups** (part III of the life-style contract) can help increase your chances for success. In the Health Assessment, you identified individuals from whom you derive comfort, support, happiness, and inner strength. These individuals are ideal members of a support group to facilitate and sustain your efforts to change behavior. The support group may provide several functions, such as giving casual reminders to follow the contract, participating with you, providing praise, listening, and monitoring your progress.

If individuals fail in their contracts, it is usually during the first six to eight weeks of the program. Failure seems to occur because they lack motivation and want to give up, and consequently they drop out of the program. **Trigger responses** (part IV of the life-style contract) can help prevent this. Sample triggers might include playing stirring music for motivation, looking at a picture of yourself when you were leaner if you are trying to lose weight, or reading appropriate literature.

In some cases, the *starting date* (part V) should be immediately, but sometimes it takes time to contact support people, purchase equipment, or take an appropriate course. Careful selection of the starting date is important, particularly when you need time to get ready.

It is a good idea to set a time within two to four weeks to *reevaluate the life-style contract* (part VI). Generally, come considerations are overlooked initially, and you might need to modify your contract to accomplish the desired outcome. Modifications will probably be a matter of when, where, or intensity (starting out gradually).

How will you know when you reach your goal? *Specifying at what point the goal will be met* (part VII) helps you determine when you will be happy with your achievement. Examples might be when you can jog thirty minutes without stopping and feel good afterwards or when you can look forward to meditation and feel benefits from practicing it.

During the process of identifying the behavior, the standard of acceptable compliance should be considered. For example, will you need to do something hourly, daily, weekly, twice weekly, and so on? If you slack off, at what point are you no longer in compliance?

Most psychologists suggest that you build in a *reward* (part VIII) when you have accomplished your goal. This is appropriate if you want to do so, but for some people the sense of accomplishment and control might be reward

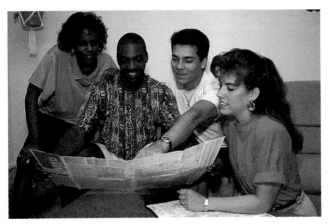

Rewards for health behavior changes should be consistent with the goal.

enough. One word of caution, however, is that rewards should not be in conflict with the accomplishment of the goal. Buying an ice cream sundae to celebrate weight loss is an example of such a conflict.

While this type of contracting is not legally binding, a signature represents commitment. Do not sign until you are ready to make a commitment and are determined to comply with the contract. The signature of a facilitator (someone to help you fulfill your contract) (part X) is another way to help promote success. Careful planning, thinking through all of the steps described, and determination to change are all necessary ingredients for success.

Are you ready to make some positive changes in your health? Use the Health Assessment you completed earlier to create your own life-style contract (fill in the blank contract in fig. 1.6).

Summary

1. Despite the availability of abundant health information, we actually know little about our health.

2. Health has been defined in many ways. In this text, we use a multifaceted concept that includes mental health, emotional health, social health, physical health, occupational health, and spiritual health. Personal life-style dramatically affects health.

3. Most individuals are inconsistent in their health behavior, and there are many motivations for health behavior. They include fear, social pressure, health habits, attitudes and values, knowledge, and cultural influences.

4. To change behavior, the biological, psychological, and cultural factors as well as the interplay among them must be understood.

5. Health and what is done about it is not simply an individual affair—it is connected to larger cultural issues. You can choose to alter many influences to arrive at a balance conducive to optimal health.

6. One health decision can have many ramifications for other health decisions. Deciding and acting on health issues involves recognition, evaluation, implementation, and review.

7. Social pressure, habits, attitudes and values, and knowledge can influence decision making.

8. Protective skills, negotiation, disruption, disorganization, and adjustment skills are parts of a model for action to promote optimal health.

9. Strength intervention includes four stages: assessing, nurturing, freeing, and optimizing.

10. Life-style contracting can systematically help with health behavior change. When preparing a life-style contract, many factors must be considered, including apperception, barriers to change, substitution, confluence, systematic enhancement, support groups, and triggers to action.

11. The best way to improve health lies in what we do or do not do—both to and for ourselves—not in what others do for us.

Commitment Activities

1. Circle the number on this continuum that you think best represents your current health status.

1	2	3	4	5	6	7	8	9	10
poor health								optimum health	

Why did you rate yourself as you did? List the conditions or behaviors that you believe prevent you from reaching a higher level of health (e.g., overeating, smoking, overwork).

_____

_____

_____

_____

_____

_____

_____

_____

_____

_____

_____

Which of these behaviors are you willing to change? As you read this text, pay special attention to conditions or behaviors you are willing to change, then commit yourself to making needed changes. For those things you are not yet willing to change, commit yourself at least to learning more about them. From time to time, reassess yourself on this continuum (Source: adapted from Marshall W. Kreuter, "An Interaction Model to

Facilitate Health Awareness and Behavior Change" in *Journal of School Health*, November 1976, pp.543–45).

2. A continuum can be used to evaluate community health. Ask community members to assess the level of health in their neighborhood or town, then identify conditions that are roadblocks to better community health. What can be done to move your community's health closer to a "10"?

3. List five of your health behaviors. Carefully examine them for inconsistencies, and ask yourself why the inconsistencies exist. For each inconsistency, consider what you can do to increase positive health behavior (create consistency). How can you reduce barriers to action? Are you willing to do so?

4. Using the outline for a life-style contract in figure 1.6, develop your own life-style contract for one or two health behaviors. It might be helpful to discuss possible parts of the plan with those who are significant in your life.

5. For the next five days, jot down daily at least three decisions you make related to your health. Then evaluate the decisions based on the information within this chapter.

6. Develop a personal model of decision making for health based on the material in this chapter and other sources. Follow the steps in your model as you make health decisions. Remember to evaluate your model occasionally and to revise it as necessary.

References

Abood, D. A., and Conway, T. L. "Health Value and Self-Esteem as Predictors of Wellness Behavior." *Health Values* 16, no. 3 (May/June 1992):20–26.

Bensley, R. J. "Defining Spiritual Health: A Review of the Literature." *Journal of Health Education* 22, no. 5 (September/October 1991):287–90.

Bergmann, B. L., and Greenberg, J. S. "A Study of the Psychosocial Profile of the Health Promoting Adult." *Journal of Health Education* 22, no. 6 (November/December 1991): 354–62.

Chapman, L. S. "Developing a Useful Perspective on Spiritual Health: Well-Being, Spiritual Potential, and the Search for Meaning." *American Journal of Health Promotion* (Winter 1987): 31–39.

Eberst, R. "Defining Health: A Multidimensional Model." *Journal of School Health* 54, no. 3 (March 1985): 99–104.

Flach, F. F. *Resilience: Discovering New Strength at Times of Stress.* New York: Ballantine Books, 1989.

Goodloe, N. R., and Arreola, P. M. "Spiritual Health: Out of the Closet." *Journal of Health Education* 23, no. 4 (May/June 1992): 221–26.

Hamrick, M. H.; Anspaugh, D. J.; and Smith, D. L. "Decision Making and the Behavior Gap." *Journal of School Health* (October 1980): 455–58.

Kreuter, M. W. "An Interaction Model to Facilitate Health Awareness and Behavior Change." *Journal of School Health* (November 1976): 543–45.

Norman, R. "Health Behaviour: The Implications for Research." *Health Promotion* 25, no. 2 (1987): 2–9.

Pelletier, K. R. "Mind-Body Health: Research, Clinical, and Policy Applications." *American Journal of Health Promotion* 6, no. 5 (May/June 1992): 345–58.

Price, J. H.; Galli, N.; and Slenker, S. *Consumer Health: Contemporary Issues and Choices.* Dubuque, Iowa: Wm. C. Brown Publishers, 1985.

Promoting Health/Preventing Disease: Year 2000 Objectives for the Nation. Washington, D.C.: Public Health Service, U.S. Department of Health and Human Services, September 1990.

Richardson, G. E., and Berry, N. F. "Strength Intervention: An Approach to Lifestyle Modification." *Health Education* 18, no. 3 (March 1987): 42–46.

Richardson, G. E.; Neiger, B. L.; Jensen, S.; and Kempfer, K. L. "The Resiliency Model." *Health Education* 21, no. 6. (November/December 1990): 33–39.

Additional Readings

Garrity, J. M. "Understanding and Supporting Health Behavioral Change." *SIECUS Report* 20, no. 1 (October/November 1991): 8–10. Describes factors that are likely to influence health behavior change and outlines ways that we can support the health behavior change of others.

Halpern, C. R. "The Political Economy of Mind-Body Health." *American Journal of Health Promotion* 6, no. 4 (March/April 1992): 288–91+. Indicates that research shows a new set of effective methods (such as meditation, yoga, supportive group therapy, and guided imagery) can assist healing; however, there are economic, political, social, and professional barriers to the use of these methods.

McGinnis, J. M. "A Healthy Campus—Forecasting from the 1990 Health Objectives for the Nation." *Journal of the American College Health Association* 35, no. 1 (January 1987): 158–70. Reviews the health status of college-age students and considers challenges for the future of college health.

Pezza, P. E. "Orientation to Uncertainty and Information Seeking About Personal Health." *Health Education* 21, no. 2 (March/April 1990): 34–36. Based on a literature review, the author explains how orientation to uncertainty may be useful in better understanding how information is acquired as a prelude to personal health decision making.

Perhaps one of the most exciting discoveries in the last two decades is the rediscovery and the medical confirmation of the power of the mind and its interaction with the body. Ancient philosophies and practices have always linked the mind and the body, but modern medicine has functioned on the idea that for every physical disease, there is a physical cause. For example, to prevent disease, you get an immunization; to prevent heart attack, you should exercise and eat a low-fat diet; and if you have a bacterial infection, then you should take penicillin.

In the early 1980s, physicians started to ask themselves why we are constantly exposed to microorganisms (viruses, bacteria, etc.) that sometimes are activated and cause disease while other times the bacteria and viruses rest in respiratory passages without any harmful effect.

At the same time, some amazing documented cases of "miraculous" healings of serious diseases began to be reported. In one such case, a Mr. Wright was given about two weeks to live by his physicians. His body was bloated with tumors the size of oranges that had to be drained of one to two quarts of fluid each day. The medical staff was merely attempting to make him as comfortable as possible until his inevitable death. Mr. Wright heard about a new experimental cancer drug called Krebiozen and told his physician that he wanted to try it. It just so happened that the hospital where Mr. Wright was dying had been selected as an experimental site for the new drug. Because the physician wanted to experiment with patients who had a better chance of survival, he was reluctant to let Mr. Wright take the drug. Mr. Wright persisted and finally received permission to use the drug. After one injection of Krebiozen, the tumors reduced to half the size in two to three days, and, within two weeks, Mr. Wright went home apparently in total remission and free of tumors.

Some time later, which happened to be a day or two after the drug Krebiozen was reported in the media to be ineffective, Mr. Wright returned to the hospital with the tumors again. The physician, knowing that something more than the drug was at work, then put Mr. Wright in a control group for a "new" Krebiozen. This meant that Mr. Wright would not receive the drug but rather an injection of sterile water. The administration was given with great ceremony by the physician and with great anticipation by Mr. Wright, who perceived the administration to be a double dose of the "new" drug. After a few days the tumors again disappeared. A few months later, renewed reports citing the ineffectiveness of Krebiozen were made public and, shortly after, Mr. Wright died (Locke and Colligan 1986).

Other case studies relate astonishing accounts of patients with multiple personalities with one personality having diabetes, tumors, or allergic reactions to certain substances. When a new personality emerged, the conditions were no longer evidenced. Tumors disappeared in a few days, symptoms of diabetes disappeared, and allergies were no longer existent (Borysenko 1987).

Studies in medical literature demonstrate longer survival rates of patients with AIDS, cancer, or heart disease if they have positive personality traits. People with optimism, hope, faith, a cause or purpose, a fighting spirit, and a determination to overcome a disease do live longer and are happier.

Intuitively, we have known for years that if your are too busy to get sick, you are not as likely to get sick. When we are experiencing the most stress or are most depressed, or when we are grieving or most upset, we tend to get sick more often. Conversely, we also know that when things are going along smoothly, when we are excited about living, when we have a cause and purpose, and when we are working toward goals, we seem to have more energy and are healthier. Why is this?

The relatively new and exciting medical field that studies this phenomenon is called **psychoneuroimmunology (PNI)** (Ader, Felten, and Cohen 1991). This is the study of the way that we think (psycho), which then affects the central nervous system (neuro), and then effects our immune system (immunology). Much of the study of the field of PNI has been to understand how the immune system is triggered. Scientists have found that "no major sector of the immune system is without a hard-wire connection to the brain" (Locke and Colligan 1986).

The total picture of the interaction of the mind and body involves a two-directional network. How we think can affect our body, and how fit our body is can affect the way we think.

Studies show that when we have a fighting spirit, are optimistic, have a cause in life, and have great hope, our immune system can be fortified. There are actually more elements available in our immune system (i.e., macrophages, T cells, and B cells) to fight the invasions of foreign microorganisms (Locke and Colligan 1986; Borysenko 1987).

A precaution about PNI is important to understand. How you think can in fact either weaken or fortify your immune system. This is *not* to suggest that you can think diseases away, but you can help the process. If you are sick, *it is important to follow a physician's treatment plan;* but you can supplement the physician's plan by believing that treatment will work, that with proper treatment you will overcome the problem, and that you feel medicines and treatments working. If you are not sick, *it does not mean that you do not need periodic physician examinations.* It means that positive thinking will help to keep you well.

Implications

Ask yourself the question, How can this information help me? At the end of each of the parts of this text is a discussion of the implications of PNI to your life-style. The essence of all the recommendations will be to help you overcome negative mind and body states and promote positive states. There are four key elements in successful adoption of positive states.

1. Live through repeated and varied new experiences in the social, emotional, cognitive, physical, and spiritual domains of living, which will be specified in later sections.

2. When making decisions, take advantage of outcomes of those decisions (positive or negative) to learn and improve your decision-making skill.

3. Through experiences and decisions, focus on understanding yourself better so that you can refine your decision-making skill.

4. Become aware of or establish a cause in life. A cause is more than a goal or something you do for yourself. A cause is generally made up of many goals that generally involve improving the condition or welfare of someone or something besides yourself (help your family, preserve the environment, help a kid or kids, help the elderly, or numerous other worthy causes).

As it pertains to the preceding section, here are some things that might help you attain optimism, a fighting spirit, hope, or a cause.

1. When you experience a setback in life, are depressed, or are anxious, talk to yourself and get excited about this mental state. You can perceive it as a great opportunity to learn a new coping skill. Turn the negative state into a positive one.

2. Consider a variety of ways to establish a cause. Think about your own environment and people you interact with, take a close look at your natural environment, visit some residents in a home for the elderly, visit some youth organizations, visit a homeless shelter, and see where you can potentially volunteer to help people or things.

3. Do something you have not done before. After you think of something, learn how, get a role model or someone to show you how, and then do it. Successful experiences might include anything in life such as trying to cook, iron, sew, make something; trying out for a play or team; visiting a different religious ceremony; trying meditation, yoga, horseshoes, tennis, etc. Take a different type of class at your school, maybe a recreation class to learn to fish, scuba, or play chess.

Sources: R. Ader, D. L. Felten, and N. Cohen (Eds.), *Psychoneuroimmunology,* 2d ed., Academic Press, San Diego, 1991; J. Borysenko, *Minding the Body, Mending the Mind,* Addison-Wesley, Reading, Mass., 1987; and S. Locke and D. Colligan, *The Healer Within: The New Medicine of Mind and Body,* E.P. Dutton, New York, 1986.

Life-Style Contract

There are several things you can do to improve your health as a result of the topics discussed in this chapter. The following is a partial list of some of the behaviors that could enhance your health status.

Health Behaviors

1. Select a personal strength area in your life and nurture it.
2. With major or minor decisions, take time to complete a decision tree or go through the steps of making a good decision.
3. Assess your risks of disease or death and determine which of those can be removed and remove them.
4. Do activities that can, over time, modify your locus of control to a more internal perspective such as imagery strategies (picture yourself in control of many situations) or consciously change a behavior. Both of these have been shown to help modify the perspective of control.

In this chapter you learned to complete a contract using strength intervention. The assumption for the example here is that a person is not receiving the strength, comfort, and support he or she should be from some activities that were strength areas.

◆

Sample Life-Style Contract

I. Behavioral selection
  A. Factors to consider before making a behavioral selection
    1. Nurturing _This is what I will do_
    2. Freeing _____
    3. Optimizing _I'll focus on relaxing_
    4. Motivation/readiness _____
    5. Apperception _The guitar helped while I was in college_
    6. Barriers to change _takes more time_
  B. Behaviors I will change (no more than two)
    Play my guitar and sing to help me relax and it makes me feel good

II. The plan
  A. General plan _I will do it when I talk to my two kids at bedtime_
  B. Substitution _Instead of just talking, I'm going to sing and play_
  C. Confluence _Time with kids and playing my guitar_
  D. Systematic enhancement _____
  E. When _8:30 p.m. - bedtime_
  F. Where _In the kids' room_
  G. Intensity _n/a_
  H. Preparation _Bring out my old songbook from several years ago and get my guitar from my folks_
  I. With whom _my two kids_

III. Support groups
  A. Who _My wife / My kids_
  B. Role _For the few times I've done it, the kids like it, so I'll have them badger me_
  C. Organized support _n/a_

IV. Trigger responses _I'll put a picture of a guitar over the kids' bed_

V. Starting date _This Wednesday_

VI. Date/sequence the contract will be revaluated _One month_

VII. Evidences of reaching goal _Relaxed evening — guitar skills_

VIII. Rewards when contract is completed _I feel so good when I play—that short escape will be reward enough_

IX. Signature of client _____

X. Signature of facilitator _____

XI. Additional conditions/comments: _____

◆

CHAPTER 2

Stress Management and Mental Health

Key Questions

- What is mental health?
- What is stress?
- What are stressors?
- What are some skills that can help you to be mentally healthy?
- What is the body's response to stressors?
- What are the points of intervention for stress management?
- Can stress be positive?
- What are some ways to manage stress effectively?
- How can you help someone who may be contemplating suicide?

Chapter Outline

The Stress Management/Mental-Health Model
External Stressors and Interdependence
   Overstimulation
   Frustration
   Environmental Stressors
   Nutritional Stressors
   Interdependence
Perceptual Control or Mental Health
   Developmental Theories
   Mental-Health Characteristics and
     Well-Being
The Stress Response
   Stress and Peak Performance
   General Adaptation Syndrome (GAS)
   Stress-Related (Psychosomatic)
     Disease
Techniques to Manage Stress and
     Fortify Mental Health
   Managing External Stressors
   Developing Mental/Perceptual Health
     Skills
   Managing the Physiological Stress
     Response
When Adversity and Stressors Exceed
     Our Ability to Cope
   Mental Disorders
   Suicide
   Psychoanalysis and Psychotherapy

M ost of us have been fearful, upset, and under stress at times in our lives and perhaps have wondered how we would ever survive an emotional or mental crisis. You may have wondered if you were "going crazy" and should seek professional help. More frequently, we are discouraged, let down, or rejected but find ways to deal and cope with our problems. On the positive side, we often experience times of excitement, sudden good news, or falling in love and reach a peak mental and emotional state, at least temporarily. Consider the following analogy to provide perspective on **stress** and **mental health** (Jola 1970).

> There I am standing by the shore of a swiftly flowing river and I hear the cry of a drowning man. So I jump in the river, put my arms around him, pull him to shore, and apply artificial respiration. Just when he begins to breathe, another cry for help. So back in the river again, reaching, pulling, applying, breathing, and then another yell. Again and

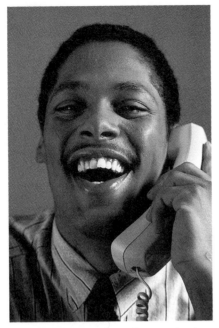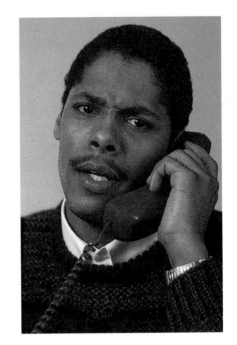

It is normal to feel emotional swings from happiness to hurt and anger.

again, without end goes the sequence. You know, I am so busy jumping in, pulling them to shore, applying artificial respiration, that I have no time to see who the "heck" is upstream pushing them all in.

Many of us find ourselves caught up in the raging river of stress, demands, pressures, and conflict and feel like we are about to drown. We are often physically, mentally, and emotionally drained and sometimes seek professional help to pull us out. Physicians give medications to help individuals relax, sleep, wake up, and remain calm as they live through their woes. Mental health professionals listen to, direct, and support individuals as they face daily the raging currents of chronic stress and crises. These professionals jump into the swiftly flowing river, pull individuals in need out, and give artificial respiration.

It is clear that **stressors,** competitiveness, and the hectic nature of society push us into these currents of stress. What is troublesome, though, is the evident weakness that leaves us incapable of resisting the push. And if we do end up in the river's currents, we often can't swim and pull ourselves out. The strong currents are part of today's society, so why haven't we developed into strong swimmers who can swim to safety when overwhelmed? Strong swimmers can enjoy swift currents as long as they are in control and know they will not drown.

This chapter provides an understanding of the relationship between stress and mental health and instruction on how to improve your coping and stress management skills. Strategies for managing adversity and external pressures are recommended. How our personal thoughts can create stress is also discussed. Stress can be posi-

tive and help us perform better, have high energy levels, be more efficient, and reach peaks of performance. Stress can also be negative in that it can result in personal problems, overloading, frustration, and dysfunction due to excessive expectations. Negative stress may result in medical or psychological problems, and positive stress may result in high-quality life experiences. This chapter describes (1) the stress-induced ups and downs of mental, emotional, and physical health, (2) what happens when we do not cope effectively, (3) techniques for managing external, perceptual, and physiological stressors, and more important (4) the process of acquiring mental health skills to improve mind, body, and soul as well as interdependence.

This chapter is a guide to mental-health swimming skills. The skills you will learn for general mental health and stress management can be used for specific challenges and issues in the remaining chapters. To assure an understanding of the relationship between mental health and stress, a stress management/mental-health model is presented. The remainder of the chapter focuses on each of the elements of the model to assure control of stress in your life and the maximization of your mental health strengths.

The Stress Management/ Mental-Health Model

Reflecting on the model for the prevention of health problems explained in chapter 1, remember that each of us is constantly bombarded with stressors, or as in the

Assessing mental health and stress is a complex task and difficult to do in limited space. The following assessment instruments represent a sampling of stress and mental-health indicators that should help you to personalize this chapter. You will be asked to refer to some of these assessments later in the chapter.

Self-Esteem Assessment

For each item write *a* in front of each statement that describes you and *b* in front of each statement that does not describe you.

_____ 1. People generally like me.

_____ 2. I am comfortable talking in class.

_____ 3. I like to do new things.

_____ 4. I give in very easily.

_____ 5. I'm a failure.

_____ 6. I'm shy.

_____ 7. I have trouble making up my mind.

_____ 8. I am popular with people at school.

_____ 9. My life is all mixed up.

_____10. I often feel upset at my home, room, or apartment.

_____11. I often wish I were like someone else.

_____12. I often worry.

_____13. I can be depended on.

_____14. I often express my views.

_____15. I think I am doing okay with my life.

_____16. I feel good about what I have accomplished recently.

Scoring/Interpretation

Determine how many matches you have with the following key. Total that number.

1. a	5. b	9. b	13. a
2. a	6. b	10. b	14. a
3. a	7. b	11. b	15. a
4. b	8. a	12. b	16. a

From the total number of matched, interpret as follows:

12–16 high self-esteem

8–11 moderately high self-esteem

4–7 moderately low self-esteem

0–3 low self-esteem

Depression Assessment

Indicate which of the following reflect what you do or how you feel. Indicate by marking an *X* in the space provided if it is like you.

_____ 1. I use drugs to relax or have fun.

_____ 2. I need to see someone about how sad I feel.

_____ 3. I have trouble making it to class.

_____ 4. I think I would be better off dead.

_____ 5. My life seems hopeless.

_____ 6. I have thought through how I would kill myself.

_____ 7. People around me would be better off if I were gone.

_____ 8. I change my moods often.

_____ 9. I'm not interested in much anymore.

_____10. I can't seem to concentrate.

_____11. I feel unloved and unwanted.

_____12. I have a quick temper.

_____13. I feel guilty.

_____14. I take things too hard.

_____15. I have been thinking a lot about death lately.

Scoring/Interpretation

If you have marked number 2, 4, 5, 6, 7, or 11, then you should talk with someone right away about your feelings and needs. You may want to talk to your instructor about where to go for help.

If you have marked any of the other responses (number 1, 3, or 8–13) in conjunction with number 15, then you should also talk with someone about how you feel.

If you have marked three or more of the remaining statements (number 1, 3, or 8–13), you may also want to seek help.

Assertiveness Assessment

Indicate what you would do in the following situations by circling *a*, *b*, or *c*.

1. A professor gives you a grade that is lower than you had expected.
   a. Ask the professor to recalculate the grade because you feel he or she is in error.
   b. Complain to the professor but accept the grade.
   c. Say nothing.

2. In a cafeteria line after waiting some time to get something to eat, a group of people recognize the person in front of you and crowd in line.
   a. Ask them to please move to the back of the line and wait like everyone else.
   b. Make a comment but not ask them to move back.
   c. Say nothing.
3. Someone near you is smoking in a nonsmoking section.
   a. Ask him or her to notice the no smoking sign and please put out the cigarette.
   b. Make a comment like, "Can't you read?" but don't ask him or her to put it out.
   c. Say nothing.
4. You have waited for ten minutes at a department secretary's office to get course information, and she is obviously making a personal call.
   a. Get her attention and say, "Can you help me?"
   b. Make heavy sighs and frustrated looks.
   c. Wait patiently.

Scoring/Interpretation

Assign the following number of points to each of your answers. Total your points.

a = 4	b = 2	c = 0

Interpret as follows:

12–16 assertive	6–11 moderately assertive	0–6 unassertive

Stress Index

To identify the types and degrees of stress you are experiencing, complete the following index. Circle the number that corresponds to your reaction to each statement. Total the numbers in each column and add them to arrive at a subtotal for each section.

	Always	Often	Sometimes	Rarely	Never
1. I get upset when I have to wait in lines.	5	4	3	2	1
2. I work by the clock to see how much I can get done in a short amount of time.	5	4	3	2	1
3. I get upset if something takes too long.	5	4	3	2	1
4. I make almost every activity I do competitive with myself or others.	5	4	3	2	1
5. I feel guilty when I am not working on something.	5	4	3	2	1
				Section subtotal	_____
6. I get upset when I can't do something my way.	5	4	3	2	1
7. I get upset when my accomplishments are dependent on the actions of others.	5	4	3	2	1
8. I get anxious when my plans become disrupted.	5	4	3	2	1
9. All good things are worth waiting for.	1	2	3	4	5
10. When I set a goal I can't reach, I simply alter it.	1	2	3	4	5
				Section subtotal	_____
11. I have been given too much responsibility.	5	4	3	2	1
12. I get depressed when I think of everything I have to do.	5	4	3	2	1
13. People demand too much of me.	5	4	3	2	1
14. I often find myself without enough time to complete my work.	5	4	3	2	1
15. Sometimes I feel that my head is spinning, or I get confused because so much is happening.	5	4	3	2	1
				Section subtotal	_____

	Always	Often	Sometimes	Rarely	Never
16. I succeed in most things and will try even when the task is difficult.	1	2	3	4	5
17. I am very comfortable being with members of the opposite sex.	1	2	3	4	5
18. I am generally comfortable around teachers, bosses, and other superiors.	1	2	3	4	5
19. I prefer that others make decisions for me.	5	4	3	2	1
20. I don't think I have too much going for me.	5	4	3	2	1
21. I am most relaxed when I am busy.	5	4	3	2	1
22. I throw away old clothes, toys, and other mementos.	1	2	3	4	5
23. I enjoy being alone.	1	2	3	4	5
24. I feel the need to belong to a social group.	5	4	3	2	1
25. I get homesick easily.	5	4	3	2	1

Section subtotal _____

	Always	Often	Sometimes	Rarely	Never
26. I often feel my stomach knotting, my mouth getting dry, and my heart pounding when I get nervous.	5	4	3	2	1
27. When I get nervous, I can feel my muscles tense, my hands and fingers shake, and my voice become unsteady.	5	4	3	2	1
28. After a crisis, I relive the experience over and over in my mind, even though it is resolved.	5	4	3	2	1
29. I know that I must resolve a crisis or it will bother me for a long time.	5	4	3	2	1
30. When nervous, I imagine the worst possible outcomes of the original crisis.	5	4	3	2	1

Section subtotal = _____

Total = _____

Scoring/Interpretation

By summing all the subtotals on the index, you estimate your overall susceptibility to stress based on social situations and personality. Interpret your score as follows:

100 or higher	High stress
50–99	Moderate stress
49 or below	You are doing well for now; keep it up

The section of the text describing the causes of stress helps you further interpret these results.

---

analogy, the swiftly flowing currents. Figure 2.1 shows the relationship between (1) stressors, which can be described as adversity, life events, and challenges, (2) mental health or perceptions, referred to as "protective skills" in the model for the prevention of health problems, and (3) the stress or physiological response to perceived stressors. The elements of the model are explained in depth throughout this chapter, but to reinforce your understanding of the relationship, a brief description of the model is provided here.

A stressor triggers the stress response. The stressor can be an emotional experience, an intellectual challenge, a social situation, a spiritual experience, environmental pollutants, and/or nutritional or physical stimulants. Stressors are daily events that may or may not be controllable. They are challenges, opportunities, or different types of adversity such as embarrassing situations or school demands.

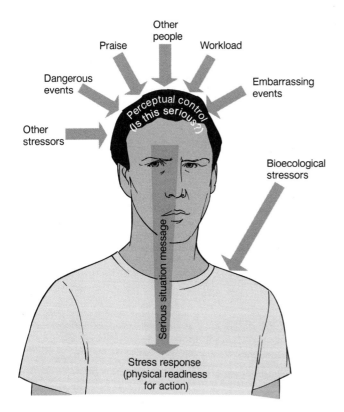

Praise

Other people

Workload

Dangerous events

Embarrassing events

Other stressors

Perceptual control (Is this serious?)

Bioecological stressors

Serious situation message

Stress response (physical readiness for action)

Figure 2.1

Stress management/mental-health model.

We live in social networks, such as families, roommates, academic classes, communities, churches, clubs, and governments. Individuals in these networks are sources of support, stressors, and interactions. When positive interactions occur within the networks, supportive relationships develop, ideas are created, and energy is produced. This positive form of the interaction is termed **interdependence.**

Our mental health or perceptions determine the conscious or subconscious interpretation of the external stressors. They decide whether the external event is a positive stressor, a negative stressor, or an unimportant external event. This decision represents perceptual control and determines whether a message is sent to the physiological system to respond to the stressor or ignore it.

If our perception is that the stressor is something to worry about, then the body experiences the **stress response.** This means the body prepares for action by increasing muscle tension, heart rate, blood pressure, strength and energy-producing hormones, diameter of the pupils, and brain-wave frequency. The body is ready to fight the potential danger or run away if necessary.

The interaction of external stressors, our conscious and subconscious perceptual control, and the resulting physiological stress response is the simple essence of stress management. There are skills and techniques to control external stressors, there are mental health skills that allow you to control your state perceptually, and when the stress response does affect you, there are skills that allow you to maximize the energy produced by the stress

response for positive gain. The remainder of this chapter describes the management, control, and skill building of each of these three dimensions of living.

External Stressors and Interdependence

As we go through our daily lives, we are constantly exposed to external life events, stressors, challenges, information, and incidentals that are barely noticed. These are picked up by our senses so that we hear, see, smell, feel, touch, and taste things around us. Some of what we sense is judged important and some not. Those close to us are sources for nurturing, support, friendship, and information and are generally deemed important. When you walk across campus among many people, generally most of those people are unnoticed by you. Those external stressors or interdependent relationships that we do deem as important create potential problems or states that require skills for optimal living. Consider some of the following specific types of stressors from external sources. Recommendations for managing each of the stressors are included later in this chapter.

Overstimulation

Overstimulation occurs when professors, bosses, spouses, children, roommates, parents, and others in our lives require us to perform certain tasks. Class assignments, readings, and work demands are constantly imposed on us, and in addition we often take tasks on that are not important. When you find yourself incapable of meeting the demands placed on you in certain situations, you are overstimulated or overloaded. Types of overstimulation include time pressures, excess responsibility or accountability, lack of support, or excessive expectations of ourselves or from others. Review your score from the Health Assessment at the beginning of the chapter. Your score on questions 11–15 of the Stress Index indicates whether you suffer from overstimulation. A section subtotal of 6–11 indicates low stress from overstimulation, 12–16 indicates moderate stress from overstimulation, and 17–25 indicates high stress from overstimulation.

Frustration

Frustration occurs when someone, something, or some personal lack of competence makes it impossible for us to attain a particular goal. The goal may be major, such as trying to get into medical school. Frustration can occur because our scores are low on the entrance examinations or because it is difficult to study quietly because of noisy roommates. Frustration is a frequent cause of distress. Your score on questions 6–10 of the Stress Index represents your tendency toward frustration. A section subtotal of 0–11 indicates that you are not easily frustrated (low stress), 12–16 indicates you are moderately frustrated (moderate stress), and 17–25 indicates you are easily frustrated (high stress).

Environmental Stressors

Environmental stressors such as pollutants and microbes activate the body's immune, circulatory, and hormonal systems to ward off invading germs. Those foreign elements, whether hidden in water pollution, air pollution, or food contamination, constitute real stressors.

We need to consider environmental stressors carefully when deciding on a place to live. Loud noises also increase stress levels. Rock concerts or constant proximity to an airport not only promote deafness but can also raise blood pressure, heart rate, hormone levels, and other symptoms of the stress response.

Nutritional Stressors

Nutritional stressors abound on the market shelves, and they are prominently and prolifically advertised. Caffeinated soft drinks, coffee, and tea; refined sugar, which causes metabolic ups and downs; salt, which may be linked to high blood pressure; foods high in cholesterol; chocolate; cigarette smoking; and other drugs are stressors.

Interdependence

In life, we grow from being totally dependent on someone through the process of becoming independent, and then we attain the optimally functioning state of interdependence. Interdependence occurs when two independent people who are fulfilling their potential of mind, body, and soul interact in a way that their combined level of happiness, productivity, and energy is greater that the simple addition of their independent states. When couples, friends, co-workers, families, church congregations, neighborhoods, cultures, communities, or nations work well together, with each member gaining from the others, the multiplying effect is extremely rewarding. There are some key skills required to experience interdependence. **Communication skills** are essential to optimal interdependent relationships.

Perhaps the most powerful communication skill is simply described as the *emotional bank account* (Covey 1989). This concept simply requires that for positive interdependence, one partner must continually make "deposits" into the other partner's emotional bank account. Deposits might include paying compliments, giving favors, keeping promises, and trustworthiness. Withdrawals are made when promises are broken, when one party takes advantage of the other, when blaming occurs, or by any other action that causes harm. The key to positive interdependence, then, is to maintain a ten to one ratio of deposits to withdrawals. In this way, one partner can afford an occasional withdrawal if the account has plenty of deposits.

Another communication skill to consider is the level of communication used: level 1 involves information giving; level 2 involves directing or sometimes arguing, level 3

<table>
<tr><td colspan="2">TABLE 2.1</td></tr>
<tr><td colspan="2">Four Levels of Communication</td></tr>
<tr><td colspan="2">

Level 1: Information giving—Sociable, friendly, conventional, and playful; emphasizes thinking and does not indulge disclosure

Level 2: Directing/arguing—Directing, persuading, blaming, demanding, defending, praising, assuming, competing, evaluating, advising, and withholding; emphasizes feeling and little disclosure

Level 3: Exploring—Tentative, elaborating, exploring, speculating, searching, pondering, wondering, proposing, reflecting, receiving; necessitates work and thinking and little disclosure

Level 4: Self-disclosing—Aware, active, congruent, accepting, responsible, disclosing, responsive, understanding, caring, and cooperative; necessitates work, disclosure, and feelings

</td></tr>
<tr><td colspan="2">Source: S. Miller et al., Connecting Skills Workbook. Copyright © 1989 Interpersonal Communication Program, Littleton, Colorado.</td></tr>
</table>

involves exploring; and level 4 involves self-disclosing. Table 2.1 summarizes the main features of each level.

For our lives to be happy, skills in communicating emotions, feelings, thoughts, and ideas effectively are important. Listening, understanding, and empathizing with others when they share feelings, emotions, and thoughts are also critical for optimal interdependent relationships. The emotions, thoughts, and other mental states that are communicated are discussed in the next section.

Perceptual Control or Mental Health

While demands, actions, stressors, and life events bombard us, our perception is consciously or subconsciously recording these events. Our interpretations, decisions, understanding, and perceptions comprise our mental health. Mental health is the capacity to cope with life situations and stress, to grow emotionally, to develop to our fullest potential, and to grow in awareness and consciousness. Mental health is feeling good about yourself, accepting your physical appearance, being content with life, and gaining inner peace. Mental health also means actively seeking experiences to promote peak mental states. The perceptual part of stress management means learning to live with those stressors that you cannot control, to manage those that you can, and to alter our perceptions of stressors.

The term *mental health* often carries a neutral or negative connotation; many associate it with such terms as *mental disorder* and *mental institution*. But just as health is seen as more than simply the absence of disease or infirmity, so mental health is viewed as a positive state rather than the absence of mental infirmity or illness. Mental health means more than the opposite of distress, anxiety, neurosis, or psychosis. Optimal mental health means acquiring skills to deal effectively with setbacks, adversity, and stressors. Effective coping skills include the ability to solve personal problems, to gain control over situations, and to do self-counseling. Also important are a cause or purpose in life and believing in yourself. When setbacks do occur, the mentally healthy person will feel discouraged, disorganized, or depressed temporarily, but ultimately he or she bounces back, more capable than before the setback. Mentally healthy people learn to grow and develop through new experiences.

Developmental Theories

How you perceive events, cope with them, make decisions, and think is a product of your experiences, your genetic makeup, and how well you have dealt with challenges and stressors previously. Many psychological theories explain the natural growth process and effective coping. Descriptions of some of these theories follow.

Erikson's Stages of Development

Erik Erikson (1963) described naturally occurring growth steps as developmental stages. He indicated that positive mental health means mastering different skills during different stages. Table 2.2 shows the eight stages that Erikson saw as important to basic development, as well as the crises (challenges) most frequently encountered in these stages.

Each stage has alternative outcomes, such as "trust versus mistrust" and "autonomy versus shame and doubt." If an individual is in the final period of the "identity" crisis or in the young adult stage, where the alternative outcomes of the crisis are "intimacy" and "isolation," he or she needs to develop communication skills and become more open so that intimate relationships can result. By intimacy, Erikson does not mean marriage, nor does he imply sexual or physical closeness. Same-sex friendships are as important as opposite-sex relationships, and emotional, intellectual, social, and spiritual intimacy are as important as physical intimacy.

Erikson's theories state that individuals need to develop friendships, communicate, share happy and sad times, give and receive, and understand how mutually shared experiences are more fulfilling than isolated ones.

Maslow's Hierarchy of Needs

Abraham Maslow (1962) indicated that individuals have certain needs and that growth occurs through the fulfillment of a **hierarchy of needs.** He suggests that certain needs must be met in order to fulfill our human potential. The needs hierarchy can be better understood with some examples. If an individual is born in a country where people are starving or dying of thirst, then the major concern is foraging for food and water. Thoughts of developing self-esteem, furthering education, working on social skills, and developing talents, except as they relate to foraging for food, are far removed. Beginning with this idea, Maslow proposed that we can arrange our different

needs in a hierarchy and must fulfill a large portion of basic needs before higher needs can be fulfilled. So, basic physiological needs (food, air, water, and sleep) must be met before we can become concerned with safety needs (shelter and freedom from danger). After meeting safety needs, we then seek to love and be loved. When love needs are met, then self-esteem (personal worth) needs can be met, which finally leads to self-actualization.

Self-actualization, which means fulfilling human potential as well as satisfying most of the basic human needs, represents the highest level of mental health according to Maslow's hierarchy of needs. These priorities are shown in figure 2.2 on page 37. Maslow stated that few people are self-actualized because of the cultural, social, and motivational constraints around our achieving this high goal. He studied the lives of Abraham Lincoln, George Washington Carver, Thomas Jefferson, Eleanor Roosevelt, and fifty-six others who were, in his estimation, self-actualized. He described them as having the following traits:

1. An accurate perception of their physical and social surroundings and a comfortable feeling with them (no fear of the unknown).
2. An acceptance of people, despite their faults.
3. Long-term goals, which they work hard to attain without letting the goals disrupt their life-styles.
4. A capacity to be spontaneous, natural, and simple.
5. The need for occasional solitude and privacy, which may appear to others as aloofness or absent-mindedness.
6. An independence of mind not greatly influenced by external forces, such as media, propaganda, or salespersons.
7. Continuous enjoyment of beauty.
8. A variety of spiritual experiences, with feelings of ecstasy, power, or a close spiritual source of strength.
9. A feeling of sympathy for all, no matter who they are or what they have done.
10. Imperfections; capacity to experience guilt, anxiety, and sad feelings.
11. A strong capacity for love and an intense closeness with a few friends.
12. An ability to look at life in unique, refreshing ways.
13. A philosophical sense of humor—seeing human life and situations that accompany it in a humorous light.
14. Process orientation (focusing on and enjoying the process of obtaining a goal) rather than goal orientation.
15. Democratic character structure (placing little emphasis on race, creed, color, or socioeconomic structure), gained by learning from and listening to all people.

TABLE 2.2

Erikson's Stages of Development

Stage	Crisis	Description
Sensory-oral	Trust versus mistrust	The baby enters the world and obtains its first major impression—whether its needs and wants will be satisfied or neglected. The relationship, primarily with the mother, largely determines whether the infant will have a trusting impression, which is accomplished by warm, close, loving, fulfilling relationships, or a sense of mistrust, which stems from neglect, being ignored, a lack of tender touching, and frequently having wants unfulfilled.
Muscular-anal	Autonomy versus shame and doubt	In the second and third years of life, the major tasks are toilet training and walking. If the child finds success and support in accomplishing these tasks, then a feeling of independence, control, pride, confidence, self-esteem, or autonomy is likely to result. On the other hand, if toilet training is mishandled and results in a traumatic ordeal, then the child may experience shame and doubt, accompanied by the lack of confidence to face and control the environment and him- or herself.
Locomotor-genital	Initiative versus guilt	The child of age four to five learns that he or she can travel and explore on his or her own. Children have a strong attraction to the parent of the opposite sex that eventually leads to some disappointment, because they ultimately lose out to the same-sexed parent. They develop a sense of what they want and develop initiative to obtain gratification. Parental rules become restrictive and, when broken, result in guilt. Serious guilt occurs when the child is made to feel guilty about self-initiated activity.
Latency	Industry versus inferiority	In the child of six to twelve years, sexual drives become relatively latent (dormant). During these years, the child seeks to be industrious and craves recognition but is also very sensitive to criticism. He or she tries to channel this industrious nature into socially accepted channels. Too much criticism will result in feelings of inferiority.
Puberty and adolescence	Identity versus role confusion	This age (twelve to seventeen years) is often described as the period of "identity crisis," in which the individual is no longer a child but not yet an adult. The stage is marked by tremendous physical growth, emotional development, social skill development, and value clarification. The adolescent who works through these crises feels comfortable with his or her unveiling identity, while unsuccessful completion of this stage promotes societal role confusion in the adolescent.
Young adult	Intimacy versus isolation	Between the ages of approximately seventeen and twenty-three years, the individual faces the challenge of developing intimate relationships with members of his or her own sex and, usually more importantly, members of the opposite sex. Intimacy implies that mutual interaction promotes creativity, energy, responsibility, and happiness. Isolation, or failure to develop intimate relationships, results in pessimism, cynicism, and unhappiness.
Adult	Generativity verses stagnation	Adults either find themselves actively engaged in raising children, developing professional careers, enhancing their moral or spiritual existence, and other generative activities that promote satisfaction, or they become engrossed in self-absorption and gratification of material needs, contributing little to others.
Maturity	Ego integrity versus despair	As older people reflect on their past, they may feel the sense of accomplishment and satisfaction that leads to ego integrity, or, if they regret having accomplished few of their goals, they may then despair because they know they cannot relive the past. People who experience ego integrity have a sense of personal dignity, believe in the value of human existence, and feel comfortable with their place in the community.

Adapted from *Childhood and Society,* Second Edition, by Erik H. Erikson, by permission of W.W. Norton & Company, Inc. Copyright 1950, © 1963 by W.W. Norton & Company, Inc. Copyright renewed 1978, 1991 by Erik H. Erikson.

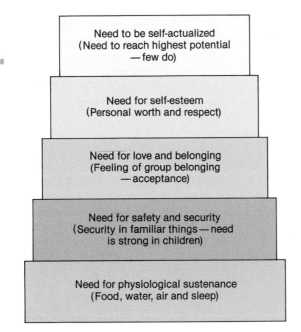

Figure 2.2

Maslow's hierarchy of needs.

Source: Data for diagram based on Hierarchy of Needs from Abraham H. Maslow, *Motivation and Personality,* 3d edition. Revised by Robert Frager et al., HarperCollins Publishers, 1954, 1987.

16. An acceptance of the cultural norms in which they live but also transcending these to reach higher norms.

17. Simple values—the ability to accept the nature of life and the value of human nature, to withhold judgment of others, and to treat everything as part of life.

18. Cooperation between head and heart rather than war between basic instincts and conscience or between lust and righteousness.

We can all strive toward the goal of self-actualization. It is productive to look at physiological, safety, love, self-esteem, and self-actualization needs to determine which needs have been fulfilled and which have not. Maslow has estimated that most people fulfill about 85 percent of their physiological needs, about 70 percent of their safety needs, 50 percent of their love needs, 40 percent of their self-esteem needs, and 10 percent of their self-actualization needs.

Erikson's and Maslow's theories help us understand human nature and why we act and feel the way we do. The theories also help us to understand the natural process of acquiring mental health coping skills. Our successes and failures in meeting our needs and dealing with life stages determine how we think and behave or, in other words, how we contribute to our personality.

Mental-Health Characteristics and Well-Being

Some of our perceptual or mental characteristics can cause us problems if not handled correctly. On the other hand, other characteristics help to fortify us against stress.

Type A and Type B Behavior Patterns

The **type A behavior pattern** is characterized by an intense sense of urgency. An individual with this behavior pattern has a need to get as much done as possible in as short a time as possible; shows aggressiveness and frequent hostility; has a high sense of motivaton and competitiveness but a short temper; has an intense achievement motive but frequently a lack of properly defined goals; and lacks concentration because of an intrusion of distracting thoughts. A person with type A behavior characteristics is likely to be highly stressed. The person with the **type B behavior pattern** takes life as it comes and does not get extremely upset at losing or not attaining a goal. Type B personalities usually set more realistic goals than type As.

The type A and type B behavior patterns were described by Friedman and Rosenman (1974), who suggested a correlation between the type A behavior pattern and cardiovascular disease. More recent literature has noted conflicting reports regarding the relationship between stress-prone type A behavior and cardiovascular disease (Fischman 1987). The controversy stems from studies that indicate that type A individuals have survived longer following a heart attack than type Bs. It appears that the traits within the type A behavior pattern that seem to carry the highest risk (four to five times greater chance of dying of a heart attack) are a mistrusting nature, harboring feelings of anger, and aggressive expression of hostility (University of California, Berkeley 1992). From the most conservative perspective, though, a person who demonstrates type A tendencies will probably experience the negative short-term results of stress, such as frustration, fatigue, overcommitment, and abrasiveness.

Review your score on the first five questions in the Stress Index. Your score for these five questions falls into one of the three groups and indicates the degree to which you are a type A or type B: 0–11 indicates you tend toward the less stressful type B personality; 12–16 indicates you have moderate tendencies toward the type A personality; and 17–25 indicates you have strong tendencies toward the type A personality.

Psychological Hardiness: The Stress-Resistant Personality

Shortly after the type A behavior pattern was identified, researchers (Kobasa, Maddi, and Kahn 1979) studied those people who exhibited type A behavior patterns but did not seem to suffer any ill effects. It was found that these people exhibited several characteristics that appeared to protect them against the effects of the type A behavior pattern. Kobasa and colleagues call this **psychological hardiness.** Flannery (1987) also describes a stress-resistant personality. The traits of the psychologically hardy are as follows:

1. Personal control: Individuals see themselves as having control over their lives as demonstrated by planning, self-directing, and not being swayed by others. They see themselves as in charge of their own destiny.
2. Commitment and task involvement: Individuals get personally involved in work, school, or relationships. They are devoted and dedicated and not easily diverted by short-term pleasures.
3. Challenge: Individuals take on assignments, problems, and opportunities with vigor. They seem to thrive on daily challenges.
4. Life-style choices: Stress-resistant individuals are willing to make life-style choices regarding diet, exercise, and relaxation and adhere to their life-styles.
5. Social supports: These individuals have positive personal relationships that buffer stressors and help them cope by providing emotional, informational, and instrumental support.

To understand the concept of hardiness, consider if you are one who sees school as a challenge, are committed to it, know that you are in control of what grades you receive, have good social support, and are experiencing a healthy life-style. If so, then you are probably insulated to some degree from the negative effects of stress. These perceptions also provide an avenue whereby you can fortify yourself and benefit from stress. The perception that stressors, whether they be relationships, tests, auditioning, competing, or joining a group, are opportunities to demonstrate control, commitment, and challenge help to make stress productive for you. Other stress-resistant factors are humor (Benson and Stuart 1992) and spiritual orientation (Moore 1992).

Self-Esteem

You can face many negative experiences and still have good mental health if you have positive **self-esteem.** It is interesting that we are not born with concerns about whether we are good or bad, smart or stupid, pretty or ugly, lovable or unlovable, but we develop these ideas from significant people in our lives. We form self-images, which are pictures of ourselves created from parents', teachers', and peers' input. Self-image is the content of our perceptions and opinions about ourselves. The positive or negative attitudes and values we see in ourselves and the evaluations or judgments we make about ourselves form our self-esteem. According to Coopersmith (1981), "Self-esteem refers to the evaluation a person makes and customarily maintains with regard to him or herself. Self-esteem expresses an attitude of approval or disapproval and indicates the extent to which a person believes him or herself capable, significant, successful, and worthy."

Self-esteem, that is, our positive feelings about ourselves, is one of the factors in increased motivation, involvement in learning, and successful performance in relationships and occupation. Those who do not have positive feelings suffer from feelings of unworthiness, inadequacy, helplessness, inferiority, and a sense that they cannot improve their situations.

Seeing yourself as helpless or devalued can lead to stress. Poor self-esteem has been shown to lead to numerous stress-related diseases and poor success in living. The "self-fulfilling prophecy" of not trying hard because you think you will fail, and therefore you do fail, works against those with low self-esteem. Struggling to raise self-esteem is usually accompanied by improved opportunities or better luck. Your score on questions 16–20 of the Stress Index indicates your level of self-esteem: 0–11 indicates high self-esteem (low stress); 12–16 indicates moderate self-esteem (moderate stress); and 17–25 indicates low self-esteem (high stress).

Anxiety Prone Personality

Some individuals see their problems as worse than they really are; such individuals are anxiety prone. For them, every stressful event seems to be a life-or-death situation. Though a torn blouse or shirt is a common mishap, it is a major embarrassment for those with an **anxiety prone personality.** These individuals have difficulty recovering from a problem and continue to relive the crisis for days and weeks after; this repeated review of the experience becomes a stressor itself.

Those who have an anxiety prone personality can sometimes detect such overt symptoms as a pounding heart, gurgling stomach, trembling hands, awkward speech, and other types of muscle tension when under pressure. To evaluate your proneness to anxiety, score your answers to questions 26–30 of the Stress Index: 0–11 indicates low stress due to the anxiety prone personality;

12–16 indicates moderate stress due to the anxiety prone personality; and 17–25 indicates high stress due to the anxiety prone personality.

Nurturing Strengths and Positive Addictions

Nurturing personal strengths is the approach used throughout this text. This approach advocates the very important principle of giving time, energy, and attention to individual strength areas or those areas that provide strength, comfort, support, and happiness. By nurturing strengths, we build resources for coping and establish havens in life where we can feel good and comforted. This principle is particularly important as it relates to mental health.

Glasser (1976) described behavior strengths as **positive addictions,** or those activities we do to give ourselves strength. Examples include activities such as meditation, exercise, or imagery. He suggests that positive addictions should include the following six elements:

1. It is something noncompetitive that you choose to do and can devote about an hour each day to it.
2. It is possible to do it easily and doesn't take a great deal of mental effort to do well.
3. It can be done alone or, rarely, with others, but it does not depend upon others to do it.
4. There is an accompanying belief that it has some value (physical, mental, or spiritual).
5. There is the belief that through persistence it will result in improvement, but this is completely subjective.
6. The activity can be done without self-criticism.

Selecting a positive addiction or nurturing personal strength areas reinforces and strengthens coping potentials.

Value-Behavioral Congruence

A strong coping approach is to align values and beliefs with behaviors. This is called **value-behavioral congruence.** Belief and value systems reflect what you feel is right, wrong, ethical, or unethical and are an important part of mental health. Values and beliefs may be of your own choosing, or they may have been imposed by family members, friends, religious leaders, or other sources and finally adopted by you. These values may be changeable or very stable. Contemplating these values and behaving in accordance with them is a key to happiness. One of the most devastating experiences for a person is to believe that something is right or wrong and then behave differently than that value dictates. Many young people, for example, enter college and experience freedom from parental influence for the first time and begin to experiment with drugs, sexual behaviors, or even dishonesty, all of which were forbidden in the protective environment of home. The resulting value-behavioral *incongruence* can be mental

debilitation and guilt. Guilt negatively influences self-esteem, the ability to study, social interactions, emotions, energy level, and other dimensions of health. There are only two realistic strategies to cope with guilt; behave in accordance with your value system or alter your values so they are aligned with your behavior. Altering your value system is generally time-consuming and painful, whereas self-discipline and commitment can alter behaviors, in most cases, almost immediately.

Self-Understanding: Personality

Each of us is unique and thinks and acts differently from everyone else. Understanding who you are, living within your natural approach to living, and then maximizing who you are are key components of happiness. It is extremely frustrating trying to be like someone else. Some of your basic nature is learned through experiences, and some of who you are is inherent. **Personality** is the product of many factors, experiences, disruptions, growth processes, and genetics. Personality is how you act, perceive, think, and feel. Your personality determines how well you can cope with the stressors, life events, and adversity that occur on a regular basis. Understanding your personality helps you to understand how and why you do the things you do. One way to understand your personality is to take a personality assessment instrument and at least understand the characteristics of personality. Personality

TABLE 2.3

Characteristics Measured by the California Psychological Inventory

Personality Characteristic	Intended Implications of Higher and Lower Scores
Dominance	Higher: confident, assertive, dominant, task-oriented Lower: unassuming, not forceful
Capacity for status	Higher: ambitious, wants to be a success, independent Lower: unsure of self, dislikes direct competition
Sociability	Higher: sociable, likes to be with people, friendly Lower: shy, feels uneasy in social situations, prefers to keep in the background
Social presence	Higher: self-assured, spontaneous; a good talker; not easily embarrassed Lower: cautious, hesitant to assert own views or opinions; not sarcastic or sharp-tongued
Self-acceptance	Higher: has good opinion of self; sees self as talented, and as personally attractive Lower: self-doubting; readily assumes blame when things go wrong; often thinks others are better
Independence	Higher: self-sufficient, resourceful, detached Lower: lacks self-confidence, seeks support from others
Empathy	Higher: comfortable with self and well-accepted by others; understands the feelings of others Lower: ill at ease in many situations; unempathic
Responsibility	Higher: responsible, reasonable, takes duties seriously Lower: not overly concerned about duties and obligations; may be careless or lazy
Socialization	Higher: comfortably accepts ordinary rules and regulations; finds it easy to conform Lower: resists rules and regulations; finds it hard to conform; not conventional
Self-control	Higher: tries to control emotions and temper; takes pride in being self-disciplined Lower: has strong feelings and emotions, and makes little attempt to hide them; speaks out when angry or annoyed
Good impression	Higher: wants to make a good impression; tries to do what will please others Lower: insists on being himself or herself, even if this causes friction or problems
Communality	Higher: fits in easily; sees self as a quite average person Lower: sees self as different from others; does not have the same ideas, preferences, and so on, as others
Well-being	Higher: feels in good physical and emotional health; optimistic about the future Lower: concerned about health and personal problems; worried about the future
Tolerance	Higher: is tolerant of others' beliefs and values, even when different from or counter to own beliefs Lower: not tolerant of others; skeptical about what they say

assessment can be accomplished through a number of personality inventories available from school counselors, psychologists, and other mental health professionals located at your university or college counseling center. Table 2.3 lists some personality characteristics.

Ego Defense Mechanisms

Psychologists have observed how individuals react when their self-esteem is threatened. Some of these coping mechanisms are healthy, and others are unhealthy. For example, daydreaming in class can help reduce boredom, but continued daydreaming may result in failing the class. Unhealthy mechanisms are those that keep us from facing reality. Several of these common coping mechanisms, called **ego-defense mechanisms,** are listed in table 2.4.

The Emotions

We need to practice continually the many skills involved in developing relationships. These skills are based on emotions, feelings, and personality traits. Basic emotions are

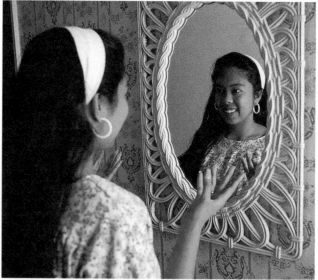

Understanding, accepting, and maximizing who you are is critical to good mental health.

TABLE 2.4

Ego Defense Mechanisms

Mechanism	Process	Example
Compensation	Covering up weakness by emphasizing desirable traits, or making up for frustration in one area with gratification in another.	If we are not considered physically attractive, we may lose ourselves in intellectual pursuits.
Denial of reality	Protecting oneself from unpleasant reality by refusing to perceive or face it.	Sexually transmitted diseases often go untreated because we deny their reality.
Displacement	Discharging pent-up feelings and emotions, which are usually hostile, on objects less dangerous than the ones that initially aroused the emotions.	The manager who is reprimanded by the boss at work in turn reprimands a spouse because a meal is late or cold.
Fantasy	Overcoming frustration by imagining that achievements have actually occurred.	Using college attendance to allow us to tell stories of great athletic or social accomplishments back home until the stories seem real.
Identification	Trying to become like something or someone else in thought or behavior; feeling increased self-worth by identifying with someone or something held in high esteem.	Wearing a football jersey similar to those worn by professionals, with a number of a favorite player.
Projection	Placing responsibility for one's own good or bad behavior on others, or attributing one's own desires to others.	"I failed that exam because Professor X is a lousy teacher."
Rationalization	Thinking up "good" reasons to justify irrational behavior; attempting to prove that one's behavior is rational and justifiable and thus worthy of social and self-approval.	When angered we may throw a dish against a wall and break it, later rationalizing that "I didn't like that dish anyway."
Regression	Retreating to an earlier developmental level that doesn't carry the responsibilities or difficulties of the current level; retreating to an age that one had enjoyed and where one had resolved the crisis associated with that stage.	Going to a park and playing on the playground equipment or developing strong emotional dependencies on a physical caretaker when distressed.
Repression	Consciously or subconsciously preventing painful or dangerous thoughts from entering the consciousness; often called "selective forgetting," although the thoughts are not really forgotten, for they "slip out" in dreams or conversations.	"Forgetting" the name of our old love until we suddenly call our new love by the old one's name!
Sublimation	Converting socially unacceptable instinctual drives or impulses into socially acceptable behaviors or personally acceptable channels.	Diverting our sexual drives into wrestling or picking someone up just in fun can seem more acceptable than premarital sex.

love, anger, and fear; all others are really combinations of these three. Jealousy, for example, is a combination of anger and love. Understanding your emotions and those of significant others is crucial to successful social interaction.

Emotions are very powerful in our lives. This is often demonstrated by actions and reactions under the influence of intense anger, fear, or love that are out of character for a person. The sway of emotions often finds us regretting our actions when emotionally distressed. By understanding emotions, we can better recognize in ourselves and in those we care about one of the forces that affects actions. Though love may be the most important emotion for healthy individuals to understand, an understanding of anger and fear is also essential.

Communication of all feelings is vital for healthy interpersonal relationships. "Relationships are not destroyed by honest expressions of anger" or any other emotion, according to Branden (1980, 140), but "relationships die every day as a consequence of anger that is not expressed. The repression of anger kills love, kills sex, kills passion."

The degree of hurt that we feel is generally proportionate to the amount of love we feel; the more we love, the more we can be hurt. The intensity of these emotions can be compared to the pendulum of a clock. As love increases, the pendulum swings in one direction, but when hurt occurs, it travels just as far in the other direction (fig. 2.3).

To cope with hurt, many of us become subconsciously or consciously angered, or we shut off the swing of the pendulum altogether by denying any emotion. "When a couple in love quarrel, it is very common to see each of them shut down, disconnect from the depth of their feelings for each other, disconnect from the depth of their love, so as to protect themselves in case things don't work out. They become impersonal" (Branden 1980, 166).

How you feel is a function of your emotions. By controlling your emotions, you can choose to be optimistic, hopeful, challenged, and excited and to have a fighting spirit. You can also decide to experience self-pity, be depressed, and sense helplessness. Consider the guidelines in the box on page 43 for controlling and maximizing your emotions through pairing. **Pairing** is the process of

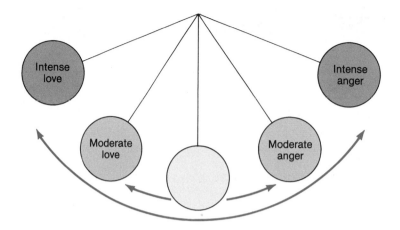

Figure 2.3

The emotional pendulum: love to hurt and anger.

storing in your brain desired emotions and then finding some trigger to access and then assume the desired emotion.

The Stress Response

When the mind perceives something as stressful, the body responds physiologically. Hans Selye (1977), a pioneer in the study of stress, defines stress as the "non-specific response of the body to any demand made upon it." In other words, stress is any physiological response of the body to demands from external environmental cues (people, situations, elements), internal mental processes (worry, fear, happiness), or physiological processes (drugs, sugar, biorhythms). In short, stress is a physiological arousal generally called the stress response. The stress response is demonstrated in a temporary state by muscles becoming tense, brain waves moving rapidly, heart rate increasing, blood pressure increasing, adrenalin and other hormones flowing through the system, and other responses that will be described later.

Stress is basically a positive element in our lives and should be used in a positive way. It is important not to become stressed to the point of becoming counterproductive and ill. Selye uses the term **eustress** to describe positive stress and the term **distress** to describe negative stress. Eustress can be labeled as a productive/healthy stress and distress as counterproductive/unhealthy stress. To conceptualize this, consider someone who has no stress at all. By the definition of stress, this would mean that there is no physiological arousal at all or that the person is essentially dead. Some physiological activity is evident during sleep or even when comatose, but twenty-four hours of sleep per day is not healthy. Stress increases with activity such as waking up, exercising, eating, communicating with others, facing daily challenges, working hard, or playing. At the same time, the activity increases health status and productivity.

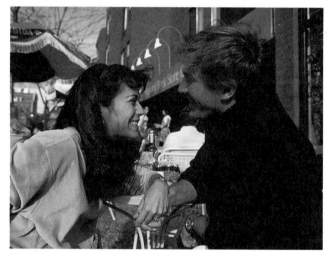

Sharing your feelings openly is an important part of mental health.

If stress levels reach a point of overstimulation, of extreme competitiveness (to the point of becoming hostile), of a life void of recreational activities, or of a lack of adequate rest, then we experience the negative aspects of stress. Figure 2.4 shows the rise in productivity and health as a result of stress. At some point, productivity and health peak, and if stress continues to increase, it results in decreased health and productivity until serious psychological and physiological health problems appear. Excessive stress in the form of opportunities, increased responsibilities, arguments, and so on becomes counterproductive.

Stress and Peak Performance

Olympic records are rarely made during practice but rather in the heat of competition, with crowds cheering in a stressful situation. An actor's best performance is with a large audience full of expectations and not during rehearsals. Many of us are most productive when we work

Controlling and Maximizing Your Emotions

Directions

1. Maximize your positive emotions.
2. Turn negative emotions into positive ones.
3. Anchor positive emotions in your brain.
4. Access positive emotions when you need them.

Clarification

1. Take advantage of your positive emotions by letting them contribute towards productivity, particularly as it pertains to working toward your cause in life and its contributing goals. Positive emotions or perceptions such as love, joy, optimism, the fighting spirit, sensitivity, warmth, calm, peace, and excitement can contribute to life-enriching activities you are trying to accomplish. When engaging in fitness, personal productivity, interpersonal growth, and power of the mind activities, associate love and excitement with those activities. For example, while preparing to exercise, imagine the love of someone encouraging you or the excitement of a job accomplishment with the exercise, recognizing that the exercise will help you be even more deserving of love or help you to be even more productive.

2. It requires strong mental and emotional control to turn negative emotions into positive actions, but many of us can do it. Negative emotions most often have destructive effects on your own mind, body, and soul as well as those around you. If you act during anger, often you regret your actions. If you fear and don't act, you often miss out on an opportunity. If you are pessimistic and doubt the positive outcome of something, then the likelihood of failure increases.

   Some negative emotions generate a terrific amount of energy due to their stressful nature. Anger and fear are the best examples. Often when we are angry, our muscles get tense, our heart rate increases and we think rapidly (although not clearly or rationally), which is a state of readiness to do something. We can choose to express that anger in a negative way by yelling at someone, destroying something, or stomping, or we can recognize anger as a powerful activator and preplan for anger. Then when it occurs, we can channel that energy into something constructive. When anger hits, rather than verbalizing yourself at that time, use that energy to exercise. Not only will you exercise more vigorously, but you will be able to think through the situations that caused you to become angry and be more rational in your actions.

   Fear of doing something, whether to approach someone, give a talk or presentation, start a business venture, or try a new skill, generates energy. If you can view that fear as an opportunity for growth (if the venture is a good thing to do) and learn to follow through, it well become easier to capitalize on that fear in the future.

   Some of the negative emotions create states of the soul that are energy draining. Guilt, helplessness, and depression generally leave you without energy or a desire to do much of anything. If you can see guilt, helplessness, depression, and other emotions as an opportunity to solve problems, learn a new coping skill, and surface after the fact much stronger, then you can almost enjoy the process.

3. Reflect back to a time when you had peak emotional states, and mentally relive those states (i.e., falling in love, being very productive, etc). Fix this mental state in your mind so that when you need to be energized or feel loving, you can go back to this memory quickly and assume that emotional state.

4. Try the following imagery strategy to acquire a desired emotional state. For example, you have had a stressful day at work and need to be loving to a child or spouse when you arrive home. Adapt this strategy to fit your needs.

   Get into a comfortable position and relax for a moment by breathing with your diaphragm. Imagine the optimal emotional state you want to have with this person. Visualize as clearly as you can your actions, what you will say, and your loving nature. Imagine the person as clearly as you can—the eyes, hair, smile. Now feel the desired emotions that you want to have when you see this person. Carry those emotions as you travel home.

Source: From G. E. Richardson, *Resiliency Training Manual.* Bountiful, Utah: Privately printed, n.d.

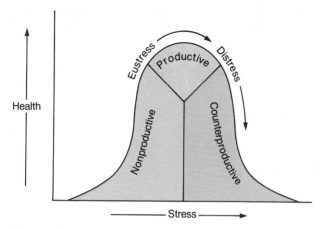

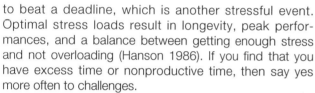

Figure 2.4

Relationship between health, productivity, and stress.

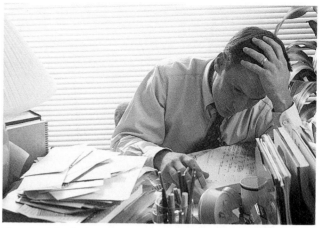

The physiological stress response is triggered by mental and social stressors.

to beat a deadline, which is another stressful event. Optimal stress loads result in longevity, peak performances, and a balance between getting enough stress and not overloading (Hanson 1986). If you find that you have excess time or nonproductive time, then say yes more often to challenges.

Laughter and enjoyment of good humor, proper diet, formation of realistic goals, an understanding of stress, practice of relaxation skills, sufficient sleep, good training for current or future jobs, living within financial means, and working hard to maintain a stable home life can all help us to reach our potential. Others have suggested that good self-esteem, effective partner communication, social support, decision-making skills, a purpose in life, good self-management skills, time to play, assertiveness skills, control of perceptions, and self-awareness are also conducive to peak performance (Detert and Russell 1987).

General Adaptation Syndrome (GAS)

The response of our bodies to stress, whether eustress or distress, occurs in three stages, which Selye (1977) called the **general adaptation syndrome (GAS):** the alarm stage, the resistance stage, and the exhaustion stage.

During the **alarm stage,** the body's defenses are called on to battle against a particular stressor. This is the **fight-or-flight response** triggered by a real or perceived threat. The hormonal stores are depleted as they are pumped into the blood, the blood vessels constrict, energy is utilized in tensing the muscles, and other fight-or-flight responses occur, as listed following:

1. A sharp increase in blood pressure (to increase availability of oxygen)
2. An increase in the blood sugar (energy for muscles)
3. Quick conversion of glycogen (stored carbohydrates) and fats into energy (sustain high energy utilization)

4. Increased respiration (to increase availability of oxygen)
5. Increased muscle tension (quick tension for greater strength)
6. Pupil dilation (visual acuity)
7. Release of thrombin (blood-clotting hormone to resist wounds)
8. Suppression of digestion (to give the body full reaction capacity)
9. Release of cortisone (to resist allergy attacks and dust)
10. Release thyroid hormone (speed up body's metabolism for energy)
11. Release of endorphine (body's own painkiller)
12. Release of cholesterol in the blood (long-distance fuel)

Figure 2.5 demonstrates the two pathways that trigger the stress response, both voluntarily and involuntarily. The involuntary response, triggered by sudden noise, touch, or other stimuli, travels through the hypothalamus in the brain (primitive and automatic response), which stimulates the sympathetic nervous system (stimulating brain system) and arouses the body for action. After the sudden involuntary response, the cerebral cortex evaluates the danger of the stimulus to determine whether a state of arousal is necessary. If it is determined that something is stressful, the voluntary pathway goes through the cerebral cortex (where we think, assess, and interpret), the **limbic system** (the emotional influence), the **hypothalamus,** the **pituitary gland** (which stimulates the adrenal glands), and the **thyroid gland** to secrete substances to trigger the stress response. If the stressor is so damaging that life cannot go on (gunshot, carbon monoxide, and so on), then the organism dies during the alarm stage, perhaps in a few moments or within a few days.

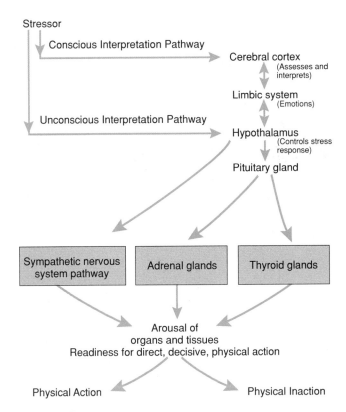

Figure 2.5

Pathways of the stress response.

No organism can maintain itself in the state of alarm forever, though, and it begins to adapt by entering the **resistance stage.** The body generates more hormones, dilutes the blood, and builds up energy stores to resist the stressor. In this stage, the body attempts to restore the balance (homeostasis) it had before the alarm stage.

Over weeks, months, and even years, if the stressor is not removed, the rejuvenated resistance begins to wear and the body enters the **exhaustion stage.** This is similar to the alarm stage in that reserves are eventually used up and the body becomes susceptible to disease with the lowered resistance. The weakest and most susceptible organs or sites are the likely targets of disease. At the exhaustion stage, the debilitating process in the body is often irreversible, and the organ becomes diseased or ceases to function.

Stress-Related (Psychosomatic) Disease

By understanding the GAS, stress has been linked to a number of diseases and psychological conditions. In particular, **psychosomatic disease** is psychological in origin and is directly associated with stress. Psychosomatic diseases are of two types. **Psychogenic psychosomatic disorders** are structural and functional disorders, such as migraine headaches, ulcers, asthma, backaches, and skin reactions that result from emotional stress (Girdano and Everly 1986). **Somatogenic psychosomatic disorders,** such as colds or

TABLE 2.5	
Some Diseases and Conditions That Have Stress as a Risk Factor	

Cardiovascular Diseases

Coronary artery disease
Hypertension (high blood pressure)
Angina (pain in the chest due to insufficient blood to the heart)

Muscle-Related Disorders

Tension headaches
Grinding and clenching of teeth
Shoulder and backaches

Allergic Diseases

Asthma
Hives
Hay fever
Allergic cold or swelling

Oral Conditions

Tooth decay
Ulcerated gums
Canker and cold sores
Tics (uncontrollable facial muscle contractions)
Habits such as thumb sucking, nail biting

Miscellaneous Diseases

Skin rash
Loss or graying of hair
Dandruff
Arthritis and rheumatoid arthritis
Overproduction of pituitary or thyroid hormones
Hypoglycemia (low blood sugar)
Infectious mononucleosis and other infectious diseases
Ulcers of the stomach or colon
Cancer
Depression
Diabetes
Gout
Warts
Premenstrual tension
Inflamation of vein walls

coronary heart disease, result when the body's resistance is reduced by emotional stress. Somatogenic psychosomatic disorders act as a catalyst for some already present organic diseases, such as cancer or arthritis, perhaps accelerating their growth. This latter concept implies that most diseases may have a psychosomatic component. Table 2.5 lists some of the diseases that have a stress component.

Psychological problems associated with distress include high levels of anxiety, irritability, fear, sleep problems, loss of appetite, overeating, inability to relax or enjoy normal activities, compulsive behaviors, ritualistic ways of coping, overdependence on alcohol or drugs, and overdependence on other people. In addition to the personal expense of destructive stress, the psychological and physical problems that affect individuals cost business millions of dollars each year in health-care costs, lowered productivity, and absenteeism (Somerville 1989).

Techniques to Manage Stress and Fortify Mental Health

As indicated, stressors are external or perceptual events or forces that may directly cause the physiological stress response. Stressors may also indirectly result in the stress response because of individual interpretation of the seriousness of the event or force. Stress management, then, is an individual's planned attempt to avoid or control certain external forces or events, reduce the seriousness of the events through mental and emotional control, or act to reduce the stress response after it occurs. If stress becomes excessive, that is, to the point of frustration and fatigue, then we need to manage stress at one of the three points of intervention: managing external stressors, developing mental/perceptual health skills, and managing the physiological stress response.

Managing External Stressors

Managing external events means dealing with specific stressors that result in frustration, overstimulation, boredom, and loneliness. It means controlling your environment and eating nonstressful foods. Managing external stressors also means taking advantage of the people and places around you. External stressors include individuals who provide you support, comfort, and happiness, so it is important to learn to deal effectively with those around you.

Managing Life Events

Managing external stressors is a function of identifying the stressors, such as noise, potentially embarrassing situations, potential arguments, or excessively difficult elective classes, and then avoiding or controlling them. We must also learn to cope with those external stressors that cannot be controlled or avoided.

For example, frustration occurs when our attempts to reach a goal are thwarted. To manage frustration, consider the following recommendations:

1. Analyze the reasons for your frustration, and determine what barriers prevent the accomplishment of a goal. Make a plan to overcome them.

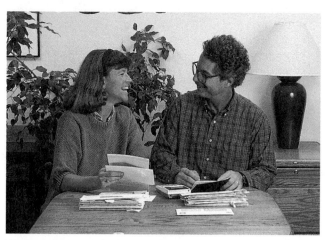

We can choose to be happy even when facing external stressors.

2. Choose alternative goals. When you cannot reach one goal, elect an accessible goal that will provide the same or similar rewards.
3. When you feel frustrated, do a relaxation exercise to rejuvenate yourself.

Another example is overstimulation, which occurs when demands or expectations exceed your capability to respond. Consider the following recommendations for managing overstimulation:

1. Establish priorities among your list of tasks to be done, allow plenty of time to accomplish each task, and follow your list.
2. Learn to say no when appropriate, and avoid overloading.
3. Delegate responsibility to others when possible or ask for help in fulfilling responsibilities.
4. Break a large task down into small parts rather than trying to do the whole thing at once.
5. Admit that you cannot do everything, and accept the fact that you are human.
6. Don't get caught up in the myths that lead to inefficiency (Semler 1989), namely thinking that the quantity of work is more important than quality, that no one else can achieve the same results as you, and that specific problems are urgent.
7. Practice time management as described in the accompanying box.

Managing Nutritional and Environmental Stressors

Some guidelines for managing nutritional and environmental stressors include the following:

1. Reduce your consumption of alcohol, tobacco, caffeine, and other drugs.
2. Avoid exposure to loud noises, such as loud stereos, airplanes, and rock concerts.

The reason many of us suffer frustration and overload is that we waste a lot of time. Careful planning and managing time effectively help to make the most of the time available each day. Day planners are popular because they provide the opportunity to plan your day and reflect on the important happenings of that day, and they provide evidence of success because of planning. Make or purchase a day planner that gives you a place to list tasks that need to be done, time slots in a day, and space to comment on the day's activities. You may be familiar with other time management approaches, for example, Franklin Institute or One-Minute Manager. If you are not familiar with other approaches, try the following steps to plan your day:

1. List all the tasks that need to be done and estimate the amount of time needed to accomplish the task. For a major task, such as a class paper, break the task down into manageable parts (literature review, introduction, subheadings, and so on).

2. Add 10 percent more time to each task for a buffer.

3. Rank order the tasks according to importance or due date.

4. Identify all available time to do the tasks. Mark out slots that are not available (classes, meetings, work commitments, time for exercise).

5. Place the tasks in available time slots according to your priorities and also in slots that maximize your potential. If you are more productive in the morning, then do your most challenging or creative work then. If you work better at night, then plan the most challenging tasks at night.

If you work better alone, then block time to be alone. Conversely, if you work better in groups, then arrange to do your most challenging tasks in some group situations. This step results in a realistic estimation of what you can get done in a day.

6. Upon completion of a task, write to the side how long it took you and other comments that will help you plan in the future.

7. Any tasks that did not get accomplished in one day should be added to the list for the next day, coupled with new tasks. Plan your next day in the same manner.

Source: From G. E. Richardson, *Resiliency Training Manual.* Bountiful, Utah: Privately printed, n.d.

3. Chart your biorhythms (natural ups and downs) each day for one month. Then plan your day around your biorhythms. Do your most challenging tasks in the morning, if you are a morning person, or in the evening if you are an evening person.

Learning Interdependent Skills

Interpersonal actions range from being totally passive to overly aggressive, with the moderate and healthy action termed **assertiveness.** Passive behavior is evidenced by a person who is withdrawn, who rarely says anything, particularly with strangers, and who is extremely shy. Aggressive behavior is shown by a person who pushes his or her opinion to the point of violating the rights of others to express freely. An aggressive individual may be hostile, not listen to other opinions, and dominate conversations. Assertive behavior is evidenced by individuals who feel comfortable enough with themselves to speak to others and make statements that represent their own feelings and thoughts. Assertive individuals have the following qualities: they are free to reveal themselves; they can communicate with people on all levels; they have an active orientation to life (go after what they want); they act in a way they themselves respect; and they sense the freedom to say no.

Assertiveness training is the process of mentally preparing and practicing assertive behaviors until they become natural. The gradual process of turning a passive person into an assertive person is generally accomplished one step at a time. Steps to assertiveness can be incorporated into an individual's life-style one step at a time (Girdano and Everly 1986):

1. Begin by greeting others.

2. When you can greet others, try complimentary statements.

3. Then, in a group, try starting statements with "I," such as "I think . . ." or "I tried . . ."

4. Try asking "why" to get additional information.

5. Share some feelings spontaneously.

6. Try disagreeing when appropriate and if you really disagree.

7. Maintain eye contact.

As you think about the levels of communication described earlier (see table 2.1), practice skills by imagining a potential or recent argument with someone. Analyze objectively the elements of the argument for all of the level 2 qualities (directing, persuading, blaming, etc.). Practice moving the level of communication to a more meaningful level.

To better understand how to move from level 2 to level 4, ask yourself, Why am I trying to blame, accuse, or deny? What are my true feelings on this? Start with "I feel this way . . . " and express your true feelings. Do not say, "I feel that your problem is . . . . " Express your own state, and let the other individual worry about his or hers. Remember that communicating at level 4 is very difficult because self-disclosure leaves you vulnerable. But, it is the most effective and efficient form of communication. To resolve and enrich relationships, work towards level 4, expressing how you truly feel about a situation and not telling the other person how he or she feels. You do not communicate on this level most of the time; only when you need to. We spend most of our time at the first level, or information-giving level.

The special value of communication is that we can openly express ourselves to those with whom we want to have a powerful relationship. Holding back, blaming, or other communication shortcomings only hinder relationships. This is the rule for business, romantic, friendship, or familial relationships. Simply being aware of these levels helps communication. As you talk with someone, think about at what level you are communicating.

If we understand what types of communication are used in different circumstances, then we have accomplished the first step in maximizing communication.

Developing Mental/Perceptual Health Skills

The process of acquiring mental/perceptual health coping skills generally occurs through the natural process of experiencing new life events, challenges, and adversity. There are also skills we can learn to approach our mental-health potential. The essence of developing positive mental-health skills includes the following:

1. Understand yourself.
2. Learn general mental-health skills and skills dealing with personal needs and challenges.
3. Actively identify and pursue your personal cause and purpose in life.
4. Engage in positive, repeated, varied, empowering, and new life experiences.

Understand Yourself

Self-understanding is really a lifelong process. The way we act, think, perceive, and react are functions of many complexities of the body, mind, and soul. Although space does not allow for a complete personality assessment, some of the personality characteristics you may have are listed in table 2.3. The essence of enriching who you are requires three general guidelines.

1. Maximize and fortify the characteristics of your personality and temperament by using skills of the mind and soul described in this chapter.

2. Live within those dimensions of personality and temperament that cannot or should not be modified.
3. Modify problematic areas of your life by using skills of the mind and soul described in this text.

The accompanying box describes some examples of temperament or personality characteristics and how you can maximize them.

Creative Personal Problem Solving

Creative personal problem solving can be defined as a cognitive-affective-behavioral process. An individual identifies and discovers an effective means of coping with problems encountered in every day living with this process. It has been shown that those with an ability to solve personal problems experience less stress (D'Zurilla and Sheedy 1991). When we make poor decisions, then we generally must deal with problems that result from our poor decisions. For example, in a romantic relationship, if one partner decides to go on a date with someone else, then the resultant problem will be to deal with the jealousy or distrust of the other partner.

The creative approach to personal problem solving incorporates both systematic and creative styles. The following systematic steps are suggested:

1. Define the problem clearly (collect as many facts as possible).
2. Generate a creative list of alternative solutions to the problem.
3. Think through the outcomes of each of the alternative solutions.
4. Make the choice for the best alternative.
5. Make preparations (acquire skills, materials, etc.) to enact the best alternative.
6. Implement the solution.
7. Evaluate the solution outcome.
8. Make modifications—learn from the experience.

It is with the second step that the creative portion of personal problem solving occurs. When thinking of solutions, write down the most logical solutions; then do some creative exercises to enhance the options. Think beyond moral, realistic, and financial limits for problem solutions; in other words, think wild and crazy. If the problem is that someone close to you got drunk and emotionally hurt or embarrassed you, then think of wild and crazy solutions, such as taking him or her to another planet or space-age laboratory where there is no ethyl alcohol and the person can be reprogrammed, throwing your friend into jail, or having Batman or the president take the person to the Bat Cave or the White House and tell your friend how hurt you are, how your friend is messing up his or her life, and how you wish he or she wouldn't drink. From these wild ideas may come some ideas that are more practical when the bounds of ethics and finances are fixed.

Skills of the Mind: Living Within Your Personality and Temperament

Many of us try to be what we are not and therefore find ourselves in frustrating, draining, and challenging situations. It is important to understand yourself and then maximize who you are.

Consider who you are and then use the following examples as general guidelines to plan your life and to live within your personality and temperament.

If You Are	You Face the Potential Problem	Your Solutions Might Be
Introverted	Working in groups (draining and nonproductive)	Do your most challenging and creative work alone
Extroverted	Working alone (draining and nonproductive)	Do your most challenging and creative work with others
Imaginative	Being compelled to do practical and repetitive work (frustrating)	Make the job you do creative, futuristic, and imagine what could be
Practical	Being compelled to do futuristic and creative work (frustrating)	Make the job you do based on facts and experience
Affective	Overrelying on feelings, relationships, and values (poor decisions)	Consider policy and rules and logical consequence before making decisions
Objective	Overrelying on facts, rules, and policy in making decisions (cold hearted)	Consider the exception to the rule and people's feelings, emotions, and circumstances
Decisive	Being too inflexible and potentially missing better options (missed opportunities)	Consider flexibility if deadline is reached and quality could be enhanced with time or other options
Open	Having trouble completing tasks because of being too flexible (poor work ethic and lack of accomplishment)	Take deadlines and goals more seriously and work towards completion
Risk taking	Venturing and losing too much (fewer resources)	Carefully consider outcomes
Conservative	Not getting ahead because of fear of venturing (stagnation—few resources)	Venture with fairly safe projects with high likelihood of success
Traditionalist	Being compelled to do actions that compromise your traditional values (guilt)	Live by your values

Source: Adapted from Richardson, G. E. *Socrates 2000: Guide to Personal Life Enrichment* (1992). Life Enrichment International, Nassau, Bahamas.

Perhaps when your friend is sober, consider visiting a holding cell for drunks, making a pact to not have alcohol at home or to limit alcohol consumption, reprogramming thinking through communication, or having someone who might have seen your friend drunk describe how he or she is hurting people.

Using a forced matrix for solutions means putting things together that normally are not put together to come up with solutions. For example, on one side of a matrix, place messages or feelings that the person who got drunk needs to hear (hurt, love, wishing he or she would quit, anger), and on the other side of the matrix, place some different ways to communicate messages (announcements at sporting events, billboards, telegraph, letters, videos, computer programs) besides talking (fig. 2.6). By pointing to the square where two ideas cross, perhaps some different ideas will be formed. Normally, you wouldn't think of making a video to tell someone you are hurt, going to a baseball game to hear an announcer make an expression of love, or even putting a message on a hotel marquee.

Meditation

There are many forms of **meditation,** including yoga. Some methods emphasize mindlessness, while others emphasize mindfulness. Some methods suggest particular sitting positions, while others suggest that the body simply be comfortable. Opinions also vary on the steps needed to reach a state of deep relaxation and contemplation: some suggest the repetition of a mantra or special sound to tune

	Hurt	Fear	Love	Anger	Wishing to quit
Sporting events			X		
Billboards					X
Telegraph					
Letters					
Videos	X				
Computer programs					

Figure 2.6

Creative personal problem solving with a forced matrix.

the mind and tune out its busy activity; others suggest that the practitioner listen carefully to the silence or the small sounds around, incorporating them into the meditation and into the body.

Whether the meditation form is Yoga, Zen Buddhist, or Tibetan, all these Eastern teachings have much to offer the West in terms of relaxation and self-awareness techniques. Most individuals find a method that suits them, and their choices seem to depend more on personality and life experience than on the higher effectiveness of one method over another. Whatever the method, however, the intent and basic practice are the same. Meditation is a way to relax the body's musculature and quiet the mind's ceaseless activity. The meditator becomes a participant observer of his or her own inner activity of consciousness by practicing being aware of being aware. This awareness seems to effect a spontaneous release of stress.

Imagery

We have a natural ability to daydream that we can use to escape our problems temporarily. By consciously using **imagery**, we can forget about our problems and let our mental and physical functions rest, if only for a few minutes. For an example of an imagery strategy, try the following:

Position yourself comfortably in a chair or flat on the floor with your legs and arms uncrossed. Take a few deep breaths, holding them for a moment and then releasing them smoothly and fully. Picture in your mind what is described in this scenario as clearly as you can, using as many senses as possible. In your mind's eye, you should see things, imagine how they would feel, look for color, see the movement, smell the smells, and so forth.

With your eyes closed, imagine that you are floating, perhaps on a cloud, and that you are rising above the place where you are now. The temperature is perfect and you have no fear as you float high in the sky looking at the views below. You find that as you are traveling, you are arriving at the ocean, and you continue to fly over

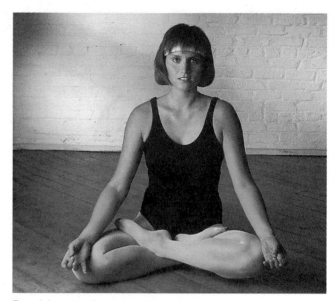

Practicing yoga is an excellent way to control stress.

the beautiful blue sea. You feel so good, so relaxed. You notice that you are coming to a small island and feel yourself gradually coming to a stop on a sandy shore. It is beautiful. Look to the sea and you can see the gentle waves pushing onto the shore. Inland you can see beautiful trees. Smell the smell of the fresh ocean breeze and hear the sound of the waves. Walk along the shore. You notice that you are barefoot and can feel the wet sand under your feet and the occasional waves lapping at your toes. Among the trees you notice a hammock tied between two trees. Walk over to the hammock and sit down, then lie down. You feel the security of the hammock around your shoulders as you swing back and forth. Feel that gentle swinging and rocking. You can see the blue sky, hear the sounds around you, and are so comfortable and relaxed.

Imagine other scenarios that may be more relaxing or comfortable for you: a mountain scene or a hot bathtub, for example.

Type A Behavior

Consider the following recommendations if you have a type A behavior pattern:

1. Use time more efficiently and effectively, and don't try to accomplish too much in one time frame. Use time management as described earlier in the chapter.
2. Talk to yourself, reduce you ego involvement, and remember that your whole reputation does not rest on any one action.
3. If easily distracted, practice concentration as you would any other skill.

4. Do thought stopping by yelling "Stop" aloud when you keep thinking about many different issues when you should be focusing on one. Remember that you can only accomplish one thing at a time. Keep a note pad and list things to be done that occur to you when in the middle of another task.
5. Use imagery for a short escape.
6. Become committed to, challenged by, and try to gain control of the tasks that you are called upon to do (hardiness).

Proneness to Anxiety

Try the following if you are prone to anxiety:

1. Do thought stopping as described for type A behavior.
2. Follow the steps to self-counseling as described in the accompanying box.
3. Learn to do imagery and deep breathing to distract yourself during your anxious thoughts.

Enhance Self-Esteem

To enhance self-esteem, try some of the following strategies:

1. Practice imagery (visualizing yourself as succeeding and doing well in activities).
2. Replace any self-defeating or self-critical statements (such as, "That was dumb" or "I can't do anything") with positive ones (such as, "I can do it if I really try").
3. Find and do those activities that result in good feelings about yourself.
4. Take time to consider accomplishments.
5. Be with people who recognize accomplishments and mutually enjoy each other.
6. Drop by the student counseling center at the college and ask to see a counselor to practice some esteem-building skills.
7. Try positive verbalization (Girdano and Everly 1986). Write down some positive personality traits that you like about yourself and reflect on those traits. Add positive traits as you identify them. With a low self-esteem, it is healthy to spend reflective time dwelling on positive traits.
8. Accept compliments from others (The Wellness Institute 1985). Saying thank you to a compliment rather than shrugging it off helps to enhance self-esteem.
9. In your daily planning, be sure to include those activities that you do well or that provide a strong likelihood of success. For example, play a game you do well, do homework in your better subjects, or make a point to talk with someone who loves you. Then enjoy that experience.

Identify and Pursue Your Personal Cause

The world seems driven by the selfish perception, What can I accomplish and get for me? rather than What can I do for us? Motivation is strongest when we work towards a cause. A cause is working towards an end or a process that requires some sacrifice, that consists of several goals, and that benefits others in addition to yourself.

Engage in New Life Experiences

New life experiences should be positive, repeated, varied, new, and empowering. The resiliency process described in chapter 1 suggests that when individuals experience new life challenges, they acquire new skills and become more competent. For an experience to promote growth, it should be positive. "Positive" means only that as a result of the experience, there is an opportunity to learn from the experience. If you try for a team and fail, this can still be a positive experience if you learn that a selected approach did not work and you now have the experience to try again with a new approach.

"Repeated" implies that there are times when we are ready to experience challenges and other times when we are not. If we are not mentally and emotionally ready to take on a challenge, than we may on a subsequent occasion. "New" and "varied" reflect the need for the experience to create a challenge rather than be something you have done before and that does not demand new skills. "Empowering" is important because you need to sense some control of the outcome and with success, reap the rewards of increased mental skills. A systematic approach to these life experiences might follow these steps:

Cause as Step 1: Consider your cause in life and how important it is to you.

Goals as Step 2: To accomplish your cause or purpose, it becomes necessary to plan a series of short-term and long-term goals that should be held constantly in mind.

Readiness as Step 3: As specific goals become clear, then you can plan and prepare mentally and physically to accomplish the goals. A specific plan should be developed to include how, when, where, with whom, and intensity of the plan.

Believe in Yourself as Step 4: Bandura (1977, 1989) believes that a critical component of behavior change or the acquisition of a goal is that the person believes/perceives that he or she is capable of making the change. You must sincerely believe that you can accomplish the tasks necessary to accomplish the goal.

Take Action as Step 5: When you are mentally ready, have a plan, and sincerely believe that you can accomplish the goal, then you implement the plan. This is the action portion and the last planned phase in the process of voluntarily subjecting yourself to

Self-counseling is the process of asking yourself the right questions, allowing time for your mind to analyze and process the questions, and coming up with answers and solutions based on your past experiences and perspectives. When you face a problem, feel depressed, or are emotionally upset, go through the process outlined here by asking yourself relevant questions such as those listed in the right column.

Process	*Questions to Ask Yourself*
1. Sort (facts and emotions)	What part of the concern is truth or fact?
	What part is emotion?
	What are the elements of the problem: What is? as opposed to What should be?
2. Understand	What is the adversity, challenge, or problem?
	What is the situation, and how do I want to deal with it?
	Why do I feel the way I do?
	How do I feel about myself as a result of facing the adversity, challenge, or problem?
	What is the belief I have about myself as a result of the situation?
	As a result of the belief I have about myself in light of the situation, how do I act differently in my everyday life?
	Are my thoughts, beliefs, and actions helping me to feel the emotions that I want to feel?
3. Consider action	Do I really need to take an action?
	Will the action be protective to me or those close to me?
	Will acting help accomplish my goals or cause in life?
	Will the action result in feelings that I want to have?
	By not taking action, will the problems be resolved or will I still be bothered?
4. Make a perspective shift	Is there a way that I can distract myself from thinking like this and think about something I like?
	Is there a way I can argue with myself to find a way out of thinking like this—argue about the adversity and the resulting negative beliefs about myself?
	If I looked at myself as another person, how would I give counsel?
5. Come to some resolve	What is the ideal resolve or action (inaction) to take?
	How close can I approximate that ideal action?

Clarification

1. Make decisions on facts rather than your emotional reaction to a situation.
2. Ask yourself positive questions that result in positive answers. If you ask negative questions such as, Why does this always happen to me? or What is wrong with me? then your brain will produce negative answers. Positive questions such as those cited or such as the following produce positive answers:

    How can I improve a relationship from this concern?

    What is wrong with the way I am thinking?

    How can I use what triggers my stress as a steppingstone for self-improvement?
3. Give your brain time to work. Sleep on it, think about it while exercising, or ponder it while showering. Soon your mind will come up with good thought processes.
4. When reflecting on taking action or modifying perspectives, consider whether the situation is something you can control. If it is, then taking action to better the situation is important. If it is a thought process, then try the following:

    Distraction—Stop the existing thought process and think about something you like. For example, if you are dieting and need to quit thinking about chocolate, pie, and ice cream, think about something else that is also pleasurable.

Disputation—Analyze the adversity that is causing the thoughts or belief you have about yourself and the consequences to your life as a result of the negative belief, then think of arguments to fight the negative belief. In the case of a diet, rather that thinking, "I am a weak person if I overeat," think, "I have done quite well for two weeks—this is like a short vacation, and I will get back on my diet now and go at least a little longer."

Distancing—Realize that your negative thoughts are just that—negative thoughts—and may or may not be facts. Try and look at the belief as something that is not part of you but something that you can look at objectively and finally throw away. In the example of the belief that "I am a weak person if I overeat," you can look at that negative thought from a distance and view it as a temporary state, one that shouldn't be part of you, and then discard that thought.

Source: From G. E. Richardson, *Resiliency Training Manual.* Bountiful, Utah: Privately printed, n.d.

disruption in order to experience growth. You should engage in your plan with great perseverance and tenacity, yet try to be sensitive to others as well.

Disruption and Disorganization as Step 6: The disruption that is likely to occur by trying to accomplish a goal or realize a dream will be mild to severe. Disruption and disorganization merely imply that you encounter a situation or challenge not experienced before. You may be discouraged.

Renew Your Cause as Step 7: It is always important, in the disruption stage, to remember and renew the cause/purpose or dream that initially motivated the planned growth process.

Introspection as Step 8: Introspection is the personal experience of assessing available personal resources to deal with a disruption. It is an opportunity to reactivate little-used skills, modify them to fit a new situation, or identify new skills necessary to resolve the disruption and reach the desired goal.

Skill Acquisition as Step 9: New, reactivated, or modified skills needed to meet the mental disruption and resulting disorganization might include creative personal problem solving, assertiveness, value/behavioral congruence, communication, self-counseling, or internalization of control. It may be that learning effective communication skills is required to resolve the disruption.

Renewed Action as Step 10: With new, modified, or reactivated skills, resilient adjustment can occur, and the initial action plan or the renewed action plan can be completed. The new skills that were necessary for resilient adjustment were likely not evident in the initial planning and became necessary during the process of growth. The action plan proceeds with the new skills and should be carried out again with tenacity, sensitivity, and/or perseverance.

Managing the Physiological Stress Response

When the stress response has occurred, and the feelings of tenseness, frustration, or measurable increases in heart rate, blood pressure, shakiness, or other symptoms occur, then several strategies can be used to reduce the stress response.

Exercise

Although fitness and exercise are discussed later in this text, it should be clear that exercise is one of the best strategies for reducing the stress response. Aerobic exercise uses the hormones in the blood generated by the stressors, fatigues tensed muscles, uses the oxygen provided from increased heart rate and blood pressure, and allows you to return to a tired but relaxed state. It cannot be overemphasized that by dealing directly with the stress response, you act in accordance with what your "fight or flight" response prepares you to do. Since fighting is generally not appropriate, then flight via walking, jogging, cycling, or swimming respond to the body's need in a direct way.

Yoga

Yoga is a practice designed to bring the body, mind, and universe into harmony through a variety of physical and mental disciplines. Many forms of yoga have been introduced to the Western world. Many Westerners now use yoga to relieve stress and as a vehicle for personal growth. The practice of yoga involves more than physical exercises; it also includes breath control, concentration, and various meditative techniques. The purpose of yoga exercises is not to increase bodily strength but to create an awareness in the practitioner of the different bodily states, such as tension and relaxation. The body's flexibility results not from straining and stretching but from learning how to relax and release muscles.

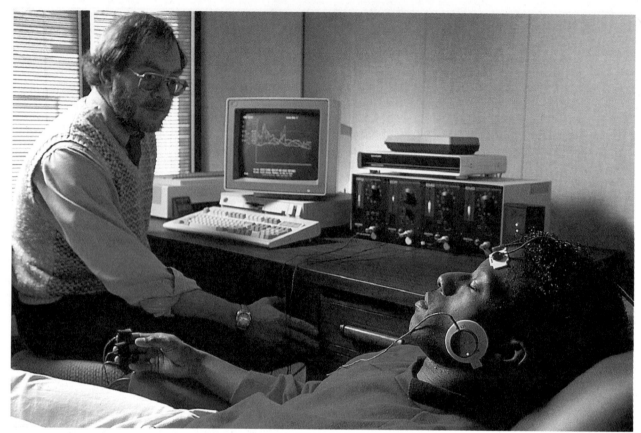

Biofeedback allows you to control stress by learning to control biological stress indicators such as heart rate, muscle tension, and temperature in body extremities.

Progressive Relaxation

The accompanying box describes how to do progressive relaxation. Progressive relaxation is a good method to deal with the stress response.

When Adversity and Stressors Exceed Our Ability to Cope

In the model for the prevention of health problems explained in chapter 1, the outcome of disruption and adjustment followed one of four tracks. The focus thus far has been on resilient adjustment or successful coping using mental health skills. Sometimes adversity and pressures exceed our ability to cope resiliently. We do not learn from the experience and return to our same routine, if possible. We may maladapt and following the event have actually fewer protective characteristics, such as a reduced zest in pursuit of goals, lower self-esteem, or reduced self-confidence. We may adjust dysfunctionally and require therapeutic help.

When there is a genetic weakness or a learned inability to cope, or when pressures are excessive, the imbalance sometimes forces individuals to seek professional help. There is no disgrace in seeking professional help.

Seeing a mental health professional is no different than seeing a physician to deal with a physical problem. By seeking professional help, individuals can build coping capabilities and maintain a mentally healthy life. If the imbalance is excessive, then serious psychological problems can result.

Some individuals cope during such an imbalance by no longer confronting reality. The following sections briefly describe some of the psychological illnesses that result when reality is not faced or when individuals escape reality by taking their own lives.

Mental Disorders

Mental disorders can be minor or major, depending on how poorly the individual handles emotional stress. Most of us suffer emotional distress at some time in our lives. For example, you may place great importance on performance in a particular examination, and if you do not do well, you may be depressed for a disproportionately long time afterward. Or, you may become so infatuated with someone that, for a time, you lose interest in everything else in your life. These are minor forms of mental distress. The first is a simple example of depression; the second, a simple example of obsession coupled with depression.

Get as comfortable as you can and close your eyes. Isolate yourself from the environment in your mind by consciously relaxing. Take a deep, cleansing breath, let it out, and then take another deep breath and hold it for five seconds. Let it out and feel the tenseness leave your body.

As you continue to take deep breaths, concentrate on the relaxation and tension relief you feel each time you exhale. Concentrate only on your breathing. Next focus on selected parts of your body. Tense and then relax the muscles in the area. This allows you to sense the difference between tensed and relaxed states of the muscles. First focus on your feet, curling your toes on both feet to flex the muscles. Flex, holding for five seconds, and relax. Recognize the marked difference from the tense to the relaxed state and feel the tenseness drain from your feet. Focus now on your lower leg muscles. Point your toes and flex your calf muscles. Flex, holding for five seconds. Now relax and feel the tension leave your calf muscles. Your feet and lower legs should now be so relaxed that they almost feel as though they are floating.

This exercise continues, focusing on the other general muscle groups of the body one by one. The progression continues with the upper leg muscles, the hands, the forearms, the biceps, the abdominal muscles, the shoulder and neck muscles, and then the facial muscles.

When we suffer from these lesser forms of mental distress, we remain very much in contact with our everyday lives and do not lose touch with reality. When depressed by unrequited love, we can usually maintain our daily lives and interact with others, even though we may not do so happily. When, before a sports event, an athlete is anxious about a performance, he or she may dream about it, wake up sweating, lose interest in food, and become irritable, but the athlete does not stop moving and acting appropriately in his or her environment.

At any stage of the life cycle, many forms of poor mental health can arise. These once were generally classified as neuroses but are now usually broken down into more specific categories. **Somatoform disorders** result when the brain determines subconsciously that the person is sick and thus the body develops physical symptoms. **Dissociative disorders** are conditions such as multiple personality (individuals actually assume different characters) or hysterical neurosis. **Adjustment disorders** are quite simply mental distress arising from an inability to cope with changes in the environment, such as an inability to study because of anxiety about an examination or an inability to adjust to limited activity brought about by physical incapacitation. **Anxiety disorders** are excessive fears called phobias, as well as panic disorders. Most of us experience some moderate phobias, or fears, such as acrophobia (fear of high places), astraphobia (fear of thunder and lightning storms), claustrophobia (fear of enclosed places), mysophobia (fear of contamination or germs), or monophobia (fear of being alone). We also probably experience moderate somatoform disorders and depression at one time or another but eventually work through them. Some individuals develop somewhat abnormal habits.

More serious are mental disorders such as **psychoses,** where individuals lose contact with the outside world. Despite widespread disagreement on the origin of these diseases, it is clear that some may be genetically predisposed and most are also subject to environmental influence. These more serious disorders include organic brain syndromes, which are controlled by actual physical disturbance in the brain through injury or other trauma, as well as **schizophrenic disorders** and **paranoid disorders.** Less extreme but equally troubling to the sufferer are personality disorders, in which the person tends to distort rather than escape reality.

Suicide

An extreme method of dysfunctional coping is **suicide,** the intentional killing of oneself. Suicide is the denial of a human being's most urgent need, self-preservation, and contradicts the value placed on human life. Roughly five thousand young people in the United States between the ages of fourteen and twenty-five will kill themselves this year (more than thirteen people per day). This is almost triple the rate of suicide thirty years ago (White, Murdock, and Richardson 1987). With reporting, masking, and interpretation problems in suicide statistics, the actual rate of suicide may be twice this figure. Add to this the number of attempts, which may be as high as one hundred per actual suicide, and a mental health problem of major proportions emerges.

Why Suicide?

The thought of suicide crosses nearly everyone's mind at some time during the life cycle. We all feel helpless or worthless at times. We simply do not get through life without the loss of a loved one or a major disappointment that leads to despair. Most of us can cope with these feelings. Why do others decide to end it all?

An impulsive person in the heat of anger, frustration, or disappointment may commit suicide without planning—someone who has perhaps been jilted by a partner or a teenager angry at his or her parents. Depression can make a person feel that life has no meaning, that special problems will never be resolved, and that the best thing to do is end it all. Someone in constant pain, especially with a terminal illness, may see suicide as an escape from suffering. Older people are most susceptible in this area.

Those who attempt suicide are trying to communicate with those around them. A person may be asking a spouse to come back; a son or daughter may be asking parents for attention. Although the attempted suicide may deliver the message, it seldom alters the situation.

The following represent items that may increase the risks of suicide.

1. Religion with no taboos against suicide. Religion is a particularly strong influence on suicide rates. Predominately Catholic nations, with strong sanctions against suicide, have lower suicide rates than mixed or predominately Protestant nations. Protestant Sweden has a suicide rate twice that of the United States and twelve times that of Catholic Ireland.

2. Urban environment. Urban standards of conduct and belief are weak compared to those in nonurban areas and create a high risk for urban residents.

3. High unemployment. Suicide rates increase and fall with economic cycles.

4. Availability of method. Access to automobiles, firearms, and potentially lethal drugs also increases risk.

5. Gender. Males are more likely to complete the suicide, and females are more likely to make an attempt at suicide.

6. Race. The order of greatest risk is white males, black and other nonwhite males, white females, then black and other nonwhite females.

7. Family relationships. Single-parent households, poor intrafamily relationships, and few siblings cause higher risks than other family situations.

8. Psychiatric profile. Depression, acting out behaviors, inability to cope with stress, a tendency toward alienation, and isolation are high risk factors (White, Murdock, and Richardson 1987).

Prevention of Suicide

Anyone who threatens to commit suicide should be taken seriously. You can try to befriend the person. The Samaritans, an international, privately funded suicide prevention agency, founded in 1953, suggests the following guidelines for befriending a suicidal person (Langone 1986):

1. Be yourself. Anything else feels phony, sounds phony, and won't be natural to you or to the person talking to you.

2. Your job is to listen. You want to make a relationship with the individual so he or she can trust you enough to tell you what is really on his or her mind.

3. What you say or don't say is not as important as how you say it.

4. Deal with the person, not just the problem. Talk as an equal, not a counselor.

5. Give your full attention, and listen for feelings as well as facts.

6. Don't feel you have to say something every time there is a pause. Silence gives you both time to think.

7. Show interest, and invite the person to continue without giving the third degree. Simple questions such as, What happened? and What's the matter? are not threatening.

8. Steer towards the pain, not away from it. The person wants to tell you; you have to provide the opening.

9. Try to see and feel things from the other person's point of view. Be on his or her side.

10. Let the person find his or her own answers, even if you think you see an obvious solution.

11. Many times there are no answers and your role is simply to listen, to be with the person, and to share the pain.

There are many suicide prevention and crisis intervention centers throughout the United States, some sponsored by schools and church groups, others by the community. A suicide prevention center is a place a person in crisis can call to get emergency advice, help, and referral. Volunteers are trained to calm the caller, assess the problem, and refer the caller to professional help. Some centers assign a team to travel to the person in crisis. Centers usually have a twenty-four-hour telephone service. Follow-up and referral services include emergency room services, outpatient clinics, inpatient programs, and educational and consultation services for the entire community.

Psychoanalysis and Psychotherapy

If anxiety, depression, or abnormal behavior becomes serious, there are many schools and kinds of psychotherapies available. Therapies range from **psychoanalysis,** in which an individual may spend years with an analyst working through unresolved developmental stages, conflicts, and traumatic experiences that may have caused the present disorder, to **family therapy,** which operates on the principle that a family is a unit with hidden rules and expectations that can sometimes hurt rather than help its members if enforced without loving awareness.

There are many sources of help for emotional problems. These include community religious leaders, physicians, counselors, licensed clinical psychologists, psychiatric social workers, psychiatrists, and licensed marriage, family, and child counselors (MFCC).

Most important, you are in control of most situations. This chapter has provided suggestions for improving your mental health skills and dealing with stress. Apply them and you will find more joy and happiness.

Summary

1. Mental health is the capacity to cope with life situations, to grow emotionally, to develop our full potential, to feel good about ourselves, and to gain inner peace.

2. Stress is a physiological response to stressors as manifested by increased heart rate, blood pressure, muscle tension, hormonal secretions, and brain-wave activity. The pathway in the brain that stimulates the stress response is either involuntary, via the hypothalamus and sympathetic nervous system, or voluntary, via the cerebral cortex, limbic system, hypothalamus, pituitary gland, and thyroid gland.

3. The difference between mental health and mental illness may be seen as a balance between coping skills and the pressures we face.

4. Eustress is positive stress, and distress is negative stress.

5. The general adaptation syndrome describes the body's response to distress.

6. The stress management/mental-health model identifies three points where stress management and mental-health skill development can occur: managing external stressors, developing mental/perceptual health skills, and managing the physiological stress response.

7. The process of acquiring mental-health coping skills is to subject yourself, voluntarily or involuntarily, to adversity, challenges, and new life events.

8. When pressures exceed the ability to cope, individuals may seek professional help with no disgrace. There are several types of health professionals who can help.

9. Suicide is often preventable if early warning symptoms are detected and befriending occurs.

Commitment Activities

1. Take fifteen minutes to sit on the campus grounds and watch people passing and greeting each other. How many people greet each other and do not seem to know each other? Take a chance today and say hello to someone you do not know. What happened? How did you feel before you did it? How did you feel afterward?

2. Keep a personal stress diary during the next three days. Note which events cause you to feel stressed and whether you feel the stress is positive or negative. Review you personal stress diary, and honestly consider how you managed and coped with the stressful events you experienced. What might you have done to better cope with the stressor?

3. Take the opportunity to go through the process of adopting a new coping skill. Challenge yourself by trying something you have not done before. Go through the process of committing yourself, preparing, feeling the disruption, and gradually learning. For example, if you have not ice skated before, try it, and then learn to at least stand up and skate around the rink. The process of seeing, trying, disrupting, and, with time, reintegrating and learning something new demonstrates the principles discussed in this chapter.

References

Bandura, A. "Human Agency in Social Cognitive Theory." *American Psychologist,* 44, no. 9 (1989): 1175–84.

Bandura, A. "Self-efficacy: Toward a Unifying Theory of Behavior Change." *Psychology Review* 84 (1977): 191–215.

Benson, H., and Stuart, E. M. *The Wellness Book.* New York: Birch Lane Press, 1992, pp. 266–85.

Branden, N. *The Psychology of Romantic Love.* Los Angeles: J. P. Tarcher, 1980.

Coopersmith, S. *S.E.I.: Self-Esteem Inventory.* Palo Alto, Calif.: Consulting Psychologists Press, 1981.

Covey, S. R. *The 7 Habits of Highly Effective People.* New York: Simon and Schuster, 1989.

Detert, R. A., and Russell, R. "Identification and Description of Content Elements for Stress Management in Health Education." *Health Values* 11 no. 1 (1987): 3–12.

D'Zurilla, T. J., and Sheedy, C. F. "Relation Between Social Problem-Solving Ability and Subsequent Level of Psychological Stress in College Students." *Journal Personality and Social Psychology.* 61, no. 5 (November 1991): 841–47.

Erikson, E. *Childhood and Society,* 2d ed. New York: Norton, 1963.

Fischman, J. "Type A on Trial." *Psychology Today* 21 no. 2 (1987): 42–64.

Flannery, R. B. "Toward Stress Resistant Persons: A Stress Management Approach to the Treatment of Anxiety." *American Journal of Preventive Medicine* 3 no. 1 (1987): 25–30.

Friedman, M., and Rosenman, M. H. *Type A Behavior and Your Heart.* New York: Knopf, 1974.

Girdano, D. A., and Everly, G. S. *Controlling Stress and Tension: A Holistic Approach.* Englewood Cliffs, N.J.: Prentice-Hall, 1986.

Glasser, W. *Positive Addiction.* New York: Harper and Row, 1976.

Hanson, P. G. *The Joy of Stress.* Kansas City: Andrews, McMeel and Parker, 1986.

Jola, I. K. "Helping—Does It Matter: The Problems and Prospects of Mutual Aid Groups." Address to the United Ostomy Association, 1970.

Kobasa, S. C., Maddi, S. R. and Kahn, S. "Hardiness and Health: A Prospective Study." *Journal of Personality and Social Psychology,* 42, (1982): 168–77.

Langone, J. *Dead End.* Boston: Little, Brown, 1986.

Maslow, A. H. *Toward a Psychology of Being.* New York: Van Nostrand, 1962.

Moore, T. *Care of the Soul.* New York: HarperCollins, 1992.

Selye, H. *Stress Without Distress.* New York: Signet Books, 1977.

Semler, R. "Senhor Semler's Planet." *Across the Board* 26 (1989): 10.

Somerville, J. "Stress Treatment Costing Billions." *American Medical News* 32 (1989): 17.

University of California, Berkeley. "How Anger Affects Your Health." *Berkeley Wellness Letter* 8, no. 4 (January 1992): 4.

The Wellness Institute. *The Lifestyle Inventory.* College Station, Tex.: TWI, 1985.

White, G. L., Murdock, R. T., and Richardson, G. E. "Adolescent Suicide." *Physician Assistant* 11, no. 5 (1987): 103–14.

Additional Readings

Crosby, R. "Self-Concept Development." *Journal of School Health* 52, no. 7 (1982): 432–36. An article that gives interesting ideas on the development of and activities to enhance self-concept.

Greenberg, J. *Comprehensive Stress Management.* Dubuque, Iowa: Brown & Benchmark, 1990. An excellent book providing an overview of stress management. This is highlighted by personal experiences and references from the author.

McGinnis, A. L. "Getting the Most Out of Life." *Reader's Digest* 139, no. 831, July 1991, pp. 17–21. A good article on turning tragedy into opportunities.

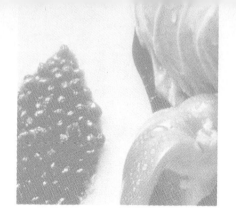

PART **II**

Nutrition, Physical Activity, and Weight-Control Choices

I N CHAPTER 3, INFORMATION IS PROVIDED AND SKILLS ARE EMPHASIZED THAT WILL HELP YOU PLAN FOR OPTIMAL NUTRITION, EAT WELL ON A BUDGET, AND UNDERSTAND DECISIONS RELATED TO FOOD ADDITIVES AND LABELING. IN CHAPTER 4, THE HEALTH BENEFITS OF PHYSICAL ACTIVITY ARE STRESSED. SKILLS NEEDED TO DEVELOP AND CONTINUE A PERSONAL FITNESS PRO-GRAM ARE EMPHASIZED. IN CHAPTER 5, IMPORTANT INFORMATION ABOUT WEIGHT CONTROL IS PRESENTED.

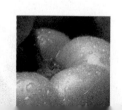

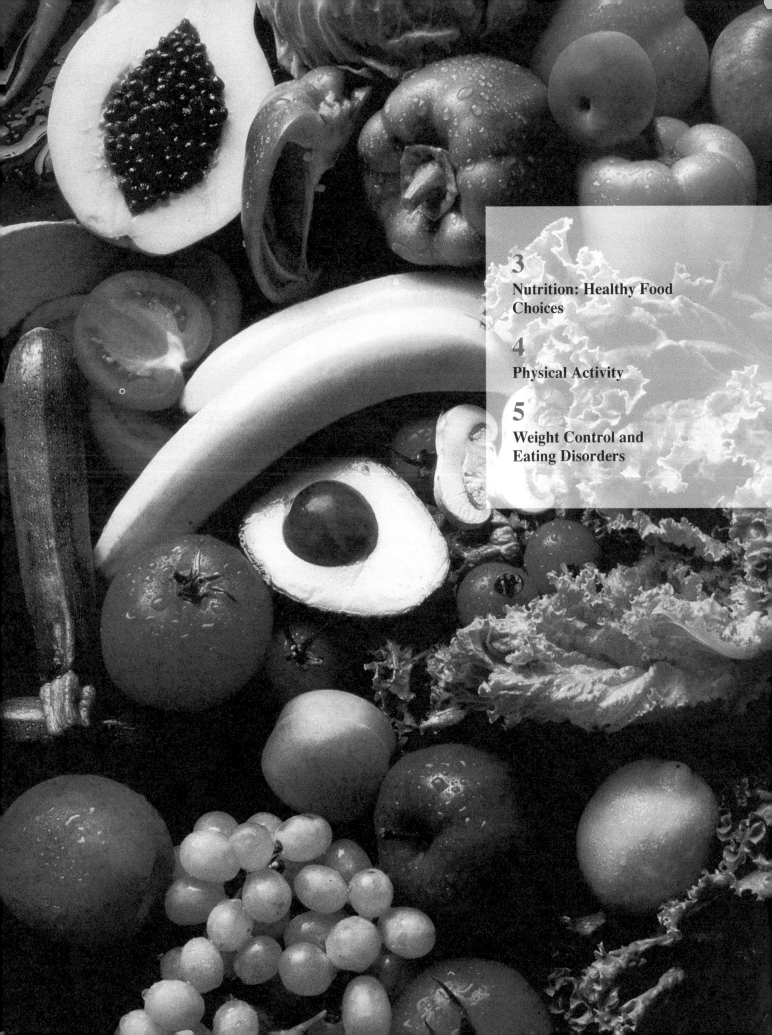

CHAPTER 3

Nutrition: Healthy Food Choices

Key Questions

- What factors affect your food choices?

- What is the nutritional status of Americans?

- What are the components of good nutrition?

- Why is it important to plan for good nutrition?

- What can you do to eat inexpensively and nutritiously?

- What are some nutritional concerns for athletes, the elderly, and vegetarians?

Chapter Outline

Factors Affecting Food Choices
Nutrition in the United States
Nutrition Basics
    Carbohydrates
    Proteins
    Fats
    Vitamins
    Minerals
    Water
Planning for Optimal Nutrition
    Food Choices
    Eating Well on a Budget
    Fast Foods/Convenience Foods
Nutrition and the Consumer
    Food Additives
    Nutrition Labeling
Special Nutritional Considerations
    Vegetarians
    Athletes
    Individuals Under Stress

This chapter helps you understand the basics of nutrition, which is the study of food and the process of receiving nourishment, and apply this information to your life. Included are a review of nutrition, suggested changes you can make to eat more nutritiously, and ways to become a more nutrition-conscious consumer. Ways in which good nutrition can enhance coping skills are also examined, along with things you can do from a nutritional perspective to increase your resiliency.

In our society, we are probably more interested in nutrition than ever before. This interest has translated into an overabundance of advertising, including much that promotes the nutritional advantages of products, whether or not those advantages exist. Since much more money is spent advertising the less nutritious foods than the more nutritious foods, we need to be informed and concerned consumers to differentiate fact from fiction.

Many college students are interested in nutrition because they want to be able to perform at their maximum level academically and/or physically. Most college students also make the majority of decisions

Nutritional Assessment

Circle Y to indicate a yes response, or circle N to indicate a no response.

Y	N	1. Do you eat breakfast every day?
Y	N	2. Do you eat three or more meals a day?
Y	N	3. Do you have small snacks such as potato chips, candy, cookies, soft drinks, and so on between meals?
Y	N	4. Do you often eat your evening meal after 7:00 P.M.?
Y	N	5. Do you usually eat a light evening meal?
Y	N	6. Do you usually eat white bread?
Y	N	7. Do you often eat sugar-coated cereals?
Y	N	8. Do you eat a variety of foods, including fruits, vegetables, meats, breads, and dairy products?
Y	N	9. When you eat meat, do you usually eat lean cuts of meat?
Y	N	10. Do you usually use margarine rather than butter?
Y	N	11. Do you usually add salt to your food?
Y	N	12. Do you usually drink whole milk?
Y	N	13. Do you often eat refined flour products (pasta, cakes, cookies, and so on)?
Y	N	14. Do you often eat refined sugar products (candy, sugar, soda, pop, and so on)?
Y	N	15. Do you usually eat two or three servings of meat or protein-rich foods a day?
Y	N	16. Do you usually limit your intake of fat (whole milk, salad dressing, gravies, fat in meat servings, margarine, and butter)?
Y	N	17. Does you diet contain more shellfish, red meat, and processed meat than poultry and fish?
Y	N	18. Do you often eat foods seasoned by or cooked in pork or other meat fat?
Y	N	19. Do you keep your calorie intake within your usual daily requirements?
Y	N	20. Is your food usually broiled, baked, or boiled rather than fried?
Y	N	21. Do you eat most of your meals at home (or in the school cafeteria)?
Y	N	22. Do you eat high-roughage foods daily (fresh fruits, bran, raw vegetables, and so on)?
Y	N	23. Do you drink six or more glasses of water per day?

Scoring/Interpretation

Give yourself one point for each of your responses that agree with the following key.

1. Y	7. N	13. N	19. Y
2. Y	8. Y	14. N	20. Y
3. N	9. Y	15. Y	21. Y
4. N	10. Y	16. Y	22. Y
5. Y	11. N	17. N	23. Y
6. N	12. N	18. N	

A prudent diet is one that is generally healthy and good for you. The following scale suggests a prudent or nonprudent diet:

18–23 Prudent diet

11–17 Moderately prudent diet

0–10 Nonprudent diet

regarding their food choices. Therefore, information on nutrition becomes more important. The results of the Health Assessment at the beginning of this chapter provide an indication of the quality of your current nutritional choices.

Factors Affecting Food Choices

Eating would be a very simple activity if we ate only when hungry and applied our knowledge of nutrition to our food choices; however, it is much more complex than that. As young children, we learned to associate food with good times and bad times. These behaviors continue in adulthood. We reach for food to feel better in times of disappointment and to celebrate in times of happiness. Food becomes a coping mechanism for some.

Although there is an almost endless number of food items from which to choose, most of us limit our food consumption to less than one hundred foods. Parents have much to do with influencing their children's eating habits.

Nutrition in the United States

Since food is so readily available in this country, Americans should have the best diets in the world. Unfortunately, easy access to food does not result in good food choices.

- American cheese consumption is on the rise, which is likely due to our consumption of pizza. Americans consumed 25 pounds of cheese per person in 1990.
- Consumption of poultry products has increased steadily since 1970. Americans consumed 64 pounds of poultry per person in 1990.
- Egg consumption has dropped from 276 eggs per person in 1970 to 187 eggs per person in 1990.

- Milk consumption has dropped from 214 pounds per person in 1970 to 88 pounds per person in 1990.
- Fruit consumption has risen from 18 pounds per person in 1970 to 90 pounds per person in 1990.
- Although coffee intake is down, caffeine levels have remained the same due to our consumption of chocolate and soft drinks.

- Sugar consumption has increased 15 pounds per person since 1970 mostly due to our consumption of soft drinks.
- Americans continue to consume more food per person than ever.
- The amount of fat in our diet continues to increase. Forty-three percent of our calories are from fat. (Note: This author quotes a higher percentage of fat intake than many others. Most figures will be in the range of 37 percent.)

Source: Candy Sagon, *L.A. Times/Washington Post*.

Many Americans have problems that relate to excessive eating rather than to dietary deficiencies.

Dietary factors are associated with six of the ten leading causes of death in the United States, including coronary heart disease, some types of cancer, stroke, noninsulin-dependent diabetes mellitus, chronic liver disease and cirrhosis, and atherosclerosis ("Institute Offers 'Clear-Cut' Diet Plan" 1992). The U.S. Department of Agriculture and the U.S. Department of Health and Human Services have published three sets of dietary guidelines. The most recent revision includes specific suggestions, including the following:

Eat a variety of foods.

Maintain desirable weight.

Choose a diet low in fat, saturated fat, and cholesterol.

Choose a diet with plenty of vegetables, fruits, and grain products.

Use sugars only in moderation.

Use salt and sodium only in moderation.

If you drink alcoholic beverages, do so in moderation.

For some Americans, these recommendations involve minor dietary modifications, while for others they involve major dietary nutritional changes (fig.3.1). Our nutritional decisions involve options related to behavioral and motivational choices and the decision-making process mentioned in chapter 1.

Healthy People 2000 (1990) lists nutrition as one of the health promotion priorities and includes twenty-one nutrition objectives. Acknowledged in the report is the correlation between poor nutritional practices and chronic diseases. The change in focus of Americans from nutritional deficiency to the emphasis on chronic disease prevention

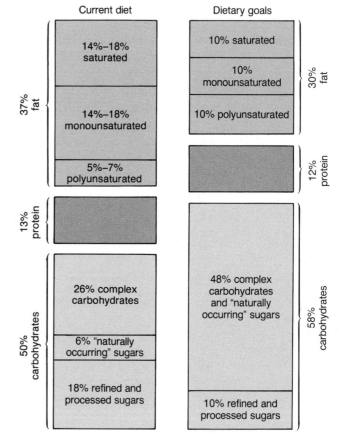

Figure 3.1

Percent of calories from different nutrients in the current American diet and in an ideal diet.

Source: Based in part from *Dietary Goals for the United States,* 1977; prepared by the Senate Committee on Nutrition and Human Needs.

and health maintenance is also discussed. The progress in this area is reflective of the impact of national concerns regarding nutrition.

Nutrition Basics

Whatever our age, to stay healthy we need to replenish our cells by ingesting food. Food passes through our digestive system, which transforms today's meal into tomorrow's energy, renewal, and growth. If too much food, too little food, or too much food of low nutritional value is consumed, our health is negatively impacted.

The process of digestion begins in the mouth. Saliva produced at the sight, smell, or thought of food contains enzymes (compounds that speed the rate of a chemical reaction without being affected by the reaction) that break down carbohydrates and mucus that moistens food. Food moves through the esophagus into the stomach, where enzymes and stomach acids mix with the food. A meal usually leaves the stomach within two to three hours of consumption and passes into the small intestine, where it stays for three to ten hours. Although the small intestine is narrow, it is actually ten feet long. The majority of a meal (95 percent) is digested in the small intestine, where enzymes from intestinal cells and the pancreas mix with food during muscular contractions. Nutrients are absorbed from the small intestine into the bloodstream for use by the cells. The remaining solid waste moves from the small intestine to the large intestine, where it remains for one to three days before the waste products are eliminated from the body.

Nutrients are the nourishing elements in food. They include carbohydrates, proteins, fats, vitamins, minerals, and water. The kinds and amounts of nutrients contained in foods vary. Note that no single food provides all of the nutrients in the amounts needed for growth and health. Over forty nutrients are needed by the body. Consequently, a diet that includes a variety of foods from all of the food groups is needed to provide the necessary nutrients.

The Recommended Dietary Allowances, or **RDAs,** are the levels of nutrient intake necessary for the maintenance of good nutrition in practically all healthy persons as determined by the Food and Nutrition Board of the National Research Council (table 3.1). The RDAs are intended to help us meet our nutritional needs through foods rather than with vitamin supplements. They are not daily recommendations but are nutrient levels needed over time and should be the average intake for vitamins and minerals in a three- to seven-day period (Guthrie 1990). You should not try to plan meals based on the RDAs. Supplements to the diet are recommended only in the few cases where deficiency is commonly observed, such as iron deficiency in women ("New Recommended Dietary Allowances" 1990).

One of the practical applications of the RDAs is their use by the U.S. Department of Agriculture to establish standards for food assistance programs, to assess nutritional status, and to evaluate food supply. These standards are referred to as the U.S. Recommended Daily Allowances (**USRDA**) and influence the way in which nutritional content of food is listed on labels.

One of the chief roles of food is to supply energy to support the body's activities. This energy comes from the nutrients in food and is measured in calories. A **calorie** is a unit for measuring the heat or energy-producing value of food when it is burned by the body. Food energy is usually expressed in terms of kilocalories or kcal. Calories are also a measure of the energy we expend in different activities.

Carbohydrates

Carbohydrates supply the energy to our bodies that is needed for daily activities. While some individuals may have previously associated carbohydrates with excess calories, many now consider complex carbohydrates, such as pasta, a positive alternative for a protein dish high in fat. Carbohydrates are also metabolized faster and more efficiently than proteins.

Carbohydrates are compounds composed of carbon, hydrogen, and oxygen. Their major function is to provide a continuous energy supply to the cells of the body. Carbohydrates supply four calories of energy per gram and can be categorized as either simple or complex. **Simple carbohydrates** are composed of one or two simple sugar units, while **complex carbohydrates** are composed of longer chains of sugar units.

Simple Carbohydrates

Sugars are simple carbohydrates found naturally in foods such as fruit and milk and in some vegetables, such as beets and peas. Sugars refined from sugar cane and sugar beets are also added to foods such as candy, soft drinks, and ice cream.

Simple carbohydrates provide immediate energy, while complex carbohydrates provide longer-lasting energy. As carbohydrates enter the body, they are changed into **glucose,** the energy source for cells. Along with proteins, vitamins, and minerals, cells use this energy to repair themselves, make new cells, and carry out their work. Glucose is found in molasses, corn syrup, honey, and fruits and is classified as a **monosaccharide** since it contains only one molecule of sugar. Fructose is a monosaccharide found in fruits. **Disaccharides** are simple carbohydrates formed from two monosaccharides. They include **sucrose** (simple table sugar), which is a combination of fructose and glucose; lactose (found in milk products), which is a combination of glucose and galactose; and maltose, which is formed by the combination of two glucose molecules.

Sugar Intake

Americans consume more than 130 pounds of sugars and sweeteners per person each year (Liebman, "The Changing American Diet" 1990). Sugary snacks are filled

TABLE 3.1

RDAs for Adult Men and Women

Category	Age	Weight (lb)	Height (in)	Protein (g)	Fat-Soluble Vitamins				Water-Soluble Vitamins							Minerals						
					Vitamin A (mcg RE)[a]	Vitamin D (mcg)	Vitamin E (mg)[b]	Vitamin K (mcg)	Vitamin C (mg)	Thiamin (mg)	Riboflavin (mg)	Niacin (mg)	Vitamin B6 (mg)	Folate (mcg)	Vitamin B12 (mcg)	Calcium (mg)	Phosphorus (mg)	Magnesium (mg)	Iron (mg)	Zinc (mg)	Iodine (mcg)	Selenium (mcg)
Males	15-18	145	69	59	1,000	10	10	65	60	1.5	1.8	20	2.0	200	2.0	1,200	1,200	400	12	15	150	50
	19-24	160	70	58	1,000	10	10	70	60	1.5	1.7	19	2.0	200	2.0	1,200	1,200	350	10	15	150	70
	25-50	174	70	63	1,000	5	10	80	60	1.5	1.7	19	2.0	200	2.0	800	800	350	10	15	150	70
	51+	170	68	63	1,000	5	10	80	60	1.2	1.4	15	2.0	200	2.0	800	800	350	10	15	150	70
Females	15-18	120	64	44	800	10	8	55	60	1.1	1.3	15	1.5	180	2.0	1,200	1,200	300	15	12	150	50
	19-24	128	65	46	800	10	8	60	60	1.1	1.3	15	1.6	180	2.0	1,200	1,200	280	15	12	150	55
	25-50	138	64	50	800	5	8	65	60	1.1	1.3	15	1.6	180	2.0	800	800	280	15	12	150	55
	51+	143	63	50	800	5	8	65	60	1.0	1.2	13	1.6	180	2.0	800	800	280	10	12	150	55

Reprinted with permission from *Recommended Dietary Allowances: 10th Edition*. Copyright 1989 by the National Academy of Sciences. Published by the National Academy Press, Washington, D.C.

[a] mcg—microgram = 1/1,000,000th gram; RE—retinol equivalent = 1 mcg retinol or 6 mcg beta-carotene
[b] mg—milligram = 1/1,000th gram

Note: Recommended Dietary Allowances (RDAs) are established by the National Research Council of the National Academy of Sciences and published by the government. The RDA for any given nutrient represents the amount considered "adequate to meet the known nutrient needs of practically all healthy persons."

with **empty calories** meaning they contain no vitamins, minerals, or protein. Your nutrition may be negatively affected when you substitute sugary items for those with nutrients. The increased use of artificial sweeteners has not curtailed sugar consumption. In fact, sugar consumption has continued to grow.

A careful reading of product labels on the supermarket shelf shows that it is difficult to select a food prepared without sugar (table 3.2). Sugar is included not only in foods that are obviously sweetened but also in sauces, some baby foods, almost all fruit drinks, salad dressings, canned and dehydrated soups, pot pies, frozen TV dinners, bacon and other cured meats, some canned and frozen vegetables, most canned and frozen fruits, yogurt, and breakfast cereals. Many of the presweetened cereals, most often advertised during children's television programming, contain nearly as much sugar in one serving (one cup) as half a can of pop ("TV Feeds Kids Steady Diet of Sugary-food Ads" 1990).

The $7 billion cereal business is getting bigger as food manufactures target children in an effort to increase their 33 percent share of the market. Although sugar-coated breakfast cereals have been available for years, manufacturers are being more aggressive with their newest wave of presweetened cereals, which incorporate themes from the most current movies, toys, and fads. The products are advertised during cartoons and may have ninja nets (Ninja Turtles cereal) or hearts, bows, and stars (Barbie cereal). One of the biggest concerns with this trend relates to the difficulty in providing children with a proper nutritional balance in their diets because of the number of calories that come from sugar. Children's cereals are 44 percent sugar, while adult cereals are 10 percent sugar ("Kid's-eye Cereals" 1990).

There are over one hundred sweet substances identified as "sugar," including fructose, dextrose, lactose, and maltose, but the word *sugar* is commonly used to refer to *sucrose.* Some sugars aren't quite as bad for the teeth as sucrose; otherwise, there is virtually no difference among them. There is no nutritional value in any of the sugars other than calories ("Honey vs. Sugar" 1992).

Although a number of diseases have been linked with excessive consumption of sugar, tooth decay is the most obvious problem. Dental caries (cavities) begin when oral bacteria lower the pH of the mouth from a normal 6.7 to 5.5 or lower. It is thought that bacteria (probably streptococci) convert carbohydrate to plaque, which deposits on the teeth. The bacteria between the plaque and the tooth enamel produce acids that dissolve tooth enamel. In this protected area, bacteria are not reached by saliva or by tooth brushing, so they continue to erode enamel. If the enamel is thin or weak, the process moves very quickly, and bacteria eat through the dentin and may enter the pulp cavity. At this point, it may be impossible to save the tooth by drilling and filling.

The more often sugar is present in the mouth, the more opportunity oral bacteria have to metabolize sugar, produce acid, and erode tooth enamel. A large amount of

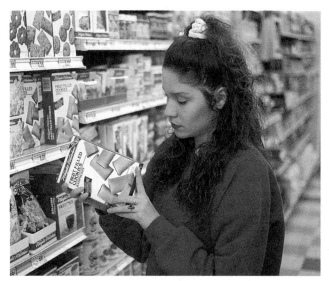
Sugar is hidden in many foods.

sugar consumed once a day is far less damaging to the teeth than a small amount consumed several times a day. Sticky snacks high in sugar are particularly harmful because the bacteria on the teeth continue to make acid and erode the enamel.

There are several things you can do to maintain healthy teeth and gums. They include (1) daily flossing, (2) regular brushing (with a soft nylon brush with rounded bristles) in a circular motion with the brush at a 45-degree angle with the gum line, (3) avoiding tooth whiteners (which erode enamel) and toothpastes or powders with sugar for flavoring, and (4) rinsing the mouth with water several times a day.

Since sugar is the most common ingredient added to food, it takes a conscious effort to reduce the intake of sugar in your diet. Some suggestions for decreasing the intake of sugar include the following:

1. Read labels for hidden sugars (look for ingredients ending in *ose*) and select products with the fewest. On foods high in sugar, it is listed as one of the first ingredients. Choose items in which sugar does not appear or appears low on the ingredient list.

2. Decrease your intake of foods and beverages containing sugar. Be aware of soft drinks and presweetened products such as cereals.

3. Select fresh fruits or fruits packed in water or their own juices rather than syrup.

4. Prepare foods at home rather than buying commercially produced foods, which tend to be high in sugars. Gradually decrease the amount of sugar added to recipes.

5. Substitute spices, such as cinnamon, for sugar to bring out the flavor of foods.

6. Explore ways to decrease sugar intake by reducing sugar added to beverages and other foods.

7. Substitute fruit for sweetened desserts or snacks.

TABLE 3.2

Refined Sweeteners in Breakfast Cereals

	Serving Size	Table Sugar Equivalent (tsp)	Sugar Calories (% of total calories)		Serving Size	Table Sugar Equivalent (tsp)	Sugar Calories (% of total calories)
General Mills				Cracklin' Oat Bran	1 oz.	2	27
Boo Berry	1 oz.	3.3	47	Nutri-Grain, Wheat & Raisins	1 oz.	2	23
Count Chocula	1 oz.	3.3	47	Bran Buds	1 oz.	1.8	40
Franken Berry	1 oz.	3.3	47	Frosted Mini-Wheats, Sugar-Frosted	1 oz.	1.8	25
Chocolate Crazy Cow	1 oz.	3	44	Frosted Mini-Wheats, Apple-Flavored	1 oz.	1.8	25
Pac-Man	1 oz.	3	44	Most	1 oz.	1.5	24
Strawberry Shortcake	1 oz.	3	44	All-Bran	1 oz.	1.3	29
Trix	1 oz.	3	44	40% Bran Flakes	1 oz.	1.3	22
Cocoa Puffs	1 oz.	2.8	40	Crispix	1 oz.	0.8	11
Lucky Charms	1 oz.	2.8	40	Product 19	1 oz.	0.8	11
Cheerios, Honey Nut	1 oz.	2.5	36	Rice Krispies	1 oz.	0.8	11
Donutz, Chocolate Flavor	1 oz.	2.5	33	Special K	1 oz.	0.8	11
Donutz, Powdered	1 oz.	2.5	33	Corn Flakes	1 oz.	0.5	7
Golden Grahams	1 oz.	2.5	36	Nutri-Grain, Corn	1 oz.	0.5	7
Buc Wheats	1 oz.	2.3	33	Nutri-Grain, Wheat	1 oz.	0.5	7
Nature Valley Granola, Fruit & Nut	1 oz.	2	25	*Post*			
Nature Valley Granola, Cinnamon & Rasin	1 oz.	1.8	22	Super Sugar Crisp	1 oz.	3.5	51
Body Buddies, Brown Sugar & Honey	1 oz.	1.5	22	Honeycomb	1 oz.	2.8	40
Body Buddies, Fruit Flavor	1 oz.	1.5	22	Raisin Bran	1 oz.	2.3	40
Kaboom	1 oz.	1.5	22	Fruit 'n Fibre	1 oz.	1.8	31
Nature Valley Granola, Coconut & Honey	1 oz.	1.5	16	Raisin Grape Nuts	1 oz.	1.5	24
Nature Valley Granola, Toasted Oat	1 oz.	1.5	18	40% Bran Flakes	1 oz.	1.3	22
Country Corn Flakes	1 oz.	0.8	11	Grape Nut Flakes	1 oz.	1.3	20
Total	1 oz.	0.8	11	Grape Nuts	1 oz.	0.8	12
Total, Corn	1 oz.	0.8	11	*Ralston Purina*			
Wheaties	1 oz.	0.8	11	Cookie Crisp, Choc. Chip Flav.	1 oz.	3.3	47
Kix	1 oz.	0.5	7	Cookie Crisp, Vanilla Wafer	1 oz.	3.3	47
Cheerios	1 oz.	0.3	4	Donkey Kong Junior	1 oz.	3.3	47
Kellogg's				Cookie Crisp, Oatmeal Flavor	1 oz.	3	40
Honey Smacks	1 oz.	4	58	Sugar Frosted Flakes	1 oz.	2.8	40
Apple Jacks	1 oz.	3.5	51	Raisin Bran	1 oz.	2.3	36
Froot Loops	1 oz.	3.3	47	Bran Chex	1 oz.	1.3	18
Cocoa Krispies	1 oz.	3	44	Crispy Rice	1 oz.	0.8	11
Sugar Corn Pops	1 oz.	3	44	Corn Chex	1 oz.	0.5	7
Frosted Flakes, Sugar	1 oz.	2.8	40	Corn Flakes	1 oz.	0.5	7
Frosted Flakes, Banana	1 oz.	2.5	36	Rice Chex	1 oz.	0.5	7
Frosted Krispies	1 oz.	2.5	36	Wheat Chex	1 oz.	0.5	7
Marshmallow Krispies	1 oz.	2.5	29	*Quaker Oats*			
Raisins, Rice & Rye	1 oz.	2.5	29	Cap'n Crunch's Crunchberries	1 oz.	3.3	43
Strawberry Krispies	1 oz.	2.5	36	Cap'n Crunch	1 oz.	3	44
Corn Flakes, Honey & Nut	1 oz.	2.3	33				

TABLE 3.2—Continued

Refined Sweeteners in Breakfast Cereals

	Serving Size	Table Sugar Equivalent (tsp)	Sugar Calories (% of total calories)		Serving Size	Table Sugar Equivalent (tsp)	Sugar Calories (% of total calories)
King Vitamin	1 oz.	3	44	Life, Cinnamon	1 oz.	1.5	22
Quisp	1 oz.	3	44	100% Natural	1 oz.	1.5	17
Cap'n Crunch's Peanut Butter	1 oz.	2.5	31	Life	1 oz.	1.3	18
100% Natural, Raisins & Dates	1 oz.	2.3	28	Shredded Wheat	1.3 oz.	0.3	3
100% Natural, Apples & Cinn.	1 oz.	2	23	Puffed Rice	0.5 oz.	0	0
				Puffed Wheat	0.5 oz.	0	0

Note: Figures for cereals include naturally occurring sugar in raisins and other dried fruits.

Copyright 1984, CSPI. Adapted from *Nutrition Action Healthletter* (1875 Connecticut Ave., N.W., Suite 300, Washington, D.C. 20009-5728. $20.00 for 10 issues).

ISSUE

Soft Drinks for Breakfast

Food manufacturers have learned that convenience is a key factor in determining what beverages we consume at breakfast. The more steps involved in preparing a product, the less likely it will be consumed. In response to this and our interest in consuming caffeine in the morning, the soft drink industry now promotes its products for breakfast. Coca-Cola advertises its drinks for consumption in the morning, Pepsi-Cola is test marketing a product called "Pepsi A.M.," which has 28 percent more caffeine than regular Pepsi, and Royal Crown Cola places coupons for free RC products in boxes of General Mills cereals ("The Pepsi (De)generation" 1990).

- **Pro:** Individuals drink soft drinks anyway, so it really doesn't matter what time of day the drinks are consumed.

- **Con:** It is irresponsible to try to replace milk and orange juice with soft drinks, particularly for children.

What could be the effects of drinking soft drinks for breakfast?

Complex Carbohydrates

Complex carbohydrates are composed of three or more simple sugars bonded together. They must be converted to simple carbohydrates before being used by the body. Complex carbohydrates include **starch, fiber,** and **glycogen.** Starches form the major part of the American diet and are found in foods such as whole-grain bread, potatoes, rice, and vegetables. Despite the negative meaning often associated with starches, they are an important part of the diet and provide high nutritional benefit.

Fiber is found in the walls of plant cells and in the tough structural parts of plants, like the stringy part of celery or the bran of wheat and other cereals. It is not digested in the small intestine. Fiber may be soluble or insoluble. Insoluble fiber speeds the passage of the food through the digestive tract and may help prevent the development of **carcinogens** (cancer-causing agents) in the colon. It may also help prevent constipation and hemorrhoids. Good sources of insoluble fiber include whole grains, since bran layers comprise the outside covering of grains.

Soluble fibers are digested in the large intestine. They may help control diabetes and lower **cholesterol,** a waxy, fatlike substance that circulates in the blood. Although the results of some studies (Kirby et al. 1981; Van Horn et al. 1986), show a drop in cholesterol levels associated with consumption of oat bran, the results of another study show no difference in the effects of eating oat bran and low-fiber refined flour (Swain et al. 1990). The researchers in the latter study, however, indicated that soluble fibers such as guar, psyllium, and pectin do lower cholesterol (Liebman, "Has the Oat-Bran Bubble Burst?" 1990).

The practical aspects of fiber intake need to be considered while researchers debate the issue. Since daily consumption of fiber in the United States is two to three times lower than levels recommended by the National Cancer Institute (ten grams versus the recommendation of twenty to thirty grams), it is probably a good idea to increase fiber consumption if appropriate (table 3.3). This increase needs to be done gradually to allow the body to adjust to the increased intake of fiber. Fluid intake also needs to be increased to prevent constipation, which may result from increased fiber intake. The known ways to lower cholesterol are to eat less saturated fat and cholesterol (Liebman, "Has the Oat-Bran Bubble Burst?" 1990).

Glycogen, the third form of complex carbohydrate, is formed in the body from extra glucose. Extra glucose is converted into fatty acids and stored by the body in the

TABLE 3.3

Fat and Fiber Content in Foods

	Fat (grams)	Fiber (grams)		Fat (grams)	Fiber (grams)
Beans, Peas, and Tofu			Nabisco Shredded Wheat (1)	1	3.0a
(A serving is 3/4 cup of cooked beans.)			Quaker Oatmeal (2/3 c)	2	2.7a
Campbell's Old Fashioned Beans	2	14.7a	Kellogg Corn Flakes or Product 19 *(1 c)*	0	1.0
Pinto beans	1	14.2a	Nabisco Cream of Wheat *(2/3 c)*	0	1.0
Kidney beans	1	13.8a	Nature Valley Oat Granola *(1/3 c)*	5	1.0
Campbell's Pork & Beans	2	13.0a	Kellogg Special K or Rice Krispies *(1 c)*	0	0.0
Black-eyed peas	1	12.3a	*Breads*		
Green Giant Chili Beans	2	11.0a	*(A serving is two slices, unless otherwise noted.)*		
Navy beans	1	9.0a	Arnold Bran'nola Dark Wheat or Original	2	6.0
Van Camp's Pork & Beans	1	7.4a	Pita bread, whole wheat *(5 in. pocket)*	1	4.4
Chick peas (garbanzos)	3	7.1a	Earth Grains 100% Whole Wheat	2	4.0
Lentils	1	5.6a	Pepperidge Farm Thick Dijon Rye	2	4.0
Split Peas	1	4.1a	Wonder 100% Whole Wheat	2	3.6
Tofu *(4 oz)*	5	1.4	Pepperidge Farm Pumpernickel	2	3.0
Soups			Roman Meal Sandwich Bread, thin	1	2.0
(A serving is 10 oz prepared.)			Pepperidge Farm Honey Wheat Berry	2	2.0
Pritikin Navy Bean	1	20.3a	Pepperidge Farm Raisin Cinnamon	3	2.0
Health Valley Split Pea	3	10.4a	Home Pride Butter Top Wheat	2	1.6
Health Valley Vegetable	1	9.1	Bagel, plain *(1)*	2	1.4
Campbell's Homestyle Bean	2	7.5a	Wonder White, Italian, or French	2	1.4
Health Valley Lentil	4	5.9a	Sara Lee Croissant *(1)*	6	0.1
Campbell's Black Bean	3	5.0a	*Crackers*		
Pritikin Split Pea	0	4.0a	*(The number of crackers in a 1/2 oz serving is shown in parentheses.)*		
Cereals			Ryvita High Fiber Crispbread *(2)*	0	4.0
(All servings, which are shown in parentheses, are 1 oz. Serving sizes for hot cereals apply to the cooked cereal.)			Wasa Fiber Plus *(1 1/3)*	1	3.7
Kellogg All Bran w/Extra Fiber *(1/2 c)*	1	14.0a	Ralston Ry-Krisp Naturals *(2 triples)*	0	3.6
General Mills Fiber One *(1/2 c)*	1	13.0a	Wasa Hearty Rye Crispbread *(1)*	0	2.6
Wheat Bran *(1/2 c)*	0	12.6a	Finn Crisp Original Rye Crispbread *(1)*	1	2.0
Kellogg All Bran *(1/3 c)*	1	10.0a	Manischewitz Whole Wheat Matzos w/Bran *(1/2)*	1	2.0
Nabisco 100% Bran *(1/2 c)*	2	10.0a	Nabisco Wheat'n Bran Triscuits *(3)*	2	2.0
Kellogg Bran Buds *(1/3 c)*	1	8.0a	Nabisco Oat Thins *(8)*	3	1.0
Ralston Bran Chex *(2/3 c)*	0	6.1	Quaker Rice Cakes *(2)*	0	0.6
Rice Bran *(1/3 c)*	6	6.1	Nabisco Triscuits *(3)*	2	0.5
Kellogg Fruitful Bran *(2/3 c)*	0	5.0	Saltines *(4)*	1	0.3
Kellogg Raisin Bran *(3/4 c)*	1	5.0	*Fruits and Juices*		
Nabisco Wholesome'N Hearty *(2/3 c)*	1	5.0a	*(A serving is one piece of fruit, unless otherwise noted.)*		
Post Fruit & Fibre *(1/2 c)*	2	5.0	Figs, dried *(3)*	1	5.3
Quaker Rice Bran Honey Crunch *(1/4 c)*	5	5.0a	Apple, large	0	4.7a
Nabisco Shredded Wheat 'N Bran *(2/3 c)*	1	4.0	Pear	1	4.3
Wheatena *(1/2 c)*	1	4.0	Apricots, dried *(10)*	0	3.6a
Kellogg Bran Mueslix *(1/2 c)*	2	4.0	Prunes, dried *(5)*	0	3.5a
Quaker Oat Bran, hot cereal *(2/3 c)*	2	4.0a	Orange	0	3.1a
Kretschmer Wheat Germ *(1/4 c)*	3	3.3	Strawberries *(1/2 c)*	1	2.0
Kellogg Nutri-Grain Wheat *(2/3 c)*	0	3.0	Raisins (1/4 c)	0	1.9a
Post Grape-nuts *(1/4 c)*	0	3.0	Banana, medium	1	1.8
General Mills Total or Wheaties *(1 c)*	1	3.0	Peach	0	1.4

TABLE 3.3—Continued

Fat and Fiber Content in Foods

	Fat (grams)	Fiber (grams)		Fat (grams)	Fiber (grams)
Cantaloupe (1/4)	1	1.1	Healthy Choice Salisbury Steak	7	2.3b
Grapefruit (1/2)	0	0.7	Le Menu Chicken Parmigiana	20	2.3b
Grapes (10)	0	0.4	Lean Cuisine Oriental Beef w/Veg.	7	1.3
Orange juice (3/4 c)	0	0.4	*Grains and Pasta*		
Vegetables			*(A serving is one cup prepared, unless otherwise noted.)*		
(A serving is 1/2 cup, unless otherwise noted.)			Bulgur (Cracked wheat)	0	8.1
Baked potato w/skin, medium (1)	0	4.2a	Whole-wheat spaghetti	1	5.9
Sweet potato w/out skin, medium (1)	0	3.4a	Aunt Jemima Buckwheat Pancake Mix (3)	8	5.0
Brussels sprouts, cooked	1	3.3a	Near East Couscous	0	3.9
Corn, cooked	1	3.1	Uncle Ben's Herbed Rice Au Gratin	8	3.6
Peas or Winter squash, cooked	1	2.9	Noodle Roni Stroganoff	34	3.6
Carrot, raw (1)	0	2.3a	Brown rice	1	3.3
Broccoli or Spinach, cooked	0	2.0	Aunt Jemima Whole Grain Waffles (2)	3	3.0
Cauliflower, cooked	0	1.4	Golden Grain Macaroni & Cheddar	30	2.8
Spinach, raw (1 c)	0	1.4	Spaghetti or macaroni	1	2.1
Tomato (1/2)	0	0.8	Aunt Jemima Original Waffles (2)	6	1.5
Green pepper, raw (1/2)	0	0.6	Rice-A-Roni Spanish Style	8	1.4
Lettuce, iceberg (1 c)	0	0.6	Uncle Ben's Converted White Rice	1	1.0
Mushrooms or Cucumbers, raw	0	0.5			
Nuts and Seeds			*Cakes, Pastries, and Muffins*		
(A serving is 1/4 cup, unless otherwise noted.)			*(A serving is one item, unless otherwise noted.)*		
Almonds, roasted in oil	18	3.8	Arrowhead Mills Apple Oat Bran Muffin	4	6.9a
Pistachios	18	3.8	Health Valley Raisin Oat Bran Muffin	3	5.2a
Peanuts, dry roasted	18	2.9	Sara Lee Blueberry or Oat Bran Muffin	8	4.0
Tahini (2 Tb)	16	2.8	Betty Crocker or Hostess Oat Bran Muffin	8	2.0
Cashews, roasted in oil	16	2.0	Dunkin' Donuts Oat Bran Donut	19	1.9
Peanut butter (2 Tb)	16	2.0	Sara Lee Dutch Apply Pie (1/6)	16	1.1
			Sara Lee French Cream Cheesecake (1/8)	18	0.8
Frozen Dinners and Entrees					
(A serving is one package.)			*Cookies, Candies, and Chips*		
Weight Watchers Chicken Divan Potato	6	8.0	*(A serving is one item, unless otherwise noted.)*		
Weight Watchers Beefsteak Burrito	12	7.0	Popcorn, air-popped (3 c)	0	3.9
Green Giant Fettucine Primavera	8	6.0	Health Valley Tortilla Chips (1 oz)	8	3.6
Lean Cuisine Spaghetti w/Sauce	7	5.6	Archway Molasses Cookie	2	2.0
Lean Cuisine Zucchini Lasagna	7	5.3	Quaker Chewy Nut & Raisin Granola Bar	6	1.6
Weight Watchers Pasta Primavera	13	5.0	Snickers Bar	13	1.4
Green Giant Rotini Cheddar	10	4.5	Fig bars (2)	2	1.3
Lean Cuisine Chicken Cacciatore	9	4.4	M & M's Peanut Chocolate Candies	12	1.3
Green Giant Tortellini Provencale	5	4.0	Graham crackers (4)	2	1.0
Lean Cuisine Chicken Parmesan	8	3.6	Archway Oatmeal Cookie	3	1.0
Celeste Cheese Pizza-For-One	25	3.6	Potato chips (14)	10	1.0
Right Course Homestyle Pot Roast	7	3.4b	Pretzels, twisted (5)	1	0.8
Lean Cuisine Filet of Fish Divan	8	3.2	Nature Valley Granola Bar	5	0.8
Weight Watchers Sweet'N Sour Chicken	2	3.0	Mars Bar	11	0.8
Lean Cuisine Szechwan Beef w/Veg.	10	3.0	*Fast Foods*		
Budget Gourmet Sirloin Tips	11	2.8b	*(A serving is two slices for pizza and one item for other foods.)*		
			Pizza Hut Supreme Personal Pan Pizza	28	9.0

aContains at least 1 gram of soluble fiber.
bCSPI estimate. All other information obtained from the manufacturers or the U.S. Department of Agriculture.

TABLE 3.3—Continued

Fat and Fiber Content in Foods

	Fat (grams)	Fiber (grams)		Fat (grams)	Fiber (grams)
Arby's Baked Potato w/Broccoli & Cheese	20	7.3[a,b]	McDonald's McD.L.T.	37	1.7[b]
Pizza Hut Cheese Pan Pizza (12 in)	18	5.0	Arby's Regular Roast Beef Sandwich	15	1.5[b]
Pizza Hut Pepperoni Thin'n Crispy (12 in)	20	4.0	McDonald's Egg McMuffin	11	1.2[b]
McDonald's Chicken Salad Oriental	3	3.0[b]	McDonald's Quarter Pounder w/Cheese	29	1.2[b]
Burger King Whopper	36	2.4[b]			
Hardee's Grilled Chicken Sandwich	12	1.9[b]			

[b]CSPI estimate. All other information obtained from the manufacturers or the U.S. Department of Agriculture.

Copyright 1990, CSPI. Adapted from *Rough It Up* which is available from CSPI, 1875 Conn. Ave., N.W., # 300, Washington, D.C. 20009-5728 for $4.95.

liver and in muscle as a source of energy. The glycoge is converted into glucose when needed and is made available to the body for ready energy.

The diet of Americans contains fewer complex carbohydrates than the diets of many people in other developed countries. It takes a concerted effort to increase the consumption of these foods. This effort is worthwhile because of the many nutrients provided by complex carbohydrates. Some suggestions for increasing the intake of these foods include the following:

1. Investigate ways to increase consumption of complex carbohydrates.
2. Use whole-grain flour when baking.
3. Substitute foods containing complex carbohydrates for foods containing simple carbohydrates.
4. Select fresh fruits and vegetables when possible (table 3.4).

Proteins

Proteins are the second most commonly found nutrient in the body next to water, they comprise about 16 percent of body weight, and they are made up of carbon, oxygen, hydrogen, and nitrogen. Proteins supply four calories of energy per gram.

Proteins are part of nearly every cell and help build bone, muscle, skin, and blood. They help protect us from disease because they are the major ingredient in antibodies. They regulate body functions because they assist in the formulation of hormones. They control chemical activities because of their role in forming enzymes. Oxygen, iron, and nutrients are transported to the cells of the body through protein.

Although their primary function is the building and repair of the body, calories from protein are used to supply energy if the supplies from carbohydrates and fats are inadequate. Proteins are not an efficient or effective source of energy because calories that may have been used in the repair and maintenance of the body are used to supply

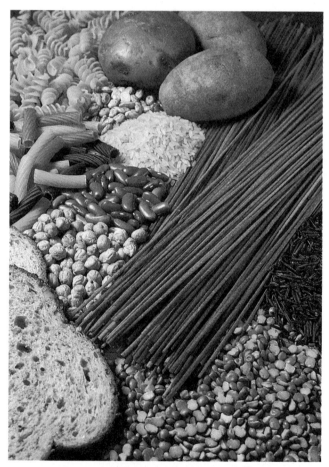

Fiber plays an important role in our diet and can be found in whole grains, fruits, and vegetables.

energy. This is of special interest to those who fast as a means of achieving weight loss, because protein in muscles may be used to provide energy if there are inadequate supplies of fats and carbohydrates.

The building blocks of protein are approximately twenty different **amino acids,** or chemical compounds. Nine of these amino acids cannot be made or synthesized in the

TABLE 3.4

The Healthiest Vegetables

Vegetable (1/2 cup cooked, unless noted)	Score	Vit. A	Vit. C	Folate	Iron	Copper	Calcium	Fiber
Sweet potato, no skin (1)	582	✔	✔	*		✔		✔
Carrot, raw (1)	434	✔	✔					*
Carrots	408	✔						*
Spinach	241	✔	✔	✔	✔	*	✔	*
Collard greens, frozen	181	✔	✔	✔	*		✔	NA
Red pepper, raw (1/2)	166	✔	✔					
Kale	161	✔	✔			*	*	*
Dandelion greens	156	✔	✔	NA	*	NA	*	*
Spinach, raw (1 c)	152	✔	✔	✔	*		*	*
Broccoli	145	✔	✔	✔				*
Brussels sprouts	128	✔	✔	✔	*		✔	
Broccoli, frozen	127	✔	✔	✔			*	*

Vegetable (1/2 cup) cooked, unless noted)	Score	Vit. A	Vit. C	Folate	Iron	Copper	Calcium	Fiber
Potato, baked, w/skin (1)	114	NA	✔	*	✔	✔		✔
Mixed vegetables, frozen	111	✔	*					✔
Winter squash	110	✔	✔	*		*		*
Swiss chard	105	✔	✔	NA	✔	NA	*	*
Broccoli, raw	100	✔	✔	*				*
Snow peas	90		✔	NA	*			*
Mustard greens	85	✔	✔	NA	NA		*	*
Kohlrabi	82		✔	NA	NA			
Romaine lettuce (1 c)	78	✔	✔	✔	NA			
Cauliflower	77		✔	*				*
Cauliflower, raw	77		✔	*				*
Asparagus	75	✔	✔	✔		*		*
Green peppers, raw (1/2)	67	*	✔					

✔ Contains at least 10 percent of the USRDA.

*Contains between 5 percent and 9 percent of the USRDA.

Note: The score for each vegetable was developed by adding up its percent of the USRDA for six nutrients plus fiber. There is no USRDA for fiber, so a value of twenty-five grams was assigned. If no number was available (NA) for a nutrient, it was assigned a value of zero. This could make the scores of some vegetables lower than they should be.

Copyright 1991, CSPI. Adapted from *Nutrition Action Healthletter* (1875 Connecticut Ave., N.W., Suite 300, Washington, D.C. 20009-5728. $20.00 for 10 issues).

body, so they must be obtained through food. These are called **essential amino acids.** Foods that contain all nine of these amino acids are known as **complete proteins.** Proteins from animal sources tend to be complete, while proteins from vegetable sources are not. Although many of the products derived from animals are good sources of protein (milk, meat, poultry, and fish products), they may be high in fats and cholesterol.

Protein is broken down and rebuilt in nearly every part of the body, with as much as 3 percent to 5 percent of the protein in the body replaced each day. Once enough protein has been eaten to supply bodily functions, the excess is broken down for energy or stored as fat. More protein is needed for females when they are pregnant or breast-feeding.

Although many of us wonder if we consume adequate amounts of protein, it is likely our intake is adequate because of the large amounts of protein in many commonly consumed foods. In the United States, children consume twice the USRDA for protein, the average middle-aged man consumes 60 percent more than the USRDA for protein, and the average middle-aged woman consumes 25 percent more than the USRDA for protein. There is growing evidence that excess amounts of protein can contribute to osteoporosis, heart disease, and certain cancers. There is also some evidence of a connection between a high protein diet and loss of renal function in later years (Roberts 1989).

The major recommendation regarding protein is to keep the amount ingested at the level recommended by the USRDA and to replace animal proteins with plant proteins. Some suggestions for doing this include the following:

1. Feature complex carbohydrate dishes as the main course for meals, and use meats and poultry as side dishes.
2. Limit the serving size when eating meat.
3. Increase consumption of plant proteins.

Fats

Although there are a number of negative associations with fat, it is essential for the proper functioning of the body. Fats protect the vital organs against injury, they provide insulation against the cold, and they depress hunger pangs. Fats supply nine calories of energy per gram. They are a concentrated source of energy when carbohydrate supplies are insufficient, such as during prolonged exercise. In addition, fats enhance the taste of food and transport the four **fat-soluble vitamins** (A, D, E, and K).

Juice or Consequences?

The expanded juice market has provided another challenge for consumers who are trying to determine nutritional content of the products they buy. While in the past the word "juice" may have been associated with a beverage that was 100 percent pure fruit juice, this is no longer the case. A product may be called "juice" when there is only 5 percent of pure fruit juice. Some suggestions that may help prevent confusion include the following:

1. Beware of products that are labeled *blend, punch, ade, drink,* or *cocktail.*
2. Read the labels and look for the presence of sugars or syrups.
3. Read the information carefully. A claim of "100 percent pure" or "100 percent natural" does not mean that a product is comprised only of fruit juice (Tonnessen 1990).
4. Be suspicious of white grape, apple, or pear juice concentrate (Schmidt 1991).

The following table may help when choosing among the real fruit juices. Note that there is significant difference in the amount of calories and minerals.

Comparison Shopping: From Apples to Oranges

Beverage (8 oz)	Calories	Vitamin C (mg)	Vitamin A[a] (IU)	Potassium (mg)
Orange juice (fresh)	111	124	496	496
Orange juice (frozen concentrate)	112	97	194	474
Orange Kool-Aid	96	6	—	8
Pink grapefruit juice (fresh)	96	94	1,087	400
White grapefruit juice (fresh)	96	94	25	400
V-8 Vegetable Juice	47	40	3,000	480
Tomato juice (canned)	32	33	1,012	400
Apple juice	116	2	2	296
Grape juice (canned)	155	trace	20	334
Cranberry juice cocktail	147	108[b]	—	61
Prune juice	181	11	9	706
Pinapple juice	139	27	12	334
Peach nectar	134	13	634	101

[a]Approximate, based on content of retinol and carotenoids.
[b]Vitamin C added.
Note: The RDA for vitamin C is 60 mg; for vitamin A 4,000 to 5,000 IU. There is no RDA for potassium; estimated safe and adequate daily dietary intake is 1,875 to 5,625 mg.
Source: Composition of Foods Agriculture Handbook No. 8, prepared by the U.S.D.A. Human Nutrition Information Service.

Triglycerides, the most common fatty substance in the blood, are the major source of dietary fat and comprise 95 percent of our fat intake. Fat is transported by the blood to the muscles, where it is used for energy (McGlynn 1990). Excess fat is stored in adipose cells (fat cells) that can increase in size fifty times to store excess fat. In addition, new adipose cells are formed when the existing cells are full (Wardlaw and Insel 1990). Fat is initially stored around organs and in muscles. By the time we can see the bulges in our bodies, these storage areas are full.

Fat cells are composed of fatty acids and glycerol. The fatty acids consist of a chain of hydrogen and carbon atoms along with a few oxygen atoms. Fatty acids may be classified as saturated, monounsaturated, or polyunsaturated, depending on the number of hydrogen atoms that are bonded to the molecule.

Saturated fatty acids contain the maximum number of hydrogen atoms (i.e., are saturated with hydrogen), are usually from animal sources, and are solid at room temperature. **Monounsaturated** fatty acids have one double bond between their carbon atoms and are found in olive and canola oils. **Polyunsaturated** fatty acids contain two or more double bonds between the carbon atoms. Safflower, corn, and soybean oils contain polyunsaturated fatty acids. The **unsaturated** fatty acids are usually liquid at room temperature and are found in plant sources. Palm oil, palm kernel oil, and coconut oil are highly saturated fats even though they are from plant sources. Vegetable oils are often hydrogenated, which is the process of adding hydrogen to polyunsaturated or monounsaturated fats. This increases their saturation. Oils may become more saturated when used repeatedly at high temperatures (Roberts 1989).

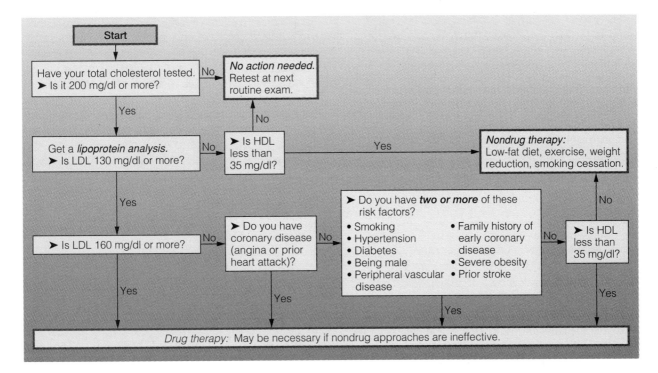

Figure 3.2
Guide to the cholesterol maze.

While cholesterol (another fatty substance in the blood) consumption has negative implications, it is actually crucial in a number of body functions. Cholesterol is a component of cell membranes, it is used to protect the nerve fibers, and it assists in the production of certain hormones, including the sex hormones. Eight hundred to 1,500 milligrams of cholesterol are produced by the body each day. The body regulates the amount of cholesterol by producing less when more cholesterol is obtained through dietary sources. This process, however, does not function properly in 25 percent to 33 percent of the population ("Fear of Eggs" 1989). Cholesterol in the blood is harmful because it accumulates on arterial walls, causing them to narrow. This can lead to atherosclerosis, the formation of fat deposits on the walls of the arteries, and sometimes to a heart attack.

Cholesterol is not soluble in water and is transported through the bloodstream with a protein carrier and triglycerides. This combination is called a **lipoprotein** (fatty proteins). There are three types of lipoproteins involved in transporting protein in the body. The **high-density lipoproteins (HDL)** are considered "good" cholesterol because they remove other cholesterol from the walls of the arteries and transport it to the liver, where it is processed and excreted (Stamford 1990). Both the **low-density lipoproteins (LDL)** and the **very low-density lipoproteins (VLDL)** are considered "bad" cholesterol because they allow the cholesterol to circulate in the bloodstream.

In fact, LDL transports two-thirds of the cholesterol in the blood ("Forget Cholesterol" 1990). It appears that the cholesterol in both the LDL and VLDL is on its way to the cells for storage. This can be harmful because the cholesterol may build up in the arteries and cause the arteries to clog, resulting in a heart attack (fig. 3.2). The distribution of the lipoproteins may be as important as the cholesterol level in the blood. A high ratio of HDL would appear to put people at lower risk of coronary heart disease (McGlynn 1990). There is evidence in research studies that oxidized LDL clogs the arteries and may encourage the likelihood of heart attacks (Liebman 1991). The antioxidant properties of vitamin C are being studied to determine if vitamin C can inhibit the oxidation of low-density lipoprotein cholesterol (Strickland 1991). Other substances being studied for their antioxidant properties include vitamin E and beta carotene ("Battling the Bad Fat" 1992).

Many individuals are looking for foods to raise their HDL. HDL levels in blood, however, are raised by getting the body to increase production of HDL. This is done by eating a diet rich in fiber, maintaining proper body weight, and exercising vigorously.

The average American consumes approximately 37 percent of total calories from fat, including 16 percent from saturated fat ("Where's the Fat?" 1990). The American Heart Association and the National Cancer Institute recommend that fat comprise less than 30 percent of total calories, with the amounts equally distributed among saturated, monounsaturated, and polyunsaturated fats. Daily cholesterol consumption, which is currently 400 milligrams to 600 milligrams daily, should be reduced to less than 250 milligrams daily. Some ways to reduce the total intake of fat and cholesterol include the following:

1. Select lean poultry and remove the skin before cooking.
2. Avoid fried foods and breaded foods.
3. Select lean cuts of red meat, such as flank, round, and rump.
4. Prepare foods by baking, broiling, boiling, or microwaving rather than frying. Use a receptacle under the food to catch the fat drippings when broiling rather than letting the food sit in the fat.
5. Select skim or low-fat milk products. If whole milk is consumed, decrease the amount of fat by mixing it with skim milk. In time, increase the amount of skim milk added until the milk is only skim milk. Select low-fat cheeses.
6. Select monounsaturated or polyunsaturated fats and oils. Check the label to be sure of the type of fats and oils.
7. Remove all visible fat from meat prior to cooking.
8. Check labels for fats and select products with less fat.
9. Include more fish in the diet.
10. Limit intake of foods from fast-food restaurants since a high percentage (40 percent to 50 percent) of calories in fast foods comes from fat (Roberts 1989).
11. Cool cooked stew or soup and remove the fat before reheating and serving (Hunter 1989).

Vitamins

Vitamins are organic substances that are essential in small amounts for chemical reactions to occur in the body. They do not provide energy, as some individuals mistakenly believe, but combine with enzymes to enable the body to use other nutrients. Vitamins are found in all foods except sugar, alcohol, and highly refined fats and oils (McGlynn 1990). The body requires only one ounce of vitamins for every 150 pounds of food consumed (Wardlaw and Insel 1990). Thirteen vitamins are absolutely necessary for good health.

Vitamins are grouped and categorized according to their solubility in either water or fat. The fat-soluble vitamins include vitamins A, D, E, and K, which are stored and transported by the fat cells of the body. Since they can be stored in the body for long periods of time, it is not essential to consume foods containing them every day. Because they are stored in the body, it is possible to have toxic levels of these vitamins if **megadoses,** which are amounts many times higher than the RDAs, are consumed.

The **water-soluble vitamins** include the eight B vitamins and vitamin C. They are not stored in the body and need to be replenished every day. Our supplies of these vitamins are continually depleted or flushed out of the system through urine and perspiration.

The vitamin content of foods is affected by processing procedures (e.g., vine-ripened items are more nutritious than those picked green), storage procedures (e.g., wilted vegetables are not as nutritious), and cooking procedures (e.g., extended cooking time usually results in a loss of vitamins).

There is a great deal of controversy as to whether or not vitamin supplements should be taken. Vitamins are related to chemical reactions within the body and are needed in precise amounts. Amounts in excess of the RDAs are wasted. If you eat a balanced diet from a variety of foods, you probably do not need extra vitamins from pills. Vitamin supplements may be recommended, however, for heavy smokers, women on oral contraceptives, heavy drinkers, individuals with specific disorders, surgical patients, and the elderly.

Minerals

Minerals are inorganic elements involved in a variety of metabolic functions. They are required in the body in varying amounts to fulfill their functions, whereas vitamins are required in very small amounts. Minerals are divided into two classifications: **macrominerals** and **trace minerals.** The macrominerals are required by the body in relatively large amounts and include calcium, magnesium, sodium, potassium, phosphorus, sulfur, and chlorine. The trace minerals are required in much smaller amounts.

Calcium

The mineral present in the largest amount in the body is **calcium.** The adult human body contains approximately 1,200 to 1,250 grams of calcium, with the vast majority of it in the bones and teeth (98 percent of it is located in the bones and 1 percent in the teeth).

Calcium is needed for growth and maintenance of strong bones and teeth. It is also needed to assist in the clotting of blood, to regulate the flow of fluids in and out of the cells, to transmit nerve impulses, and to maintain the normal excitability of the heart muscle as well as other muscles. In addition, calcium may play a preventive role in several cancers, in **hypertension** (high blood pressure) ("Yet Another Reason to Drink Your Milk" 1992), and in **preeclampsia** (a mild form of hypertension in pregnant women) (Oestreicher 1990). Calcium is constantly moving in and out of bones, with as much as 20 percent of the calcium in the bones replaced in the course of a year. Calcium is the major mineral most likely to be in short supply in the American diet, especially in females. Those who eat high-fiber diets need to include extra amounts of calcium since fiber decreases the body's ability to absorb calcium by as much as 20 percent (Edell 1992).

Adequate supplies of calcium need to be maintained throughout life. It is especially important for college students to maintain their intake of calcium, since many consume soft drinks in place of milk. This may be a problem because of both the decreased calcium intake and the excretion of calcium that results from consumption of fluids high in phosphorus, such as colas.

TABLE 3.5

Are You at Risk for Osteoporosis?

Factors That Increase Risk	Factors That Decrease Risk
Substantial Evidence:	*Preliminary Evidence:*
Increased age	Increased childbirths
Surgical removal of ovaries	Diabetes
Use of corticosteroidal drugs	Use of thiazide diuretics
Alcohol use	Moderate exercise
Cigarette smoking	Asian ethnicity
Low dietary calcium	
Obesity	
Black ethnicity	
Use of estrogen	

Source: National Institutes of Health, Draft Summary Statement, Research Directions in Osteoporosis, 1987.

ISSUE

Should Restaurants Be Required to Tell Customers They Use MSG?

MSG (monosodium glutamate) is a flavor enhancer that is added to a wide variety of foods. MSG is added to foods because it is less expensive than other products. A small percentage (1 percent to 2 percent) of the population is sensitive to MSG. These individuals indicate that they develop headaches, pressure, burning sensations, and paranoia when they consume MSG. In 1993, manufacturers were required to list MSG on labels ("Who's Afraid of MSG?" 1992).

- **Pro:** There is a health risk associated with consumption of MSG. Those who eat in restaurants have a right to know if they are at risk.
- **Con:** This is just one more hassle for business. There is no concrete evidence that this is a problem. It is not fair to require any more regulations for businesses.

What needs to be done before consumption of MSG is considered a health risk? What do you think the consumer should know about MSG?

One of the results of calcium deficiency is **osteoporosis,** a loss of bone material that may result in loss of bone mass. Bones may become brittle and be more likely to break. Those with bulimia, an eating disorder characterized by binge eating often followed by vomiting, may be subject to an early onset of osteoporosis since their mineral consumption is often low. There is a rapid loss of dense bone mass right after menopause (the cessation of menstruation), which makes postmenopausal women more susceptible to osteoporosis. Estrogen therapy increases calcium absorption, and postmenopausal women who do not receive supplements of estrogen have the lowest rates of calcium absorption (Wardlaw and Insel 1990). Postmenopausal women seem to be most likely to suffer from osteoporosis, though osteoporosis has also been diagnosed in men (Orwoll et al. 1990) and in premenopausal women as young as thirty-five. Other risk factors are shown in table 3.5.

The most promising way to reduce the risk of osteoporosis in later years appears to be the intake of calcium throughout the growing years ("New Recommended Dietary Allowances"1990) and for several years after menopause is completed. The decrease in estrogen at menopause results in a 15 percent lower bone mass. Since calcium is released from the bone at this time, dietary calcium will not make an impact until the process has stabilized (Ostreicher 1990).

Current research supports intake of calcium through the diet rather than calcium supplements, with low-fat or skim milk one of the best sources of calcium (Clark 1990). Because weight-bearing activities are important in maintaining strong bones, activities such as jogging, walking, running, and dancing are recommended to maintain strong bones ("Weight-Bearing Exercises Help Prevent Bone Weakness" 1990). You may also want to monitor your intake of protein, since there is evidence that high-protein diets might contribute to osteoporosis ("New Recommended Dietary Allowances" 1990).

Sodium

Sodium and chloride are the components of table salt, with sodium composing 40 percent of the salt molecule by weight. While sodium intake would be approximately 500 milligrams a day if no processed foods were eaten and no salt were added to food, the typical sodium intake of Americans is 3,000 milligrams to 7,000 milligrams per day (Wardlaw and Insel 1990). Seventy-seven percent of sodium comes from processed foods (Mattes and Donnelly 1991).

Sodium is needed in the body to regulate the acid-base balance, to maintain the osmotic pressure of body fluid, and to preserve the normal irritability of muscle and the permeability of cells. Only 200 milligrams of sodium are needed per day, the equivalent of one-tenth of a teaspoon.

Although most of us can adjust to different levels of sodium intake, approximately fifteen to twenty million people are sodium sensitive (Williams 1990). These individuals have a tendency to develop hypertension, which is a persistent elevation of blood pressure above the normal level. Since we have no way of knowing who is or who will become sodium sensitive, it is advised that the entire population reduce sodium intake ("Too Much Salt?" 1990). There is no known disadvantage to moderate sodium restriction (*Healthy People 2000* 1990). It is doubtful that you will consume too little sodium because the body prevents this by craving salty food (Edell 1991). Hypertension is rare in populations with low sodium consumption.

It is impossible to tell in advance who will develop hypertension. There are some risk factors, however, that indicate a higher risk for developing hypertension.

1. Race. Blacks are two times as likely to develop hypertension as whites. Blacks tend to develop hypertension at a younger age, and it tends to be more severe than in whites.

2. Family history. Those with a family history of hypertension tend to be at higher risk. Limited use of sodium is a good idea if hypertension runs in a family.

3. Obesity. Hypertension is more prevalent among the obese than among lean people. Although weight loss is one of the most effective ways to reduce blood pressure, reduction of sodium intake is also recommended.

4. Age. Blood pressure tends to rise with age. Reduction of sodium intake is recommended among older adults.

Individuals with any of these risk factors are advised to limit sodium consumption.

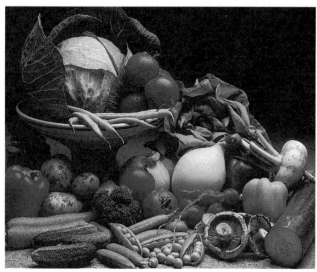

Whereas fresh vegetables are low in sodium, frozen and canned vegetables often have large amounts of added sodium.

Americans have acquired a taste for sodium and add it to foods out of habit. It is typical to see someone salt food before sampling. Reducing sodium consumption may take a special effort because many are accustomed to the taste and because sodium is so prevalent in food products. Although foods from vegetable origin are low in natural sodium, many foods from animal origin are high in natural sodium. These foods include meat, fish, poultry, milk, and eggs. Some suggestions for reducing sodium consumption include the following:

1. Reduce or eliminate salty foods in your diet, such as cured or processed meats.
2. Reduce or eliminate salt added to foods.
3. Experiment with the flavor of other seasonings on foods rather than using salt.
4. Read labels and select low-sodium products.
5. Select fresh produce over frozen or canned. A half cup of cooked peas has 2 milligrams of sodium, while a half cup of cooked frozen peas has 70 milligrams, and a half cup of canned peas has 185 milligrams.
6. Limit your intake of processed foods.
7. Consider sodium intake when selecting foods at fast-food restaurants. Items such as triple cheeseburgers can contain between 1,354 milligrams and 1,953 milligrams of sodium (Roberts 1989).

Potassium and Iron

Two other minerals of special interest are potassium and iron. Potassium works with sodium to maintain a normal heartbeat and to nourish the muscles. Although sodium and potassium work together and must be in balance, sodium is associated with raising blood pressure, while potassium is associated with lowering it. Excessive ingestion of salt depletes the body's reserves of potassium, and the amount of sodium in the heart and muscles increases when potassium amounts are low. Potassium deficiencies may cause irregularities in heartbeat, insomnia, and nervous disorders. Good sources of potassium include all vegetables, oranges, whole grains, and sunflower seeds.

Iron deficiency is one of the most common nutrient deficiencies. The main function of iron is to make hemoglobin, the part of the blood that transports oxygen from the lungs to the tissue. A daily intake of 18 milligrams of iron is recommended for women, and an intake of 10 milligrams is recommended for men. Pregnant women should increase their daily intake by an additional 15 milligrams ("New Recommended Dietary Allowances" 1990). Iron needs increase during menstruation, pregnancy, periods of rapid growth, or whenever there is a loss of blood.

Although animal organs are good sources of iron and are the sources most readily absorbed, they contain high amounts of saturated fats. Better nutritional choices are leafy green vegetables, whole grains, dried fruits, and legumes.

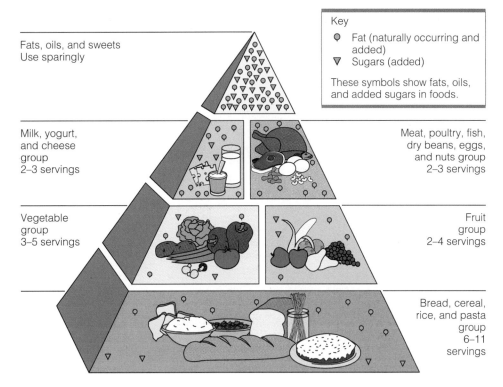

Figure 3.3
Food Guide Pyramid: A guide to daily food choices.
Source: USDA.

Water

Water is the most important nutrient of all. You can survive for weeks without other foods but only a few days without water. This is because the body cannot conserve or preserve water as well as the other nutrients. **Dehydration,** which is the removal of water from the tissues of the body, can result within hours and can be fatal.

Water transports the other nutrients to all cells, carries wastes away, and regulates body temperature. Approximately two-thirds of our body weight is composed of water. The bodies of females contain approximately 50 percent to 55 percent water, while the bodies of males contain approximately 55 percent to 60 percent water. An adult needs approximately ten cups of water per day.

The body uses protective measures to maintain its water level. After eating a meal high in sodium, you may be thirsty. This is the body's way of diluting the sodium to reduce the high level of it and prevent reactions from the body organs. When there is too much water in the body, the brain signals the kidneys to remove more water in the urine.

Each day, approximately 2.5 liters to 3 liters (approximately five to six glasses) of water are lost through urination, perspiration, and breathing. We take in water in three forms: in water and other liquids, in foods (foods such as melons and fruits contain 90 percent water), and as a product of cell oxidation. Water leaves the body through the kidneys, the lungs, the feces, and the skin.

The normal means of acquiring water are sufficient under typical circumstances. You need to monitor your intake of fluids, however, especially in situations where loss of water may exceed intake, such as in hot weather and/or during vigorous activity. Thirst cannot be relied upon as an indicator of water need because there is usually a delay between our need for water and the feeling of thirst. It is important to note that the thirst mechanism usually shuts off prior to rehydration, so you need to continue to drink water even if you are no longer thirsty.

Planning for Optimal Nutrition

We must eat a variety of foods to have a balanced diet. This takes some planning, particularly for college students who are responsible for making the majority of their food selection decisions and who may have limited time and/or money. It is not an impossible task to eat a healthful diet, though more than half of the adults in the United States do not ("Just What Is A Balanced Diet, Anyway?" 1992).

Food Choices

The Food Guide Pyramid released by The U.S. Department of Agriculture in 1992 replaces the four basic food groups (fig. 3.3) ("Pyramid Scheme Foiled" 1992). In the new pyramid, foods are divided into six groups based on the similarity of nutrients. There is a wide variety of foods within these groups, and the portions recommended are

Buying nutritious processed foods for kids is not easy. Experts convened by the Center for Science in the Public Interest determined that foods marketed for children closely resemble junk foods. The panel was unable to find a cookie, frozen dessert, granola bar, hot dog, or luncheon meat that met the group's standards. Many of kids' foods have excessive amounts of fat, sodium, and sugar, which contribute to heart disease, cancer, and high blood pressure in later life. Refer to the following list for the best of the processed foods (Duston 1992):

• Breakfast cereals: Alpen (no salt or sugar added), Kellogg's Nutri-grain Wheat; old-fashioned or quick oats; Post Grape-Nuts, Weetabix, Wheatena.

• Cheese: Weight Watchers Low Sodium American.

• Chips, Pretzels, Popcorn: Arrowhead Mills Blue or Yellow Corn Curls (unsalted); Baja Bakery Rice & Bean Tortilla Bits Light; Guiltless Gourmet No Oil Tortilla Chips; Skinny's Corn Chips; Weight Watchers Microwave Popcorn, unsalted pretzels, all brands.

• Cookies: None.

• Frozen dinners: None

• Canned or shelf-stable entrees: Fungle's Fun Foods, Health Valley Fast Menu, Hormel Health Selections Sweet and Sour Chicken.

• Frozen entrees: Health Choice spaghetti with meat sauce or macaroni and cheese; Tyson Looney Tunes Pasta.

• Fast-food meals: None.

• French fries: McCain Classic Cut, Golden Steak Fries or Crinkle Cuts; Ore Ida Home Style Wedges, Dinner Fries, Golden Crinkles, Cottage Fries, Pixi Crinkles, or Lites Crinkle Cuts.

• Frozen Desserts: None.

• Frozen Dessert Bars: FrozFruit Orange, Cantaloupe, Mango, Strawberry Lemon, Raspberry, Pineapple or Fruit and Yogurt.

• Fruit Beverages: Orange, grapefruit, fortified apple, or fortified grape juice.

• Fruit snacks: Nature's Choice Real Fruit Bars.

• Granola Bars: None.

• Hotdogs: None.

• Luncheon Meats: None.

• Milk: Skim or 1 percent low fat.

• Pizza: Rice Crust Soy Cheese; Soypreme French Bread Garden Patch or Whole Wheat Cheese Style; Special Delivery Soya Kaas or Cheese; Tree Tavern Pizsoy.

• Soup: Campbell Low Sodium Split Pea, Low Sodium Chicken with Noodles or Low Sodium Tomato: Hain Split Pea No Salt; Pritikin Split Pea, Lentil, Minestrone, or Vegetable; Spice Hunter Quick and Natural.

relatively small. Fats, oils, and sweets should be eaten sparingly because they tend to be high in calories and low in nutrients. It's a good idea to avoid these items, particularly when trying to lose weight. Foods within a specific group may have similar nutrients but may vary significantly in their overall nutritional value. It is a good idea to choose foods that are lower in sodium, fat (particularly saturated fat), and sugar and higher in fiber and complex carbohydrates.

Alcohol is not included in the new pyramid. Although it does contain calories, alcohol has no nutrients. It was shown in a recent study that consumption of alcohol makes the body burn fat more slowly and throws off the body's normal disposal of fat (Suter, Schultz, Jequier 1992).

Nutritious meals can be planned and prepared with minimal effort. Select ample fruits and vegetables because they can be eaten raw and are especially good snacks. A bit of advance planning allows for more nutritious and more economical eating.

Eating Well on a Budget

College students face some unusual challenges regarding food and eating well. Some are away from home for the first time and in a situation where foods are served at specific times, while others are in living situations that require they fix their own foods. In either event, students face the challenge of trying to eat well on a budget and without a great investment of time.

When living in housing where meals are prepared and served at specific times, you can do several things to eat well and economically. Find out the serving times and obtain a copy of the menu for the week or month. Plan to eat at the serving times rather than missing meals and spending money on fast-food meals or snacks. Review the menu before meals and determine what items to select. When reviewing the menus, consider the food groups and select foods that are the most nutritious choices, despite the temptation to do otherwise. If it is difficult to select nutritious choices, talk with those in charge of the food service and make some positive recommendations. They are likely to be receptive to ideas like a salad bar if they know there is student interest. Since meals are often included in the total cost of the housing, you have a right to be served healthy foods and get your money's worth for your investment.

Resist the temptation to go to a fast-food restaurant to save time if you live in an environment where meals are not provided. Plan a menu for a week that features low-cost foods. Skim milk and nonfat dry milk are good choices among dairy products; fresh produce in season is the

Although it may be more difficult to eat nutritiously at fast-food restaurants than at home, there are ways to reduce the fat and calories. Here are some suggestions:

McDonald's

- Order the filet of fish sandwich without tartar sauce to eliminate one-third of the calories and two-thirds of the fat.
- Order the fat-free apple bran muffins instead of the Danish pastry.
- Skip the mayo when ordering the McD.L.T. to save yourself 135 calories and 15 grams of fat.

Burger King

- Hold the mayo on the Whopper to skip 150 calories.
- Skip the mayo on the broiled chicken sandwich and eliminate 90 calories.

- Save 270 calories by choosing the Light Italian dressing rater than the regular dressings.

Taco Bell

- Skip the fried shell that holds the taco salad to remove half the fat and half the calories.
- Note that a bean burrito has half the fat of an order of nachos even though they have the same amount of calories.

Pizza Hut

- Order the pizza without the cheese to skip 40 percent of the calories and 85 percent of the fat.
- Ask for extra veggies on your pizza.

Kentucky Fried Chicken

- Remove the skin from the fried chicken to cut calories in half and remove two-thirds of the fat. Note that the extra crispy chicken has 45 percent more fat.

- Skip the fries since they have more fat and calories than three orders of mashed potatoes and gravy.

Wendy's

- Avoid the potato salad, the cheddar chips, the pasta salad, and the cole slaw at the salad bar.
- Skip the chocolate chip cookies, since they contain more fat and the same number of calories as a single hamburger.

Baskin Robbins

- Choose a sugar cone rather than a waffle cone to reduce calories and fat.
- Order sorbet or daiquiri ice rather than ice cream.
- Vanilla and Very Berry Strawberry are low in calories compared with the other flavors of ice cream.

---

best bet in the fruits and vegetables group; dried beans and peas are usually more economical than meat, poultry, and fish; and store-brand whole and enriched grain products are the best choices in the breads and cereal category.

When shopping, buy in bulk and use coupons. Determine the cost savings in money and time when shopping at several stores. Select the store where the prices are best, even though it may mean bagging your own groceries. Check with other students for ideas on saving money and eating well. They may be able to indicate the best places to shop and provide some great tips for saving money.

Fast Foods/Convenience Foods

Fast foods are a way of life for most Americans. Fast foods can refer to the foods served by the chain restaurants that line our highways and also to the trendy microwave meals sold in the frozen-food section of grocery stores. Many fast foods are high in fat, sodium, simple carbohydrates, and calories. While it is probably acceptable to eat these foods occasionally, a steady diet of burgers, fries, and cokes is not recommended.

The food group most likely to be lacking in a fast-food meal is the fruits and vegetables group. Fast-food restaurants, however, often include salad bars and fruit bars to appeal to the health-conscious consumer. If the salad or fruit bar is chosen resist the temptation to add high-calorie

and high-fat dressings and toppings if nutrition is your concern. Be sure to include several selections from the fruits and vegetables group at the next meal if you don't choose the salad or fruit bar (table 3.6).

Nutrition and the Consumer

Being a nutrition-conscious consumer involves many things. You must be knowledgeable about food additives and able to interpret labels, evaluate nutritional claims in advertising, determine sound sources of nutrition information, and apply this information when making nutritional decisions.

Food Additives

Food **additives** include items such as food coloring, salt, and sugar. They are intended to serve four purposes: (1) maintain or improve nutritional value, (2) maintain freshness, (3) help in processing or preparation, and (4) make foods more appealing. These additives are better controlled now than at any time in history. The FDA has the authority to regulate additives on the basis of safety, but they have no power over the number or necessity of additives in a product. The informed and selective consumer has the real power.

TABLE 3.6

The Best, the Worst, and (Some of) the Rest

		Calories	Fat (tsp)[a]	Sodium (mg)[b]	Gloom[c]
	Breakfast Foods				
	McDonald's English Muffin w/butter	169	1	270	9
	McDonald's Hotcakes w/Butter & Syrup	413	2	640	20
	McDonald's Egg McMuffin	293	2¾	740	25
	McDonald's Biscuit w/Sausage & Egg	529	8	1,250	57
	Burger King Croissan'wich w/Sausage	538	9¼	1,042	61[d]
W	Hardee's Big Country Breakfast (Sausage)	1,005	16¼	1,950	97
	Burgers				
	McDonald's Hamburger	257	2¼	460	17
	McDonald's Quarter Pounder w/Cheese	517	6¾	1,150	45
	Wendy's Big Classic w/Cheese	640	9	1,310	56[d]
	McDonald's McD.L.T.	674	9½	1,170	56
W	Wendy's Triple Cheeseburger	1,040	15½	1,848	85[d]
	Jack-in-Box Ultimate Cheeseburger	942	15¾	1,176	88
	Chicken Sandwiches				
B	Carl's Jr. BBQ Chicken Sandwich	320	1¼	955	17
B	Hardee's Grilled Chicken Sandwich	330	2¾	1,240	25
	Jack-in-the-Box Grilled Chicken Fillet Sandwich	408	3¾	1,130	29
	Wendy's Chicken Breast Fillet Sandwich	430	4¼	705	27[d]
	Arby's Chicken Breast Sandwich	403	5¾	1,019	33
W	McDonald's McChicken Sandwich	490	6½	780	39
W	Arby's Roast Chicken Club Sandwich	610	8½	1,500	53
	Mexican Foods				
B	Jack-in-Box Chicken Fajita Pita	292	1¾	703	16
	Taco Bell Chicken Fajita	226	2¼	619	18[d]
B	Taco Bell Bean Burrito w/Green Sauce	351	2¼	763	17[d]
	Taco Bell Taco	183	2½	276	16[d]
	Taco Bell Steak Fajita	234	2½	485	18[d]
	Jack-in-Box Beef Fajita Pita	333	3¼	635	22
	Taco Bell Super Combo Taco	286	3½	462	23[d]
W	Taco Bell Taco Light	410	6½	594	39[d]
	Salads (no dressings added)				
B	McDonald's Chicken Salad Oriental	141	¾	230	7
B	Burger King Chicken Salad	140	1	440	9
	McDonald's Chef Salad	231	3	490	21
	Hardee's Chicken Fiesta Salad	286	3¼	533	26
	Jack-in-Box Mexican Chicken Salad	442	5¼	1,500	41
	Taco Bell Taco Salad w/out Shell	520	7	1,431	47[d]
	Wendy's Taco Salad	660	8½	1,110	45[d]
W	Taco Bell Taco Salad w/Shell	941	14	1,662	75[d]

[a]To covert teaspoons of fat to grams, multiply by 4.4.
[b]The recommended daily sodium intake for an adult is 2,400 mg.
[c]CSPI's "Gloom" rating ranks foods according to their fat, sodium, cholesterol, and vitamin and mineral content. The higher the number, the worse the food.
[d]"Gloom" rating was estimated without full information on fat content from manufacturer.

W = 1989 Worst, **B** = 1989 Best

Note: All information obtained from manufacturers.

Copyright 1989, CSPI. Adapted from *Fast Food Eating Guide* which is available from CSPI, 1875 Conn. Ave., N.W., # 300, Washington, DC 20009-5728 for $4.95.

ISSUE

Food Irradiation

Radiation of food is a process that kills bacteria and extends shelf life. The first commercial food irradiation plant was built in Florida. It shipped irradiated food to grocery stores for the first time in 1992. The strawberries that were shipped looked and tasted fresh for three weeks longer than normal.

- **Pro:** Radiation is a safe way to prevent food-borne illnesses that may result from eating fruits, vegetables, pork, and poultry. In addition, foods stay fresh much longer.
- **Con:** Radiating food changes its molecular structure, which decreases the nutritional value and may increase the risk of cancer and birth defects. Note that Maine, New York, and New Jersey don't allow the sale of irradiated foods.

Do you think that preventing food-borne illness and extending shelf life justify this process? Would you eat food that has been irradiated?

Source: James Martinez, AP, *Birmingham News/Birmingham Post Herald,* January 25, 1992.

Nutrition facts

Serving size: 1/2 cup (114g)
Servings per container: 4

Amount per serving

Calories: 260 — Calories from fat: 120

	% Daily Value*
Total fat 13g	**20%**
Saturated fat 5g	**25%**
Cholesterol 30mg	**10%**
Sodium 660g	**28%**
Total carbohydrate 31g	**11%**
Sugars 5g	
Dietary fiber 0g	**0%**
Protein 5g	

Vitamin A 4% • Vitamin C 2% •
Calcium 15% • Iron 4%

*Percentages (%) of. Daily Values are based on a 2,000 calorie diet. Your Daily Values may vary higher or lower depending on your calorie needs.

Nutrient		**2,000 Calories**	**2,500 Calories**
Total fat	Less than	65g	80g
Sat. fat	Less than	20g	25g
Cholesterol	Less than	300mg	300mg
Sodium	Less than	2,400mg	2,400mg
Total Carbohydrate		300g	375g
Fiber		25g	30g

1g fat = 9 calories
1g carbohydrates = 4 calories
1g protein = 4 calories

Figure 3.4
New nutrition labeling became effective in 1993, when labels such as this one replaced those in use since 1973.

Nutrition Labeling

It is important to read the nutrition label on a product to select the most nutritious foods. The FDA has developed a labeling program to help us identify the nutrient content of the foods we buy (fig. 3.4). All labels with nutrition information must follow the same format, and any food that has an added nutrient or makes a nutritional claim must have a nutrition label.

Information on the label includes the following:

1. the serving size and number of servings in the container;
2. the calories per serving and the number of calories from fat in each serving;
3. the percent of Daily Value (percentage of the day's allotment of the nutrient comes from this food) of total fat, saturated fat, cholesterol, sodium, total carbohydrates, sugars, dietary fiber, and protein in a serving;
4. a general guide to the amount of various nutrients (fat, saturated fat, cholesterol, sodium, total carbohydrates, and fiber) you should limit yourself to each day on a 2,000 calorie and a 2,500 calorie daily intake;
5. the number of calories in one gram of fat, carbohydrates, and protein.

Nutrition labeling can help you serve better meals and save money. By reading and comparing labels, you can select the most nutritious foods and track calories. Individuals on special diets recommended by their physicians can use nutrition labeling to help avoid restricted foods.

The food labels used by the Food and Drug Administration from 1973 to 1993 were developed when nutrient deficiencies were a major concern. The labels were difficult to understand because they weren't presented in a helpful format and because they contained information of little relevance to most of us.

The labels introduced in 1993 reflect some of the health concerns of the American public and make it easier for consumers to shop wisely. The USRDA for protein, thiamine, riboflavin, and niacin were eliminated. The newer labels are required for all foods that are sources of nutrients, whereas the previous labels were required only when a food was fortified or when a nutritional claim was made. Foods such as fruits and vegetables now have nutritional information available ("Nutritional Labels for the

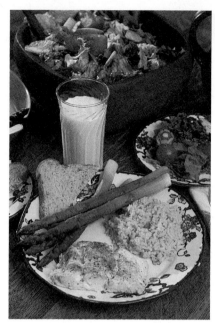

It is important to choose a variety of foods.

'90s" 1990). Even candy bars are required to have nutritional labels ("Unmasking Labels that Hide the Fat" 1992).

A plan proposed by the FDA includes regulating standard serving sizes. Some companies use a very small serving size to compute the contents of a food. This way the nutritional information on the food may look much better than it really is. For example, Diet Coke is advertised as having less than one calorie per serving. The serving, however, is six ounces, which is half a can. Most people drink the whole can, therefore, six ounces is not an accurate serving size.

There are standard definitions for terms used to describe products such as "high fiber," "light," "low sodium," "cholesterol," or "low fat" (Pacelli 1990). For example, products advertised as "light" or "lite" must have at least one-third fewer calories than the norm for that product. They must have at least 50 percent less fat if more than half the calories come from fat ("Unmasking Labels that Hide the Fat" 1992). "Low fat" products must have three or fewer grams of fat per serving. These definitions help you more accurately judge the nutritional value of different products.

Just because a product is advertised as being low in fat does not mean it is low in other ingredients you may wish to avoid. "Lite" versions of mayonnaise and salad dressings often contain large amounts of sodium. Lite mayonnaise can have as much as 170 percent more sodium than regular mayonnaise (Hold the Mayo?" 1992).

After the FDA began defining certain terms, some food manufacturers began labeling their foods with words that have not been defined. An example is the term "healthy." Many of the foods with "healthy" on the label are anything but. The FDA is considering defining implied claims like "healthy," much to the aggravation of the Grocery Manufacturers Association. You may wish to look at the number of products labeled "healthy" the next time you are in a grocery store (Hurley and Schmidt 1992).

Because there is so much misinformation in the field of nutrition, it is important for the consumer to be wary. Consider the following guidelines when determining whether or not a source of information is credible:

1. Is one food or product promoted as the only one needed for good health?
2. Is the person promoting the product likely to experience personal gain?
3. Is there a variety of foods from the food groups recommended in the plan?
4. Is the person selling the plan or promoting the product someone associated with reliable health information?
5. Is the person promoting the product a good role model?

Special Nutritional Considerations

The nutritional information discussed in this chapter applies to the majority of healthy adults. There are several groups whose nutritional considerations merit special discussion. These groups include vegetarians, athletes, and individuals under stress.

Vegetarians

The majority of nutrients consumed by **vegetarians** is from plant sources. Vegetarian diets are increasingly popular and are chosen for a number of reasons.

The types of vegetarian diets include vegan, lacto vegetarian, and lacto-ovo vegetarian. Vegans eat only plant foods. The vegan diet is the most difficult to adhere to and balance from a nutritional perspective. Lacto vegetarians eat plant foods and dairy products. Low-fat or skim milk products should be used in the lacto vegetarian diet to keep it low in fat. Lacto-ovo vegetarians eat dairy products, eggs, and plant foods. This is the most common form of vegetarian diet in America.

All types of vegetarian diets can be nutritious if care is taken in food selection. Vegetarians typically have lower weights, less constipation, lower blood pressure levels, less risk for heart disease and certain cancers, and more favorable levels of blood cholesterol than the majority of the population. There are some risks, however, associated with a vegetarian diet. Vegetarian diets may be lacking in vitamins (including vitamin D, vitamin B-12, and riboflavin), minerals (including zinc, calcium, and iron), and amino acids.

The greatest concerns regarding vegetarian diets relate to lack of vitamin D and vitamin B-12 and the need for enough calories to meet energy needs. Lack of calories to meet energy needs is usually a problem for child vegetarians rather than adult vegetarians. Special efforts are needed to ensure that children consume adequate calories to meet the energy needs of their growing bodies.

Vegetarian women who become pregnant usually do not need to alter their diets if they are lacto or lacto-ovo vegetarians. Vegans need to assure they receive adequate amounts of protein, vitamin B-6, iron, calcium, zinc, and a vitamin B-12 supplement.

Although there once was a concern that vegetables and grains lacked essential amino acids, we now know that these foods contain amino acids in varying amounts. To obtain high-quality protein from plant sources, essential amino acids must be present in a specific pattern so they can be used by the body as high-quality proteins. Because vegetable foods contain varying amounts of the essential amino acids, vegetable protein foods must be combined so that one food provides what the other is missing. The foods can be eaten three to four hours apart and still complement each other. Vegetarians who consume a wide variety of foods are likely to obtain the needed amino acids. The following list shows how to pair vegetable protein foods with other vegetable protein foods to achieve high-quality proteins:

1. Legumes (dried peas, beans, lentils, peanuts) with grains (wheat, oats, rice, corn). Example: peanut butter on whole wheat bread.
2. Legumes with seeds. Example: pea soup with sesame crackers.
3. Legumes with nuts. Example: mixed dry-roasted soybeans and walnuts.

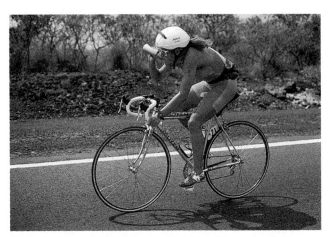

Water is the best fluid replacement drink for most activities.

The concept of complementing proteins is controversial among some vegetarians, who feel a vegetarian diet can provide all of the essential amino acids in amounts far exceeding the RDA (Moran 1989). It will be interesting to monitor the resolution of this controversy.

Athletes

Most athletes are interested in all factors that help them improve their performance, including nutrition. This is true of the professional athlete, as well as the average American involved in fitness activities. To achieve top performance, a well-balanced diet must be consumed. Top performances are not the result of eating certain foods.

There is a great deal of misinformation about nutrition and physical performance. One area involves protein. Since muscles are made of protein, it was assumed that a high-protein diet would build muscles. On the contrary, muscles are built from exercising specific muscle groups, not from certain foods. Protein is needed for building tissue, but athletes do not need additional supplies since most Americans consume more protein than they need.

Athletes must consume adequate supplies of complex carbohydrates to provide needed energy, since they are the primary fuel needed by the muscles during exercise. Complex carbohydrates provide energy at a slow and gradual pace, while simple carbohydrates cause a rapid drop in blood sugar. Carbohydrate consumption for athletes involved in heavy training should be approximately four hundred grams per day. It is best to consume a large portion of the carbohydrates within two hours after the end of training because glycogen synthesis is the greatest then (Wardlaw and Insel 1990).

Extra calories may be needed by athletes to meet the demands of training. The best advice for supplying these demands is to increase the portions of a well-balanced diet. It is a poor idea to consume products high in fat or protein to add these extra calories.

Fluid replacement is extremely important for athletes, particularly those involved in endurance sports. Athletes involved in endurance activities may lose six to eight

Making Healthy Nutrition a Part of Your Life

Nutritional choices influence every aspect of your life because these choices influence how you feel. How you feel impacts your mind, body, and soul and the interdependence of these factors. For most of us, eating nutritiously requires some specific changes and a certain amount of commitment to maximize the benefits.

Complete the following activities to assess to what degree you possess health skills related to nutrition. Successful completion of all of these activities indicates that you have the prerequisites needed to make nutritious food choices a part of your life-style. Or, use this information to develop a nutritious life-style.

Mind

Decide if eating nutritiously is important to you and why it is important. Determine what you want to accomplish as a result of making nutritional changes.

Body

Evaluate your present eating habits. Consider how you feel as a result of your food choices. Determine your areas of strength and your weaknesses. Consider how the positive and negative aspects influence your health.

Soul

Determine if the benefits associated with eating nutritiously are related to the values you hold. Consider the immediate as well as long-term benefits.

Interdependence

1. Share the benefits of eating nutritiously with someone who is important in your life. Discuss ways in which nutrition impacts all areas of your life.

2. Determine changes to improve your nutrition. Evaluate what is needed to complete these changes successfully.

3. A certain level of commitment is needed to implement any long-term changes successfully. Review what you can do in other areas of your life to encourage that commitment and assist with the changes.

---

pounds per hour, which is mostly water weight. A 3 percent weight loss can hamper performance, while a 7 percent loss could have a detrimental affect on the functioning of the heart and circulatory system (McGlynn 1990).

Water is still considered the best fluid replacement drink; however, some of the more recent studies have shown that glucose solutions may be better than water for fluid replacement during prolonged exercise (activities that last longer than ninety minutes), providing the concentration of glucose is less than 12 percent. The absorption rate is decreased at the 12 percent level, and the athlete may experience gastrointestinal distress (Powers and Howley 1990). It is recommended that athletes consume two cups of fluid fifteen minutes before an event and one cup of fluid every fifteen minutes for sports events that last longer than thirty minutes (Wardlaw and Insel 1990). Salt tablets are never recommended as a means of replacing sodium lost during exercise since they increase the likelihood of dehydration.

Individuals Under Stress

Diet is related to stress in several ways. Certain foods may produce a response similar to the stress response. Nutrients can be depleted during stressful times, and consumption of certain foods may worsen stress-related diseases.

Pseudostressors are substances in the diet that may produce effects similar to stress for certain individuals. These products may have a negative impact on health and interfere with normal functioning by replicating sympathetic nervous system stimulation. Reactions may include an increase in the metabolic rate and a release of stress hormones that increase heart rate and metabolism (Greenberg 1990). Dietary stressors include products containing caffeine, such as colas, coffee, tea, chocolate, and some over-the-counter drugs. Although the reaction varies in each individual, some may find they are nervous and unable to sleep after consuming these products. Those who react this way should limit the intake of these products, particularly in the evening, and check product labels.

Stress can impact nutrition by depleting certain nutrients, particularly vitamin C and the B complex vitamins. These vitamins are used to produce the hormone cortisol during periods of stress and are also used by the body to process products high in refined sugar. A diet deficient in these vitamins may result in depression, anxiety, nervous disorders, weakness, and sleep disturbances.

Consumption of large amounts of sugar over a short time may result in elevated levels of blood sugar, followed by periods of hypoglycemia (low blood sugar). This source of dietary stress may result in trembling, anxiety, dizziness, fatigue, and lethargy but can easily be modified by a reduction in the amount of simple carbohydrates consumed.

Consumption of too much or too little of certain nutrients may worsen diseases related to stress. The likelihood of heart disease is increased when a diet high in saturated fats is consumed, allowing cholesterol to increase in the blood and accumulate on the wall of the arteries.

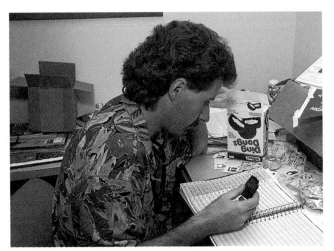
The stress of a job need not be heightened by eating dietary stressors such as sugar and caffeine.

If you are under prolonged stress, you may be more susceptible to the effects of stress because your immune system is weakened. Consequently, nutritional patterns become even more important during stressful times. Those under stress tend either to significantly reduce their intake of food or to eat snack food of low nutritional value. To work through a difficult time, it is especially important to eat a well-balanced diet and to utilize the stress products through exercise. Good nutritional practices can enhance the coping skills that are protective skills. While nutritional choices may not appear to make an immediate impact on health, they have short-term as well as long-term effects. Good nutritional choices help ensure that you are in a strong physiological position to deal with the stressors you encounter.

Summary

1. Acknowledged in the *Healthy People 2000* objectives for the nation is the correlation between poor nutritional practices and chronic diseases.

2. Guidelines exist to improve the nutrition of Americans.

3. Useful elements of food are called nutrients and include carbohydrates, proteins, fats, vitamins, minerals, and water.

4. Needed levels of nutrients are indicated in the RDA.

5. Food supplies energy that is measured by kilocalories.

6. Americans need to eat more complex carbohydrates and fewer simple carbohydrates.

7. Protein intake is likely to be more than adequate in most individuals.

8. Fat supplies nine calories per gram, while proteins and carbohydrates supply four calories per gram.

9. HDL removes cholesterol from the walls of the arteries.

10. Vitamins do not provide energy but are needed for chemical reactions to occur in the body.

11. Inadequate supplies of calcium are associated with osteoporosis.

12. Fifteen to twenty million Americans are sodium sensitive.

13. Water is the most important nutrient of all.

14. The Food Guide Pyramid has replaced the basic four food groups. Foods are divided into groups based on the similarity of nutrients.

15. There are a number of things students can do to eat well on a budget.

16. An occasional fast-food meal is fine, as long as needed nutrients are made up at the next meal.

17. Food additives allow us to store foods for long periods.

18. Ingredients on labels are listed in order of concentration in the product.

19. Vegetarians need to be especially careful about getting needed amounts of vitamin B-12.

20. The best fluid replacement drink for most activities is water.

Commitment Activities

1. Collect sample menus from local restaurants that advertise meals that are heart healthy, "lite" dishes, diet plates, or low in sodium. Analyze these to determine if the meals are more nutritious than the other offerings.

2. Develop a list of changes to improve your nutrition. Discuss these with the food supervisor to see which ones could be implemented (if living in a dormitory).

3. Develop a list of guidelines and recommendations for selecting nutritious meals when eating out. Be sure the ideas are general enough to apply to restaurants serving a wide variety of foods.

4. Plan a trip to a local supermarket. Be a comparison shopper and use a product checklist that is developed by the class. Compare brands, sizes, and nutritional content and check the results with other members of the class.

References

"Battling the Bad Fat." *Harvard Health Letter* 17, no. 3 (January 1992):6–7.

Clark, N. "Milk: Destroying the Myths." *The Physician and Sportsmedicine* 18, no. 2 (1990):133.

Duston, "Food Aimed at Kids Mostly Junk, Group Says." Associated Press release in the *Birmingham News,* August 3, 1992, pp. 1a, 6a.

Edell, D. "Calcium and Fiber at Odds." *Edell Health Letter* 11, no. 1 (December/January 1992):4.

Edell, D. "Your Built-in Salt Sensor.". *Edell Health Letter* 10, no. 2 (February 1991): 4.

"Fear of Eggs." *Consumer Reports* 54, no. 10 (1989): 650–52.

"Forget Cholesterol?" *Consumer Reports* 55, no. 3 (1990): 152–56.

Greenberg, J. *Comprehensive Stress Management,* 3rd ed. Dubuque, Iowa: Wm. C. Brown, 1990, p. 78.

Guthrie, H. "Recommended Dietary Allowances 1989." *Nutrition Today* (January/February 1990):43–45.

Healthy People 2000: National Health Promotion and Disease Prevention Objectives. U.S. Department of Health and Human Services/Public Health Service, 1990 pp. 56, 93–95.

"Hold the Mayo?" *Consumer Reports on Health* (April 1992):30.

"Honey vs. Sugar" *Consumer Reports on Health* (January 1992):8.

Hunter, B. T. "Strategies to Reduce Dietary Fat." *Consumers' Research,* 72, no. 4 (1989):29–31.

Hurley, J., and Schmidt, S. "Food Labels Get 'Healthy'." *Nutrition Action Healthletter,* 19, no. 6 (July/August 1992):8.

"Institute Offers 'Clear-Cut' Diet Plan to Reduce Disease Risk." *Health Education Reports* (February 27, 1992):2.

"Just what Is a Balanced Diet, Anyway?" *Tufts University Diet and Nutrition Letter,* 9, no. 11 (January 1992):3.

"Kid's-eye Cereals." *Nutrition Action Healthletter* (June 1990):3.

Kirby, R. W.; Anderson, J. W.; Sieling, B.; Rees, E. D.; Chen, W. L.; Miller, R. E.; and Kay, R. M. "Oat Bran Intake Selectively Lowers Serum Low-Density Lipoprotein Cholesterol Concentrations of Hypercholesterolemic Men." *American Journal of Clinical Nutrition,* 34 (May 1981):824–29.

Liebman, B. "The Changing American Diet." *Nutrition Action Healthletter* (May 1990):8

Liebman, B. "The Clogging of an Artery." *Nutrition Action Healthletter* (March 1991):9.

Liebman, B. "Has the Oat-Bran Bubble Burst?" *Nutrition Action Healthletter* (January/February 1990):4.

Mattes, R. D., and Donnelly, D. "Relative Contributions of Dietary Sodium Scores." *Journal of the American College of Nutrition* 10, no. 4 (1991):383–93.

McGlynn, G. *Dynamics of Fitness,* 2d ed. Dubuque, Iowa: Wm. C. Brown Publishers, 1990, pp. 18, 157, 158, 210.

Moran, V. "Protein Complementing." *Vegetarian Times.* (February 1989):23–25.

"New Recommended Dietary Allowances." *Consumers' Research* 73, no. 1 (1990):25–27.

"Nutritional Labels for the '90s." *Changing Times* (June 1990):100.

Oestreicher, A. "Calcium Credited with Many Routes as Protective Factor," *Medical World News* 31, no. 4 (1990):22–23.

Orwoll, E. S., Oviatt, S. K.; McClung, M.; Deftos, L.; and Sexton, G. "The Rate of Bone Mineral Loss in Normal Men and the Effects of Calcium and Cholecalciferol Supplementation." *Annals of Internal Medicine* 112, no. 1 (1990):29–34.

Pacell, L. C. "FDA to Take Hard Look at Food Labels.: *The Physician and Sportsmedicine* 18, no. 4 (1990):29.

"The Pepsi (De)generation." *Nutrition Action Healthletter* (January/February 1990):16.

Pollner, F. "Heart Association, Feds Set for New Kind of Food Fight." *Medical World News* 3, no. 21 (1990):42.

Powers, S. K., and Howley, E. T. *Exercise Physiology: Theory and Application to Fitness and Performance.* Dubuque, Iowa: Wm. C. Brown Publishers, (1990), pp. 476, 484.

"Pyramid Scheme Foiled." *Nutrition Action Healthletter* 19, no. 6 (July/August, 1992):3.

Roberts, C. "Fast Food Fare and Nutrition." *Consumers' Research* 72, no. 12 (1989):30–33.

Schmidt, S. "Stripped-Juice Tease." *Nutrition Action Healthletter* (October 1991):9.

Stamford, B. "What Cholesterol Means to You." *The Physician and Sportsmedicine* 18, no. 1 (1990):149–50.

Strickland, D. "Vitamin C Seen to Help Prevent CAD." *Medical World News* 32, no. 8 (1991):11.

Suter, P. M.; Schutz, Y.; and Jequier, E. "The Effect of Ethanol on Fat Storage in Healthy Subjects." *New England Journal of Medicine* 326, no. 15 (April 1992):983–87.

Swain, J. F., Rouse, I. L.; Curley, C. B.; and Sacks, F. M. "Comparison of the Effects of Oat Bran and Low-Fiber Wheat on Serum Lipoprotein Levels and Blood Pressure." *New England Journal of Medicine* 322, no. 3 (1990):147–52.

"TV Feeds Kids Steady Diet of Sugary-food Ads." *Tufts University Diet & Nutrition Letter* 9, no. 9 (1990):7.

Tonnesen, D. "The Big Fruit-Juice Squeeze." *Health* 22, no. 1 (1990):32–33.

"Too Much Salt?" *Consumer Reports,* 55, no. 1 (1990):48.

"Unmasking Labels That Hide the Fat." *Kiplinger's Personal Finance Magazine* 46, no. 2 (1992):92.

Van Horn, L. V.; Liu, K.; Parker, D.; Emidy, L.; Liao, Y.; Pan, W. H.; Giumetti, D.; Hewitt, J.; and Stamler, J. "Serum Lipid Response to Oat Product Intake with A Fat-Modified Diet." *Journal of the American Dietetic Association* 86, no. 6 (1986):759–84.

Wardlaw, G. M., and Insel, P. M. *Perspectives in Nutrition.* St. Louis: Times Mirror/Mosby College Publishing, 1990, pp. 305, 384, 388, 389.

"Weight-Bearing Exercises Help Prevent Bone Weakness." *Health Education Reports* (June 7, 1990):4–5.

"Where's the Fat?" *Consumer Reports 55*, no. 3 (1990):158–59.

"Who's Afraid of MSG?" *Consumer Reports on Health* 4, no. 1 (1992):6.

Williams, M.; *Lifetime Fitness and Wellness—A Practical Approach,* 2d ed. Dubuque, Iowa: Wm. C. Brown Publishers, 1990, p. 115.

"Yet Another Reason to Drink Your Milk." *Tufts University Diet & Nutrition Letter* 9, no. 11 (January 1992):1.

Additional Readings

"FDA's Proposal for New `Daily Values' for Nutrients." *FDA Background* (February 12, 1992). The changes in the revision of the food label are discussed.

Liebman, B. "The Name Game." *Nutrition Action Healthletter* (March 1992):8. Shows some of the actual ingredients in products.The products shown contain far less of the ingredients advertised than one might expect.

Physical Activity

Many college students participated in physical activities while growing up. Generally, the emphasis in school was on learning skills, and little attention was given to the relationship of health to physical activity.

In spite of the potential benefits of regular physical activity, few Americans engage in it. In fact, the U.S. Centers for Disease Control reports that only about 36 percent of high school students get enough exercise ("CDC Finds That High School Kids May Do Less Vigorous Exercise" 1992). As for adults, almost 60 percent get little or no exercise ("First the Good News" 1992).

Less than 10 percent of the U.S. adult population exercises at the level recommended by the 1990 national health objectives: "Exercise which involves large muscle groups in dynamic movement for periods of twenty minutes or longer, three or more days per week, and which is performed at an intensity of 60 percent or greater of an individual's cardiorespiratory capacity." As children become older, move through adolescence, and enter early adulthood, fewer of them exercise with each year of increasing age *(Promoting Health/Preventing Disease: Year 2000 Objectives for the Nation* 1990).

Why should you be active? What is physical fitness, and what are its benefits? In this chapter, these questions are answered. A description of how to develop a personal exercise program and a discussion about how physical activity is related to life-style are included.

Physical Fitness and Its Benefits

What Is Physical Fitness?

Physical fitness has many components. Traditionally, they have included agility, balance, cardiorespiratory capacity, coordination, flexibility, muscular endurance, power, reaction time, speed, and strength. More recently, physical fitness includes five components: muscle strength, muscle endurance, flexibility, body composition (i.e., degree of fatness), and cardiorespiratory muscle endurance ("American Academy of Pediatrics Statement" 1987). Although a high level of fitness in all of the traditional components is ideal, to get the health benefits of physical activity, only muscle strength, muscle endurance, flexibility, a favorable body composition, and cardiorespiratory endurance are needed. Most of the other components are concerned with physical skills that are not basic to health.

Some individuals think of fitness as a state of being. We prefer to think of it as a way of life. While it is best to develop an active life-style as children and continue the pattern throughout the life cycle, it is never too late to start exercising. Even people in their fifties, sixties, seventies, and eighties can benefit from physical activity. In fact, regular physical activity, of the right type, retards much of the usual loss of physical capacity associated with age (Kasch et al. 1990)

Physical activity must be continued throughout life, or fitness will be lost and health impaired. It is fairly simple to adjust the exercise prescription as needs change, but people must continue to be active.

Health Benefits of Physical Activity

Those who exercise regularly report that they feel better, have more energy, and often require less sleep. Regular exercisers often lose excess weight while improving muscular strength and flexibility. Greater body satisfaction is associated with increases in exercise participation (Davis and Cowles 1991), as are psychological benefits such as enhanced self-esteem, greater self-reliance, decreased anxiety, and relief from mild depression.

Some fear that repeated vigorous exercise, such as running, aerobics, and tennis, will harm their joints. A five-year study by the Stanford Arthritis Center found that runners putting in an average of twenty-seven miles per week over five to forty years were no more likely than sedentary nonrunners to develop early signs of arthritis in their hips or knees (*Health Education Reports,* 1990).

Sustained exercise improves the efficiency of the heart and increases the amount of oxygen the body

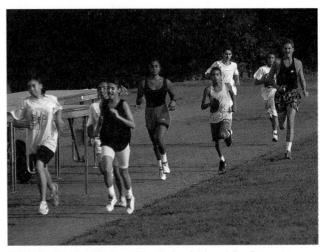
Obtaining the health benefits of physical activity does not demand a high level of skill.

can process in a given period of time. Evidence strongly suggests that when exercise is an integral part of daily activities it helps prevent coronary artery disease, helps maintain blood pressure within safe limits, controls body weight, and contributes to the control of diabetes ("Physical Exercise" 1990). Even modest exercise (such as brisk walking for thirty to forty-five minutes at three to four miles per hour, six to seven times a week) cuts the risk of cardiovascular disease (Phillips 1990).

There are also nutritional benefits from exercise. It helps control obesity, helps suppress the appetite, helps conserve lean tissue instead of fat tissue, and enables the physically active person to have a healthier quantity and quality of fats in the blood (Shephard 1989).

Additional benefits from exercise are continually added to an already long list. For example many individuals with arthritis are now encouraged to increase exercise levels. In addition to the usual health benefits, they can obtain improved joint mobility and pain control through physical activity (Samples 1990). In addition, physical activity may reduce the risk of colon cancer (Cremmons 1990) and increase bone mass (Cooper 1989). Countless investigators in many parts of the world have come to the same conclusion: physical activity does benefit health.

As discussed, quality of life is probably far more important than quantity; however, strong evidence indicates that premature death rates are significantly lower among the physically active. This is true with or without consideration of hypertension, cigarette smoking, extremes or gains in body weight, or early parental death (Paffenbarger et al. 1986). Exercise helps increase the length of life as well as the quality of life. In fact, there is no single group that can benefit more from exercise than the elderly (Allison 1991).

Exercise compensates for the changes that accompany aging in several ways. It helps prevent the loss of muscle and can even help regain lost muscle. It helps preserve bone mass, prevent brittle bones, and even build bone. It boosts the resting metabolic rate and therefore

Physical Fitness

Should You Exercise?

Mark any of the following that apply to you:

_____ Your physician said you have heart trouble or a heart murmur, or you have had a heart attack.

_____ You frequently have pains or pressure—in the left or mid-chest area, left neck, shoulder, or arm—during or right after you exercise.

_____ You often feel faint or have spells of severe dizziness.

_____ You experience extreme breathlessness after mild exertion.

_____ Your physician said your blood pressure is too high and is not under control. Or you do not know if your blood pressure is normal.

_____ Your physician said you have bone or joint problems such as arthritis.

_____ You are over age sixty and are not accustomed to vigorous exercise.

_____ You have a family history of premature coronary artery disease.

_____ You have a medical condition not mentioned here that might need special attention in an exercise program (asthma, insulin-dependent diabetes).

Scoring/Interpretation

None of these factors will prevent you from exercising, but if you checked any of the items, you should first receive medical clearance from your physician to exercise.

Flexibility Assessment

Place a box on the floor. It should measure twelve to fifteen inches high, any width, and at least eighteen inches long. On top of the box place a ruler with the zero point of the ruler at the edge of the box farthest from the wall. Sit down facing the box with feet flat against the side of the box and legs fully extended.

Slowly reach (stretch) with hands extended toward the edge of the box and beyond if possible. The maximum stretch must be held for a three count. With the ruler "zeroed" at the edge of the box, determine how many inches you may lack reaching the edge (a negative score) or how many inches past the edge onto the ruler that you can reach.

Scoring/Interpretation

	Women	Men
Normal range (inches)	+4 to +10	–6 to +8
Average	+2	+1
Desired	+2 to +6	+1 to +5

Muscular Endurance Test

Lay down on a mat on your back with your hands interlocked behind your head. Your knees should be bent at ninety degrees and your feet should be held by your partner. Do sit-ups for one full minute, touching elbows to your knees and then returning to the starting position. Do as many sit-ups as you can for one full minute. The score is the number of sit-ups you are able to do during that period. (Be careful not to pull on your head or neck while doing sit-ups.)

Scoring/Interpretation

Rating Scale for One-Minute Sit-up Test					
			Age		
Rating	20–29	30–39	40–49	50–59	60–65
Males					
Excellent	47	40	35	30	29
Good	41	35	30	25	24
Average	35	29	25	20	18
Fair	29	24	19	15	13
Poor	9	5	2	0	0
Females					
Excellent	42	37	30	21	20
Good	36	31	25	17	16
Average	30	26	20	12	11
Fair	24	20	15	8	6
Poor	3	1	0	0	0

J. Gavin Reid/John M. Thomson, *Exercise Prescription for Fitness*, © 1985, p. 126. Adapted by permission of Prentice-Hall, Inc., Englewood Cliffs, NJ.

Initiation/Continuance of Exercise

Section I: Exercisers

This tool is designed to determine the likelihood of your continuing to exercise throughout your life, which is a desirable attribute. Check all that apply to you. If you do not currently exercise, then skip to section II.

_____ 1. I exercise alone or enjoy exercising alone if no one else is around.

_____ 2. It is difficult for me to get motivated to exercise.

_____ 3. I exercise only because someone else encourages me to do it or I am in an organized sport.

_____ 4. Exercise is a high priority in my life.

_____ 5. I exercise all year around, not just certain seasons.

_____ 6. I am unhappy or fidgety when I miss an exercise session.

_____ 7. My role model (hero) exercises.

_____ 8. I enjoy exercise.

_____ 9. I am hooked on exercise.

_____ 10. I plan to exercise all my life if possible.

Scoring/Interpretation

1. = 2	6. = 2
2. = –2	7. = 2
3. = –2	8. = 2
4. = 2	9. = 2
5. = 2	10. = 2

Total your score for the statements you checked and interpret it as follows:

    10 to 16 = High likelihood of continuing exercise
    4 to 9 = Moderate likelihood of continuing exercise
    0 to 4 = Low likelihood of continuing exercise

If you scored low, then after reading this chapter you may be able to make some changes in your attitude and increase the likelihood of your continuing an exercise program throughout your life.

Section II: Nonexercisers

The purpose of this tool is to determine the likelihood of your starting an exercise program. Mark all that apply to you.

_____ 1. I am really motivated to start an exercise program.

_____ 2. I used to exercise and liked it.

_____ 3. I've been wanting to start for a long time but wasn't sure how to start.

_____ 4. I'm willing to try and start but doubt I will stick to it.

_____ 5. I am not sure exercise will help me much.

_____ 6. I don't like to exercise.

_____ 7. The benefits of exercise are not worth the time and effort.

_____ 8. I tried once and quit because I didn't like it.

Scoring/Interpretation

1. = 2	5. = –2
2. = 2	6. = –2
3. = 2	7. = –2
4. = –2	8. = –2

Total your score for the statements you marked and interpret it as follows:

    2 to 6 = High likelihood of starting an exercise program
    0 to –2 = Moderate likelihood of starting an exercise program
    –3 to –10 = Not likely to start an exercise program

By reading this chapter, it is hoped you can realize the benefits of exercise and become motivated to start. After reading the chapter, retest yourself on this if you scored low on likelihood of starting an exercise program.

---

aids in weight control and improves aerobic capacity as in younger people ("Can Exercise Turn Back the Clock?" 1992).

To summarize, the health benefits of regular exercise include the following:

1. improved physiological functioning;
2. improved appearance;
3. increased efficiency of the heart and lungs;
4. increased muscle strength and endurance;
5. reduced stress response;
6. protection from lower back problems;
7. possible delay in the aging process;
8. maintenance of proper body weight;
9. possible reduction of the risk of coronary heart disease;
10. naturally induced fatigue and relaxation (McGlynn 1990).

A physically fit person has greater ability to tolerate the challenges of daily life. It is important to note that the physical and psychological benefits of physical activity combine to enhance resiliency, as discussed in chapter 1. Physical activity is valuable in treating depression and enhancing feelings of well-being and self-esteem ("Physical Exercise" 1990). It also increases resistance to stress, anxiety, and fatigue (Williams 1990). The physically fit person is better able to adapt through resilient reintegration (see chapter 1) when disruption and disorganization occur in life. Physical activity is an excellent example of a protective factor that enhances all of the components of health.

To understand what health benefits might be gained from physical activity, it is necessary to know how exercise affects the human body. Specifically, understanding two general physiological principles will help you to have realistic expectations. The first one, the **principle of specificity,** means "you get what you train for." In other words if you want to become stronger, it is imperative to train for strength and not for endurance. If you want to improve your ability to run long distances, it is important to lengthen the distances you regularly run. One physical capacity is not significantly improved by working on another. For example, doing many sit-ups daily won't improve abdominal strength as effectively as doing fewer sit-ups with a weight held behind the head. Doing more sit-ups improves endurance, not strength.

Related to the principle of specificity is the **overload principle,** which states that to improve a physical capacity, a stress must be placed on the relevant part of the body. For example, if increased strength is desired, you must work with increasing amounts of weight. If increased endurance is the goal, you must perform the activity more times or for a longer period.

Anabolic steroids are growth-stimulating chemicals—some of which are found naturally in the body. They were developed synthetically to promote tissue growth in those who experienced atrophy because of prolonged bed rest. It did not take long for some individuals to wonder if anabolic steroids might help develop muscle mass and strength in athletes.

Steroids do not directly improve performance in aerobic activities such as long-distance running, skiing, or swimming. While they may help build lean body mass and improve strength in individuals involved in intense training activities, such as weight lifting, the real possibility of harmful side effects greatly outweighs the questionable increase in performance. Anabolic steroids have been associated with adverse effects on the liver, cardiovascular system, reproductive function, and psychological status.

Sources: G. McGlynn, *Dynamics of Fitness.* Copyright © 1990 Wm. C. Brown Communications, Dubuque, Iowa; and S. K. Powers and E. T. Howley, *Exercise Physiology.* p. 88. Copyright © 1990 Wm. C. Brown Communications, Dubuque, Iowa.

These principles help explain how improvement in three major systems of the body—the muscular, cardiovascular, and respiratory systems—can take place.

Unfortunately, there is a third principle, the **law of reversibility,** that must also be considered. A significant reduction of working capacity begins to occur within days after training is stopped. The saying "use it or lose it' definitely applies to physical fitness. A gradual decline of performance capacity results and a decrease in size (atrophy) of muscle cells. Therefore, continued physical activity is necessary to maintain the benefits achieved.

Fitness of Major Body Systems

Fitness of the Muscular System

From a physiological standpoint, a strength overload seems to lead to **hypertrophy,** which means muscle fibers become larger and stronger. An endurance overload probably results in an improved blood supply to the working muscles. These are positive changes because they improve the health and functioning of the muscles.

The overload and specificity principles shed some light on the issue of isometric versus isotonic muscular activity. This issue has been debated for many years. **Isometric activities** involve exerting muscular force against an immovable object so that there is muscular contraction but no joint movement. **Isotonic activities,** by contrast, involve exerting muscular force throughout the range of motion of a joint, such as lifting a heavy object. You can gain strength with either method, but it appears that isotonic activities are more practical for most people, and, from a health standpoint, it makes more sense to use a full range of joint motion. Isometric activities increase strength *only* at the specific joint angle at which training is done and may also cause potentially dangerous blood pressure fluctuations. Isotonic activities, on the other hand, develop strength throughout the entire range of motion and are applicable to everyday motions. To develop muscular endurance, isotonic activities are preferable because movement is needed to achieve the health benefits of physical activity.

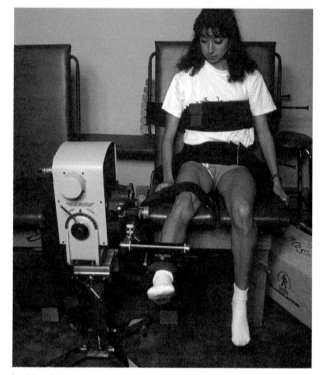

Isokinetic contractions are obtained with specialized equipment.

A third type of muscle contraction is an **isokinetic contraction.** A muscular contraction is isokinetic when the speed of the contraction is kept constant against a variable resistance. Specialized equipment allows muscles to encounter maximum resistance throughout a complete range of motion. While isometric, isotonic, and isokinetic methods can all produce significant gains in strength in relatively short periods of time, research seems to indicate that the isokinetic form of resistance training is superior to the other methods for strength gains (Brown 1986). Equipment needed for isokinetic contractions is quite expensive and probably only available at a well equipped fitness center. Isokinetic contractions, however, do increase strength throughout the full range of motion and result in less injury and soreness than either isometric or isotonic exercise (McGlynn 1990).

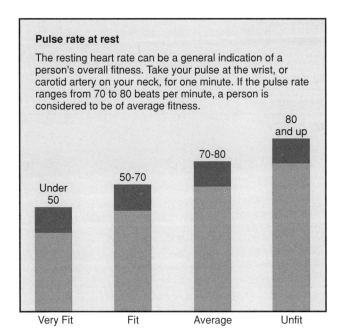

Pulse rate at rest

The resting heart rate can be a general indication of a person's overall fitness. Take your pulse at the wrist, or carotid artery on your neck, for one minute. If the pulse rate ranges from 70 to 80 beats per minute, a person is considered to be of average fitness.

80 and up

70-80

50-70

Under 50

Very Fit   Fit   Average   Unfit

Figure 4.1
Checking pulse rate.

Fitness of the Cardiovascular System

The heart is a muscle, so it becomes stronger by using it. As it becomes stronger, it doesn't need to work as hard to pump blood. This is why those in good physical condition tend to have low resting pulse rates. A resting pulse rate of seventy to eighty beats per minute is average, but it is not unusual to find physically fit people with resting rates around forty to fifty beats per minute (fig. 4.1). A low pulse rate allows the heart more rest and more time to fill with blood between beats so it can better perform its task as a pump. As the heart muscle becomes stronger, it also becomes better able to withstand potential problems. If a heart attack (condition where the heart muscle receives insufficient blood) should occur, a strong heart can deal with it much better.

Coronary is a general term referring to a heart attack that occurs because of a problem with the **coronary circulation.** Because the heart receives no benefit from the blood that flows through it, it needs to have its own circulation system (coronary circulation), which is strengthened by regular, total body, physical activity.

Increased circulatory efficiency, better coronary circulation, and more rest and strength for the heart all combine to enable the circulatory system to better resist cardiovascular disease and cope with problems that do develop. These valuable benefits can be obtained from a physically active life-style. Table 4.1 summarizes cardiovascular training effects.

Fitness of the Respiratory System

As you regularly perform strenuous physical activity, your respiratory system develops more efficiency and an

TABLE 4.1

Cardiovascular Training Effects

Cardiovascular Training Increases	Cardiovascular Training Produces	Cardiovascular Training Decreases
Tolerance to stress	Lower resting heart rate	Obesity-adiposity
Arterial oxygen content	Physical conditioning of muscles	Arterial blood pressure
Electron transport activity	Greater oxygen utilization	Heart rate
Efficiency of the heart	Greater stroke volume	Vulnerability to dysrhythmias
Blood vessel size	Lower heart rate for submaximal work	Stress response
Efficiency of blood circulation		Need of heart muscle for oxygen

increased work capacity. A variety of related changes occur for this to happen, including the following:

1. *Greater possible maximal oxygen intake.* This means the body's cells can take in a greater amount of oxygen. We already breathe in far more oxygen than needed, but cells develop the capacity to use more of this oxygen.

2. *Decreased oxygen debt for the same work.* The muscular contractions involved in physical activity are made possible because of a chemical conversion process fueled by oxygen. After strenuous physical activity, we need oxygen in higher quantities for the chemical processes to "recharge." As fitness improves, the same work requires a smaller **oxygen debt.** Oxygen debt is the amount of oxygen used during recovery from physical activity above the amount normally used during that same time at rest.

3. *Ability to withstand a higher oxygen debt.* Aside from requiring a smaller oxygen debt for the same work, the fit person can withstand a higher oxygen debt. The combination of these two factors enables the fit person to do more physical work with less discomfort than the relatively unfit person.

4. *Decreased oxygen requirement.* As the body becomes more efficient, it needs less fuel to do the same work. Because less oxygen is required for a given amount of physical work, oxygen debt for the same work is lower, the body can withstand a higher oxygen debt, and greater maximal oxygen intake is possible; thus, the respiratory system of a fit person functions far more efficiently than that of an unfit person. This capacity is the keystone of health benefits derived from physical activity.

Physical activity is not a cure-all. The improvements in physical functioning, the psychological rewards, the

Benefits of Physical Activity

Are the benefits of physical activity worth the effort required both to accommodate the activity (by reorganizing daily living patterns) and to perform the activity?

- **Pro:** Physically active people feel the benefits they get are worth the effort it takes. They report sleeping better, feeling more energetic, losing weight, dealing more effectively with stress, and being physically stronger with greater endurance.
- **Con:** Some people have gotten along fine for years with little or no physical activity. They need to earn money, complete certain chores, and spend time with loved ones. Their schedules are full, and they don't feel that they have the time it takes to be physically active.

Are the benefits worth the effort?

TABLE 4.2

Norms for the 1.5 Mile Run for Seventeen- to Twenty-Five-Year-Old Adults

Percentile	Males	Females
99	7:21	8:42
90	8:53	11:23
80	9:13	12:00
70	9:27	12:25
60	9:42	12:46
50	10:00	13:14
40	10:16	13:44
30	10:34	14:17
20	10:54	14:38
10	11:30	15:23

From Larry Brown, *Lifetime Fitness,* 3d edition. Copyright © 1992 by Gorsuch Scarisbrick Publishers, Scottsdale, Ariz. Reprinted with permission.

tendency toward prevention of many diseases, and the use of physical activity for certain types of rehabilitation and treatment, however, combine to make exercise one of the more powerful health influences over which we have control. When establishing a life-style conducive to health, few activities give so much return for the investment as exercise.

Developing a Physical Activity Program

Once the commitment is made, the first step in developing an exercise program is to determine your present physical fitness level and how much strenuous activity your body can take.

Medical Checkups and Stress Tests

Some experts stress the need for a medical checkup and perhaps an exercise stress test before beginning an exercise program. If you choose to have a checkup, your physician should examine your cardiovascular system and check your blood pressure, muscles, and joints.

As part of a medical checkup, or perhaps in place of it, you may decide to take an exercise stress test. Some authorities question the benefit or necessity of stress tests. Of course, individuals with obvious circulatory or other physical problems should seek medical advice before beginning an exercise program or taking a stress test. Others may opt for a self-test, such as those in tables 4.2 and 4.3. Although these tests are easy to administer and score, use caution. It is not wise to push hard to score as well as you can—particularly if you have not been exercising regularly. The tests should be viewed as a rough indicator of present condition and nothing more.

Capacity for intense physical activity relates more to general health and present fitness level than to age. Strenuous physical activity can be performed safely and successfully by persons in their fifties, sixties, and beyond, if common sense is used.

For a long time there was an unwritten rule that females weren't supposed to be as active as males. But females need physical activity as much as males and are not immune to the consequences of inactivity. Of course, some females may be more successful at certain types of activity than some males, but individual differences are more important than gender differences.

Designing a Cardiovascular Fitness Program

When your initial activity level has been determined, the next step is to design a program of activities. This includes scheduling exercise and deciding on intensity, duration, frequency, type of activity, and what accessories to use.

Schedule

A haphazard exercise program is likely to yield haphazard results. There is nothing magical about which days of the week or the time of day to exercise, but a regular schedule is necessary to obtain or maintain desired results. If a training session is missed, doubling the intensity of the next session will not make up for it.

When scheduling a good exercise program, remember to add in time for warming up and cooling down. Warming up helps the body gradually adjust to activity. Specific warm-up activities will depend on the type of strenuous activity to be performed, but in general, mild total activity followed by stretching will help the body get ready to exercise. Cooling down, a gradual slowing of activity, is helpful for similar reasons. When running, for

Myths About Females and Physical Activity

1. *Myth:* If women exercise, they will develop large muscles, as men do.

   Fact: Men develop large muscles from some types of physical activity, but women generally do not. This is because women have much lower levels of the hormone testosterone.

2. *Myth:* Biological differences between males and females prevent females from developing high levels of fitness.

   Fact: There is little if any difference between males and females in this respect. Everyone can develop high fitness levels if they take appropriate steps.

3. *Myth:* Women cannot exercise for long periods of time.

   Fact: Women have a higher percentage of body fat than do men (approximately 15 percent to 20 percent versus 10 percent to 15 percent in men). This difference makes them particularly suited for endurance activities.

4. *Myth:* Women should not exercise during menstruation.

   Fact: Generally, there is no reason why activity patterns should be any different during menstruation. In fact, some women who experience discomfort during menstruation find that physical activity helps relieve the discomfort. Regarding menstruation, however, it should be noted that severe, prolonged training, such as long-distance running, is associated with the cessation of menstruation and the absence of ovulation (American College of Sports Medicine 1979). Whether this happens because of exercise intensity or reduction of body fat is not known, but this situation is not harmful. Incidentally, heavy exercise should not be relied on as a contraceptive method.

5. *Myth:* Physical activity is harmful to women's breasts.

   Fact: Activity itself is not harmful to women's breasts. Women would be wise, however, to use a good sports bra for proper support.

6. *Myth:* Pregnant women should not exercise.

   Fact: While it might not be a smart time to begin training for the Boston Marathon, there is generally no reason why a pregnant woman cannot continue an established exercise program. Even those who have not been physically active can safely participate in an appropriately designed program. In fact, maternal exercise does not decrease blood flow to the fetus as was once thought (Gauthier 1990).

TABLE 4.3

1.0 Mile Walk Categories for Thirty- to Sixty-Nine-Year-Old Healthy Adults

Category	Males	Females
Excellent	<10:12	<11:40
Good	10:13–11:42	11:41–13:08
High average	11:43–13:13	13:09–14:36
Low average	13:14–14:44	14:37–16:04
Fair	14:45–16:23	16:05–17:31
Poor	>16:24	>17:32

From J. Rippe et al., "One Mile Walk Time Norms for Healthy Adults" in *Medicine and Science in Sports and Exercise,* 18(2):521, 1986. © by the American College of Sports Medicine. Reprinted with permission.

example, you might slow to a moderate jog, then a fast walk, then a slow walk, and, finally, use some stretching exercises after the run.

Intensity

Perhaps the most important consideration in planning a personal exercise program is the intensity of activity. The appropriate intensity is enough exercise to condition the muscles and cardiovascular system without overextending the body. Each individual's "target zone" is 60 percent to 80 percent of his or her individually measured **maximal aerobic power**—the point where, despite harder efforts, the heart and circulation cannot deliver more oxygen to the tissues without approaching exhaustion (Zohman 1983). Below the 60 percent level, there is little fitness benefit unless the individual has been bedridden for awhile. (Lower levels are good for health, however, even if fitness benefits are not realized.) Of course, those at lower fitness levels must start at a lower intensity and work up gradually.

There is a relationship between aerobic power and heart rate as well as between age and maximal attainable heart rate. Figure 4.2 shows target zones for people of different ages. Usually, about twenty to thirty minutes in the **target zone** (not counting warm-up and cool-down time) provides a significant conditioning effect on the cardiovascular system.

You can determine if you are in your target zone by counting your pulse. Place your hand over your heart or on the carotid artery (side of the neck): find the beat within a second, count for ten seconds, and multiply by six. Through trial and error, you can find the correct exercise intensity needed to put the pulse in the target zone. It is important to count the pulse immediately upon stopping exercise because the rate changes very quickly.

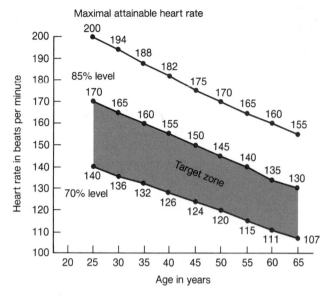

As we grow older, the heart rate which can be reached during all-out effort falls. These numerical values are "average" values for age, and one-third of the population may differ from these values. It is quite possible that a normal 50-year old man may have a maximum heart rate of 195 or that a 30-year-old man might have a maximum of only 163. The same limitations apply to the 70 percent and 85 percent of maximum lines.

Figure 4.2

Target zones for physical activity.

From L. Zohman, M.D., Beyond Diet: Exercise Your Way to Fitness & Heart Health, CPC International, Englewood Cliffs, New Jersey.

Recognizing that some individuals may have trouble exercising at the intensity needed to reach the target zone, and also realizing that others may only be willing to exercise at lower intensities, some experts feel that too much emphasis is placed on developing and maintaining cardiovascular fitness. The opinion that low-level physical activity may help reduce the likelihood of heart disease is gaining support. In fact, beneficial effects on cholesterol and blood pressure occur from as low as 40 percent to 50 percent of maximal heart rate, and a target heart rate of 50 percent to 60 percent of maximum seems best for hypertensive people (Bankhead 1991). Also, participating successfully in low-level physical activity may encourage a person to increase the intensity gradually (Kasper 1990).

With any physical activity, it is important to progress slowly. It is unwise, and perhaps even dangerous, to increase exercise intensity or duration too fast.

Duration

Your long-range goals and present level of fitness will influence exercise duration. Beginners might not be able to maintain the target rate for the recommended twenty to thirty minutes. In this case, it is wise to increase exercise time (at the target heart rate) gradually until twenty to thirty minutes are possible. Longer periods of time will not provide greater health benefits. Longer work periods

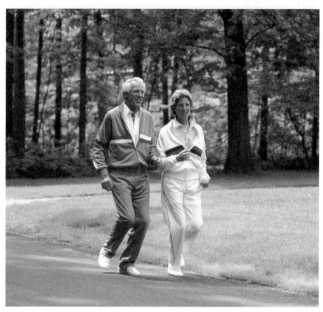

At least a simple self-test is essential prior to beginning a physical activity program.

are necessary, however, for those interested in improving performance in certain activities.

There is a trade-off between intensity and duration. For example, high-intensity activity is more likely to result in injuries, soreness, and dropping out of the activity. From the standpoint of health, it makes sense to encourage medium-level intensity and longer duration activity.

Frequency

Some individuals attempt to store the benefits of exercise by exercising strenuously only on weekends. Unfortunately, this doesn't work and can even be dangerous. Benefits from exercise begin to be lost after even two or three days without activity. Three is the *minimum* number of times per week to exercise, but daily activity is best. (Weight training, done on alternate days, is an exception.)

It is unwise to exercise to the point of exhaustion. Simply following the suggestions given for intensity, duration, and frequency are sufficient.

When designing a personal fitness program, remember the guidelines of the American College of Sports Medicine (ACSM), a medical and scientific organization that provides information on sports medicine and exercise science ("ACSM Guidelines for Fitness Updated" 1990):

1. Train three to five days a week.
2. Work out at 60 percent to 90 percent of maximum heart rate. (Note that the 90 percent level is only for those in top shape. Most of us should not exceed the 80 percent level.)
3. Exercise aerobically for twenty to sixty continuous minutes. (Note the key word, *continuous.*)
4. The activity can be anything that uses large muscle groups and is rhythmical and aerobic in nature.

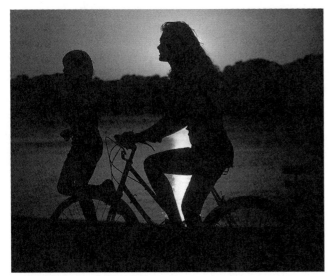

The health benefits of activity can be obtained in various ways.

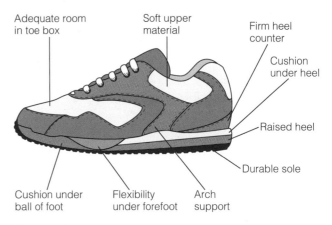

Figure 4.3
What to look for in a running shoe.

Choosing Suitable Activities

About half of the population in this country currently exercises, and there are activities available to suit everyone. Among the most popular are aerobics, jogging or running, walking, swimming, cycling, rope skipping, and weight training. The potential benefits from different types of activity are similar, so individual preference is a major factor. You should choose an activity you like so you will stick with it. Different activities can easily be combined, and occasionally started and stopped, as long as an overall program is followed.

Aerobics

The term **aerobics** means any form of total body activity performed at a rate below that needed to produce oxygen debt. In other words, this means longer, moderately intense activity rather than shorter, high-intensity activity. In practice, the term has been used synonymously with aerobic dance for many years. This is changing, however, as many forms of aerobics have emerged—even to the point of aerobics being a serious sport for some.

The amount of stress the body receives from aerobics, mostly the joints and bones, is referred to as the impact. Originally, most aerobics classes emphasized high-impact activities. Then low-impact aerobics became popular, but they often did not provide sufficient activity for the cardiovascular system. More recently, middle-impact aerobics have become popular. The idea is to keep the stress on the body down but still have a strenuous workout.

Countless variations of aerobics can be found. These include step training or step aerobics (activity variations designed to move the body up and down off steps from four to twelve inches high), sports dance (aerobics using simulated sports moves), cross-training (aerobics combined with other forms of exercise such as weight training),

interval training (alternating low-intensity and high-intensity exercise in the same workout), and circuit training (aerobic floor exercise combined with other types such as stationary bikes, climbers, ski machines and strength training machines in an alternating fashion). Aqua-aerobics is also growing in popularity (Malanka 1990).

As with other forms of physical activity, it is important to progress slowly in aerobics. One wise health decision is to be sure your aerobics instructors are properly trained.

Jogging or Running

As we define these terms, *running* is just faster than *jogging.* If you are physically ready to begin a running program, the most important consideration is to secure proper shoes. They may seem expensive, but proper running shoes are a necessity (see fig. 4.3 for some basic requirements). It is recommended that running shoes have the following characteristics ("Shoes for Sports" 1986):

1. well-cushioned heels, slightly raised to absorb impact, flared to provide stability, and rounded or beveled at the back to make forward movement easier;

2. a firm back portion of the shoe to stabilize the hindfoot and an Achilles pad to prevent irritation of the Achilles tendon as the foot moves up and down;

3. a flexible, cushioned midsole thicker than the sole of regular sneakers and with a surface that provides adequate traction;

4. enough room in the toe box so toes do not touch the end since they need enough room to move up and down;

5. a well-padded tongue to prevent irritation of the tendons along the top of the foot.

It isn't easy to tell how long running shoes last. All of them lose a significant amount of resiliency after around four hundred miles of running. Shoes should be replaced if they clearly feel less cushiony than they did when new.

Visually, the only reliable sign of a worn-out shoe is a large amount of uneven wear located anywhere on the sole ("Running Shoes" 1992). Beyond good shoes, the only necessary ingredients are comfortable clothing and a desire to run.

Fitness is improved by increasing the distance run or by covering the same distance in less time. Most individuals find it more fun to vary or combine the two. Slow but steady progression is important in all forms of physical activity, and progress can be tracked with a chart and periodic measurement of heart rates at rest and immediately following activity.

Walking

Walking has become increasingly popular as a form of total body physical activity. If your goal is to burn off calories, walking can be effective. In fact, you will burn as many calories walking a mile as running a mile. The overload principle, however, reminds us that efficiency of the cardiovascular system is improved in direct proportion to the overload placed on it. In general, walking does not produce the same overload as running (although as the walking pace becomes faster and the running pace becomes slower, there is a point where the overloads are the same).

Walking does not stress the joints as much as running or aerobics. It is probably easier for most people as well. In addition, it can be done almost anywhere and requires no skills or major equipment.

Serious walkers might want to purchase walking shoes. Since walking isn't just slow running, a walker's shoe is different from a runner's shoe. A walker's shoe benefits from some cushioning, but too much can actually promote wobbling of the feet while walking. Walkers need more flexibility in the sole and shoes that facilitate the heel-to-toe roll of a normal walking foot. Some walking shoes have a beveled heel or rocker profile—they're slightly rounded at the bottom like the runners on a rocking chair. Walking shoes must be comfortable, since walkers are often in their shoes longer than runners.

Details such as a padded collar and Achilles notch are helpful ("These Shoes are Made for Walking" 1990).

Water Activity

Swimming, like running, must tax the cardiovascular system and raise the heart rate to appropriate levels to provide real benefits; just paddling or floating is inadequate. Improvements in distance or time are as appropriate to strive for in swimming as in running. One advantage to swimming is that you usually don't need to worry as much about a cool-down period, because the coldness of the water keeps the body temperature from rising.

Other physical activity in water has become popular. Walking, running, and aerobics in water provide a safer and in many ways more effective workout than the same exercises on land. Because of the resistance in water, water workouts can burn calories faster and work your heart harder than similar land-based exercises—and also be easier on the joints. It would be a mistake, however, to substitute water workouts for all land exercises because weight-bearing exercise is needed to help prevent bone loss ("Fitness Update" 1991).

Cycling

Cycling can be done outside, with a rolling bicycle, or inside, with a stationary bicycle. Besides making sure that the bike is safe, it is crucial to adjust the seat height and handlebars correctly. With the toe on the pedal, there should be a small bend at the knee when the pedal is in the fully down position. Handlebars should be positioned so that the body is relaxed and leaning slightly forward. The effects of altering distances covered and times traveled are similar to those in running and swimming.

Rope Skipping

Rope skipping is a great exercise that is inexpensive and allows mobility. In addition, both arms and legs are used, and many jumping patterns can be utilized. For best results, grip the rope at armpit level when the loop is touching the floor or ground. Shorter or longer ropes make skipping more difficult.

Weight Training

Weight training builds muscle strength and endurance and should not be confused with weight lifting, which is a competitive sport using standardized lifts. In weight training, barbells and dumbbells provide resistance to the action of the muscles being trained. To develop strength, a relatively heavy load should be used for few repetitions; to develop muscular endurance, increase the number of repetitions and lighten the load. As strength increases, apply progressively greater loads; as muscular endurance increases, progressively increase the number of repetitions. From the standpoint of total health, it is unlikely that a weight training program by itself will provide sufficient benefits to the circulatory system. It can be a fine addition, however, to another program designed to strengthen the circulatory system.

Before wearing weights around your ankles and/or wrists while exercising, consider the risks involved. Ankle weights can increase the risk of stress fractures of bones in the lower extremities and feet and inflammation of the Achilles tendon—the tendon in the back of the ankle. Gravity triples the effect of an ankle weight on the foot and increases the tendency for feet to roll inward to handle the stress.

Wrist weights, when worn properly, are safer than ankle weights. Weights heavier than one-half to two pounds increase the risk of straining or tearing tendons that stabilize the shoulder joint and may increase your chances of developing bursitis (inflammation of the lubricating sac that surrounds a joint).

Walking with a normal arm swing with hand-held weights of five pounds or less is not enough to provide health benefits (Owens 1989). So, why use wrist or ankle weights at all with so many apparent risks and little possible benefit? Simply exercising a little faster can increase your overload, and therefore your heart rate, without any of the risks of hand or ankle weights.

Steps to Develop a Personal Fitness Program

For best results a fitness program must be personal. Here are some steps to increase your chances of success:

1. *Make it personal.* The program should be designed to fit your needs and goals rather than to compete with someone else.
2. *Proceed gradually.* You may want to progress quickly, but give your body a chance to adjust to the new activities.
3. *Set reasonable goals.* Don't expect too much too fast.
4. *Pick activities that you will continue.* Consider your interests and skills as well as available facilities.
5. *Consider medical and physical concerns when selecting appropriate activity.*
6. *Expect some soreness.* Some muscle soreness is natural and is nothing to worry about; if the soreness is extreme, you're probably ignoring step 2.
7. *Use total body activity.* Emphasize activities for the circulatory and respiratory systems—that is where most of the health benefits are.
8. *Be regular.* The weekend athlete has highly questionable exercise habits that put an unnecessary strain on the body. Participate in vigorous activity at least three or four times per week for at least twenty to thirty minutes each time. (Review information on target heart rate to help you determine what is "vigorous.")
9. *Use several ways to exercise if possible.* You will be less likely to become bored if you have different ways to exercise.
10. *Determine and use the target heart rate* (see fig. 4.2). This is a good guide to activity intensity.

Factors Influencing Choice of Program

A number of factors influence the type of activity program you choose. For example, you need to consider your body condition and fitness level. An obese person might find swimming a more appropriate activity than tennis at first. But regardless of body condition, everyone receives similar benefits from fitness activities.

1. Are facilities available for aerobic exercise (which promotes cardiovascular health)?

   Aerobic exercise facilities include treadmills, exercise bicycles with a resistance control, stair-climbing machines, a long swimming pool (at least sixty feet), and a running track or a large empty room that can be used for run/walk/jog sequences.

2. Are members encouraged to attend three or more times weekly for the fitness exercising?

   Some clubs permit members to attend as often as they wish yet subtly discourage regular attendance for fear of overloading the facility. Visit the facility on the days and at the times you wish to exercise to make sure that they are not oversubscribed.

3. What kind of training do the instructors have?

   An instructor with a degree in exercise physiology or physical education probably knows the principles of aerobic conditioning exercise and can work with you on an effective program. Are the instructors certified in first aid and CPR?

4. What kinds of exercise classes are offered?

   Classes that feature running, swimming, fitness dancing, and other aerobic activities usually indicate a good facility for developing and maintaining cardiovascular fitness. Classes in yoga, weight lifting, or calisthenics may promote muscle building or flexibility but usually do not promote cardiovascular fitness.

5. Are other health programs available?

   If a facility offers diet consultation, smoking cessation, or other supplementary programs, it is health-oriented, and its exercise classes are probably geared to cardiovascular fitness.

6. Are adequate dressing and storage facilities available?

   Lockers should be provided with keys so that you may safely leave your valuables. The dressing room areas should be clean.

7. Is it preferable to join a club that is part of a chain?

   Only if the chain is oriented to cardiovascular fitness.

8. Is a good facility expensive?

   Not necessarily. If it meets the standards detailed, a facility in the "Y" system is often adequate and inexpensive. Posh surroundings are not necessary, although they may add to your comfort.

Emotional temperament is also important. Some individuals are better suited to distance running, circuit training, or rope skipping than, say, weight training. Also consider motor ability and motor educability (some individuals learn physical skills easier and faster than others). If you want to play tennis or another activity requiring a certain level of skill, take a realistic look at your present and potential skill levels. If you select activities that demand skills you do not possess, you are likely to get more frustrated than fit.

Availability is an obvious consideration. It is difficult to play racquetball if there are no courts in the community. If you want team sports to be part of your program, you need people to participate and a way to organize the activities.

Training Facilities

Some individuals like to exercise at home, and others prefer to use training facilities. Advantages of using a training facility include socializing, having a regular place to change and shower, the availability of exercise equipment and trained instructors, the opportunity to participate in organized sports, and the promotion of self-discipline. Disadvantages include a possibly inconvenient location, the need to go to a set place (perhaps at a set time), the cost, and a feeling of obligation. If a training facility is used, carefully check out the quality of the program, the instruction, and the equipment.

Your Personality

When your fitness program matches your personality, you are more likely to stay with it. While picking a particular activity simply for its psychological effect isn't enough, it may be an important consideration. At the same time, how you perform an activity may be just as important as the activity itself. For example, a runner who wants to relax and get physical benefits at the same time might choose to leave the stopwatch at home to avoid being too competitive.

Personality factors such as sociability, spontaneity, discipline, aggressiveness, competitiveness, mental focus, and risk taking can be used to determine the likelihood of an individual staying with an activity. For example, compared to running, walking is more spontaneous, less aggressive, and takes less discipline. Racket sports are high in sociability, spontaneity, competitiveness, and focus but low in discipline. Swimming is fairly high in discipline and low in sociability, spontaneity, and aggressiveness. If you're having trouble sticking to a fitness program, these ideas may help explain why (Gavin 1989).

Maintaining a Fitness Program

The success of a fitness program depends on keeping at it. If you begin an exercise program with unrealistic expectations, you may become frustrated and give up when

Fitness for Life

Being physically active is a way of life—influenced by and influencing mind, body, and soul and their interdependence. To get and keep benefits from total body activity, appropriate physical activity must become a part of your basic life-style. To do this, certain health skills are needed.

The following activities will help you determine if you have the needed health skills related to fitness. You will also see how they relate to the mind, body, and soul. If you can successfully complete all of them, you will have the prerequisites for a sound personal fitness program. Then, the rest is up to you.

Mind

Decide on goals and objectives for your personal fitness program. What do you want to accomplish and why?

Body

Determine your present fitness level. Do it in at least two different ways so you know where you should start in a personal training program.

Soul

Consider why a personal fitness program is important to you. How does it relate to what you value in life and what you want to accomplish in the short term as well as the long run.

Interdependence

1. Explain the health benefits of physical activity to a friend. Be sure to include information about the effects of physical activity on the muscular, cardiovascular, and respiratory systems as well as effects on mental health.

2. Outline a fitness program that meets your personal goals and objectives. Be sure to consider facilities needed, personality factors, and what can be done to assure that you follow and continue the program.

3. Finally, describe how you can help "guarantee" success. And, how will you know when you have been successful?

Just one more step is needed once you have the skills—do it!

---

those expectations aren't soon met. Personal factors such as not being a smoker, being of normal weight, having a white-collar occupation, being self-motivated, perceiving the ability to find the time, and having no medical restrictions increase the likelihood of maintaining a fitness program. Situational factors such as social support, convenience of a facility, and using low-intensity or moderately vigorous exercise (as compared to more strenuous programs) also help program continuation (Sallis 1986).

Social norms can play an important role in maintaining a fitness program. For example, healthy adults who think their physicians want them to exercise are motivated to do so. In contrast, adults who see their personal physicians as opposed to exercise (even though they want to do it) are less likely to be physically active (Godin and Shephard 1990).

Warm-up and Stretching

It has generally been assumed that warm-up activities are necessary before participating in physical activity. Because of this, some individuals warm up vigorously before participating in tennis, basketball, running, or other activities. This can do more harm than good.

Generally, it make sense to warm up with activities that are the same as or similar to what will be done. If you plan to run, jog slowly to warm up. If you are going to play racquetball, hit the ball easily for a few minutes or play a few easy practice points. This helps the body prepare itself.

Stretching is often misunderstood. People commonly stretch vigorously before activity because they think it will loosen them up; however, brisk toe touches, for example, actually tighten muscles instead of stretching them. This is because when one set of muscles extends quickly, the opposite set naturally contracts. To avoid tightening muscles, it is important to stretch in a slow and steady manner. This allows for greater relaxation of the opposing muscle group, improves flexibility, and reduces the chances of injuring a muscle while stretching. The benefits of stretching before a physical activity are controversial, but those who want to stretch should first do a mild form of total body activity to raise the body temperature and then use only static stretching (no bouncing or bobbing).

Most individuals stretch incorrectly and for the wrong reasons. To improve flexibility, it probably makes more sense to stretch *after* physical activity than before. Stretching can also help the muscles recover from activity. Remember that a mild, total body activity provides a better warm-up than stretching.

Improvement Patterns

Many of us are impatient and want quick results. While some benefits from exercise may appear after a couple of days, significant improvement takes a couple of weeks. Also, we may move backward before we get better. The initial overload stresses the body, and performance declines as internal forces are mobilized. This decline only lasts a few days in most cases, but retrogression can occur again at any time during training—the result of disease, poor nutrition, too little rest, or lack of motivation.

Muscle Soreness

Some become discouraged when initiating a physical activity program, because muscles become stiff and sore at first. Experts are not sure about the exact reason for this. Some think soreness is due to microscopic tearing of the muscle fibers. Others feel that sore muscles result when waste products given off during chemical reactions in the body begin to collect in the muscle tissues and circulatory system. Mild activity, such as slow, rhythmic stretching exercises or even walking, stimulates the blood flow through sore areas and helps remove the waste products. Muscle soreness is common, but as the body gets more used to activity, it is usually greatly reduced or even eliminated.

Getting the Desired Results

Misconceptions about the effects of certain activities can be discouraging. Some of us have used activity to try to remove fat from a certain part of the body (termed **spot reduction**), but this isn't really possible. When we lose weight, fat is lost from the entire body, even though the loss from some spots may be especially obvious.

If you perform activities for a certain part of the body, be sure the desired muscles are doing the work. For example, men commonly do arm curls, hoping to strengthen their triceps (muscles in the back of the upper arm), but that exercise is of little benefit to those muscles.

Care is needed not to confuse total body activity with activity for certain parts of the body. For example, most bending, stretching, and other calisthenic exercises benefit certain body parts but not the overall circulatory and respiratory systems. This is fine as long as activities are consistent with expectations.

Staleness

Sometimes we get bored with an activity program and feel "stale." It seems that no matter what we do, we feel tired and slow and don't get any better. For some, it might be wise to consider more rest or even some time off from strenuous physical activity. For most individuals, however, *staleness* can probably be avoided by providing variety in the physical activity program. This might mean using different types of activity, exercising in different places, or running various distances at different speeds. No one is sure what causes staleness, but most often it goes away by itself.

Some Cautions About Exercise

With all of its positive benefits, it is still wise to follow some precautions to help avoid problems while exercising. These include the following:

1. Wearing a rubber or plastic suit can be dangerous. The elevated body temperature caused by these suits can cause heat exhaustion. Also, weight lost

from this practice is water weight, which is quickly regained when fluids are consumed again.

2. Gravity inversion devices can be dangerous. Significant blood pressure increases have been found in individuals exercising upside down. Since blood pressure increases while exercising anyway, further research is needed to determine the safety of gravity inversion devices.

3. Never end an exercise period with a wind sprint (an all-out burst of speed over a relatively short distance). Taper off slowly when ending exercise.

4. Exercises such as deep-knee bends, the "duck walk," and holding the knees partially flexed for periods of time can cause knee joint injury.

5. Toe touching can cause lower back injury. This is particularly true if you have weak abdominal muscles.

6. Doing sit-ups (which should be done with knees bent) by placing the hands behind the head can be dangerous because a pulling action can injure the spine. A good alternative is to fold the arms on the chest.

Maintenance

It may seem easier to maintain a desired fitness level than to get there, but maintaining optimal fitness requires regular activity. By being realistic about personal qualities, selecting activities that make sense, and using the target zone principle, a personal exercise program can provide satisfying results. Program maintenance is easy if you remember the following:

1. Pick rhythmic, repetitive activities that challenge the circulatory system at an appropriate intensity.

2. Do activities that are fashionable as long as you like them. The "in" thing to do might be easier to continue.

3. Pick activities you enjoy, that are suited to your needs, and that can be done year-round.

4. Make the activity more like play than work. For example, sharing activity with friends and/or using music while exercising might be helpful.

5. Wear clothing appropriate for the exercise, considering temperature, humidity, proper footwear, and comfort.

6. Warm up and cool down.

7. Follow your program regularly, at least three times per week throughout the week.

Excuses for not being active are perhaps already running through your mind. Without motivation, no amount of

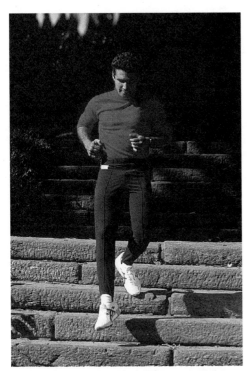

While traveling, you may need to be especially creative and determined to maintain physical activity patterns.

information will lead you to physical fitness, but most excuses for inactivity are pretty flimsy.

- "I don't have time." We each waste at least a few hours each week, and that's all the time you need. Make time for what you want to do.
- "I don't have a place to exercise" or "I don't have anyone to exercise with." Many forms of exercise require no special place, and while it might be nice to have another person along, physiological benefits are not influenced by the presence of someone else. In fact, many people report that their solitary exercise gives them time to think and be alone.
- "I'm too old." People of all ages need physical activity to keep their bodies functioning properly, and anyone can participate in a physical activity program.
- "I'm too weak." Using the target zone principle, it is simple to design a program for any individual need.
- "It's boring." Vary the pace, the time of day, the type of activity, the clothes you wear, or anything else if you need more variety.
- "It's too cold/hot/humid/late/early/windy to exercise." Honestly reevaluate your motivation and your exercise program if you often turn to this type of reasoning. If you value an active life-style, none of these excuses will prevent activity.

Creating an Active Environment

Many of us actually go out of our way to be sedentary. To counteract this tendency, the environment must be reorganized to provide activity. For many, this means an adjustment in life-style.

Adjusting Life-Style and Environment

One way to adjust life-style is by altering daily routines to encourage more exercise. For example, when traveling a relatively short distance, walk instead of driving. Coffee breaks can be replaced with exercise breaks, the stairs can be used instead of elevators or escalators, and creative thinking can result in other possibilities.

You can also encourage exercise by finding an apartment conducive to walking to school or by altering your home environment. Move the phone a few steps, and place objects on higher shelves to encourage stretching to get them. Other opportunities to stay active around the home include washing the car, raking leaves, and shoveling snow instead of paying others to do these tasks.

Rewards

Rewards related to activity can also be helpful. For example, an exercise chart shows progress, thereby reinforcing motivation to continue. Using exercise time to be active with other people can be a social reward. After reaching a personal goal, a reward of a new warm-up suit, a weekend vacation, or some other appropriate prize might be a motivator. Access to physical activity might be made easier by buying exercise equipment. This might include buying a few weights or installing a basketball basket so you won't have to make a trip to the gym.

Exercising While Traveling

Exercising while traveling can present unique problems, but these can be overcome with a little creativity. When staying at a hotel, safe places to jog can usually be found, or the exercise rooms that are becoming more common in hotels can be used, or even hotel stairways can be used for a good workout. When traveling by car, you can take a short jog or walk at a rest stop.

Most of us are locked into daily routines, and it can be difficult to modify existing behaviors. After the possibilities for modification are assessed, personal needs are considered, and a realistic decision is made about which behaviors can be modified, then action must be taken. Just thinking about exercising does little to improve physiological functioning.

Summary

1. Physical fitness has many components; however, those most necessary for health are cardiorespiratory capacity, body composition, flexibility, muscular endurance, and muscular strength.

2. Health benefits of regular physical activity include improved physiological functioning, a more positive self-concept, reduced stress response, maintenance of proper body weight, possible reduction of the risk of coronary heart disease, possible delay in the aging process, and protection from lower-back problems.

3. As a result of total body physical activity, the cardiovascular system functions more efficiently. Flow of blood at the capillary level increases, the heart becomes a stronger muscle, there is a lower resting pulse rate, and coronary circulation is improved.

4. As a result of total body physical activity, the respiratory system functions more efficiently. There is greater possible maximal oxygen intake at the cell level, a decreased oxygen debt for the same work, an ability to withstand a higher oxygen debt, and a decreased oxygen requirement.

5. Developing a physical activity program involves determining present level of fitness, considering an exercise schedule, and deciding on intensity, duration, frequency, type of activity, and accessories.

6. Factors to consider when maintaining a fitness program include realistic expectations, warm-up and stretching, improvement patterns, muscle soreness, staleness, and maintenance.

Commitment Activities

1. Cultural factors make it more or less likely that we will lead physically active lives. Unfortunately, for most of us, there seem to be more cultural factors interfering with physical activity than supporting it. Identify the cultural pitfalls that make it more difficult for you to lead a physically active life by making use of total body activity. Divide your list into two parts—those you can't do much about and those over which you have control. Then, for a two-week period, see if you can begin to eliminate cultural pitfalls to physical activity.

2. One factor that can interfere with participation in physical fitness activities is the availability of facilities. This might mean simply a place to shower or a safe place to run. Within your community, assess the general availability of exercise facilities. For example, can those in local industries be active during their lunch hours if they so desire? Are local recreation facilities available during evenings and weekends? Are there attempts to provide facilities to meet a variety of needs? Are there safe places to walk, jog, swim, and ride a bike? If the answers to these questions are yes, great! If not, you have another challenge—what can be done about it?

3. Develop a fifteen-minute presentation on the benefits of regular exercise that you could make to a commercial organization. Your presentation should include probable benefits to the company as well as those to the individual workers. What kind of a beginning program would you recommend?

References

"ACSM Guidelines for Fitness Updated." *Running and FitNews* 8, no.7 (July 1990):1.

Allison, M. "Improving the Odds." *Harvard Health Letter* 16, no.4 (February 1991):4–6.

"American Academy of Pediatrics Statement on Physical Fitness and the Schools." American Academy of Pediatrics Committee on Sports Medicine and Committee on School Health, 1987.

American College of Sports Medicine. "Opinion Statement: Participation of the Female Athlete in Long Distance Running." *Medicine and Science in Sports* 11, no. 4 (1979):9.

Bankhead, C. "Intensity of Exercise Now Debate Focus." *Medical World News* 32, no.9 (September 1991):22–23.

Brown, H. L. *Lifetime Fitness.* Scottsdale, Ariz.: Gorsuch Scarisbrick, 1986, p. 38.

"Can Exercise Turn Back the Clock?" *Consumer Reports on Health* 4, no. 3 (March 1992):21.

"CDC Finds That High School Kids May Do Less Vigorous Exercise." *Health Education Reports* 14, no.3 (February 6, 1992):5.

Cooper, K. H. "The Basics of Bone." *Health* 21, no. 4 (April 1989):81.

Cremmons, A. N. "Activity May Reduce Risk of Colon Cancer." *The Physician and Sportsmedicine* 18, no. 1 (January 1990):61.

Davis, C., and Cowles, M. "Body Image and Exercise: A Study of Relationships and Comparisons Between Physically Active Men and Women." *Sex Roles* 25, nos. 1/2 (July 1991):33–44.

"First the Good News: Smoking Rates Down, But Americans Too Fat." *Health Education Reports.* 14, no.6 (March 26, 1992):3–4.

"Fitness Update." *Consumer Reports on Health* 3, no. 12 (December 1991):94.

Gauthier, M. M. "Maternal Exercise and Uterine Blood Flow." *The Physician and Sportsmedicine* 18, no.1 (January 1990):61.

Gavin, J. "Your Brand of Sweat." *Psychology Today* (March 1989):50–57.

Godin, G., Shephard, R. J. "An Evaluation of the Potential Role of the Physician in Influencing Community Exercise Behavior," *American Journal of Health Promotion* 4, no. 4 (March/April 1990):255–59.

Health Education Reports 12, no. 8 (April 12, 1990):5.

Kasch, F. W.; Boyer, J. L.; Van Camp, S. P.; Verity, L. S.; and Wallace, J. P. "The Effect of Physical Activity and Inactivity on Aerobic Power in Older Men (A Longitudinal Study)." *The Physician and Sportsmedicine* 18, no. 4 (April 1990): 73–83.

Kasper, M. J. "Emphasis on Cardiovascular Fitness as a Barrier toward Mobilizing the Sedentary Individual." *Health Education* 21, no.4 (July/August 1990):41–45.

Malanka, P. "Aerobics Rebound." *Health* 22, no. 3 (March 1990):59–65.

McGlynn, G. *Dynamics of Fitness.* Dubuque, Iowa: Wm. C. Brown Publishers, 1990.

Owens, S. G.; Al-Ahmed, A.; and Moffatt, R. J. "Physiological Effects of Walking and Running With Hand-Held Weights." *Journal of Sports Medicine and Physical Fitness* 29, no. 4 (December 1989):384–87.

Paffenbarger, R. S., et al. "Physical Activity, All-Cause Mortality, and Longevity of College Alumni." *New England Journal of Medicine* 314, no. 10 (6 March 1986): 605–13.

Phillips, P. "Modest Exercise Program Proven to Cut Risk of CVD." *Medical World News* 31, no. 5 (12 March 1990):20.

"Physical Exercise: An Important Factor for Health." *The Physician and Sportsmedicine* 18, no. 3 (March 1990): 155–56.

Promoting Health/Preventing Disease: Year 2000 Objectives for the Nation. Washington, D.C.: Public Health Service, U. S. Department of Health and Human Services, September 1990, 521.

"Running Shoes." *Consumer Reports on Health* 4, no. 1 (January 1992):5.

Sallis, J. F. "Exercise Adherence and Motivation." *Focal Points.* 2 (1986):3.

Samples, P. "Exercise Encouraged for People With Arthritis." *The Physician and Sportsmedicine* 18, no. 1 (January 1990):123–27.

Shephard, R. J. "Nutritional Benefits of Exercise." *Journal of Sports Medicine and Physical Fitness* 29, no. 1 (March 1989):83–88.

"Shoes for Sports: Choose Carefully." *Better Health* 3, no. 4 (April 1986):1–2.

"These Shoes are Made for Walking." *Consumer Reports* 55, no. 2 (February 1990):88–93.

Williams, M. H. *Lifetime Fitness and Wellness.* Dubuque, Iowa: Wm. C. Brown Publishers, 1990, pp. 48–49.

Zohman, L. R. *Exercise Your Way to Fitness and Heart Health.* CPC International (public service booklet), 1983.

Additional Readings

Bloch, G. B. "The Thinking Woman's Workout." *Health* 22, no. 1 (January 1990):56–58+. Describes a trend in health clubs called interval circuit training (ICT). The routine enhances many components of fitness.

Boughton, B. "More Clues But No Proof Yet That Exercise Lifts Mood." *Medical World News* 32, no. 10 (October 1991):12. Provides an overview of research studies designed to determine the effects of exercise on psychological health.

Poppy, J. "Moves Made to Fit." *In Health* (May/June 1990):60–72. Examines a variety of activities and gives strengths and limitations of each. It also outlines what is needed to get started.

CHAPTER 5

Weight Control and Eating Disorders

Key Questions

- What is the significance of body composition?

- What is the difference between being overweight and obese?

- How is body composition assessed?

- What are the possible causes of obesity?

- What is the best way to control your weight?

- What are the symptoms and dangers of anorexia and bulimia?

- What are practical suggestions for someone who is underweight?

Chapter Outline

Weight Control and Health
Overweight or Overfat?
    Determining Body Weight
    Determining Body Composition
Factors Affecting Obesity
    Heredity
    Exercise
    Eating Habits
    Fat Cell Theory
    Set Point Theory
Successful Weight-Control Techniques
    The Role of Diet in Weight Control
    The Role of Exercise in Weight
       Control
    The Winning Combination
Methods of Weight Control
    High-Risk Weight-Loss Procedures
    What's Right for You?
Eating Disorders
    Anorexia Nervosa
    Bulimia
Special Concerns for Those Who Are
      Underweight

Many Americans strive for the perfect physique created by the media yet have a difficult time achieving that goal. The media have defined a norm for us that is unrealistic. Very few of us can achieve this look, regardless of how much we diet and exercise.

The diet business is a big one. At any given time, forty-eight million adult Americans are on a diet (fig. 5.1) and spend $35.8 billion annually on diet and diet products (Thompson 1990). Diet clinics are plentiful, and low-calorie foods are popular items. Despite the interest in diet products and services, very few individuals have long-term weight-control success. Only 3 percent to 5 percent of dieters keep off the weight they lose. Weight loss can only be considered successful when the weight is kept off for three to five years.

Americans know how to control their weight but continue to select foods that are contradictory to weight loss. For example, many individuals concerned about dietary fat or cholesterol still purchase ice cream, butter, and high-fat cheeses each week

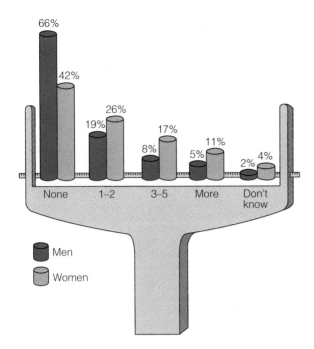

Figure 5.1

The number of times people tried to lose weight in 1991.

(Thompson 1990). It is important for us to internalize knowledge and modify attitudes before behavior change can take place.

Authors of diet books and diet plans often take advantage of the ignorance and misinformation of the American public by promising quick and easy plans. To evaluate these plans effectively, it is important to have sound knowledge of nutrition, exercise, and weight control.

In this chapter, possible causes of obesity are identified and ways to make new decisions about eating habits and exercise are explored. Undesirable methods of weight control are discussed, and eating disorders are described. The relationship between weight control and coping skills is discussed, along with the role of resiliency in the weight-control process.

Weight Control and Health

The percentage of overweight adults in the United States has steadily increased over the last several decades, making the problem of excess body fat a serious one in this country. Obesity affects 10 percent to 40 percent of school children, with 80 percent of obese children becoming obese adults. Thirty-four million adult Americans (20 percent of adults) are considered obese (Manson et al. 1990).

Cosmetic reasons may be a primary motivation to lose weight. Other factors to consider, however, include the health risks associated with extra weight in the form of storage fat. Extra body fat is associated with over twenty-

TABLE 5.1			
Risks of Being Overweight (increase in risk for disease)			
	20% to 30% Overweight	40% or More Overweight	Deaths per Year
Cancer			
Male:			
Colon/rectum	26%	73%	29,100
Prostate	37%	29%	26,100
Female:			
Breast	16%	53%	39,900
Cervix	51%	139%	6,800
Endometrium	85%	442%	2,900
Gallbladder	74%	258%	5,300
Ovary	0%	63%	11,600
Diabetes			
Male	156%	419%	14,859[a]
Female	234%	690%	21,928[a]
Heart Disease			
Male	32%	95%	289,461
Female	39%	107%	251,857
Stroke			
Male	17%	127%	61,697
Female	16%	52%	92,630

[a]This figure does not include the many diabetics who die of heart disease.

Sources: *Journal of Chronic Diseases, 32: 563,* 1979; *Personal Communication,* John Lubera, American Cancer Society; Kathy Santini, National Center for Health Statistics, *Nutrition Action Healthletter,* January 1987, p. 7.

six health conditions (Williams 1990), including heart disease, diabetes, hypertension, and cancer. There is now definite evidence that loss of even half of excess weight prevents the development of type II diabetes ("Link Between Weight Loss and Diabetes II Prevention" 1992).

Maintaining desirable body weight is also an important factor in self-concept and emotional health, since most of us feel better physically and mentally when we attain a certain weight. Positive weight-control practices enhance protective coping skills, while negative weight-control practices are very disruptive to both the mind and the body (table 5.1).

Overweight or Overfat?

The traditional method of determining your weight in pounds or kilograms is not necessarily the best indicator of whether or not you are overweight. A more accurate measurement is your percentage of body fat.

Weight Control

Weight control is a complex experience compounded by many factors that will be described in this chapter. The purpose of this assessment tool is to examine the risk factors that lead to obesity. Often after high school, we reduce our energy expenditure, maintain our calorie consumption, and begin to gain weight gradually. This assessment helps you recognize the risks of becoming overweight in the next few years.

Biological Factors

1. By looking at your parents or grandparents when they were younger, would you say you had a genetic predisposition to obesity?
   a. yes
   b. no
   c. I don't know

2. How has your weight changed over the last two to three months?
   a. stayed the same
   b. lost some weight
   c. gained some weight
   d. up and down but basically the same
   e. I don't know

3. My metabolic rate is
   a. slow or low.
   b. fast or high.
   c. about average.
   d. I don't know.

4. Which of the following statements applies to you?
   a. I can eat a lot and not gain much weight.
   b. I eat less than those around me and still I gain weight.
   c. If I eat moderately, my weight stays about the same.

Behavioral Factors

5. Which of the following applies to you?
   a. I do not exercise regularly.
   b. I exercise some.
   c. I exercise regularly.

6. My eating habits are best described as which of the following? (Mark all that apply.)
   a. I deprive myself, then binge.
   b. I overeat regularly.
   c. I reward myself with food treats.
   d. I carefully monitor my diet and know how to count calories.
   e. I don't pay much attention to how I eat, just what comes naturally.

Psychological Factors

7. Indicate which of the following describes you. (Mark all that apply.)
   a. I have a lot of distress in my life.
   b. I am often bored.
   c. I am often lonely.
   d. I repress or can't feel emotions (such as anger, affection, fear, sadness, and so on).
   e. I tend to punish myself for my behaviors.
   f. I am often depressed.
   g. I am anxious or nervous.
   h. I am often frustrated.
   i. I feel resentment toward someone or something.
   j. I am often angry.
   k. I am defensive about my appearance or my actions.
   l. I am or was deprived of love.
   m. I am a passive person (nonassertive).
   n. I have a poor self-concept (self-esteem, self-worth, self-identity, self-image, self-confidence).
   o. I don't think I have a good-looking body.
   p. I don't think I am sexually attractive.

Environmental Factors

8. Which of the following applies to you?
   a. I had an unstable childhood.
   b. My family is not very supportive.
   c. My friends are not very supportive.
   d. I feel a lot of pressure to be thin and fit.

Scoring/Interpretation

Score each question as follows and then total your score.

Biological Factors

1a = 4	3a = 4
1b = 0	3b = 0
1c = 2	3c = 2
2a = 2	3d = 2
2b = 0	4a = 0
2c = 4	4b = 4
2d = 2	4c = 2
2e = 2	

Behavioral Factors

5a = 4	6b = 4
5b = 2	6c = 4
5c = 0	6d = 0
6a = 4	6e = 2

Psychological Factors

7a–p = 1 point for each response

Environmental Factors

8a–d = 3 points for each response

Each of the areas assessed are risk factors associated with obesity. The following interpretation assesses risk for each area (biological, behavioral, psychological, and environmental) and gives an overall risk assessment.

Biological

11 or more = high risk
6–10 = moderate risk
0–5 = low risk

Behavioral

12 or more = high risk
7–11 = moderate risk
0–6 = low risk

Psychological

11 or more = high risk
6–10 = moderate risk
0–5 = low risk

Environmental

8 or more = high risk
4–7 = moderate risk
0–3 = low risk

Overall Risk (total all scores)

40 or more = high risk
20–39 = moderate risk
0–19 = low risk

Determining Body Weight

The traditional method of determining body weight is to measure body mass with a scale. Based on this, overweight is defined as being 10 percent over desirable weight, and obesity is defined as being 20 percent over desirable weight. The reference most frequently used has been the Metropolitan Life height and weight table, in which the recommended weights are based on the mortality rates of people who purchase life insurance. This table is being used less frequently because of the problems associated with it, including the increase in the recommended weights in the 1983 revision of the table, with which many disagree.

The difficulty with using body mass to determine weight is that there is no means of determining what proportion of pounds are fat (adipose tissue) and lean tissue (muscle, cartilage, skin, bone, connective tissue, and nerves). Individuals considered overweight according to the charts often have a high amount of body fat. Those with a high percentage of lean tissue (such as body builders or football players), however, may also be classified as overweight on the charts even though most of their weight is from lean tissue. On the other hand, someone may have a low percentage of lean tissue and not be classified as overweight because he or she falls within the normal range of the charts. A more accurate measurement assesses the percentage of body fat.

Determining Body Composition

Body composition is the percentage of **fat** versus **lean tissue,** with body fat classified as essential fat or storage fat. **Essential fat** is necessary to stay alive and is needed to maintain normal body functioning. It is stored in the

ISSUE

Achieving the Ideal

Americans value having a perfect body, which usually means being slim and well-shaped.

• **Pro:** The emphasis on slimness is healthy. In view of all we know about the dangers of obesity, this cultural value makes us aware of what we eat and of the wellness we can experience if we exercise and eat correctly. Individuals feel better and live longer if they maintain a slim body.

• **Con:** The societal emphasis on slimness is based on fashion and causes much unhappiness to many individuals—both over- and underweight. We should accept others as they are and neither judge nor try to change them, even indirectly, through espousing these values.

What is your opinion of society's emphasis on slimness?

heart, lungs, muscle, bone, liver, spleen, kidneys, intestines, and central nervous system. Women usually have higher levels of essential fat (12 percent) than men (3 percent) to accommodate hormonal and reproductive functions.

Storage fat is the extra fat maintained by the body in the fat cells. Once the fat cells are formed, they never disappear but only shrink in size when the amount of storage fat is lower (Wardlaw and Insel 1990). Consequently, fat babies often become fat adults. The location of this fat varies in each individual, although men tend to store extra fat in their midsection, and women tend to store fat in their

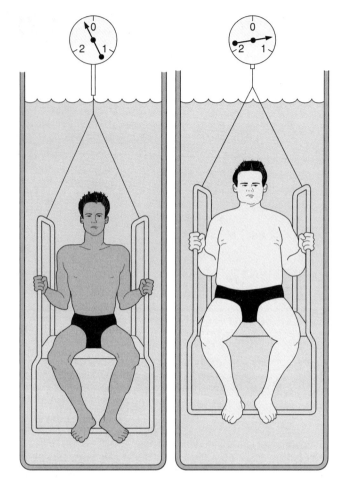

Figure 5.2

The underwater weighing method of estimating body density and proportion of fat to lean tissue. The scale weights of these two men are the same; under water, however, the leaner man on the left is shown to weigh *more* than the fatter man on the right, because lean tissue is heavier than water.

buttocks, hips, and thighs prior to menopause. After menopause, women tend to store fat in the abdomen. The waist-to-hip ratio is important, because there is a correlation between disease and fat stored in the midsection. The waist-to-hip ratio can be computed by dividing the waist measurement by the hip measurement. A ratio above .80 for females and above .95 for males may put individuals at risk for a number of diseases, including heart disease, high blood pressure, and diabetes (Thompson 1990).

Some storage fat is needed to protect the internal organs and insulate the body from cold, but it is not needed in excess amounts. Most experts recommend that body fat should not exceed 10 percent to 20 percent for males and 15 percent to 25 percent for females (Powers and Howley 1990). In one study, researchers were commissioned to estimate average body fat based on data compiled by the National Institute of Health Information. It was found that the average body fat for women is 31 percent, which is above the optimal range, and the average

for men is 19 percent, which is within the optimal range ("How Fat Is America?" 1992). Problems associated with excess weight usually refer to excess amounts of storage fat. The goal of weight-loss programs should be the reduction of storage fat, not the reduction of muscle or lean tissue.

One of the most precise ways of determining body fat is **hydrostatic weighing,** also known as underwater weighing. The results of hydrostatic weighing indicate a person's overall density compared to water and a comparison of body weight to body volume. The density figure determined by hydrostatic weighing is used in a specific calibration to determine the percentage of body fat (fig. 5.2). Underwater weighing is a precise method of determining body fat and does require a laboratory and expensive equipment. It is the criterion against which all other methods are compared.

The skin-fold technique is the most common method for determining the percentage of body fat. Calipers are used to measure the amount of **subcutaneous fat,** which is fat beneath the skin. Since approximately 50 percent of the body's fat is located beneath the skin, the percentage of body fat can be estimated from these measurements. There are numerous sites that can be measured, including the abdomen, the back of the upper arm, the thigh, and the back. This technique is subject to error because of the difficulty in obtaining accurate measurements. Measurements from three or four sites throughout the body, however, provide a more precise percentage than measurements from one or two sites. Dehydration can affect the results by 10 percent to 15 percent (McGlynn 1990).

Although there is no single authoritative source for determining the gradations of fat based on body composition, references for these definitions are provided in table 5.2.

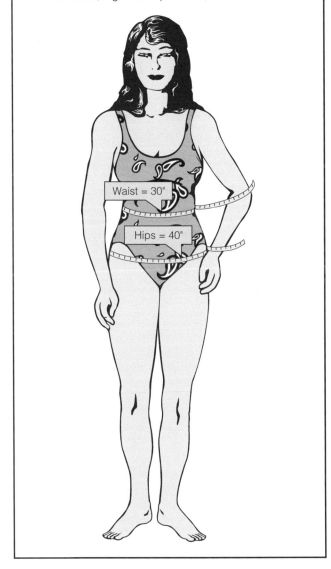
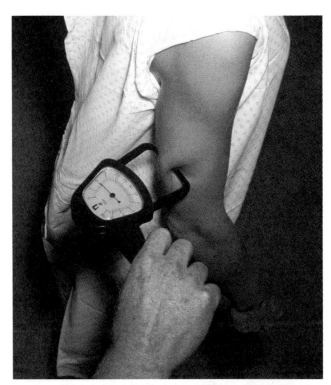

Subcutaneous fat may be accurately measured if carefully done.

may not be accurate. Obese individuals may have a genetic susceptibility to obesity and may have to work harder than individuals of normal weight to weigh less.

Our distribution of body fat may closely resemble the distribution of fat in our biological parents (Nash 1987). For example, a female whose mother has large arms is also likely to have large arms. Researchers studying identical twins have concluded that genetic influences on body-mass index are substantial, and the childhood environment has little or no influence on this (Stunkard et al. 1990). Scientists studying the long-term effects of over-feeding in identical twins attributed the similarity of weight gain and fat distribution in the twins to genetic factors (Bouchard et al. 1990).

The genetic link to obesity is not a guarantee that those who have a history of obesity in their families will be heavy. Attainment of lower fat levels and fewer pounds can be done even though it may be challenging.

Factors Affecting Obesity

Several theories explain the possible causes of obesity. These are related to heredity, exercise, eating habits, fat cell theory, and set point theory.

Heredity

There is increasing evidence of a genetic relationship to body fatness. For years, heavy individuals have been told they weren't working hard enough to keep off the fat. This

Exercise

Exercise may be the most important key to weight control. It is important for exercise to be done regularly for the results to be permanent.

Energy is supplied to the body through food in the form of calories. One pound of body fat contains approximately 3,500 calories. If more calories are consumed than are burned, fat is gained. Conversely, if fewer calories are consumed than burned, weight is lost. Exercise is the only safe way to increase the number of calories burned ("Diet

One of the most important factors related to exercise is doing it on a regular basis. The best time to exercise is whenever you can. To lose weight, however, the best time to exercise is either before breakfast or before dinner. Exercising before breakfast is recommended because the levels of insulin in the blood are low, causing the body to burn fat rather than carbohydrates. Exercising prior to dinner may suppress the appetite and relieve stress. Since many of us eat to relieve stress, this may be especially beneficial.

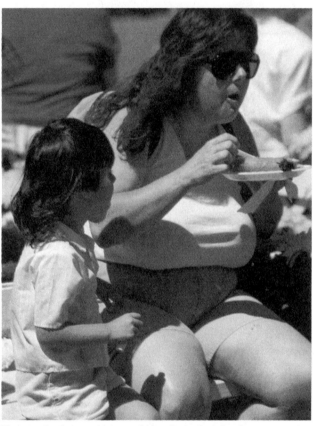

Those who have a history of obesity in their family may want to watch their weight carefully.

TABLE 5.3

Calories Burned per Hour by Selected Activities

Activity	Body Weight		
	100 lb	*150 lb*	*200 lb*
Mopping floors	144	216	288
Swimming (20 yd/min)	192	288	384
Tennis (beginner)	192	288	384
Weeding	228	342	456
Golf (carrying clubs)	270	405	540
Aerobic dancing (low impact)	276	414	552
Walking (4.5 mph)	288	432	576
Snow shoveling	312	468	624
Calisthenics	360	540	720
Jogging (5 mph)	360	540	720
Aerobic dancing (high impact)	372	558	744
Bicycling (13 mph)	426	639	852
Swimming (55 yd/min)	528	792	1056
Cross-country skiing (8 mph)	624	936	1248
Running (8 mph)	624	936	1248

Get In Shape, Stay In Shape. "Calories Burned per Minute." Copyright 1989 by Consumers Union of U.S., Inc., Yonkers, NY 10703-1057. Excerpted by permission from CONSUMER REPORTS BOOKS, 1989.

vs. Exercise: What's Best?" 1992). Exercise raises the **basal metabolic rate,** which is the speed at which our body burns its fuel. Therefore, there is a double benefit from exercise: the burning of calories during exercise and the increase in the rate at which calories are burned after exercise (table 5.3).

In addition to exercise, your general activity level is also important. Some ways to increase your activity level may include walking stairs instead of taking the elevator or parking at the far end of the parking lot instead of near the door. Labor-saving devices, such as self-propelled vacuum cleaners, may hinder weight-control efforts by decreasing caloric output.

Eating Habits

The foods we eat are an important factor in controlling weight. Research evidence shows that diet is even more important than previously thought. For years it was thought that fat individuals craved the sugar in certain foods, but it may be the fat in food that is craved, not the sugar. A study in which participants rated the taste of milkshake-like drinks showed that obese individuals preferred drinks higher in fat and lower in sugar than those of normal weight (Drewnowski et al. 1985). Other researchers have shown that overweight individuals like food that is flavorful and highly textured in addition to being high in fat (Simon 1989). Those who enjoy these qualities in food may find themselves dissatisfied when they severely reduce their calories. One solution may be to eat foods that are flavorful yet low in fat and calories.

The fact that the obese may crave fat is even more devastating considering that fat provides energy in a form the body most readily stores rather than burns. The energy in complex carbohydrates is almost never turned into body fat (Barnett 1986).

The psychological factors associated with eating may also be a problem. Food is a focus for many of the social events in life and may be associated with celebrating good times as well as surviving bad times. Food can become very destructive if it becomes the focus of life and is used as a coping mechanism.

There is some evidence that personality type is a factor in food selection. Extroverts may have a more difficult time with weight management than introverts because they are stimulated by external stimuli.

Research shows that alcohol may play an important role in weight control. Researchers found that alcohol makes the body burn fat more slowly and throws off the body's normal disposal of fat. The fat that is not burned is stored in the areas where people tend to put on weight. Participants in the study consumed three ounces of pure alcohol a day and burned about one-third less fat (Suter, Schutz, Jequier 1992).

Fat Cell Theory

Adipose tissue is increased by filling existing fat cells with fat, known as **fat cell hypertrophy,** and/or by increasing the total number of fat cells, known as **fat cell hyperplasia.** Proponents of the fat cell theory state there is an increased number and size of adipose cells in the obese. There is disagreement whether the number of fat cells becomes fixed early in life or whether the number increases throughout life. Once the fat cells develop, though, they never decrease in number but may shrink in size if the stores of extra fat are decreased. It is believed that the extra fat cells influence the body to keep the cells full in an attempt to prevent the body from going into a perceived state of starvation (Nash 1987).

Set Point Theory

The set point theory is based on the concept that the body has an internal control mechanism that helps it maintain a certain level of body fat. This explains why weight tends to return to a certain level after a loss or gain in pounds. There is support for this theory when the impact of dieting on metabolism is considered. Extreme restriction of calories depresses resting metabolism by as much as 45 percent (Katch and McArdle 1987). Since dieting alone may slow metabolism and inhibit efforts to lose weight, it is ineffective. The one thing that can lower the set point is regular aerobic exercise. The difference between thin individuals and many heavy individuals may be the thin person's higher activity level, not lower caloric intake.

It appears that individuals who have the most difficult time attaining normal weight and keeping off the weight they lose are those who became obese as children (Nash

1987). Consequently, it makes sense to try to prevent the problem of obesity from developing in the young.

Successful Weight-Control Techniques

We have discussed the importance of exercise in the control of weight. Exercise and diet are the primary factors in maintaining a stable weight.

The Role of Diet in Weight Control

Many diets are considered a temporary eating plan that must be tolerated for several days or weeks until a few pounds are shed. One of the unfortunate results of completing such a diet may be the eating binge that follows as a reward.

Our approach to dieting must be changed for any hope of long-term success with weight loss. A diet must refer to eating habits that are permanent changes. Don't waste time on dieting if you don't have a commitment to lifetime weight control. Those who continually diet and allow their weight to yo-yo may be causing some of the health problems previously blamed on obesity ("Fear of Fat" 1985). The health effects of losing and regaining weight are most obvious in people thirty to forty-four years of age (Lissner et al. 1991).

Repeated dieting may actually cause the body to become fatter (Liebman, 1987). When the body is continually denied food through dieting, the metabolism is slowed as if it were reacting to a famine. The body learns to gain weight back quickly and hold on to it when food supplies are denied again. To make matters worse, it is indicated in studies that regained weight contains a higher percentage of body fat ("Fear of Fat" 1985).

Food Selection

It is important to pay close attention to the amount and the kind of food you eat to alter your food habits. Good nutrition is a prime consideration when contemplating any type of weight reduction. Reasons for this include the following:

1. It becomes more difficult to make nutritious food selections when fewer calories are consumed.
2. Selection of nutritious foods allows for an easy transition from weight loss to weight maintenance.
3. Poor nutrition during weight reduction can have serious and even fatal results.
4. Nutritional choices are especially important when nutritional needs are high, as during pregnancy.
5. Food choices can affect factors that influence weight control, such as diuresis, appetite, and satiety (Nicholas and Dwyer 1986).

It is important that a balanced diet limit intake of fat and simple carbohydrates. Our diet should not exceed the recommended amount of protein (12 percent of total calories).

Food Purchasing

1. Plan meals in advance, and buy only what is on the list.
2. Don't shop when hungry.
3. Buy low-calorie snack foods.
4. Make nutritious food selections that include many complex carbohydrates.

Food Preparation

1. Don't sample foods while preparing them.
2. Prepare only the amount needed.

3. Serve food in the kitchen rather than using serving plates on the table.
4. Use small plates.
5. Do not add high-fat items, such as sauces, to foods.

Eating

1. Drink a glass of water thirty minutes before eating.
2. Eat only in one place.
3. Cut the food into small pieces.
4. Eat slowly.
5. Review the food selections at a party before eating anything.

Activity

1. Walk whenever possible. Be sure to wear comfortable shoes that provide support.
2. Look for ways to increase activity in daily activities. Take the stairs rather than the elevator, and park at the far end of the parking lot.
3. Schedule a time for activity in each day. Start slowly, and set realistic goals.
4. Substitute another behavior for break times.

Calories consumed from products high in fat are more likely to be converted into fat than calories consumed from carbohydrates or protein (Gurin 1989). If your diet is high in fat, you are more likely to be fat than someone who consumes less fat. Food preparation methods are also important. Avoid fried foods, sauces, and creamed dishes. Condiments such as butter and sour cream can more than double the calories in a food item.

To consume adequate nutrients and to prevent metabolism from slowing too significantly, caloric intake should not go below 1,000 to 1,200 calories per day. Caloric intake below that amount likely prevents consumption of enough food to supply needed nutrients.

Goals

One of the biggest frustrations facing those who want to lose weight is the amount of time it takes. It doesn't matter that the extra pounds and fat were added over several months or years. When individuals are ready to lose weight, they want it off immediately. Therefore, it is important to set realistic goals. Do not plan to lose more than one-half to one pound per week, since weight loss is more likely to be permanent if weight is lost slowly. Any diet that promises more weight loss than this in a week is not a good one. Keep in mind that the weight-loss process isn't always steady, and several plateaus may be encountered where no weight loss occurs.

Changing Attitudes and Behaviors

If you are interested in permanent weight control, it is helpful to review your attitudes toward food and eating and determine what prompts you to eat. This is useful since food is often eaten in response to factors other than hunger. Identifying those factors and when and why they occur provides an opportunity to substitute other behaviors as part of the behavior modification process.

Permanent changes are necessary for long-term success with weight control. One of the easiest changes relates to the feeling of hunger. The **appestat,** located in the hypothalamus of the brain, sends an indicator of hunger, and the **satiety center,** also located in the hypothalamus, sends an indicator of fullness. There is a twenty-minute delay from the time the body is full to the time it signals it is full. Therefore, drinking a glass of water or eating a piece of fruit twenty to thirty minutes before mealtime activates the satiety center. The result of this is that we eat less because we feel full. There is no magical property in the particular fruit we eat to cause this reaction.

As you decrease your calorie intake, better nutritional decisions must be made. When consuming several thousand calories per day, it is easier to ingest the needed nutrients. The accompanying box lists some modifications that may be needed when shopping, eating, and exercising to maintain a healthy weight.

Behavior modification is also a requirement of any successful weight-loss program. While the process of changing behavior so you eat less and lose weight appears simple, the behavior modification process involved in weight control is far more difficult. This is most likely explained by the biological resistance to losing weight and helps demonstrate why those on very low calorie diets who don't change their exercise behaviors usually regain the majority of weight they lost through dieting (Gurin 1989).

The Role of Exercise in Weight Control

Exercise plays a very important role in losing pounds and in keeping them off. Researchers who compared the effects of weight loss by diet and by exercise found that

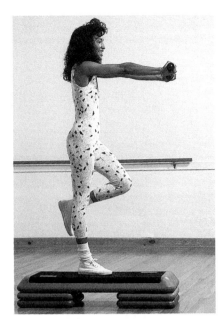

Exercise burns calories and raises the metabolic rate.

the group that exercised only lost a higher percentage of calories from fat and had more success keeping off the weight than the group that dieted only (Liebman 1987).

One of the concerns about exercising is its impact on appetite. Moderate exercise, however, suppresses appetite rather than increasing it. You may want to exercise immediately before a meal to take advantage of this effect.

A benefit of exercise is that it strengthens muscle tissue. Since muscle tissue requires more calories to maintain, there is the added benefit of burning additional calories as the percent of lean tissue increases. Although one type of tissue cannot change into another type of tissue (i.e., fat cannot change to muscle), fat cells can decrease in size as fat stores are decreased.

The Winning Combination

The ultimate goal of any weight loss program should be the loss of body fat, not just body weight. Those who combine diet and exercise lose more weight ("Exercise and Diet in Weight Loss" 1990) and are more likely to keep it off (table 5.4). Exercise and sound eating habits result in a steady weight loss that can be maintained on a permanent basis; however, exercise and dietary changes also need to be maintained. Fad diets advertise large amounts of weight loss immediately, but much of this weight is from body fluids and lean tissue.

Methods of Weight Control

There are many schemes for losing weight. The creators of these diets attempt to explain scientifically why their particular diet plan works when others have not. When you con-

ISSUE

Regulation of Weight-Loss Facilities

Weight-loss facilities are under no regulatory commission. Some feel there should be certain guidelines regarding the employees they hire and the methods they endorse.

- **Pro:** Issues related to the health concerns of the population should be regulated. It is unthinkable that these businesses are under no guidelines.
- **Con:** This is a free country, and people in business should be able to do whatever they wish.

Based on the information in this chapter, which side would you support?

sider that nearly 90 percent of Americans think they are overweight and 80 percent of fourth-grade girls are dieting, it is apparent that Americans need to be educated about sound methods for losing weight.

It is impossible to evaluate every weight-control plan because of the vast number available to the public. Some of these are very inexpensive, while others are very costly. The cost of a twelve-week outpatient weight-loss program can range from $108 to $2,120 (Speilman et al. 1992) (refer to table 5.5 for the cost per kilogram of weight lost). When contemplating a weight-control plan, consider the following:

1. Does the plan include a balanced diet with foods from all food groups?
2. Are the recommended foods easy to locate?
3. Are the recommended foods more expensive than regular foods?
4. Are the recommended foods ones the entire family can eat?

TABLE 5.5

Cost per Kilogram of Active Weight Loss (twelve weeks)

Program	80 kg (137% IBW,[a] female) (127% IBW,[a] male)	91 kg (157% IBW, female) (146% IBW, male)	114 kg (197% IBW, female) (182% IBW, male)	136 kg (236% IBW, female) (219% IBW, male)	Extra Costs (puchased outside clinic)
Very low calorie diets: Medically supervised, multidisciplinary team approach					
HMR™	$17.50	$15.00	$12.00	$10.00	Low-calorie beverages and sweeteners
Medifast™	$14.00	$12.00	$9.50	$8.00	Low-calorie beverages and sweeteners
Optifast™	$22.00	$19.00	$15.00	$12.50	Low-calorie beverages and sweeteners
United Weight Control™	$25.50	$22.50	$18.00	$15.00	Low-calorie beverages and sweeteners
Nutrient-balanced hypocaloric diets: Allied health and lay-staffed programs					
Diet Center™	$9.00	$8.00	$10.00	$12.50	Most foods and beverages
Jenny Craig™	$23.00	$20.50	$16.50	$13.50	Fresh produce, beverages
Nutri/Systems™	$19.00	$16.50	$14.50	$12.00	Fresh produce, beverages
Registered Dietitian	$15.00	$13.50	$10.50	$9.00	All foods and beverages
Weight Watchers™	$2.50	$2.00	$2.00	$1.50	All foods and beverages
Support groups: Volunteer staffed or self-help programs					
TOPS	$0.07	$0.06	$0.05	$0.04	All foods and beverages
OA	$0.00	$0.00	$0.00	$0.00	All foods and beverages

[a]Ideal body weight

From Amy B. Spielman et al., "The Cost of Losing: An Analysis of Commercial Weight-Loss Programs in a Metropolitan Area" in *Journal of the American College of Nutrition,* 11:36–51, 1992. Reprinted with permission of the author and publisher.

5. Are the recommended foods ones you would want to continue eating after losing weight?

6. Does the plan suggest some magical chemical combination that burns off fat?

7. Does the plan suggest that calories don't count?

8. Is any mention made of evaluating body fat?

9. Is exercise a part of the plan?

10. Does the plan recommend exercise at least three times per week?

11. Does the plan suggest changing diet and exercise habits on a permanent basis?

12. Will anyone benefit financially through the sale of this plan?

If you answered yes to numbers 1, 2, 4, 5, 8, 9, 10, and 11, and no to numbers 3, 6, 7, and 12, you may have found a good weight-control plan. If not, you may wish to reconsider.

High-Risk Weight-Loss Procedures

Some individuals are so desperate to lose weight that they try anything, including procedures that might be injurious to their health. These procedures include insertion of a gastric balloon, gastroplasty (stomach stapling), intestinal bypass, jaw wiring, and liposuction. Except for liposuction, surgical procedures for weight loss are rarely done, though there is some indication of an increase in gastrointestinal surgery for severe obesity ("Obesity Surgery Regaining Favor" 1991). Unfortunately, these procedures don't teach good nutritional or exercise practices.

What's Right for You?

Sometimes it's tough to know where and how to start a weight-control plan. It's best to begin by deciding on a strategy. Decide if you have a need and a desire to lose weight. Next, do some self-assessment. Consider what foods are your favorites and which activities you enjoy and would do on a regular basis. Then, do some reading. Go to the library and see what diet books are available. Look for one that takes a practical approach and includes exercise along with a variety of foods from all the food groups, limiting the intake of fat to 30 percent of total calories.

It's helpful to review your diet history. Do you experience an occasional increase in pounds that requires a minor adjustment or are the pounds out of control, requiring a more formalized program? A medically supervised program is recommended for those who have more than 50 pounds to lose, who have a family history of obesity, and who have health problems such as diabetes (Hamilton 1990).

Ensure your success by determining the ingredients that will encourage success. Once your decision is made to proceed, the following guidance can help:

1. Set realistic goals. Determine practical amounts of weight to lose and be realistic about the time line you set. Plan on no more than a one-half- to one-pound weight loss each week, and be prepared for some plateaus along the way.
2. Plan a nutritious diet that includes moderate amounts of your favorite foods. Don't eliminate all favorite foods from the diet.
3. Eat a number of small meals rather than one large meal during the day. You will probably consume fewer calories, and you will feel less deprived. Be sure to monitor the portion size.
4. Keep busy, and don't focus on dieting.
5. Include some type of exercise each day. Start slowly, and set goals that are attainable.
6. Increase your normal level of activity. Walk briskly rather than slowly, and walk rather than ride.
7. Consider eating habits and behaviors, and don't eat unless you're hungry. Think of positive behaviors to substitute for the behaviors that influence your eating.
8. Find others who are supportive of your weight-loss plan.
9. Develop ways other than eating to deal with stress.

10. Consider food decisions before social occasions. Since food is a focal point of most social gatherings, consider how to deal with this.
11. Accept some disappointments and setbacks.
12. Celebrate successes, but learn to do so without food as the focal point.

Eating Disorders

Anorexia nervosa and bulimia are highly publicized eating disorders. Although these disorders are more frequently reported among white, upper-class females, increasing numbers are being reported among other groups (Balentine et al. 1991). Most patients with eating disorders are difficult to treat and may be chronic cases that require professional help (Yates 1990). Unfortunately there is no single effective approach (Gilbert 1986). Both disorders can be treated in the short run, though long-term success is not guaranteed (Mitchell 1990).

Anorexia Nervosa

The condition in which caloric intake is severely limited is **anorexia nervosa.** Anorexia (loss of appetite) nervosa (of the nerves) refers to the suppression of the appetite rather than loss of appetite. It has been described as self-induced starvation or dieting gone out of control. Anorexics have a focused goal of thinness and willingly starve themselves and overexercise to reach that goal (Bruch 1986). There was a time in our society when we thought it was impossible to be too thin. We now know that extreme thinness can be harmful and even fatal.

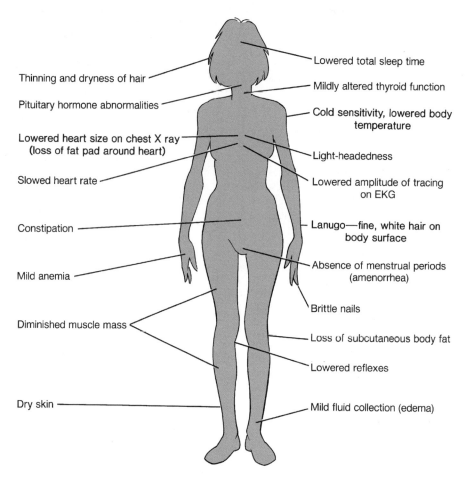

Figure 5.3

Possible signs and symptoms accompanying weight loss in eating disorders.

Reprinted by permission. In Eating Disorders Information Packet, *The National Anorexic Aid Society of Harding Hospital, Columbus, Ohio, 1990.*

Most anorexics are white females under twenty-five years of age who developed the condition in early adolescence or early adulthood. Anorexia mainly affects well-educated females from prosperous homes (Bruch 1986). Although the condition affects females 95 percent of the time, cases are reported among men, such as models, who are dependent on their thin physique for employment. The frequency of anorexia in males may be more prevalent than previously thought. In an assessment of attitudes about weight and dieting among college students, 17 percent of males indicated that the most powerful fear in their lives was gaining weight or becoming fat (Collier et al. 1990).

Weight loss in anorexics is usually achieved through fasting and extremely limited caloric consumption. Other methods used may include diuretics, laxatives, vomiting, strenuous exercise, and diet aids. The body tries to maintain essential functions when calories are severely restricted.

Less vital functions are slowed or stopped to preserve the functioning of the brain and heart. Anorexics may experience lowered body temperature, **amenorrhea,** which is the absence of menstruation, and lowered blood pressure and respiration (fig. 5.3). Anorexia results in death in approximately 10 percent of cases.

One of the most difficult things to understand about anorexia is the self-perception of the anorexic. Regardless of how much weight is lost, the anorexic still feels too heavy. Most anorexics continue dieting, and 79 percent still consider themselves overweight several years after hospital treatment (Yates 1990). Other characteristics of anorexia include an overly high activity level and the denial of hunger.

Many approaches are used in the treatment of anorexia, though the prognosis is not good. Drug therapy is used in 25 percent of cases, and behavior modification is used in 45 percent of cases. Most specialists recommend some

If you suspect a friend has an eating disorder, it is important for your friend to receive professional help. Although there are no specific procedures to follow, there are a number of guidelines you might consider.

Observe your friend's behavior. Anorexia is usually easier to spot than bulimia because of the drastic physical changes associated with the weight loss. The anorexic may try to conceal the weight loss by wearing bulky clothes. He or she may refuse to eat food, withdraw from friendships, and engage in wild, obsessive exercise patterns. Bulimia may be more difficult to recognize because

you may not see obvious personality or physical changes. Watch for purchases of enormous quantities of food that disappear immediately. Another clue may be regular trips to the restroom immediately after meals.

Express your concern and encourage the person to seek professional help. The anorexic usually denies there is a problem and indicates that he or she is in total control. The person may think others are jealous of his or her ability to control weight. It is especially important to maintain your support and concern, even though it may not seem wanted.

The bulimic is more likely to be receptive to your comments, though he or she usually denies there is a problem. Your expression of concern and support is extremely important.

If your friend refuses to seek help, request assistance. Although the anorexic is more likely to require hospitalization, both the anorexic and the bulimic may need this. Some helpful resources include your instructor for this class, the student health center, the counseling department and student services center at your school, and the county health department. Remember, your friend probably won't get better without outside help.

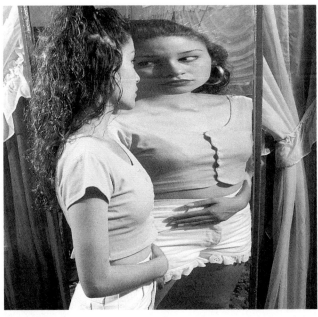

The anorexic may feel fat regardless of how much he or she weighs.

period of hospitalization to ensure weight gain (Gilbert 1986). The prognosis for anorexics is worse than for bulimics (Mitchell 1990).

Bulimia

Bulimia is an insatiable appetite characterized by binge eating. It has been confused with anorexia nervosa because periodic binging is common to both disorders; however, a number of the characteristics are very different.

Ninety-five percent of all bulimics are females. Bulimics tend to be close to normal weight and may appear to have normal eating habits. Bulimia usually begins in adolescence or early adulthood (Brey 1992). During their secretive eating binges, bulimics may consume 10,000 or more calories within a few hours. Afterwards, they try to purge the food through a variety of methods, including vomiting, laxatives, diuretics, and exercise. The anorexic may use these methods to lose weight, while the bulimic may use these methods to maintain weight. After the binge and purge are completed, the bulimic may feel depressed and discouraged about the behavior.

Bulimics tend to have a pattern of restrictive dieting followed by binging. To overcome bulimia, a normal eating pattern that eliminates dieting must be established. Although bulimia may remain hidden from others, the bulimic is more likely than the anorexic to seek treatment; however, the individual may expect immediate results and become frustrated with therapy (Yates 1990). The anorexic may request treatment only when others insist upon it. Warning signs may alert family and friends to both of these conditions (table 5.6).

Special Concerns for Those Who Are Underweight

Although you may find it hard to believe, being underweight is a problem for close to 10 percent of the population (Williams 1990). Some of the health problems associated with being underweight include the risk of delivering low birth weight babies, surgical complications, and extended recovery from illness. Females are considered underweight when their body fat is 12 percent or lower,

Healthy Weight

Attaining and sustaining a healthy weight can influence the mind, body, and soul and the interdependence of all of these factors. Attaining and sustaining healthy weight requires a lifetime commitment. The specific health skills needed to do this are all interrelated.

The following activities will enable you to assess whether you have the health skills related to attaining and/or sustaining healthy weight, along with the readiness to do this. You may also see the relationship among the mind, body, and soul related to healthy weight.

Mind

Consider the influences that make attaining and/or sustaining healthy weight important to you. Ask yourself if there are any motives for trying to attain and/or sustain healthy weight. Determine what your goals are related to healthy weight. What do you want to accomplish and why?

Body

Assess your weight and determine if you currently are at a healthy weight. Use more than one method, if possible, to assess your body weight. Consider what natural means

are available to achieve healthy weight (cutting down on junk food, exercising more, skipping seconds, passing on dessert).

Soul

Consider if attaining and/or sustaining healthy body weight is important to you. Determine if this is in harmony with the things that hold value to you. Assess if the behavior needed to achieve this is in harmony with your basic values and beliefs.

Interdependence

1. Explain the benefits of healthy weight to someone who is important in your life. Share information on the health benefits of attaining and/or sustaining healthy weight.

2. Develop a plan that meets your personal goals and objectives for attaining and/or sustaining healthy weight. Consider all of the factors that may impact this. Determine ways to deal with those factors that may be negative.

3. Describe what can be done to encourage success. Indicate the things needed to overcome temporary setbacks. Share this information with a friend.

---

and males are considered underweight when their body fat is 3 percent or lower. The underweight may be highly concerned about the effect of their weight on physical appearance and feel that they look skinny or scrawny.

Those who suffer from this condition should try to determine the cause. In some instances, it may be due to a medical condition, or it may be due to poor eating habits, nervous tension, or a genetic tendency. Once a person has determined that being underweight isn't a medical problem, there are a number of things that can be done. First, schedule regular mealtimes. Thin individuals may prefer more frequent meals of smaller portions rather than fewer meals of large portions. Caloric intake should be increased by adding complex carbohydrates to the diet. Unfortunately, a thin person is often told to add high-calorie foods such as milkshakes and other high-fat items to the diet. This is poor advice. A thin person should never add poor-quality food to the diet. The health risks associated with a high-fat diet affect the thin as well as the obese. Thin individuals should also plan regular exercise. Exercise adds contour and shape to the body by adding lean tissue. Thin individuals are likely to look better and feel better when exercise is a regular part of their life-styles.

TABLE 5.6	
Warning Signs	
Anorexia Nervosa	Bulimia
Significant or extreme weight loss of 15 percent or more with no known medical illness accounting for the loss.	Mood swings.
Reduction in food intake, denial of hunger, and decrease in consumption of fat-containing foods.	Excuses made to go to the restroom after most meals.
	Large amounts of food bought, which suddenly disappears.
Excessive exercise (hyperactivity).	Unusual swelling around the jaw.
Intense fear of gaining weight.	Laxative or diuretic wrappers found frequently in the trash can.
Ritualistic eating habits.	
Critical attitude towards others.	Weight within normal range, although person eats large amounts of food, often high in calories, (a binge).
Highly self-controlled behavior.	
Self-perception of being too fat, even when this is not true.	

Reprinted by permission. In *Eating Disorders Information Packet,* The National Anorexic Aid Society of Harding Hospital, Columbus, Ohio, 1990.

Summary

1. Only 3 percent achieve permanent weight loss despite the large number of individuals trying to lose weight.

2. We need to make permanent life-style changes to achieve permanent weight loss.

3. Extra body weight is a risk factor in heart disease, hypertension, diabetes, and cancer.

4. Body composition determines the percentage of lean and fat tissue.

5. Body fat can be determined by hydrostatic weighing and skin-fold measurement.

6. Males are considered obese when their body fat percentage exceeds 20 percent, while females are considered obese when their body fat percentage exceeds 25 percent.

7. Possible causes of obesity relate to heredity, exercise, eating habits, the fat cell theory, and the set point theory.

8. Dieting may cause our bodies to become fatter because the body retains fat to protect it from perceived starvation.

9. Caloric intake should not go below 1,000 to 1,200 calories to consume needed nutrients.

10. The best weight-control plans combine exercise and diet.

11. Weight-control plans that promise incredible results should be carefully studied.

12. People with eating disorders need professional help.

Commitment Activities

1. Vending machines are found in most of the buildings on a university campus. See if those on your campus contain any nutritious foods. Work with your class in developing a plan to include nutritious foods that are low in calories in these vending machines.

2. Menus in student residence halls could be modified for those who want to control their weight. Work with the dietitian to create a "diet bulletin board" that lists specific calories in foods at each meal (e.g., what lunch foods would be part of a daily intake of 1,200 calories?).

3. Medical science is continually improving care for individuals suffering from chronic diseases. Speak with faculty from your home economics department to see what advances may have been made during the past year. Invite someone from the nutrition department of your university or from the local health department to speak to your class about specially prescribed diets.

4. Many communities have food programs that help people of various ages. Find out what is available in your community. Look into the WIC (Women, Infants, Children) Programs, Child Nutrition Programs, Food Stamps, Meals on Wheels, and Elderly Feeding Program. Investigate the educational program that each provides.

References

Ballentine, M.; Stitt, K.; Bonner, J.; Clark, L. "Self-Reported Eating Disorders of Black, Low-Income Adolescents: Behavior, Body Weight Perceptions, and Methods of Dieting." *Journal of School Health* (November 1991):392–96.

Barnett, R. "Why Fat Makes You Fatter." *American Health* (May 1986):38–41.

Bouchard, C.; Tremblay, A.; Despres, J.; Nadeau, A.; Lupien, P. J.; Theriault, G.; Dussault, J.; Moorjani, S.; Pinault, S.; and Fournier, G. "The Response to Long-Term Overfeeding in Identical Twins." *New England Journal of Medicine.* 322, no. 21 (1990):1477–82.

Brey, R. "Eating Disorders and Eating-Disordered Behavior Among College Females." *Eta Sigma Gamman* 10, no. 1 (July 1992):64–72.

Bruch, H. "Anorexia Nervosa: The Therapeutic Task." In *Handbook of Eating Disorders,* ed. K. D. Brownell and J. P. Foreyt. New York: Basic Books, 1986, p. 331.

Collier, S. N.; Stallings, S. F.; Wolman, P. G.; Cullen, R. W. "Assessment of Attitudes about Weight and Dieting among College-Aged Individuals." *Journal of the American Dietetic Association.* 90, no. 2 (1990):276–78.

"Diet Vs. Exercise: What's Best?" *Consumer Reports on Health* 4, no. 1 (January 1992):1–3.

Drewnoski, A., et al. "Sweet Tooth Reconsidered: Taste Responsiveness in Human Obesity." *Physiology and Behavior* 35 (1985):517.

"Exercise and Diet in Weight Loss." *Nutrition Today* 25, no. 1 (February 1990):4.

"Fear of Fat." *Consumer Reports* (August 1985):455–57.

Gilbert, S. *Pathology of Eating: Psychology and Treatment.* New York: Routledge and Kegan Paul, 1986, pp. 129–32.

Gurin, J. "Leaner, Not Lighter." *Psychology Today* (June 1989):33, 34.

Hamilton, K. "The Bulge Stops." *Health* 22, no. 5 (1990):54–55.

"How Fat Is America?" (press release), Diet Center, January 8, 1992.

Katch, F. I., and McArdle, W. D. *Nutrition, Weight Control, and Exercise,* 3d ed. Philadelphia: Lea and Febiger, 1987, pp. 130,134, 162.

Liebman, B. F. "Is Dieting a Losing Game?" *Nutrition Action Healthletter* (March 1987):10.

"Link Between Weight Loss and Diabetes II Prevention." *Health Education Reports* (July 16, 1992):6.

Lissner, L.; Odell, P.; D'Agostino, R.; Stokes, J.; Kreger, B.; Belanger, A.; and Brownell, K. "Variability of Body Weight and Health Outcomes in the Framingham Population." *New England Journal of Medicine* 324, no. 26 (1991):1839–44.

Manson, J. E.; Colditz, G. A.; Stampfer, M. J.; Willett, W. C.; Rosner, B.; Monson, R. R.; Speizer, F. E.; and Hennekens, C. H. "A Prospective Study of Obesity and Risk of Coronary Heart Disease in Women."

McGlynn, G. *Dynamics of Fitness,* 2d ed. Dubuque, Iowa: Wm. C. Brown Publishers, 1990, p. 44.

Mitchell, J. E. "The Treatment of Eating Disorders." *Psychomatics.* 31, no. 1 (1990):1–3.

Nash, J. "Eating Behavior and Body Weight: Physiological Influences." *American Journal of Health Promotion* (Winter 1987):5–7.

New England Journal of Medicine 322, no. 13(1990):882–88.

Nicholas, P., and Dwyer, J. "Diets for Weight Reduction: Nutritional Considerations." In *Handbook of Eating Disorders,* ed. K. D. Brownell and J. P. Foreyt. New York: Basic Books, 1986, pp. 123, 124.

"Obesity Surgery Regaining Favor." *Medical World News* 32, no. 5 (1991):37.

Powers, S. K., and Howley, E. T. *Exercise Physiology: Theory and Application to Fitness and Performance.* Dubuque, Iowa: Wm. C. Brown Publishers, 1990, p. 338.

Simon, C. "The Triumphant Dieter." *Psychology Today* (June 1989):48–52.

Sitton, S. C., and Miller, H. G. "The Effect of Pretreatment Eating Patterns on the Completion of a Very Low Calorie Diet." *International Journal of Eating Disorders* 10, no. 3 (1991): 369–72.

Speilman, A.; Kanders, B.; Kienholz, M.; and Blackburn, G. "The Cost of Losing: An Analysis of Commercial Weight-Loss Programs in a Metropolitan Area." *Journal of the American College of Nutrition* 11, no. 1 (1992):26–41.

Stunkard, A. J.; Harris, J. R.; Pedersen, N. L.; and McClearn, G. E. "The Body-Mass Index of Twins Who Have Been Reared Apart." *New England Journal of Medicine* 322, no. 21 (1990):1483–87.

Suter, P. M.; Schutz, Y.; and Jequier, E. "The Effect of Ethanol on Fat Storage in Healthy Subjects." *New England Journal of Medicine* 326, no. 15 (April 1992):983–87.

Thompson, T. "Shape Up Diets." *Health* 22, no. 5 (1990):51–53.

Wardlaw, G. M.; and Insel, P. *Perspectives in Nutrition.* St. Louis: Times Mirror/Mosby College Publishing, 1990, pp. 237, 243.

Williams, M. *Lifetime Fitness and Wellness—A Practical Approach,* 2d ed. Dubuque, Iowa: Wm. C. Brown Publishers, 1990, pp. 129, 155.

Yates, A. "Current Perspectives on the Eating Disorders: II. Treatment, Outcome, and Research Directions." *Journal of the American Academy of Child and Adolescent Psychiatry* 29 (January 1, 1990):1–8.

Additional Readings

Baer, J. T., and Taper, J. "Amenorrheic and Eumenorrheic Adolescent Runners: Dietary Intake and Exercise Training Status." *Journal of the American Dietetic Association* 92, no. 1 (January 1992):89–90. The authors report on an assessment of the dietary status of amenorrheic and eumenorrheic adolescent females. Since there are health risks associated with training vigorously and consuming a low-energy diet, the authors emphasize the need to consume an appropriate energy intake to support performance as well as growth.

Kuczmarski, R. J. "Prevalence of Overweight and Weight Gain in the United States." *American Journal of Clinical Nutrition* 55, no. 2 (February 1992):495S–502S. The results from the Second National Nutrition Examination Survey (NHANES II) are discussed in this article. Data on overweight and weight gain in the United States are summarized by several demographic characteristics.

"Lose Weight with Big Meals." *Consumer Reports on Health* 4, no. 2 (February 1992). Researchers at Columbia University found that women burned more calories when eating a large amount of food than when eating the same amount of food in small portions over several hours. They theorize that the digestive system needs to work much harder to digest the large amount of food and burns more calories in doing so.

Psychoneuroimmunology (PNI) is the study of the powerful interaction of the mind, the central nervous system, and the body's immunological system. The positive mental states of a fighting spirit, optimism, hope, and faith can actually fortify immune systems. The brain has the capability to self-medicate and to release a variety of mental and physical painkillers and motivating substances (neuropeptides) when the demand is there. One way for the body to help in acquiring the positive mental states is through fitness, nutrition, and weight control.

In this section, we have discussed the optimal body states of eating a good diet (low fat, low sugar, high fiber, balanced nutrition), being physically fit (cardiorespiratory, strength, and flexibility), and maintaining optimal weight. The maintenance of optimal body states is much more than a physical phenomenon; it also dictates a state of mind.

During aerobic exercise, many people report the second-wind phenomenon or the endorphine rush after thirty minutes or more of exercise. The mental state during the physical peak state lasts for about two to four hours after this occurs and is a state of increased mental alertness and improved problem-solving skills. Most people suffering moderate and temporary depression generally work out their problems during the exercise period.

Think for a moment about your eating and the mental states associated with eating. Remember when you have just had a big meal and stuffed yourself—perhaps on Thanksgiving. How did you feel an hour after that meal? Were you mentally alert, energetic, and performing optimally? Or were you fatigued, tired, and sleepy?

Studies show that those who exercise, eat right, and maintain ideal weights function better mentally in their older years. The interaction is powerful. Based on this interaction, try some of the following experiences to help your mental state based on things that you do for your body.

1. After you have been exercising over a period of time and can subjectively feel the benefits of exercise and prior to your next exercise session, ask yourself some questions that will require some creativity or problem-solving capabilities (aerobic dancing, when you have to follow the instructions of a leader, may not be the best for this activity). The questions need to be constructed just right. During your exercise, try to solve the problems or answer the questions. Some sample questions, which need to be adapted to your own life, follow:

   a. How am I going to get my studying (project) completed so that when I go on spring break or other vacation, it will be done?

   b. What creative and effective way am I going to let someone special know that I am interested in him or her?

   c. How am I going to show the relationship among these four identified factors?

   The type of exercise has to be one where you do not have to think consciously about what you are doing. Walking, swimming, jogging, and cycling are good if you often find yourself in a "trance" when you do the exercise. Generally what happens is that as soon as you finish exercising, you can sit down to a computer or pencil and paper and write down the solution because it will come. Your brain is like a computer that processes the information in the best way that you can, and it functions better during exercise. The experience at least provides direction as to where you have to go to get the answer.

2. When you find yourself in a frustrating situation, when you cannot see a way through your problems, when you are saying things you do not mean, or when you are thinking irrational thoughts, stop for a moment and contemplate the difficult situation. Take the opportunity to exercise for thirty minutes or more. When you return, compare the two mental states. It will amaze you if you can resolve the situation upon your return.

3. Use your mind to enhance your exercise capability. Compare the ease of exercise when you think positively (creatively, problem solving, spiritually, or other positive states) with states when you are thinking about getting through exercise and continually trying to keep yourself going. You will likely find active mental processes help make the exercise easier.

4. When you exercise or eat, focus on the process of your body's fortifying the immune system. Imagine that the rapid metabolism is carrying out germs and fortifying the macrophages, T cells, and other elements of the immune system. Think, too, of how the body exercise is burning off calories and making you feel better. Feel the sense of self-esteem, accomplishment, and feeling good.

5. Make exercising and nutritious eating a cause in your life.

By reading and working through the activities in the last three chapters on nutrition, physical activity, and weight control, you should have a good understanding of the following:

1. Basic nutrients and their importance to health
2. Practical health decisions that can promote good nutrition
3. Problems that can result from faulty health decisions about nutrition
4. Nutritional needs of special groups
5. The components of physical fitness and the health benefits of regular physical activity
6. The effects of total body physical activity
7. Practical ways to make health decisions about the development of a personal fitness program
8. Health problems associated with being overweight
9. Health decisions related to selection and use of a weight-control plan
10. Eating disorders
11. The most effective and healthy ways to control body weight

You have also had an opportunity to assess your feelings about issues related to nutrition, physical activity, and weight control. Health-producing behaviors are enhanced by wise decisions in these three areas.

Since health decisions about nutrition, physical activity, and weight control are so basic to total health, it is appropriate to consider ways to strengthen your well-being related to these areas. The model for the prevention of health problems presented in chapter 1 provides the framework for considering the relevance of the issues presented in this section.

The following list includes some sample behaviors related to nutrition, physical activity, and weight control. These are only possibilities, and there may be others that are more appropriate for you.

1. Develop an eating plan that promotes your overall health. For example, eat breakfast every day, eat a well-balanced diet, avoid sugar-coated cereals. Those who eat meals at regular times and don't skip meals may be better able to handle the structure of a low-calorie diet (Stitton and Miller 1991).
2. Examine your diet for the past week, and determine ways it might be better. Develop a plan to improve the quality of your diet.
3. Consider what might be done to improve the quality of your nutrition when you eat away from home. Plan ways to implement what needs to be done.
4. Devise a way to help a relative or close friend improve personal nutrition. Include information they need to know and ways you will help them.

5. Begin an aerobic fitness program (jogging, swimming, aerobic dance, cycling, etc.) and stick with it for at least three months. Assess your results.
6. Set a goal to compete in or complete a five- or ten-kilometer run and develop a plan to help you do it.
7. Pick a friend or relative who is sedentary and devise a way to help him or her become physically active using aerobic activities.
8. Take action to relieve psychological problems (boredom, loneliness, depression, frustration, resentment, etc.) associated with overeating by seeking professional help and taking action.
9. Choose and implement a good weight-control plan as described in the text.
10. Develop a plan to maintain your desired body weight in a healthy way.
11. Think of a situation related to nutrition, physical activity, or weight control that has caused disorganization or disruption in your life. For example, a failed diet plan, an aborted physical activity program, or an inability to control binge eating. Develop a plan to promote resilient reintegration (see chapter 2 for a review of these terms) in your life to prevent potential health problems related to nutrition, physical activity, or weight control in the future.

Life-Style Contracting Using Strength Intervention

I. Choosing the desired health behavior or skill

A. Keeping in mind the purposes in life and goals you identified in the mental health chapter (chapter 2), consider one or two health behaviors related to nutrition, physical activity, or weight control (from the list here or of your own creation) that will help you reach your goals. To assess the likelihood of success, ask yourself questions similar to those used in previous sections, such as:

1. Is my purpose, cause, or goal better realized by the adoption of this behavior?
____ yes ____ no

2. Am I hardy enough to accomplish this goal? (This means I feel I can do it if I work hard, I am in control of what needs to be done, I am committed to do it, and the goal is a challenge for me.) ____ yes ____ no

3. Is this a behavior I really want to change and that I feel I can change? ____ yes ____ no

4. Do I first need to nurture a personal strength area? ____ yes ____ no
(If yes, be sure to include this as part of the plan.)

5. Do I need to free myself from a bad habit in order to accomplish this goal?

____ yes ____ no (If yes, be sure to include this as part of the plan.)

6. Have I considered the results of the assessments in the chapters on nutrition, physical activity, and weight control?

____ yes ____ no

(These results may be helpful in developing a plan.)

Yes answers to the first three questions are a must to be successful. It might be wise to consider a different behavior if you cannot honestly answer yes to these questions. Your answers to questions 4–6 ought to provide information for consideration in your plan.)

    B. Behaviors I will change (no more than two)

_____

_____

II. Life-style plan

    A. A description of the general plan of what I am going to do and how I will accomplish it. (Consider apperceptive experiences—successes you have had in the past—since they may help you develop the best ways to carry out this plan.)

_____

_____

_____

_____

_____

_____

    B. Barriers to accomplishment of the plan (lack of time, feelings of others, frustration from previous failures, hesitation to take action, motivation, etc.).

      1. Identify barriers _____

_____

      2. Means to remove barriers (use problem-solving skills or creative approaches such as those described in the mental health chapter) _____

_____

_____

_____

    C. Implementation of the plan.

      1. Substitution (putting positive behaviors in place of negative ones) _____

_____

2. Confluence (combining activities for time efficiency if possible) _____

_____

3. Systematic enhancement (using a strength to help a weakness) _____

_____

4. When _____

5. Where _____

6. Preparation _____

7. With whom _____

III. Support groups

    A. Who _____

_____

    B. Role _____

_____

    C. Organized support _____

_____

IV. Trigger responses _____

_____

_____

V. Starting date _____

VI. Date/sequence the contract will be reevaluated _____

_____

VII. Evidence of reaching goal _____

_____

VIII. Rewards when contract is completed _____

_____

IX. Signature of client _____

_____

X. Signature of facilitator _____

XI. Additional conditions/comments _____

_____

_____

_____

_____

_____

_____

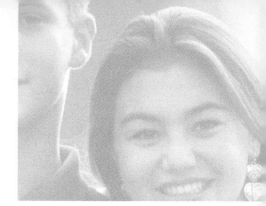

PART **III**

Sexual Choices

C HAPTER 6 PRESENTS A CON-
CEPT OF TOTAL SEXUALITY,
WHICH PROVIDES THE BASIS
FOR UNDERSTANDING YOURSELF AND OTH-
ERS. CHAPTER 7 STRESSES HUMAN SEXUAL
RESPONSE AND VARIOUS SEXUAL BEHAV-
IORS—FOCUSING ON THE FACT THAT SEXUAL
FEELINGS AND BEHAVIOR ARE INFLUENCED
BY MANY FACTORS. CHAPTER 8 DESCRIBES
CONCEPTION AND THE BIRTH PROCESS.

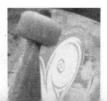

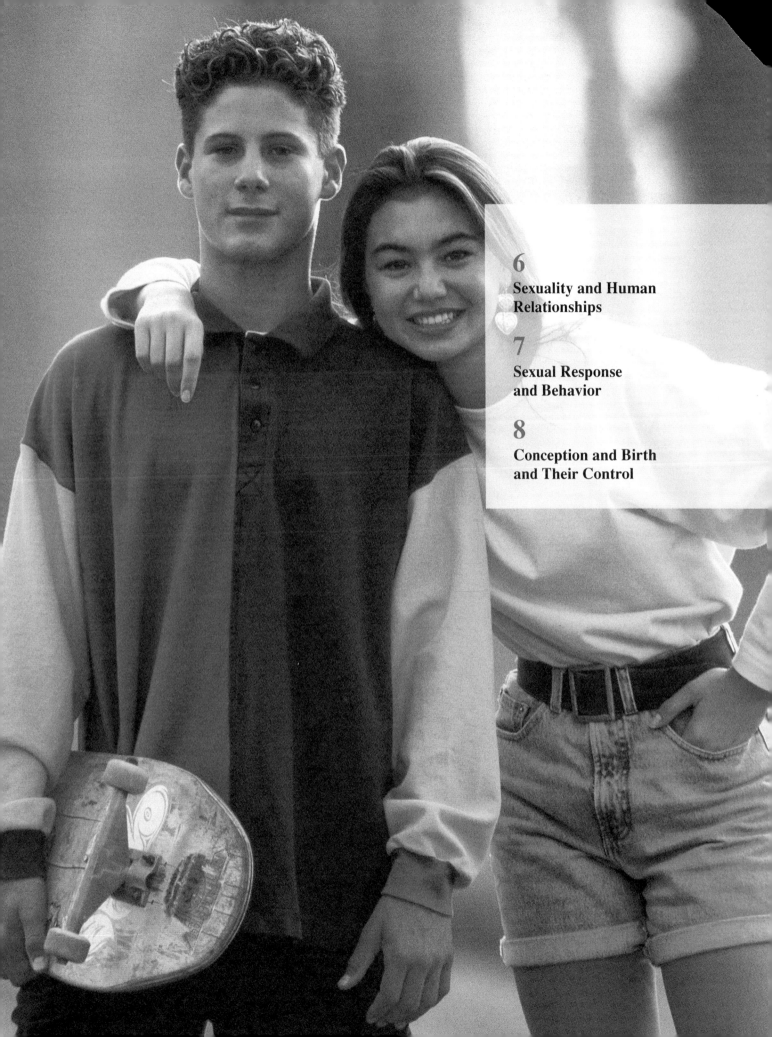

CHAPTER 6

Sexuality and Human Relationships

Key Questions

- How can human sexuality be defined?

- Has sexual behavior before marriage always been common?

- What factors influence selection of a mate?

- What can be done to improve communication?

- How can individuals be better parents?

- Are married couples very active sexually?

- How does sexuality relate to older individuals, those who are ill, and the disabled?

Chapter Outline

 W hat do you really want to know when it comes to sexuality? It is often thought that we most often want to know about sexual functioning, sexual activities, or sexual morality. While all of these aspects are important and of interest, they are not the major areas of interest related to sexuality.

Dr. Ruth Westheimer, the well-known lecturer and radio and television talk show personality, has received letters from male and female listeners and viewers since 1981. She notes that many of the letters are not specifically on sexual issues. Concerns about the care and raising of children, family relationships, and companionship needs put 41 percent of the letters into the relationship category, with only 33 percent concerning sexual issues ("Educating America" 1987). Individuals are concerned about human relationships and how sexuality relates to these relationships. Consistent with this interest and need, it is appropriate to consider what sexuality involves.

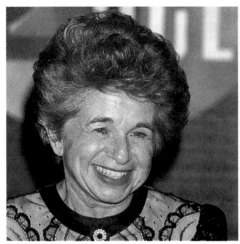

Dr. Ruth Westheimer addresses concerns and provides information about sexuality to many people.

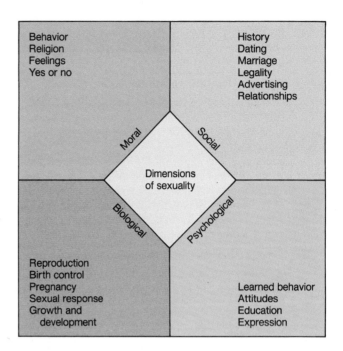

Figure 6.1

The four dimensions of human sexuality.

Sexuality Throughout Life

When we hear **sexuality,** our thoughts often turn to individuals lying in bed participating in sexual acts, particularly sexual intercourse. This narrow view reflects the same limited vision shown when we view health as merely absence of illness. Yet, unless you have spent a great deal of time studying the topic of sexuality, the sound of the word often excites interest or makes us feel slightly uncomfortable and shy—no matter how sexually experienced we are. But shyness and titillation are timid and immature responses to this powerful force in life. Sexuality is an essential part of each stage of the life cycle, and a thorough understanding of sexual natures and impulses, and of harmonious ways to express them, is vital to maintaining good health.

The Four Dimensions of Human Sexuality

Sexuality has four interacting dimensions: (1) social, (2) psychological, (3) moral, and (4) biological. Each of these dimensions influences and is influenced by the other three (fig. 6.1).

The **social dimension of human sexuality** includes the cultural factors that influence your thoughts and actions, including historical influences, dating, interpersonal relationships, and all the sexually related beliefs and behaviors learned from the environment. In contemporary society, these cultural influences include advertising, radio, television, and literature, in addition to the traditional influences of family, school, and church.

The **psychological dimension of human sexuality** reflects attitudes and feelings toward ourselves and others. It is probably the clearest example of learned aspects of sexuality resulting from past experience. From birth, we get myriad signals about how to think and act. We may learn that some words are "wrong" or "dirty" and that certain body parts are "untouchable" or "unmentionable." We even learn to be careful about what conversational topics are proper with certain people.

The **moral dimension of human sexuality** is the basic question of right or wrong: Should I or shouldn't I? Yes or no? This dimension might be based on particular religious thinking or perhaps on some basic philosophy. Daily, we face dilemmas that require moral decisions that affect and are affected by concepts of total human sexuality.

This dimension is a good example of how one dimension of sexuality can influence another. For example, it is known that sex guilt, that is, guilt about moral conduct in sexual situations, is related to sexual behavior. Since women may express greater sex guilt than men, and since those with stronger religious values seem to experience more sex guilt, consideration should be given to addressing religious values and the appropriateness of sexual activity as part of a relationship (Fox and Young 1989). Problems in one dimension of sexuality can lead to problems in another dimension. For example, guilt could lead to problems with a relationship.

The **biological dimension of human sexuality** is the one we usually think of first. It involves such considerations as physiological responses to sexual stimulation, reproduction, puberty, changes resulting from pregnancy, and growth and development in general.

Each dimension of sexuality relates to the others. For example, psychological stresses can influence the biological functioning of a woman's menstrual cycle. Moral feelings might affect psychological reactions, and biological functioning could impact social relationships. It is a mistake to assume that any one dimension is more important than another: all four constantly work together—ideally, in harmony. The relationship among the social, psychological, moral, and biological dimensions constitutes an individual's

Sexuality and Human Relations

A number of internal and external forces in your life influence the decisions you make regarding sexual behavior. What you do may be in harmony with some of these forces and in conflict with others.

Directions: Give a value to the following forces in your life as they pertain to your sexual behavior (i.e., what makes you sexually active or what makes you refrain from sexual activity). For those who are married, apply this tool to a specific sexual behavior such as the degree of fidelity to your spouse or the degree of sexual activity with your spouse.

a = a major force influencing my sexual behavior

b = a moderate force influencing my sexual behavior

c = an insignificant force influencing my sexual behavior

1. Religious influence	a	b	c
2. Family influence	a	b	c
3. How it feels when we kiss and hug	a	b	c
4. My own self-image (how I think I look to others)	a	b	c
5. My sense of right or wrong	a	b	c
6. Radio, television, or movies	a	b	c
7. How it feels to touch someone	a	b	c
8. How I learned to act	a	b	c
9. The way I feel inside	a	b	c
10. Literature (books, magazines) or music	a	b	c
11. Pleasure	a	b	c
12. My judgment	a	b	c
13. My sense of what I should and should not do	a	b	c
14. Friend's influence	a	b	c
15. Physical stimulation	a	b	c
16. Introversion or extraversion (how outgoing I am)	a	b	c
17. My morals or values	a	b	c
18. The expectations/relationship I have with boyfriend/girlfriend. (For marrieds, consider friends other than spouse.)	a	b	c
19. Fear of or anticipation of pregnancy	a	b	c
20. Desire to feel good about myself	a	b	c

Scoring/Interpretation

a = 1

b = 2

c = 3

Total values as follows from top to bottom of the four columns.

Column A	Column B	Column C	Column D
1. __	2. __	3. __	4. __
5. __	6. __	7. __	8. __
9. __	10. __	11. __	12. __
13. __	14. __	15. __	16. __
17. __	18. __	19. __	20. __
Totals __	__	__	__

Column A represents the degree to which your morals/values or beliefs influence your sexual behavior and decisions.

Column B represents the degree to which social forces influence your sexual behavior.

Column C represents the degree to which biological factors influence your sexual behavior and decisions.

Column D represents the degree to which psychological forces influence your sexual behavior and decisions.

The relative influences can be compared directly with each other to see which area is the strongest or if they are equal. You may interpret the results as follows:

11–15 major influence

6–10 moderate influence

1–5 insignificant influence

total sexuality. It is important to remember that sexuality relates more to what we are and not just to what we do. Although human sexuality is divided into dimensions for examination, it is in fact an indivisible whole.

Sexuality and Decisions for Well-Being

Surveys indicate that at any given time in a college classroom, a great number of students are thinking about something related to human sexuality. Chances are, too, that many do more than just think about sexuality. Probably around three-fourths of the readers of this text are likely to have participated in sexual intercourse, and almost all are likely to have participated in some form of sexual behavior (DeBuono et al. 1990; Flax 1992). In addition, there is a great deal of uncertainty about sexual knowledge among college students (Valois and Waring 1991). Myths, misinformation, and misconceptions about sexuality persist, in part because many of us are embarrassed to admit what we aren't sure of or just don't know. It is important, however, to separate fact from folklore so you can enjoy a healthy life ("Test Your Sexual I.Q." 1992).

Besides being the focus of much thought and behavior, sexuality influences interpersonal relationships, forms the basis of family life, and determines the reproduction of the species. Thus, sexuality is directly related to well-being

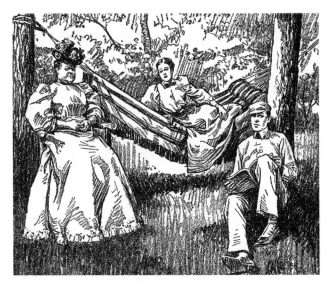

We have viewed premarital sexual behavior differently throughout history. For example, courting in the 1890's had to be done under the careful supervision of an alert chaperone.

ISSUE

Sexual Intercourse Before Marriage

There are many feelings about sexual intercourse before marriage. Some of the pros and cons are as follows.

• **Pro:** Premarital intercourse is okay as long as the individuals involved participate freely; no harm is done if they have freedom of choice, and those involved can stop any time they desire. Participating in premarital intercourse shows maturity, satisfies curiosity about sexual behavior, and can be a valuable learning experience in present or future relationships.

• **Con:** Premarital intercourse is only acceptable if there is a certain level of commitment between those involved, perhaps a strong emotional commitment or even engagement. Intimate relationships can be satisfying without intercourse. Also, some feel that intercourse should occur only after marriage and is wrong before marriage under any circumstances.

Should individuals engage in sexual intercourse before marriage?

in many ways. Being accurately informed about sexuality is, of course, crucial to future health and to making wise consumer decisions about it.

Premarital Heterosexual Behavior

Even though we emphasize total sexuality and its dimensions, we recognize that many individuals focus on specific sexual behaviors—particularly premarital heterosexual behavior. Because of this, it is appropriate to briefly consider patterns of premarital sexual behavior.

Early Patterns of Premarital Sexual Behavior

Many history books give the impression that early generations of Americans were sexually chaste before marriage. Careful reading between the lines, though, reveals that this was not the case. In the late 1700s in Massachusetts, one in three women in a particular church confessed "fornication" to her minister (Reiss 1973); the actual amount of participation was probably higher. Males on the Western frontier relied heavily on prostitution for sexual gratification. And the women's liberation movement of the 1870s, designed mainly to ensure that women would have the right to vote, revealed numerous extramarital sexual affairs. Also, the first vulcanized rubber condom was displayed at the Philadelphia World's Fair in 1876. These apparently isolated events call into general question the supposed sexual purity and innocence of our ancestors.

Recent Changes in Premarital Sexual Attitudes and Behavior

Studies done between 1920 and 1945 indicate that the greatest increase in rates of premarital intercourse occurred in the first two to three decades of the 1900s

(Bell 1966). The so-called sexual revolution began early in this century, not in the 1960s and 1970s as many think. During most of the first sixty-five years of this century, well over half of men seem to have had premarital sexual intercourse.

The first national poll of young teenagers' views on sex, pregnancy, and birth control revealed that more than half of all American teens were sexually active by the age of seventeen, but only one-third of all parents talked to their children about birth control. Two-thirds of all sexually active teens never used birth control or used it only occasionally. Only 33 percent used it every time they participated in sexual intercourse. Of those who had participated, more than one-third of all the girls and half of the twelve- and thirteen-year-olds felt pressured into their first sexual intercourse ("Teens Speak Out on Sex and Birth Control" 1987).

More recently, about 78 percent of high school males and females who had participated in sexual intercourse said they used some form of birth control during their most recent sex act. Fewer than half, however, said the method used was a condom (Flax 1992).

The average age to have sexual intercourse for the first time in the United States is 16 years for girls and 15.5 years for boys. Every thirty seconds a teenage girl becomes pregnant, and every thirteen seconds a teenager contracts a sexually transmitted disease. There are an estimated one million teenage pregnancies a year, and three million teenagers—one out of six—will contract a sexually transmitted disease each year (Sroka 1991). Worldwide, sexual intercourse occurs more than one hundred million times daily, resulting in nearly one million pregnancies and about 350,000 cases of sexually transmitted diseases ("Briefly Noted" 1992).

Approximately 50 percent of American adolescents do not use contraceptives the first time they engage in intercourse. Half of premarital pregnancies occur within the first six months after initiation of sexual intercourse ("How Healthy Are America's Adolescents?" 1990). Clearly, there are many implications related to interpersonal relationships.

Family Formation

Some argue that the institution of marriage is dying out, and the divorce rate has certainly climbed. The divorce rate does seem to have leveled off—about one in every two marriages ends in divorce. At the same time, married men and women are generally happier and less stressed than the unmarried (Coombs 1991).

Others argue that the quality of relationships cannot be measured with statistics. There may be more divorces, but this might mean that couples are ending poor-quality relationships and entering into higher-quality ones. What *do* these observations mean? Central to any such discussion is how a mate is selected and what marital options exist.

Mate Selection

Many factors are important in choosing a mate. The single most important factor is what is perceived as "love." At the same time, love seems most likely to occur between two individuals with certain similar and complementary backgrounds and traits.

In this society, the important **similarity factors** in mate selection seem to be social class, proximity of geographical location, intelligence, age, race, ethnic group, and religion. For example, we tend to choose mates of about the same education level, which is usually related to social class.

There are also **complementary factors.** For example, a person who needs to be dominant in personal relations might select a relatively submissive mate, or someone who derives satisfaction from giving sympathy and emotional support might find a mate who derives satisfaction primarily from getting such sympathy and support.

Whether likenesses, differences, or some combination of the two are the primary reasons for mate selection, certain factors do seem to contribute to marital success (Saxton 1983):

1. *Childhood background.* Characteristics such as parents who were happily married, a happy childhood, lack of conflict, and infrequency and mildness of punishment.

2. *Age at marriage.* Earlier marriages seem to be less stable than later ones.

3. *Vocational preparedness.* We need sufficient training to undertake our own support and perhaps that of a family.

4. *Emotional maturity.* Relative independence and self-direction are important.

5. *Present interests and values.* Shared interests and values that seem to correlate most highly with marital happiness are sexual behavior, romantic love, children, and religion.

6. *Length of engagement.* A fairly long engagement (six to fourteen months) seems to be most effective.

7. *Adequate sexuality education.* Because sexual conflicts after marriage are major contributing factors to unhappiness, it seems clear that adequate sexuality education promotes marital happiness.

Obviously, we do not go through life with a checklist designed to rate potential mates, but you should know what characteristics are important in the choice of a mate. In spite of some changes, the profile of the American wife remains rather traditional. The vast majority (93 percent) of married women live with their husbands in their own households. Wives are usually a few years younger than their husbands. Four-fifths of all wives have at least a high school education and over one-seventh hold a college degree. Fifty-five percent of all married women are either employed or seeking work ("Profile of the American Wife" 1987).

Reasons for getting married are many and varied, but certain factors emerge as particularly important ("Why Do Couples Get Married?" 1990):

1. *Mutuality*—couples are more likely to marry if they are equally involved and are both in love.

2. *Interdependence*—being equally involved is significant since interest in others causes break-up.

3. *Self-ratings*—women who rate themselves higher on attractiveness, intelligence, and creativity are less likely to get married; however, men who rate themselves as desirable are more likely to get married.

4. *Individual readiness*—how much more schooling, career development, and other readiness factors are important.

5. *Social networks*—this includes how well individuals know their partners, parental approval, and acceptance by friends.

6. *Similarity in parents' level of marital satisfaction.*

There are also reasons why some women don't get married ("Why Some Women Don't Get Married" 1990). Some of these reasons could also apply to men:

1. Fear of loss of freedom.

2. Fear of making the wrong choice of mate.

3. Building a career takes lots of time.

4. Marriage can infringe on the ability to get ahead in the business world.

5. Haven't found the right person to marry.

6. Unwillingness to be emotionally or physically abused, flatter a man's ego unless the compliments are merited, act docile and submissive, or subjugate her needs to his.

7. Need someone to respect, enjoy, and communicate with on many levels and not just someone to pay the bills.

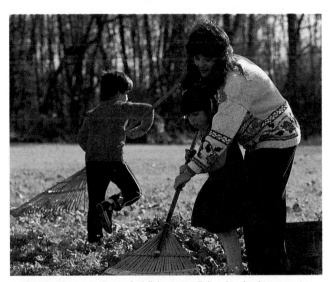

An increasing number of children are living in single-parent families.

Forms of Family Living

The typical family today is quite different from the family of the past. People living fifty to one hundred years ago may well have been part of an **extended family,** a family in which parents and children live with other relatives—a grandparent, for example, or an uncle or cousin. Now it is more likely that people grow up in and are likely to form a **nuclear family,** a family in which only parents and their children live together. Compared with many families of the past, people today are more likely to live some distance away both from where they grew up and from where relatives live.

The general shift from extended to nuclear families is just one of the changes that has altered modern family life. There appears to be less communication among family members than in the past, for example, due to television. The automobile has enabled family members to engage in activities away from each other and from home. The changing status of women in society, increased use of technology in the home, and economic constraints have also had a significant impact on family life.

In response to societal trends—and due to dissatisfaction with the traditional nuclear family—new forms of family structure have emerged. In many families, both husband and wife now work *and* share household and/or childrearing responsibilities. Other families are **single-parent families** because of divorce, separation, death, or choice. These families are increasing in number and are becoming more workable than in the past. The stigma of divorce has lessened due to its increasing prevalence, and women are more able to maintain families by themselves because of increased job opportunities.

Relatively high divorce and remarriage rates have drastically changed the profile of the American family in the past few decades. It is predicted that by the year 2000, the **stepfamily,** a family wherein one or both parents have children from a previous marriage, will be the predominant family structure in the United States and actually outnumber the nuclear family. Of all married-couple families with children under the age of eighteen, 40 percent are expected to become stepfamilies before the youngest child reaches age eighteen. Because this type of family structure is relatively new in large numbers, many questions about it remain unanswered. Some research indicates stepfamilies have more adaptability, but less cohesion, than nuclear families (Pill 1990).

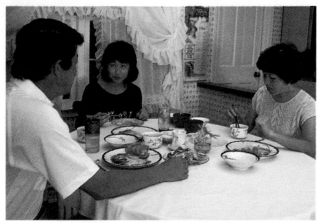
Listening is an important part of successful communication.

Other forms of family relationships are much less common than those mentioned, but it is still of interest to consider them. For example, in an increasing number of marriages, the partners have made a conscious decision not to have children. Other partners, both heterosexual and homosexual, are not marrying but **cohabiting,** that is, living together without being married. Many of these couples have also chosen to remain childless.

Most cohabitation is very short-lived; two out of five such relationships are disrupted within a year. In addition, unions formed by cohabitation, including marriages preceded by cohabitation, are much more likely to dissolve than unions formed by marriage. Cohabitation rates are highest among women, whites, persons who did not complete high school, and those from welfare-receiving or single-parent families ("Rising Prevalence" 1990).

Other types of male-female liaisons include **swinging,** which refers to a marital arrangement in which both partners include others sexually. Swinging seems to be more preferred by men than by women. Some couples find that sexual experimentation with others enhances their sexual activity with each other. Others believe that sexual activity should be enjoyed with a variety of people. Some individuals like the opportunities for female and male homosexual behavior, group sexual activity, and a greater degree of openness between marital partners. Many others feel that swinging is immoral and destructive to relationships.

Another type of liaison within the basic marriage form is the **contractual marriage,** in which each partner agrees to review the marriage contract periodically. At the time of review, couples make agreements that provide direction for the next time period. These contractual arrangements are legally binding as long as they do not contradict existing laws. As a variation, prospective marital partners sometimes agree to certain conditions on which the relationship will be based; for example, the man may agree to do the housecleaning and cooking, while the woman may agree to work outside the home and help with the laundry and childrearing chores.

A relatively new liaison is the **commuter marriage,** in which spouses set up separate households and live apart for periods of several days a week to months at a time. The main reason for doing so is pursuit of individual careers in different locations. Career development and satisfaction are the major benefits of this life-style, along with increased independence, greater self-sufficiency, and enhanced appreciation for spouse or family. Drawbacks include lack of emotional support and companionship. It is usually viewed as a temporary life-style, which enables the meshing of career aspirations and family goals (Groves and Horm-Wingerd 1991).

Family Communication

Regardless of the form intimate relations take, communication is critical. Poor communication is usually associated with a lack of listening, an attempt to win, an inability to demonstrate understanding of another's viewpoint, and a rigidity that prevents consideration of alternative solutions. (Recall the levels of communication explained in chapter 2 on mental health.)

Language and Sexuality

One factor that can contribute to communication problems is language—particularly language related to sexuality. Problems may arise when individuals do not have the same communication system and use different verbal comments, vocal styles, or nonverbal behavior. The basis for this is the lack of a precise sexual language.

At least four language systems have been developed for other purposes, but they are also used to communicate about sexuality. There are certain terms that parents often prefer to use with young children. This **child language** might be used to refer to body parts, bodily functions, or as terms of endearment. Because of this, children often grow up not knowing "proper" anatomical terms and feeling that such words are inappropriate to use.

As we grow up, we learn **street language** from peers and those who are a little older. These words seem to be power-laden and are the language of graffiti. This language can be used to impress others, but it is often socially unacceptable.

Euphemisms make it possible to avoid explicit terms while communicating with others. These include such expressions as "making love," "sleeping together," and "that time of the month." **Medical-scientific language** is concrete and technical and includes such words as "penis," "vagina," and "defecate."

An awareness of various language systems can help promote better communication. You can develop a wide tolerance for language choice, try to talk in the language system of the other person when possible, and change language choice when desirable. For effective communication, we must be sure we are speaking (and understanding) the same language (Cashman 1980).

Resolving Interpersonal Conflict

Successful resolution of interpersonal conflict requires being prepared to work on a level 4 in communication (see table 2.1). Recall that level 4 communication requires that you take some risks, be open to others' input, reveal more of yourself, and be honest, among other things.

Active Listening

Reflective listening, or **active listening,** is paraphrasing the other person's words to be sure the meaning was received. It can also include describing feelings left unspoken. This shows an understanding of where the other person is coming from. For example, you might say, "Let me see if I understood what you said. Is it correct to say that you . . ." or you could say, "Is this a correct summary of your feelings?" (and then give the summary). Reflecting the words and thoughts of others shows them you care enough to understand their views. Once speakers appreciate this caring, they are more receptive to listening and understanding your viewpoint. The net result is that each speaker not only better understands the other's point of view but also is less insistent that his or her viewpoint is the only valid one.

Identifying Your Position

Besides reflecting the other's words and thoughts, it may also be necessary to identify your position—where you are coming from. It is easier for others to understand your position if you can explain your feelings. At the very least, stating your thoughts and feelings about a situation aids communication.

Exploring Alternative Solutions

Another way of resolving interpersonal conflict is to **brainstorm** alternative solutions. The first step is to list all possible solutions without evaluating them. This allows for creativity without judgment. Then, evaluate these alternatives until a solution is reached. With this technique, it initially appears that no one wins, but in fact everyone wins.

Parenting

You don't have to be a genius or a great scholar to be a good parent. A strong desire to do a good job, a sincere acceptance of children as human beings with needs, feelings, and rights of their own, and a warm and loving heart are important. Yet, the decision to become a parent should not be taken lightly. In addition to the well-being of the parent and the child, there are also financial considerations. For example, the average cost of raising a child in Midwestern urban areas from birth to age eighteen is over $105,000 ("Cost of Raising A Child" 1991).

Unfortunately, some people mistreat their children. Perhaps there should be a special "Bill of Rights for Children" that would provide them a reasonable start in life. The accompanying box provides some suggestions that might be included.

Sexuality Education of Children

All parents are sexuality educators of their children, whether they choose to be or not. The way parents verbally and physically treat infants contributes to early sexuality education. The love given to a tiny infant is part of the process of sexuality education, as is the way parents respond when their children explore their own bodies.

Many parent-child activities through the years have implications for sexuality education. Examples are toilet training, the use (or lack of use) of terminology for body parts and certain physical activities, showing affection to children or in front of children, the way parents regard the status and roles of men and women, how parents treat and value one another, and the way parents handle children's questions about topics related to sexuality.

It is not uncommon for someone to ask: At what age should parents talk to their children about sexuality? Unfortunately, this question misses the whole point. Since sexuality has many dimensions and since we are sexual beings from birth, aspects of sexuality education are needed at all ages. It is not simply a matter of deciding to talk to the child at a certain age. Sexuality education is an ongoing process.

Children deserve to be provided with sexuality education in an acceptable manner. It is up to parents to cover the real concerns of young people. For example, masturbation is one of their biggest concerns. They should learn that masturbation is, most of the time, a normal expression of sexuality at any age. It is also important for young people to learn that while behavior can be "abnormal," thoughts in and of themselves are not. Everyone experiences a variety of thoughts and has sexual fantasies.

Boys need to understand about penis size, because size has no impact on function and size doesn't vary that much anyway. In addition, young people should realize that one or a few homosexual experiences don't make a person homosexual.

Young people are also curious about how to tell if they're really in love. Parents should never trivialize a child's love affair, but they can help children understand that there are different types of love (Gordon 1986).

Sexuality education has many benefits, including increased knowledge and improved self-concept. Among sexually inexperienced adolescents, it can even help postpone the first act of sexual intercourse ("Sex Education Can Delay Sexual Activity, Study Says" 1992).

In actual practice, sexuality education for children isn't much different from education in general. The basic principles of parenting, communication, and discipline apply in the same way no matter what the topic or situation. Sometimes the sensitive nature of sexuality makes it seem like the topic requires special handling, but sound parenting skills allow parents to provide children with a good education about sexuality.

Important Family Factors

There are a number of important factors parents can promote within a family that make a difference in the health of that family (Manning 1992). For example, encouraging family communication, using family time well, and providing adequate affection are likely to result in children who feel wanted and loved. The degree of parental support is also important. It can make a big difference if parents support their children in an excessive manner (such as making excuses for them when they are wrong) or if they expect their children to be responsible for their actions.

Independence is also an important factor. At one extreme, some parents allow little individuality and respect for autonomy. At the other extreme, independence and individuality can be considered valuable. Abuse is also a factor. Dealing with stress by using psychological crutches such as drugs, alcohol, and physical abuse can have a significant influence on family health.

Finally, the degree of parental control can be important. Parents can behave so they are viewed as authoritarian and strict; or, they can appear totally indifferent and ineffective in regard to discipline. Which combinations, and degrees, of these factors do you think are most important?

Sexual Behavior in and Outside Marriage

Again recognizing that behavioral statistics do not reflect the totality of sexuality, they can nonetheless be interesting. Here are a few for your consideration.

Marital Sexual Activity

In recent decades, two general social changes in regard to marital sexual activity have had a great impact, particularly on women. First, since more reliable contraceptives are available, conception is no longer beyond the control of sexual partners. The second change—and the one to be discussed here—is the growing realization that women have as much right as men to expect sexual satisfaction. How is sexual satisfaction achieved?

Communication about sexual matters is vitally important to a sexually harmonious marriage. The old assumptions that men naturally know how to perform sexually and know what women desire simply have no basis in fact. For instance, many women see their need for cuddling and closeness as more important than their need for intercourse. Some women may "exchange" intercourse for intimate body contact because such contact helps meet their needs for relaxation and security. These needs can be met only if the partners openly communicate.

What is known about the frequency of marital intercourse? Doddridge, Schumm, and Bergen (1987) report that the average frequency of marital intercourse for couples in their twenties and thirties is about 2 to 3 times per week. The rate drops off steadily throughout the life cycle. By the middle thirties and early forties, average coital rates are 1.5 to 2 times per week. Beyond age fifty, these figures drop to once a week and less. This means that married couples in their early twenties, on the average, have intercourse together about 150 times per year, while married couples in their forties do so about 100 or fewer times per year. Certainly there are couples who participate in sexual activity much more and much less than the average at every stage. Each person and each couple are different.

When and Why Should Individuals Have Children?

Traditionally, individuals have been free to have children whenever they desired. This is still basically true, and it is viewed as a fundamental right to have children.

• **Pro:** You should be able to have children whenever you desire and to have as many as you wish. It is not right for someone to tell others when they can have children or under what circumstances. This should remain one of the freedoms associated with living in the United States.

• **Con:** Before individuals have children, there should be strong evidence that they will be good parents. They should know parenting skills, understand children, and be able to afford to raise children. There should also be limits on how many children one couple may have. While this is a free country, the rights of children and those outside of the family must also be protected.

Should people always be free to have children?

Because couples tend to place great emphasis on the frequency of sexual activity in marriage, they must communicate their expectations. They can gain perspective by comparing rates of sexual activity with the frequency of other things they do. For example, they eat regular meals about one thousand times per year and travel to and from work or perhaps run errands once a day. By comparison, marital intercourse does not occur with great frequency.

While couples may be interested in how frequently others engage in sexual activity, using this information to bolster arguments is not effective. Informing your partner that most couples "your age" have intercourse 2.5 times a week does nothing to resolve growing problems of sexual distance creatively. Couples must work out acceptable levels, forms, and frequency of sexual activity for *themselves,* not for anyone else. What is relevant is that they communicate sexual needs and expectations and reach a satisfactory agreement about their sexual activity together. After all, quality and meaningfulness are more important than frequency of sexual activity.

Agreeing on frequency, length, and timing of sexual activity requires that partners communicate and negotiate. Difficulties with sexual language often cause communication problems. While we have developed a public language about sexuality, few have a private language for communicating about sexual behavior. Think, for example, of phrases designed to initiate or turn down sexual activity. An initiating phrase might be, "I think I'll take a shower," while a turn-down phrase might be, "I have to leave for work early tomorrow." Note which phrases are straightforward and which sidestep or hint. Why do you think we have difficulty being direct about sexual relations?

The Ethics of Affairs

People disagree about the pros and cons of affairs. Here are a few common reasons given for and against them.

• **Pro:** Sexual activity outside the primary relationship is justified for various reasons, including the need for variety, a poor sexual relationship, or a poor relationship in general.

• **Con:** Keeping sexual activity within a relationship is one of the most important characteristics of a primary relationship, regardless of whether the relationship is a happy one. Outside sexual activity is never appropriate.

How do you feel about affairs?

Extramarital Sexual Relations

In some circumstances, such as swinging, both marriage partners openly acknowledge each other's extramarital sexual involvements. Extramarital sexual activity, however, is usually secretive. It is often assumed that those who engage in extramarital sexual activity are having affairs and are emotionally involved in ongoing sexual relationships. Most extramarital sexual activity, however, is more casual; relatively few people have serious affairs.

How often does extramarital sexual activity occur? It is difficult to obtain accurate statistics on an activity that is generally not openly acknowledged. For men, the frequency of extramarital activity appears to decrease with age, while for women, it appears to increase. A conservative estimate is that 50 percent to 75 percent of men participate in extramarital sexual activity at some point during their marriages. It is generally accepted that the incidence for women has increased significantly—perhaps doubled—since 1950, when sexuality researcher Alfred Kinsey noted his figure of 26 percent (McCary 1982; Wyatt, Peters, and Guthrie 1988).

A number of social factors—such as religious beliefs, earlier patterns of sexual activity, and women's rights—tend to affect the incidence of extramarital sexual activity. Those who participate in premarital sexual intercourse, for example, are more likely to participate in extramarital sexual activity. The high divorce rate also may be related to higher rates of extramarital sexual activity. As conviction has grown that women should have more sexual rights than in the past, women have become more active seekers of sexual pleasure outside the marriage. Affluence is also a factor—the more money a person has, the greater the time and opportunity for extramarital sexual activity. Finally, the changing role of women in the labor force is a factor—women today have a greater sense of autonomy than in the past, and working women have almost as much opportunity for extramarital sexual activity as working men;

home demands, however, are still often stronger for the working woman than the working man, which lessens opportunities.

Postmarital Sexual Behavior

There are few studies on the sexual behavior of postmarital (widowed, separated, or divorced) individuals, but they seem to indicate that men continue to be as sexually active as they were during marriage, while women temporarily become less active after a marriage ends (depending on circumstances surrounding the ending) and then return to previous levels or reach even higher levels of sexual activity.

There are proportionately many more people today in a postmarital state than before. Higher divorce rates alone could account for this, but the ability of medical science to keep some people alive longer also contributes. Those who engage in postmarital sexual activity might discuss these relationships with their children so children can try to understand and communicate their reactions to their parents' relationships. Such communication contributes to the overall health of the family.

Myths and Facts About Sexuality and Aging

As we have discussed, we are sexual beings at all ages. Children are often taught that older individuals are supposed to be **asexual,** that is, without sexuality. This can sometimes become a self-fulfilling prophecy—as older individuals age, they feel they should be asexual themselves. But sexuality involves feelings, self-concept, and relationships, as well as physical activity; so how could anyone be truly asexual? The myth that aging leads to asexuality persists, however.

What are the facts about aging and sexuality? Contrary to common belief, although physiological response may become a little slower and possibly less intense with age, the average person in good health maintains sexual interest, desire, and activity throughout the life cycle. The major hindrance to sexual activity in older people seems to be attitude, not the body. Such factors as monotony, preoccupation with career, mental or physical fatigue, overindulgence in food or drink, physical or mental infirmities, and fear of unsatisfactory sexual performance can hinder sexual activity. Most of these factors, however, are strongly influenced by attitudes.

To deal with negative attitudes, it is wise to remember six rules on human sexuality and aging (Cross 1989):

1. *All older people are sexual.*
2. *Older people have a particular need for a good sexual relationship.* Because of other factors that might have caused difficult adjustments (such as retirement, loss of friends and loved ones, loneliness,

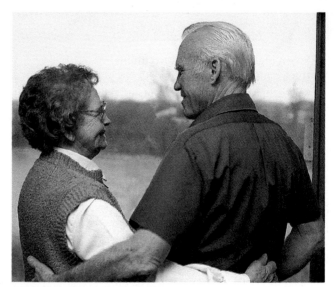
Sexuality is important throughout life.

reduced income, etc.) the warmth and security of a good sexual relationship can be very helpful.
3. *Sexual physiology changes.* Aging can result in slower physiological responses and change in appearance, but people with a healthy attitude can adapt to these changes.
4. *Social attitudes are often frustrating.* Society still tends to deny the sexuality of the aged, but younger people, and those who work with the aged, can be helpful in understanding the need for total relationships for people of all ages.
5. *Use it or lose it.* Sexual response is a physiological function that tends to deteriorate if not used. Regular sexual activity should be understood as healthy.
6. *Older folks do it better.* The elderly have the advantage of considerable experience, lots of time, and a mellowness that enables them to roll with the punches. There is no need for pressure to "perform" or to "prove oneself." These factors can lead to better (more enjoyable) sexual activity than at younger ages.

Attitudes toward **menopause,** which is the period of cessation of menstruation, are often negative; however, only a small number of women actually need medical help at this time, and most experience no loss of sexual satisfaction—provided that their attitudes don't get in the way. Menopause occurs because of decreased production of estrogen by the ovaries. (The female menstrual cycle is discussed in detail in chapter 8.) Some women experience "hot flashes" during menopause. This is usually reported as an intense feeling of heat or a sensation that the room suddenly became much warmer.

While most women do not experience severe symptoms during menopause, estrogen replacement therapy is available through a physician if such help is needed.

Promoting Healthy Relationships

Many skills combine to help produce healthy relationships. Within families and other relationships, we must first be comfortable with our sexuality. Then, we have to understand our needs and desires as well as those of our partner or other person in a relationship. We must possess good communication skills. In addition, we need knowledge and understanding of the sexuality of others—regardless of the type of individual or the group from which they come.

While promoting heathy relationships is not as easy as baking a cake, we can copy the process. It is common to use a recipe for guidance when baking a cake. As an important action step, develop your own recipe for promoting healthy relationships. Organize your recipe into categories for mind, body, soul, and interdependence as appropriate by considering the following statements and questions. Compare your recipe with those written by others. How do the ingredients you used compare to those used by others? How does your emphasis on (or amount of) each ingredient compare to others?

Mind

I need to understand where my concept of sexuality came from.

Body

I need to consider how my perceptions of my body and attractiveness of others have an impact.

Soul

How do the things I value most in life relate to my feelings about others?

Interdependence

How do I react as a result of what others do—physically and intellectually?

Doctors may prescribe other drugs for relief of menopausal symptoms such as difficulty sleeping, headache, or depression. As the proportion of women nearing menopause increases, it is likely that we will learn even more about the mysteries surrounding this stage of life (Willis 1988).

There are many myths about **hysterectomies,** the surgical removal of the uterus, but generally, the subjective level of the woman's sexual response before surgery continues unchanged, with reassurance and adequate information. In many cases, a hysterectomy does not interfere with basic hormonal production, and it is the hormones that influence feelings and drives, not the presence or absence of a uterus. Many women, however, do experience a change in the orgasmic sensation: uterine contractions are no longer part of the clitoral-vaginal response.

Unfortunately, while combating all the myths about sexuality and aging, older individuals may search for some nutritional element to aid sexual performance. No food or chemical has ever been proven to improve sexual performance; any apparent effects are only psychological.

While numerous men at some time in their lives experience prostatic problems (problems related to the prostate gland) and may even need surgery, their sexual activity does not usually end. Men who functioned well before surgery usually continue to do so afterward. There are exceptions, of course, but medical personnel and counselors can greatly help by encouraging positive attitudes as they discuss this matter with their patients or clients.

It is the mind, then, and not the body that tends to interfere with sexual activity at any age. An awareness of this will help you to be better equipped to resolve sexuality-related problems both now and later in life. This is another wonderful example of a mind-body relationship.

Sexuality in Special Groups

In addition to older individuals, the sexuality of other groups has been neglected or misunderstood. Myths abound regarding sexual activity among physically disabled people, mentally disabled people, and ill people.

Physically Disabled People

For the purposes of this discussion, physically disabled individuals are those with any kind of physical difficulty, including changes in body contours due to accident or disease or changes in body functioning that might relate to sexuality. While trying to see that basic needs are met, some have neglected the fact that the disabled are sexual beings. Concerns related to sexuality are often basic as well and need attention.

Depending on the type of disability, various areas of concern need attention, including the feeling of a loss of control over body functions, the inability to care for personal needs, the fear of being less of a person, and the feeling of unacceptability. Almost always, the general issue of a disabled person's body image is fundamental. Education and counseling about body image are important and ideally should also involve the sexual partners of disabled persons.

Certain aspects of sexual functioning are important to know about individuals who are paralyzed (Woods 1975).

1. Some components of the human sexual response cycle, such as erection, are mediated by spinal cord reflexes. Therefore, it is unnecessary to have pathways from the brain to the sex organs. For example, stimuli resulting from pressure or tension in the pelvic organs or from touch excite impulses that can cause erection.

2. The level of the spinal cord lesion and the degree of interruption of nerve impulses influence the nature of sexual functioning in the patient with spinal cord injury. For example, the local reflexes important in female orgasm are thought to be integrated into the lumbar and sacral regions of the cord.

3. Gratification can be experienced from sexual responses other than those emanating from the sex organs during the human sexual response cycle. Many handicapped individuals develop other areas of stimulation.

4. Adaptation of previous sexual practices may be necessitated as a result of spinal cord injury. For example, sexual activity may need to take place in different positions. Sexual aids may be helpful.

Physically disabled individuals are an important part of society. In recent years, much needed attention has been given to many of their needs, but there is still a failure to recognize and appreciate the sexuality of the physically disabled.

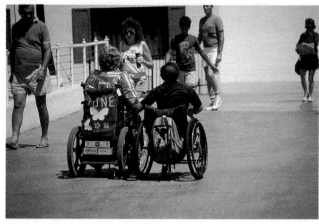

It's important to remember that disabled individuals are sexual beings too.

Mentally Disabled People

As with the physically disabled, until recently we have generally neglected the sexuality of mentally disabled individuals. Attention given to their sexual behavior was usually directed toward restricting that behavior, on the assumption that they were not interested in or could not handle sexuality. Fortunately, we now realize that mentally disabled individuals are sexual beings. They, too, need understanding and help in dealing with their sexuality. Often, there is a need to be explicit when working with mentally disabled people because they have lower reasoning levels. For example, educating the mentally disabled often requires showing them the actual positions for coitus with pictures and films so they fully understand.

Institutionalized mentally disabled individuals who are allowed to have sexual relationships can build feelings of affection and tenderness. As we increasingly recognize the rights of mentally disabled persons to participate in sexual activity, even institutionalized, severely disabled individuals are able to live happier, fuller lives.

Ill People

Most of us have little experience with the very young, the aged, the physically disabled, or the mentally disabled. Almost everyone knows someone who is ill, however, and everyone becomes ill on occasion. The ill are another group whose sexuality has mainly been ignored.

In the past, both patients and medical personnel avoided any mention of sexual topics, no doubt because both were too embarrassed to do so. Now, questions about sexual history are often asked in addition to regular questions about medical history. And doctors, patients, and partners are encouraged to discuss, when relevant, how illness or other medical problems affect sexual functioning.

Diabetes, neurological disorders, gynecological disorders, inflammation of the male's prostate gland, castration, rectal surgery, and heart attacks usually have a direct effect on sexual functioning. But those with nonrelated physical problems often develop sexual problems because of psychological factors. Some, for example, feel guilty when they get sick and try to determine where the guilt lies. Since the topic of sexuality is a leading producer of guilt, they may consciously or unconsciously avoid sexual activity. They may even allow illness to restrict their sexual life simply because they failed to ask medical personnel whether restriction was actually necessary (again note the interrelationship between physical and psychological aspects of total health).

To reduce sexual problems associated with illness, those who are ill need to feel that sexuality is appropriate to discuss and be aware of guilt feelings. In addition, in all cases of illness, they should learn when they can safely return to normal sexual activity to avoid detrimental effects on their relationships as well as on their self-concept. Those who are ill also need to realize that sexual problems can be expressed through physical symptoms; a person who asks for an examination of the genital area because of a supposed concern about cancer may actually be seeking an "acceptable" way to talk about a sexual difficulty.

If we understand this relationship between illness and sexuality, we can help reduce the incidence of problems in medical settings and increase the acceptance of everyone when illness is present, either in or out of the hospital.

Summary

1. Sexuality has four interacting dimensions: (1) social, (2) psychological, (3) moral, and (4) biological.

2. Sexuality relates more to what we are and not just to what we do and is directly related to human health.

3. There has been a great deal of premarital sexual behavior for decades and perhaps even centuries.

4. Some feel the quality of family life is deteriorating while others feel we are entering into more high-quality relationships.

5. Both similarity factors and complementary factors influence mate selection.

6. Successful family communication involves feeling at ease with language about sexuality, using active listening, identifying our position, and exploring alternative solutions.

7. Successful parenting demands considering the rights of children, personal feelings about children, and the sexuality education of children.

8. The quality and meaningfulness of marital sexual activity is more important than the frequency of sexual activity.

9. Many factors can contribute to the likelihood of extramarital sexual activity.

10. Many myths exist about sexuality and aging.

11. Myths abound regarding the sexuality of physically disabled people, mentally disabled people, and ill people.

Commitment Activities

1. Traditional concepts of sexuality have been somewhat narrow-minded. As discussed in this chapter, a total concept of human sexuality involves many components. In the coming months, try to become more aware of your own prejudices in terms of human sexuality. In your thoughts and dealings with others, reduce the use of words and images that portray your behavior as superior or "normal" in comparison with that of others. Also, try to reduce comments that might reflect stereotypes about sexuality.

2. Although it is clear that we are sexual beings at all ages, the sexuality of older people has often been neglected. Visit a home for older people in your community. Talk with an administrator to see what provisions are made for sexuality at the home. Is privacy promoted? Are conjugal visits allowed? Are programs held on sexual topics?

3. Many factors play roles in determining whom we date and perhaps marry. Certainly love must be predominant, but numerous other factors also enter the picture. List the factors you consider most important in a person you would like to date and in a person you would like to marry. Is there any difference in your two lists? What will you do now and in the future to make your lists coincide with reality? In other words, how can you be sure you will end up with a person who meets your qualifications?

4. The sexuality of mentally and physically disabled people has often been ignored in training programs for individuals who work with these groups. Determine what is being done with the topic of sexuality in training programs for those who work with the mentally or physically disabled in your area. Is it adequately covered for those who work in hospitals, clinics, or other facilities? If not, prepare suggestions for what might be done.

References

Bell, R. R. *Premarital Sex in a Changing Society.* Englewood Cliffs, N.J.: Prentice-Hall, 1966.

"Briefly Noted." *Health Education Reports* 14, no. 14 (July 16, 1992):7.

Cashman, P. H. "Learning to Talk About Sex." *SIECUS Report* 9, no. 1 (September 1980):1+.

Coombs, R. H. "Marital Status and Personal Well-Being." *Family Relations* 40 (January 1991):97–102.

"Cost of Raising a Child." *Youth Indicators 1991.* Washington, D.C.: U.S. Government Printing Office, 1991 p. 49.

Cross, R. J. "What Doctors and Others Need to Know." *SIECUS Report* 17, no. 3 (January/February 1989):14–16.

DeBuono, B. A.; Zinner, S. H.; Daamen, M.; and McCormack, W. M. "Sexual Behavior of College Women in 1975, 1986, and 1989." *New England Journal of Medicine* 322, no. 12 (March 22, 1990).

Doddridge, R.; Schumm, N.; and Bergen, M. "Factors Related to Decline in Preferred Frequency of Sexual Intercourse Among Young Couples." *Psychological Reports* 60 (1987):391–95.

"Educating America: What People Really Want to Know About Sex." *Sexuality Today* 10, no. 25 (May 25, 1987):2–3.

Flax, E. "Most High-School Students Sexually Active, C.D.C. Finds." *Education Week* 11, no. 17 (January 15, 1992):10.

Fox, E., and Young, M. "Religiosity, Sex Guilt, and Sexual Behavior among College Students." *Health Values* 13, no. 2 (March/April 1989):32–37.

Gordon, S. "What Kids Need to Know." *Psychology Today* (October 1986):22–26.

Gordon, S., and Wollin, M. M. *Parenting: A Guide for Young People.* New York: Oxford Book Co., 1975, pp. 25–26.

Groves, M. M., and Horm-Wingerd, D. M. "Commuter Marriages: Personal, Family, and Career Issues." *Sociology and Social Research.* 75, no. 4 (July 1991):212–17.

"How Healthy Are America's Adolescents?" *Target 2000.* Chicago: American Medical Association, April 1990.

McCary, J. L. *McCary's Human Sexuality.* Belmont, Calif: Wadsworth, 1982.

Manning, T. M. "Definition of Family Factors That Make A Difference." Presentation at national meeting of the Association for the Advancement of Health Education, Indianapolis, Ind., April 1992.

Pill, C. J. "Stepfamilies: Redefining the Family." *Family Relations* 39, no. 2 (April 1990):186–93.

"Profile of the American Wife." *Statistical Bulletin* 68, no. 2 (April–June 1987):18–21.

Reiss, I. L. "Changing Trends, Attitudes and Values on Premarital Sexual Behavior in the U.S." In *Human Sexuality and the Mentally Retarded,* ed. F. F. De La Cruz and G. D. La Veck. New York: Brunner/Mazel, 1973.

"Rising Prevalence of Cohabitation in United States May Have Partially Offset Decline in Marriage Rates." *Family Planning Perspectives* 22, no. 2 (March/April 1990):90–91

Saxton, L. *The Individual, Marriage, and the Family,* 5th ed. Belmont, Calif.: Wadsworth, 1983.

"Sex Education Can Delay Sexual Activity, Study Says." *Education Week* 11, no. 17 (January 15, 1992):11.

Sroka, S. R. "Common Sense on Condom Education." *Education Week* X, no. 25 (March 13, 1991):39–40.

"Teens Speak Out on Sex and Birth Control." *Sexuality Today* 10, no. 19 (February 23, 1987):3–4.

"Test Your Sexual I.Q." *Consumer Reports on Health* 4, no. 2 (February 1992):12.

Valois, R. F., and Waring, K. A. "An Analysis of College Students' Anonymous Questions About Human Sexuality." *Journal of the American College Health Association* 39 (May 1991):263–68.

"Why Do Couples Get Married?" *Behavior Today* 21, no. 39 (September 24, 1990): 4–5.

"Why Some Women Don't Get Married." *Behavior Today* 21, no. 39 (September 24, 1990):5–6.

Willis, J. "Demystifying Menopause." *FDA Consumer* 22, no. 6 (July/August 1988):24–27.

Woods, N. F. *Human Sexuality in Health and Illness.* St. Louis: Mosby, 1975.

Wyatt, G.; Peters, S.; and Guthrie, O. "Kinsey Revisited, Part I: Comparisons of the Sexual Socialization and Sexual Behavior of White Women Over 33 Years." *Archives of Sexual Behavior* 17 (1988):201–39.

Additional Readings

Chillman, C. S. "Promoting Healthy Adolescent Sexuality." *Family Relations* 39, no. 2 (April 1990):123–30. Explores adolescent sexuality as a central and positive part of the total well-being of young people from the ages of about ten to twenty years.

"Premarital Sexual Experience among Adolescent Women." *Morbidity and Mortality Weekly Report* 39, nos. 51 and 52 (January 4, 1991): 929–32. Gives statistical data about premarital sexual experience of 8,450 adolescent women and compares rates at different times.

Tiedje, L. B., et al. "Women with Multiple Roles: Role-Compatibility Perceptions, Satisfaction, and Mental Health." *Journal of Marriage and the Family* 52, no. 1 (February 1990):63–72. Examines alternative models of how women combine perceptions of role conflict and enhancement. Contains information about how women who combine the roles of a mother, spouse, and professional perceive their multiple roles.

CHAPTER 7

Sexual Response and Behavior

Key Questions

- What happens as a result of sexual stimulation?

- What sexual variations are "normal"?

- What sexual behaviors are illegal?

- What forms of sexual behavior are dangerous to others?

- What are the facts about homosexuality?

- How common is rape and other forcible sexual behaviors?

- What are the effects of pornography and prostitution?

Chapter Outline

Human Sexual Response
  Phases of Sexual Response
  Other Theoretical Models of
    Sexual Response
  Sexual Dysfunction
Sexual Behavior
  Variations in Sexual Practice
  Psychosexual Variations
  Variations in Partners
Sexual Abuse
  Rape
  Other Forms of Sexual Abuse
Commercial Sexual Behavior
  Prostitution
  Pornography

This chapter provides information you may have wondered about since your body first responded sexually. Even though basic biology is discussed, keep in mind that responses are influenced by many other factors—again illustrating the interrelationships among the dimensions of human sexuality.

Sexual relationships involve all dimensions of human sexuality; however, our particular body chemistry is an important factor. Tennov (1989) describes **limerence** as the quality of sexual attraction based on chemistry and sexual desire. It is passionate love based on sexual attraction. It is a powerful feeling that can overcome basic reasoning. It is what makes us feel sexually "turned on." Relationships that are initially based on limerence can develop into deeper, long-lasting relationships, but it is important to distinguish between love and limerence. "Crushes" experienced in the adolescent years are based on limerence. Limerence is also used in the advertising media to sell products. It is likely that relationships that are only based on limerence, and not on communication and love, will be relatively short-lived.

Sexual Response and Behavior

A. Sexual Behavior Communication

Note: Respond only as it pertains to your sexual activity. If you do not participate in any sexual activity, skip to section B. In regard to communication about sexual issues with your partner, mark all of the following that apply to your relationship.

_____ 1. I tell him or her what feels good.

_____ 2. I tell him or her what hurts, if anything.

_____ 3. I avoid frequent sexual encounters because I do not like them.

_____ 4. I let myself just go with my feelings and behave like I want to act during sexual encounters.

_____ 5. We have talked and resolved about how often to have sexual activity.

_____ 6. Sexual activity is a problem for us.

_____ 7. I have told him or her what I want during sexual activity.

_____ 8. My partner and I enjoy holding hands, kissing, and just talking as much as we do sexual activity.

_____ 9. It is important that each time we express love or date that it culminate in sexual intercourse to be a really meaningful experience.

B. Acceptance of Homosexuals

Mark all that apply.

_____ 1. I am very comfortable talking to homosexual men and women.

_____ 2. I have no negative feelings toward homosexuals.

C. Assessment of Date Rape

Note: This section is for those who are single and dating. Mark all that apply.

_____ 1. When dating, most of the excitement is to see what degree of intimacy I will be able to reach with this person (i.e., how far we will go).

_____ 2. I test how far I will go (physical intimacy) with someone by progressive fondling (hold hands, to arm around waist, rubbing back, chest, or breast and genitals) to see at what point the person will stop me.

_____ 3. When dating, I generally go with others or go somewhere public until I know someone.

_____ 4. I ask around about someone before I go out with him or her.

_____ 5. I make it very clear what my values are about physical intimacy when dating before difficult situations arise.

_____ 6. I have tried to coerce or talk someone into having sexual activity with me.

D. Prevention of Rape

Indicate which of the following you generally do.

_____ 1. I am sure that my windows and doors are locked and my home secure.

_____ 2. I list my address in the phone book.

_____ 3. I try to walk in lighted places.

_____ 4. I occasionally hitchhike.

_____ 5. I am careful not to let people know I will be alone.

_____ 6. I do not let unknown people into my home without identification.

_____ 7. I store my valuables in hidden and safe places.

_____ 8. I am aware of surroundings and suspicious movements when alone.

_____ 9. I try to travel with someone when possible.

_____ 10. I have thought through what I would do if anyone ever tried to rape me.

Scoring/Interpretation

A. Score as follows:

1. = 2	4. = 2	7. = 2
2. = 2	5. = 2	8. = 2
3. = –2	6. = –2	9. = –2

Total your score on this assessment tool and interpret as follows:

6 to 10 = healthy sexual relationship

0 to 5 = moderately healthy sexual relationship

–1 to –6 = need to improve communication skills

B. If you marked both responses, then you have an accepting attitude toward homosexuality. If you marked only one, then you have a moderately accepting attitude. If you did not mark either, then your attitude might be considered poor and you should perhaps make an effort to get to know someone who is gay and recognize his or her strengths.

C. Score as follows:

1. = 3	3. = –2	5. = –3
2. = 3	4. = –3	6. = 5

Interpret as follows:

3 to 11 = You are potentially infringing on someone else's right to live within his or her value system and legal rights. You may be "date raping" or attempting date rape.

0 to 2 = You have tendencies to infringe on someone else's right to live within his or her value system.

–1 to –3 = You are practicing moderately healthy dating precautions to avoid date rape.

–4 to –8 = You are practicing healthy dating precautions to avoid date rape.

D. Score as follows:

1. = 2	5. = 2	8. = 2
2. = –2	6. = 2	9. = 2
3. = 2	7. = 2	10. = 2
4. = –6		

Interpret as follows:

8 or higher = very good measures to prevent rape
0 to 8 = moderately good measures to prevent rape
–1 to –8 = poor measures to prevent rape

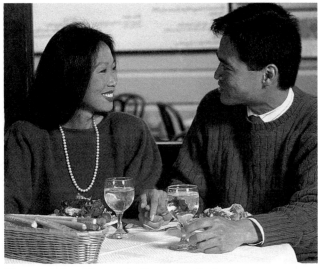

Strong relationships are built on many factors.

Human Sexual Response

The research of William Masters and Virginia Johnson (1966) revolutionized the Western world's views of general sexual behavior. Masters and Johnson gave us information about the phases of human sexual response, which is basically biological. Biological, of course, does not mean "automatic" or "machinelike." Sexual responses are influenced by such factors as human relationships, mental stress, and individual beliefs. At the same time, this biological information is basic to the understanding of our overall responses.

Masters and Johnson first studied more than eight hundred people in a laboratory situation, where the sexual response of subjects could be monitored. They studied male and female responses during masturbation, intercourse, and mechanical stimulation. They discovered that the physiological response was essentially the same regardless of the type of stimulation used.

Phases of Sexual Response

Masters and Johnson (1966) discovered that human sexual response is an ordered sequence of events that can be divided into four phases: (1) excitement, (2) plateau, (3) orgasm, and (4) resolution. Contrary to earlier thinking, they also found far more similarities than differences between male and female responses. Figures 7.1 and 7.2 show relaxed external genitalia, and figures 7.3 and 7.4 illustrate associated changes.

Excitement

In the **excitement phase** of human sexual response, in men blood flows into the erectile tissue of the penis faster than it flows out, and the penis becomes erect. In women, the vagina quickly responds to stimulation by secreting lubrication (like a sweating inside the vagina). Interestingly, male erections and female lubrication also occur during sleep approximately every eighty to ninety minutes.

In women, the clitoris, vaginal lips, nipples, and breasts tend to enlarge, while the vagina lengthens and the uterus elevates. In men, the testicles elevate. In both sexes, a skin flush over the upper body and face may develop. Additional changes might include increased muscle tension throughout the body, increased heart rate, and increased blood pressure. Men often experience tensing and thickening of the scrotal skin.

Plateau

During the **plateau phase**, the changes that occurred in the excitement phase intensify. The penis and vagina become larger. The sex flush often becomes well developed and may spread over much of the body. The woman's *labia minora* often change color, ranging from bright red to a deep wine color. The man may experience a preejaculatory emission of two or three drops of fluid. If a pregnancy is not desired, extreme caution is needed because sperm have been found in this fluid.

Orgasm

Orgasm, usually the shortest stage of the sexual response, is quite similar in men and women. Both sexes experience muscular contractions in the pelvic area that may last from a few seconds to about a minute. Muscular contractions and spasms may also occur in other parts of the body. Respiration, heart rate, and blood pressure all increase. The main difference between men and women is that men ejaculate and women do not, although some

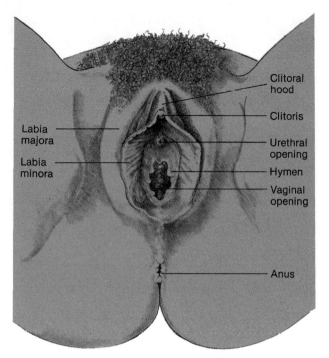

Figure 7.1

External genitalia of the human female.

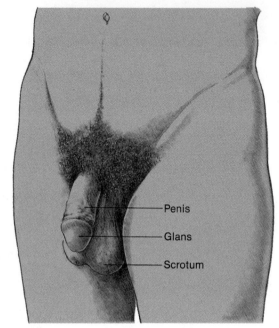

Figure 7.2

External genitalia of the human male.

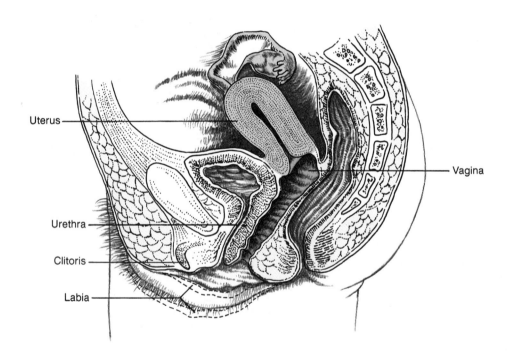

Figure 7.3

Some of the biological changes associated with female orgasm. The shape of the vagina changes so that the upper portion expands and the lower portion contracts to one-half of normal.

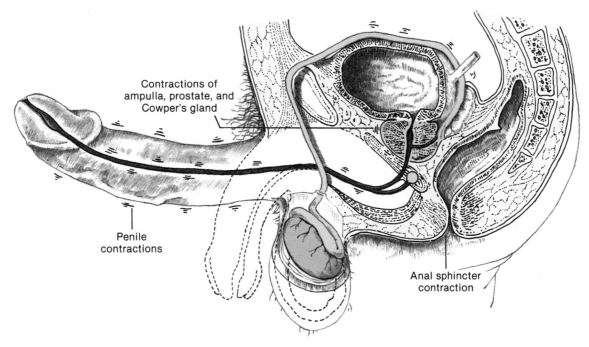

Figure 7.4
Some of the biological changes associated with male orgasm.
The penis becomes engorged with blood and the testicles
rise.

Contractions of
ampulla, prostate, and
Cowper's gland

Penile
contractions

Anal sphincter
contraction

The G Spot Controversy

Even though Masters and Johnson claim that there are not separate vaginal and clitoral orgasms, some researchers feel females have a G (Grafenberg) spot—a patch of erectile tissue in the front wall of the vagina, directly behind the pubic bone—that acts something like a second clitoris. This is supposedly an erogenous zone for women; when this spot is stimulated by deep pressure, it is supposed to produce a vaginal orgasm distinctly different from a clitoral orgasm. Some researchers even report that sufficient stimulation of the G spot results in a form of female ejaculation. Other researchers feel that this remains unproven ("G Spot/Female Ejaculation Researchers Vindicated by new Research" 1983).

A survey of 2,350 U.S. and Canadian women showed that many of the women felt that the G Spot exists in the vaginal barrel. This area is reported to be a potential source of orgasm independent of clitoral stimulation. Women who reported sensitive area orgasms were also more likely to report a spurt of fluid at the moment of orgasm (Davidson, Darling, and Conway-Welch 1989; Darling, Davidson, and Conway-Welch 1990).

controversial research indicates that certain women may experience a form of ejaculation as well if certain types of stimulation are used. (See the accompanying box on the G spot controversy.) Men usually experience expulsive contractions of the entire length of the *penile urethra* for several seconds. After several contractions, they are reduced in frequency; however, minor contractions continue for several more seconds. Contractions of secondary organs also facilitate the ejaculatory process.

In contrast to some earlier thinking that vaginal and clitoral orgasms were different, Masters and Johnson claim there is only one kind of female orgasm—a sexual one. This doesn't mean that women might not prefer different types of stimulation—just that the response is the same. Masters and Johnson also found that penis size makes *no difference* in either a man's sexual ability or a woman's sexual response.

In most males, the erection usually subsides after orgasm and cannot again be attained until some minutes or even hours have passed. The period during which a man is unable to have another erection is called the **refractory period.** This period continues until sexual tension returns to the level of early stages of excitement. Many women, however, are biologically capable of multiple orgasms within a relatively short period of time. There have been few investigations of this phenomenon, but in one study, 42.7 percent of the female respondents had experienced multiple orgasms (Darling, Davidson, and Jennings 1991).

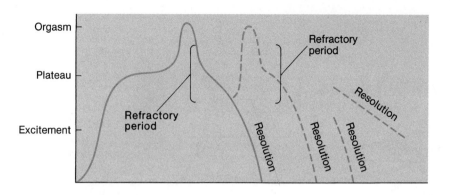

Figure 7.5

The typical male pattern of response. The dotted line indicates the possibility of a second orgasm and ejaculation after the refractory period.

William H. Masters and Virginia E. Johnson, *Human Sexual Response* (Boston: Little, Brown, 1966), p. 5.

Resolution

During the **resolution phase,** in both sexes the body tends to return to its preexcitement stage. In addition, women often experience a widespread film of perspiration unrelated to the degree of physical activity. Men may experience a similar perspiration, but it is usually confined to the soles of the feet and palms of the hands. This stage may last ten to fifteen minutes if orgasm has occurred or a much longer time if it has not. Figures 7.5 and 7.6 show the male and female cycles of sexual response.

Other Theoretical Models of Sexual Response

Two other models of human sexual response should be mentioned. Watch for similarities and differences among the models.

Kaplan's Triphasic Model

Kaplan (1979) conceptualizes human sexual response as consisting of a *desire* phase, an *excitement* phase, and a *resolution* phase. She feels it is possible to function well in one or two phases while having problems in the other. The unique component of **Kaplan's triphasic model** is the desire phase: a psychological, prephysical sexual response stage that is ignored by Masters and Johnson.

Zilbergeld and Ellison's Model

Zilbergeld and Ellison (1980) were concerned that the Masters and Johnson model focused exclusively on physiological aspects. **Zilbergeld and Ellison's model** consists of five components: (1) *interest or desire* (how frequently a person wants to participate), (2) *arousal* (how excited a person gets during sexual activity), (3) *physiological readiness* (e.g., erection or vaginal lubrication), (4) *orgasm,* and (5) *satisfaction* (a person's evaluation of how he or she feels).

Sexual satisfaction is a qualitative rather than a quantitative component. The quality of shared feelings is far more important than the number of orgasms experienced. It is also possible that a person can achieve sexual satisfaction without the "peak" experience of orgasm every time.

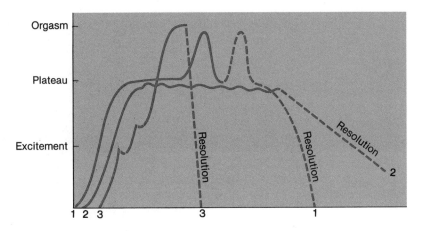

Figure 7.6

Three types of female response. Pattern 1 is multiple orgasm. Pattern 2 is arousal without orgasm. Pattern 3 involves a number of small declines in excitement and a very rapid resolution.

William H. Masters and Virginia E. Johnson, *Human Sexual Response* (Boston: Little, Brown, 1966), p. 5. Reprinted by permission of the authors.

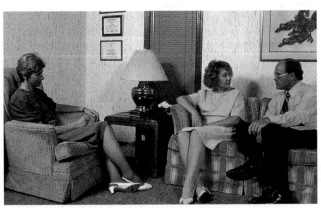

There are many sources of help for those with sexual dysfunction.

Sexual Dysfunction

Sexual dysfunction is a chronic inability to respond sexually in a way satisfying to the individual. While many prefer not to use these terms, female sexual dysfunction has traditionally been called **frigidity** and male sexual dysfunction has traditionally been called **impotence.** These conditions do not apply to those situations in which individuals are temporarily uninterested in sexual behavior or unable to respond sexually due to exhaustion, too much alcohol or other chemical substance, anger, and so on. The key word in the definition is *chronic*—that is, a consistent, long-term inability to respond (Greenberg, Bruess, and Mullen 1993).

About half of all married couples experience chronic sexual dysfunctions. Many never seek treatment; however, there has been a greater number of people seeking treatment in recent years (Greenberg, Bruess, and Mullen 1993).

The underlying cause of any sexual dysfunction may be either physical or psychological, but most experts agree that psychological causes are much more common. Because of this, sexual counseling has become prevalent in recent years. Sexual counseling is of extreme help for many, but it has also caused consumer difficulties because it is a major area of health quackery. The guidelines in chapter 16 are helpful when making a health decision related to sexual dysfunction.

Sexual Behavior

Many variations in sexual behavior are classified as abnormal, perverse, or problematic. We avoid these labels because most sexual behaviors can be seen as points on a continuum; it is difficult to judge when some specific variation becomes "abnormal" or "perverted." Exhibitionism is an example. Did you give some thought to the clothes you are wearing today? You probably chose them because you wanted to look nice; yet few would call you an exhibitionist for doing so.

Variations in Sexual Practice

Over the centuries, numerous variations in sexual practice have developed. Among the most common are masturbation, oral-genital contact, and sodomy.

Masturbation

Generally, **masturbation** is self-stimulation for sexual pleasure. Historically, many people considered it evil and detrimental to health. Even today, misconceptions about the supposed negative effects of masturbation persist.

Common myths are that masturbation leads to mental-health problems, causes skin problems, or makes a male unable to have children. Other myths indicate that only males masturbate or that masturbation ceases after a person gets married. None of these is true.

It has been suggested, only half jokingly, that 99 percent of all males masturbate at some time in their lives and the other 1 percent lie! Probably 65 percent to 75 percent of females masturbate at some time. As one way to learn about bodies and feelings, masturbation can play an important role in healthy growth and development. In fact, children often masturbate unknowingly by exploring their bodies. In addition, masturbation provides a safe sexual outlet for many individuals.

Oral-Genital Contact

There are two basic types of oral-genital contact—fellatio and cunnilingus. **Fellatio** is defined as oral (mouth) contact with a male's genital area; **cunnilingus** is oral contact with a female's genital area. This is an excellent example of behavior that some individuals think is disgusting and others think is erotic and desirable. Some individuals fear contact with such a "dirty" area of the body as the genitals; scientifically, however, this fear is unfounded. The genitals can be just as clean as any other area of the body; indeed, it has been suggested that if oral-genital contact is unclean, it is because of the many germs in the mouth!

Sodomy

The term **sodomy** refers specifically to anal intercourse but has been used often to refer to almost any form of sexual behavior someone happens to think is not "normal." Some states have laws that define sodomy as any sexual activity between anyone other than a married couple: some even outlaw certain sexual practices between married persons even though the couple participates in the activity in the privacy of their own home. In some states, the laws apply only to homosexuals, but in other states they apply to everyone. Such groups as the National Gay and Lesbian Task Force and the American Civil Liberties Union, however, have intensified lobbying efforts to encourage states to repeal antisodomy laws.

Psychosexual Variations

In addition to the practices just discussed, various sexual options are scientifically known as paraphilias. **Paraphilia** means love (*philia*) beyond the usual (*para*). There are about thirty different paraphilias, and each one exists as a fantasy and as a practice.

There is a great difference between a sexual practice that is engaged in simply as a variation and does not adversely affect anyone else and a practice that is engaged in compulsively and excludes consideration of others. For example, everyone has looked at other peo-

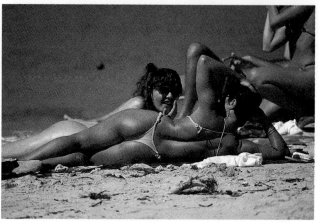

Laws and opinions vary from state to state and individual to individual. Would you call this exhibitionism?

ple's bodies in a locker room, but few compulsively seek opportunities to watch others undress in the privacy of their own homes.

Voyeurism, or **scopophilia,** refers in a general sense to obtaining pleasure from watching others undress or engage in sexual behavior. Voyeurs, often shy, lonely, and lacking social skills, commonly fantasize about having sexual relations with those they watch and often masturbate while fantasizing. Voyeurs derive satisfaction from the fear of being caught, the anonymity of the person being watched, and the fact that the person does not know he or she is being watched. Generally, voyeurs are not violent and, in fact, are fearful of any contact with those they observe.

Exhibitionism is achievement of sexual gratification by exhibiting the body (particularly the genitals) to observers. The exhibitionist, commonly called a "flasher," receives gratification because of the victim's (observer's) response. Exhibitionists might achieve orgasm by the very act of exposure, but more likely they either masturbate while exhibiting or later.

While it is often thought that exhibitionists are violent and aggressive, they are usually the opposite. It is rare for exhibitionists to do more than display the genitals. They do not want contact with the individuals to whom they exhibit themselves. While it may be difficult to do, generally the best response is to ignore an exhibitionist and continue usual activities. In this way, the exhibitionistic behavior is not reinforced.

Troilism refers to having sexual relations with another person while a third person watches. In one respect, it combines elements of exhibitionism and voyeurism.

A sexual fixation on some object other than another human being is known as **fetishism.** Almost anything can be the object of fixation—a knee, a shoe, silk, leather, and so on. As with other sexual behaviors, the fetish can exist on a continuum. In some cases, for example, a person might simply be attracted to a certain object; however, in other cases a person might not be able to sexually respond unless the object is present.

Frottage is the act of obtaining sexual pleasure by simply rubbing or pressing against another person. This is likely to occur in crowds, on elevators, and in buses and subways. It is even possible the frotteur will achieve orgasm. Normally, no additional contact or other form of behavior follows.

Masochism is sexual gratification from experiencing pain, while **sadism** is sexual gratification from inflicting pain on another person. For the masochist, the pain involved must be planned as part of an overall experience; accidentally hitting a finger with a hammer is not the kind of experience a masochist wants. Sadists, who make good partners for masochists, do not seem to be as common as masochists.

Sadism and masochism are good examples of sexual behaviors in which we need to differentiate between fantasy and behavior. For example, many more individuals report sexual fantasies involving masochism and sadism than actually participate in such behavior. It is possible to enjoy a sexual fantasy without wanting to participate in it in real life.

An extremely high sex drive that dominates the lives of certain women is known as **nymphomania.** Most women who enjoy very frequent sexual activity, however, do not approach nymphomania. A similar sex drive in men is called **satyriasis.**

Bestiality, or **zoophilia,** is sexual contact with animals. Bestiality is most common among those who live on farms. It most likely occurs during adolescence, and most individuals make a transition to more common adult sexual relations with humans.

Transvestism is sometimes confused with *transsexualism* or with *homosexuality.* A **transvestite** prefers wearing clothes of the opposite sex and is likely to achieve sexual gratification from doing so. A transvestite, however, is not likely to be interested in a sex-change operation or in relating sexually to members of the same sex. In most instances, transvestites actually have "normal" heterosexual relationships in every way except for their tendency toward cross-dressing when alone or with an understanding partner. Historians have reported hundreds of stories of life-long cross-dressers whose true behaviors were disclosed only after death (Heller 1992).

A **transsexual** believes he or she is "trapped" in the body of the wrong sex. This is not to be confused with homosexuality: transsexuals want to relate sexually to the opposite sex only if they can be in a body of the "proper" sex themselves; homosexuals want to relate sexually to the same sex. While it is an uncommon procedure, surgery and chemical therapy can be combined to change a person's gender, but only after much psychological testing and investigation.

Variations in Partners

Homosexuality—sexual attraction and/or relations between members of the same sex—is probably the most talked about variation in sexual behavior today. It is impos-

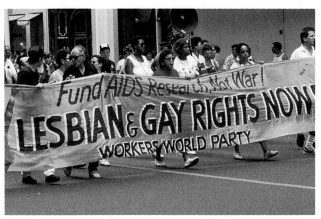

Homosexuality is probably the most talked about variation in sexual behavior today.

sible to know at what point individuals know that they have homosexual interests. Statistically, about 10 percent of the population, including friends, classmates, teachers, and sports heroes, are homosexual.

Many heterosexuals don't think homosexuals have legitimate feelings and rights. Such thinking results from a fear called **homophobia,** which arises because *homophobes* accept one or more myths about homosexuality, such as the myth that homosexuals look different from others. Actually, only about 10 percent of all homosexuals are what could be called "visible homosexuals."

Another myth is that homosexual males are effeminate and weak, while homosexual females are masculine and physically strong. In fact, sexual preference has nothing to do with one's body type or style of movement. Similarly, no relationship has been demonstrated between occupational and sexual preference. Male homosexuals are found in all occupations—from football player and truck driver to artist and corporation executive—as are female homosexuals.

The myth that homosexuals lurk at street corners and seduce innocent children into lives of homosexuality also exists. In reality, more heterosexuals than homosexuals take advantage of children. Either situation is intolerable, but it is certainly unfair to blame only homosexuals for such behavior. A related myth is that homosexuals are unfit to be teachers. There is nothing about homosexuality that affects teaching ability.

Some believe the myth that all homosexuals are mentally disturbed. The American Psychiatric Association and American Psychological Association do not list homosexuality as an emotional disorder. Apart from the social persecution and difficulties encountered, most homosexuals are happy with their life-styles and partners and lead well-balanced lives.

A related notion is that homosexuals develop their sexual preference because of problems in their family relationships. Obviously a poor family relationship can hinder anyone's development, but this theory of homosexual origins has not been substantiated. Many homosexuals do not regard their sexual preference as a "problem" at all, and researchers, so far, have been unable to explain what causes any sexual preference.

Homosexuals are often considered poor security risks. This thinking is based on the assumption that homosexuals are subject to blackmail. While there was probably some foundation for this idea in the past because of heterosexual persecution, today more tolerant and open attitudes make this possibility less likely. Furthermore, why would a publicly proclaimed homosexual be any more susceptible to blackmail than anyone else?

Most heterosexuals have been taught that homosexuality is a second-class condition, and therefore they accept disparaging myths about homosexuals. As is readily seen, however, there is no solid foundation for any of these myths about homosexuality.

Bisexuality, or **ambisexuality,** refers to those who enjoy sexual relations with members of both sexes. It is now widely believed that most individuals, left to their natural ways, are bisexual to some extent; so it seems to be the socialization process that produces exclusively heterosexual behavior. Some bisexuals are evenly divided between homosexual and heterosexual feelings, but most tend to lean one way or the other.

Sexual Abuse

Most sexual behaviors are normally engaged in by personal choice. When any one of these behaviors involves some degree of forcing one individual's will on another, it can constitute **sexual abuse.** Some specific forms of sexual abuse—rape, obscene telephone calling, pedophilia, and incest—are unfortunately common in society. While accurate statistics are hard to obtain, it appears that sexual abuse is increasing in the United States.

Rape

The legal definition of **rape** differs from state to state, but a practical definition is "forcible sexual intercourse." When a male or female is forced to have sexual intercourse against his or her will, a rape is committed. Sometimes, only the persons involved can tell when this is happening.

Some individuals feel that there is no such thing as rape—that a woman, for instance, cannot be raped unless she cooperates. This is complete nonsense. A rapist may knock a woman unconscious, tie her up, physically injure her, use a knife or gun for persuasion, or simply make strong threats. That the majority of rapes do not involve physical injury beyond the sexual assault does not mean that those raped weren't forced; nor does it mean that those raped weren't injured psychologically.

Conservative estimates indicate that a woman is raped every seven minutes and that a half million rapes occur each year in the United States (Mahoney 1984; Seligmann 1984; Tanzman 1992). The number of American women who have experienced attempted

---

ISSUE

Legislating Sexual Behavior

Historically, laws were passed to regulate such private sexual behavior among consenting adults as oral-genital contact and homosexual activity. Surprisingly, many of these laws are still on the books. They date back to early England and Puritan New England, they differ from state to state, and they are rarely enforced, but they are slow to be changed.

- **Pro:** These laws should be retained because we have a societal and moral obligation to prohibit unacceptable behavior. People should not be allowed to participate in such activity, and if we repeal these laws, we are condoning perversion.

- **Con:** Private sexual behavior among consenting adults is not a matter for the law. As long as there is legal consent, we have no reason to attempt to control personal sexual behavior. In fact, such laws are an inappropriate invasion of privacy.

Should there be laws about sexual behavior?

---

or completed rape is thought to be from 20 percent to 25 percent (DeVisto et al. 1984; Mims and Chang 1984; Tanzman 1992). In 1992, the National Victim Center reported that 683,000 adult women were raped in the United States in 1990. In addition, the center indicated that more than twelve million American women have been raped at least once in their lives, 61 percent of those raped were younger than eighteen at the time of the attack, and in 80 percent of cases the woman knew her rapist. Although rape is not as common as we may have been led to believe, the number is increasing alarmingly every year. Even one rape is one too many.

Of all the factors that influence a woman's decision to report a rape, the relationship between the woman and the rapist is the most important. Women raped by men they knew were less likely to make a report because they questioned their role and responsibility in the attack, while women in a classic rape (i.e., attacked by a stranger) had all the evidence they needed to convince both themselves and others that they had been raped (Williams 1984). It also seems more likely that a rape is reported if the offender did not have a right to be present where the assault occurred, if serious injury resulted from the assault, and if the individual raped was married (Lizotte 1985). In 90 percent to 95 percent of rapes, the rapist and rape survivor are of the same race, and most of the time they even live in the same neighborhood.

To better understand the motivations behind rape and to be able to assist rape victims more effectively, it is important to recognize that rape is a forcible violent act, not primarily a sexual one. Most rapists rape to be aggressive, to show their power, or to belittle the individual, not

It may be impossible to act in a way that guarantees you will never be raped; however, you can easily develop some protective habits to lessen the chances.

At home:

1. When returning home, have your key ready and enter immediately.
2. Be sure that doors, door frames, window frames, locks, and hinges are secure.
3. Keep valuables out of sight, outside your house (perhaps stored at a bank), if possible.

4. Have good lighting in all interior and exterior areas.

While on the street:

1. Be aware of the surroundings and environment.
2. Be alert to suspicious or unusual movements.
3. Walk in well-lighted places, avoid deserted areas, and do not take shortcuts through dark areas.
4. Walk on the left side of the street, facing traffic, so you can see oncoming cars.
5. Never hitchhike.

Personal precautions:

1. Keep doors and windows locked.
2. In the telephone directory, list only your last name and initials.
3. Be cautious how you handle telephone calls; for example, never let a stranger know you're home alone.
4. Never let an unknown person enter your residence without proper identification.
5. Have an emergency plan in mind, just in case.

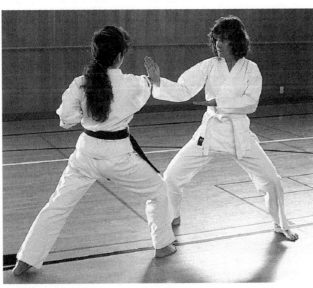

It is wise for women to learn techniques of self-defense.

to obtain what we usually think of as sexual satisfaction (Fein 1981). In fact, it is unlikely that sexual satisfaction even occurs. Families of rapists often conform closely to the stereotypical American nuclear family, in which the husband is the breadwinner and the wife attends to children and the home. Rapists have been found to be more hostile toward women, to have underlying anger motivations, to use dominance as a motive for sexual interaction, and to have underlying power motivations (Lisak 1991). Unfortunately, when many of us respond to the crime of rape, we tend to focus on its sexual rather than violent aspects. Those who are raped and their loved ones need help through difficult times in the same way as those who experience other violent crimes. Viewing rape as a violent rather than sexual act may aid a rape survivor's subsequent adjustment.

Date rape is much more common than most of us realize—probably the most common form of rape. Barry Burkhart, who has studied the topic since 1975, concluded the following ("Date Rape Is Occurring Too Often, AU Professor Says" 1987):

1. Twenty-five percent of women say they have had coerced intercourse, but only 15 percent meet the legal definition of rape. (In another study, it was estimated that 20 percent of college women had experienced attempted intercourse and 10 percent had experienced completed intercourse [Ward et al. 1991]).
2. Only 29 percent of men denied any form of sexually aggressive behavior and 15 percent had intercourse against the woman's will (but none described it as rape).
3. Sixty-one percent of the men admitted they had fondled a woman against her will, 42 percent had removed clothing, and 37 percent had touched a woman's genitals against her will.
4. Thirty-five percent of men had ignored a woman's protest, 11 percent had used physical restraint, 6 percent had used threats, and 3 percent had used physical violence to coerce sexual contact.
5. Fifty percent of the men admitted to forced sexual activity.

Burkhart reported that men who admitted to forced sexual activity could not be characterized as "sick" individuals. Most of the men were ordinary, not deranged perverts, and were doing what they thought they were supposed to do. Most of the offenders were very active in heterosexual relationships but simply saw women as objects of sexual pleasure. The women were likely to blame themselves and didn't view their treatment as strange or unusual.

More than 80 percent of the rapes on college campuses are committed by someone with whom the victim is acquainted; about 50 percent are committed on dates, and heavy drinking of alcohol and acquaintance rape often go together (Abbey 1991). Although women are fearful of walking alone on campus at night, the most common sexual assault is not the stereotypical rape attack but instead one that occurs as part of the "normal" social environment on the campus (Ward et al. 1991).

Both males and females can help prevent date rape. Males need to be aware of social pressures, to communicate with potential partners, to realize that being turned down is not a personal rejection, to accept an answer of no as meaning just that and not assume that previous permission for sexual contact applies to the present situation, and to realize that a woman does not want sexual activity just because she is dressed attractively or even in a way that might seem "sexy." Females also need to communicate clearly, to be assertive, to pay attention to what is happening, to be aware that nonverbal actions might send an unintended message, and to try not to put themselves in vulnerable situations ("Acquaintance Rape" 1986).

Other Forms of Sexual Abuse

Erotic phone calling (or letter writing) is a form of erotic distancing. The person obtains sexual pleasure from a distance and not from direct contact with another person. Obscene telephone callers receive sexual gratification from making gross remarks over the telephone, usually suggesting that the receiver of the call meet them to have sexual relations (even though the caller could never go through with this). The obscene letter writer is hoping for sexual gratification as well.

In none of these cases is the offender likely to be violent or follow up on the calls or letters, but the suggestions may be violent and should be reported. The recommended response to obscene phone calls is to say nothing and hang up.

Pedophilia is a form of sexual behavior in which an adult uses a child as the sexual object. Although actual physical force may not be used, a child is unlikely to be able to resist effectively physically, emotionally, or psychologically.

Boys as well as girls are often sexual abuse victims. Experts believe that about 2.5 percent to 5 percent of the male population is sexually victimized in childhood or early adolescence, which translates to about forty-six to ninety-two thousand new cases of sexual abuse of boys each year. It is thought that as few as one in twelve boys who are sexually abused come to the attention of a professional ("One in Twelve Sexually Abused Boys May Be Getting Professional Attention" 1982).

Either sex can be a pedophiliac, but males are most commonly the offenders. Unlike other men, child molesters associate sexual feelings with frustration, tension, and a sense of maladjustment and deviance. The child molester's apparent fear of women, his emotional immaturity, and his preoccupation with sex apparently make him turn to children for sexual gratification (Johnston 1987).

Incest is sexual behavior between persons too closely related to marry legally. The most commonly reported form is father-daughter, but in practice, brother-sister incest probably occurs more frequently. About 10 percent of all girls are involved in some sexual encounter with a male relative; boys are less frequently involved in sexual activity within families. The United States has laws prohibiting incest, but it still occurs in all social classes, geographic areas, and ethnic and racial groups. Legal action is seldom taken.

Although the number of reported cases of incest in the United States is quite low, it probably occurs far more frequently than most of us realize. Because the experience occurs within the family, outsiders are not likely to be aware of it. Additionally, shame and guilt make it probable that family members will hide incest.

It is estimated that one in four girls and one in seven boys in the United States will have suffered some form of *sexual molestation* by the age of eighteen. At least half (and possibly as many as 80 percent) of all sexually abused children are abused by individuals known to them. Parents and other relatives are responsible for 30 percent to 50 percent of all cases of sexual abuse ("Intrafamily Sexual Abuse—Incest" 1982).

At least 25 percent of all women and 10 percent of all men in this country experienced some abuse as children, ranging from sexual fondling to intercourse. Boys who are abused are far more likely to turn into offenders; girls are more likely to produce children who are abused. Abuse victims seem to be easy targets for someone because they don't know how to take care of themselves. This may be due to poor self-image, a lack of assertiveness, or the feeling they deserve to be punished (Kohn 1987).

Other interesting relationships are being uncovered related to sexual abuse. For example, nearly 66 percent of teenage girls who become pregnant were sexually abused as children. Compared with teenagers who became pregnant but who had not been abused, the abused girls became sexually active at a younger age, were more likely to have used drugs and alcohol, and were less likely to use birth control (Flax 1992).

Preventing child sexual abuse demands attention. Programs exist to educate children and adults to distinguish between appropriate and inappropriate touch, to say no to unwanted or uncomfortable touch, to tell a trusted adult if inappropriate touch occurs, and to identify their family and community support systems. In addition, college students are encouraged to consider risks related to certain behaviors, the selection of a mate who will not abuse their children, and ways in which they can protect children from sexual abuse (Olson 1985).

It is estimated that many sexually abused children may reach adulthood with no conscious memory of the abuse. Many different events can trigger the recall of these memories. If you feel you may have been abused as a child, it is wise to seek help from a professional who has experience treating adult survivors of childhood sexual abuse. If you know someone in this situation, encourage them to seek help.

Sexual harassment is probably one of the oldest forms of sexual abuse but has only recently received much attention. There are varying ways to define sexual harassment, but definitions usually include verbal abuse, sexist remarks, unwanted physical contact, leering or ogling, demand for sexual favors in return for some favorable treatment, and actual physical assault. In 1991, the topic of sexual harassment received more attention from the media and the general public than ever before during the confirmation hearings of Judge Clarence Thomas as a U.S. Supreme Court justice. For days the media featured the sexual harassment charges leveled against Judge Thomas by Professor Anita Hill. The hearings prompted many people to discuss the topic and brought attention to the prevalence of sexual harassment. In addition, a number of issues were raised, such as what constitutes sexual harassment, is it proper to make sexual harassment charges years after the alleged harassment, and how does one decide who is telling the truth when sexual harassment charges are made?

Either males or females can be sexually harassed; however, females are more likely to be harassed. On college campuses, about 25 percent to 33 percent of female students and 40 percent to 50 percent of female faculty members have experienced sexual harassment (Shavlik 1992).

Each of us is responsible for what we do and how we handle what others do to us. Open and honest communication is needed to solve a sexual harassment conflict. A continuum of how sexual harassment responses are actually handled include avoidance (ignoring and doing nothing), delusion (going along, stalling, or making a joke of it), negotiation (a direct request to the harasser to stop), and confrontation (aggressively telling the harasser to stop or taking formal actions) (Gruber 1989).

Each person must examine his or her interactions with others with greater sensitivity to be sure interactions are based on mutual respect, not stereotypes, faulty assumptions, or the erroneous opinions of others. We must form a new social contract based on mutual respect and regard for one another as human beings (Shavlik 1992).

Commercial Sexual Behavior

Some sexual activities exist mainly because of their relationship to money. Prostitution and pornography are perhaps the two most prominent examples, and they have become major social issues as well.

Prostitution

Prostitution is a much studied, but not greatly understood, sexual variation. In a general sense, the term refers to any situation in which one person pays another for sex-

---

ISSUE

Should Prostitution Be Legal?

Prostitution is illegal in most states, but some individuals wonder if the cost of law enforcement is worth it. Others feel present laws are unfair because they penalize the prostitute and not the customer.

- **Pro:** Those who would legalize prostitution feel that the money presently used for enforcement could be used for other things. They also argue that prostitution is a *victimless* crime since the customer and the prostitute are willing participants.

- **Con:** Those who argue against legalized prostitution feel the activity is immoral, that it contributes to the spread of sexually transmitted diseases, and that it is closely related to drug use and other crimes.

What is your opinion about prostitution?

---

ual gratification. The debate over whether or not prostitution should be legal and what the effects of legalization would be continues.

Adolescent prostitution is an increasing problem in the United States. During the past decade, there was a 183 percent increase in female prostitutes and a 245 percent increase in male prostitutes among youth twelve to sixteen years old. There are between 600,000 and 900,000 female adolescent prostitutes and at least 300,000 male adolescent prostitutes under the age of sixteen. They commonly come from broken homes or have poor relationships with their parents. Prostitution is used as a means of economic survival (Nightingale 1985). There are reports of children setting up their own prostitution rings while still living at home to earn spending money.

Therapy programs for prostitutes are usually not successful for many reasons, particularly because many prostitutes do not feel they can receive help. One innovative treatment program has various components: self-help groups for women and families, a treatment group for adolescents, individual counseling, outreach, and advocacy. A female prostitute who successfully underwent therapy started the self-help program for other prostitutes (Hynes 1983).

Pornography

What is **pornography?** No answer to this question satisfies everyone. Some feel that pornography, like beauty, is in the eye of the beholder. Others feel that any pictures or words related to sexuality are disgusting. We must decide how we feel based on personal beliefs as well as on the "facts" about pornography.

The Skill of Understanding

In the areas of sexual response and behavior, perhaps the most important skill is the skill of understanding. This means understanding how the body functions during sexual response and factors that influence this response. It means understanding variations of sexual behavior in a nonjudgmental way. It also includes understanding abusive sexual behavior and other behaviors that might be classified as negative to help prevent them and help others deal with them.

Personal characteristics related to the mind, body, and soul and their interaction contribute to the development of the skill of understanding. For example, knowledge, flexibility, and objectivity are a must. Honestly assess your present level of achievement in each of these areas.

Mind

Are you flexible when discussing sexual response and behavior? For example, are you willing to listen to various viewpoints? Can you accept the fact that not everyone wants to behave just as you do? Do you take the attitude that "my mind is made up so don't confuse me with the facts," or do you consider new information and respect different opinions?

Body

Do you have adequate knowledge about human sexual response and various sexual behaviors? (One good way to test yourself is to pretend you are going to teach someone about these topics and see if you have enough knowledge to do so.)

Soul

Are you objective when discussing homosexuality, pornography, prostitution, incest, rape, and human sexual response? Can you be objective on some of these topics but not on others? (One indication is your degree of emotional response when discussing these topics. Of course, this response relates to what you value.)

If you desire to deal successfully with the many topics in this chapter, the skill of understanding is a must. Assess yourself in the three areas listed as well as their interdependence, and, if needed, develop a plan to improve your abilities in each area.

According to a report sponsored by the U.S. government (*Report of the Commission on Obscenity and Pornography* 1970) and a review of this report (Money and Athanasiou 1973), the following conclusions were made: convicted sex offenders generally have been exposed to *less* pornographic and sexuality education materials during their lives than many "nonoffenders"; exposure to pornographic materials does not seem to alter a person's sexual behavior in the long run; and a person is only stimulated by portrayal of ideas or acts that turned him or her on in the first place—that is, pornographic materials do not seem to plant ideas in the mind that were not there all along. In addition, there is little, if any, difference in the response of males and females to pornographic materials, and continued exposure to pornographic material tends to lead to boredom and indifference.

In contrast to the 1970 commission study, in July 1986 the Attorney General's Commission on Pornography (often called the Meese Commission after Attorney General Edwin Meese) published its 1,960-page report, which linked hard-core pornography to sex crimes and made ninety-two recommendations for federal, state, and local governments to crack down on the $8 billion industry in the United States. Many experts have questioned the findings of the Meese Commission. For example, the Society for the Scientific Study of Sex indicated that the commission's "evidence for a direct link between exposure to sexually explicit material, pornography, or violent pornography to consequences such as sexual violence, sexual coercion, or rape [is] incomplete and inadequate" ("SSSS Sees Meese Commission as Having Dire Effect on Future Sex Research" 1986). Many opposed to the commission's conclusions strongly indicate that it is not sex but violence that is an obscenity in our society (Donnerstein and Linz 1986).

There are many and varied opinions about pornography. Some religious groups indicate that it propagates perverse sexual behavior and is immoral. Some women believe it promotes the power of males or leads to teenage psychological problems. On the other hand, producers of pornography argue that their products have positive effects. Many individuals purchase pornography for use in the privacy of their homes and cannot understand why a private matter is a public problem (Leong 1991).

There is no debate, however, when it comes to the topic of child pornography. Unanimous opposition to this form of pornography is apparent.

Summary

1. Limerence is the quality of sexual attraction based on chemistry and sexual desire.

2. Human sexual response is predictable and consists of certain phases.

3. A series of biological changes occurs in each phase of human sexual response.

4. Many variations of sexual behavior exist. Variations in sexual practice include masturbation, oral-genital contact, and sodomy.

5. Psychosexual variations include voyeurism, exhibitionism, troilism, fetishism, transvestism, frottage, masochism, sadism, nymphomania, bestiality, and transsexualism.

6. Many myths exist about homosexuality, and some individuals have strong feelings about homosexual behavior.

7. Sexual abuse incudes obscene phone calling, rape, pedophilia, incest, and sexual harassment.

8. Date rape is the most common form of rape.

9. Commercial sexual behavior includes prostitution and use of pornography.

Commitment Activities

1. Because scientific knowledge about human sexual response has become available only recently, you already know more about human sexual response (having read this chapter) than most people. Here's a chance to apply your knowledge in a practical way.

   Assume that a fourteen-year-old boy shares with you his concern about the way he feels when reading sexually oriented books, looking at sexually explicit pictures, or while on a date. He is wondering if there is something wrong with him because of the way his body seems to react. What would you tell him? Suppose a girl of a similar age and with similar concerns comes to you. What would you tell her?

2. Many feelings exist about variations in sexual behavior. We often find it hard to be objective about sexual behaviors we don't understand or agree with. Evaluate your own feelings about the many sexual behaviors discussed in this chapter. Are they based on emotions or facts? From now on, try to better understand the feelings and behaviors of others and also be more sensitive to your own negative feelings about certain sexual behaviors.

3. Services exist in most communities for survivors of sexual abuse. It helps to know about them in the event you or someone you care about needs them. Evaluate the services for survivors of sexual abuse in the community in which you live or attend college. Be sure to include services of law enforcement agencies, hospitals, clinics, health departments, and voluntary groups. Which services would you recommend to someone who needs them?

4. Various community services are available for those with concerns or problems related to human sexual response, sexual orientation, or other aspects of sexual behavior discussed in this chapter. Make a list of such services available on your campus and in the community. Learn about each of the services. Which ones would you recommend to a friend who needs help?

5. Incest is a problem in most societies. Many experts think the best answer to this problem is prevention. Develop a plan for the prevention of incest. Be sure to include components that might be used in school and community educational programs.

6. Over the next weeks, spend some time each day clarifying where you believe you are on the continuum between exclusive heterosexuality and exclusive homosexuality. How comfortable do you feel about your position? What can you do about it?

References

Abbey, A. "Acquaintance Rape and Alcohol Consumption on College Campuses: How Are They Linked?" *Journal of American College Health* 39 (January 1991):165–69.

"Acquaintance Rape: Is Dating Dangerous?" American College Health Association pamphlet, 1986.

Darling, C. A.; Davidson, J. K; and Conway-Welch, C. "Female Ejaculation: Perceived Origins, the Grafenberg Spot/Area and Sexual Responsiveness." *Archives of Sexual Behavior* 19, no. 1 (February 1990):29–47.

Darling, C. A.; Davidson, J. K.; and Jennings, D. A. "The Female Sexual Response Revisited: Understanding the Multiorgasmic Experience in Women." *Archives of Sexual Behavior* 20, no. 6 (December 1991):527–40.

"Date Rape Is Occurring Too Often, AU Professor Says." *Birmingham News,* March 23, 1987, p. 3b.

Davidson, J. K.; Darling, C. A.; and Conway-Welch, C. "The Role of the Grafenberg Spot and Female Ejaculation in the Female Orgasmic Response: An Empirical Analysis." *Journal of Sex and Marital Therapy* 15, no. 2 (Summer 1989):102–18.

DeVisto, P.; Kaufman, A.; Rosner, L.; Jackson, R.; Christy, J.; Pearson, S.; and Burgett, T. "The Prevalence of Sexually Stressful Events among Females in the General Population." *Archives of Sexual Behavior* 13 (1984):269–76.

Donnerstein, E. I., and Linz, D. G. "The Question of Pornography." *Psychology Today* 20, no. 12 (1986): 56–59.

Edell, D. "Sex Ruled Safe for Sports." *Edell Health Letter* 9, no. 4 (April 1990):3.

Fein, J. *Are You a Target?* Belmont, Calif.: Wadsworth, 1981, pp. 2–3.

Flax, E. "New Study Links Past Sex Abuse, Teenage Pregnancy." *Education Week* 11, no. 24 (March 4, 1992):9.

Greenberg, J.; Bruess, C.; and Mullen, K. *Sexuality: Insights and Issues.* Dubuque, Iowa: Wm. C. Brown Publishers, 1993.

Gruber, J. E. "How Women Handle Sexual Harassment," *Sociology and Social Research* 72, no. 1 (October 1989):306.

"G Spot/Female Ejaculation Researchers Vindicated by New Research." *Sexuality Today* 9, no. 5 (May 1983):1, 3.

Heller, S. "Scholar Finds Cross-Dressing Is a Central Part of Human Culture." *Chronicle of Higher Education* 38, no. 20 (January 22, 1992):A7–A8.

Hynes, J. "Prostitution: Creative Programming for a Vulnerable Profession." *Sexuality Today* 6, no. 15 (January 31, 1983):1.

"Intrafamily Sexual Abuse—Incest." *Family Life Educator* (Winter 1982):12–14.

Johnston, S. A. "The Mind of a Molester." *Psychology Today* 21, no. 2 (February 1987):60–64.

Kaplan, H. S. *Disorders of Sexual Desire.* New York: Simon and Schuster, 1979.

Kohn, A. "Shattered Innocence." *Psychology Today* 21, no. 2 (February 1987):54–64.

Leong, W. "The Pornography 'Problem': Disciplining Women and Young Girls." *Media, Culture, and Society* 13 (1991):91–117.

Lisak, D. "Sexual Aggression, Masculinity, and Fathers." *Signs: Journal of Women in Culture and Society* 16, no. 2 (1991):238–63.

Lizotte, A. J. "The Uniqueness of Rape: Reporting Assaultive Violence to the Police." *Crime and Delinquency* 31, no. 2 (April 1985):169–90.

Mahoney, E. "Editor's Note," *Current Research Updates* 2 (1984):8–12.

Masters, W. H., and Johnson, V. E. *Human Sexual Response.* Boston: Little, Brown, 1966.

Mims, F., Chang, A. "Unwanted Sexual Experiences of Young Women." *Psychosocial Nursing* 22 (1984):7–14.

Money, J., and Athanasiou, R. "Pornography: Review and Bibliographic Notations." *American Journal of Obstetrics and Gynecology* 115 (January 1973):130–46.

Nightingale, R. "Adolescent Prostitution." *Seminars in Adolescent Medicine* 1, no. 3 (September 1985):165–70.

Olson, M. "A Collaborative Approach to the Prevention of Child Sexual Abuse." *Victimology: An International Journal* 10, nos. 1–4 (1985):131–39.

"One in Twelve Sexually Abused Boys May Be Getting Professional Attention." *Sexuality Today* 3 (May 1982):1.

Report of the Commission on Obscenity and Pornography. Washington, D.C.: U.S. Government Printing Office, 1970.

Seligmann, J. "The Date Who Rapes." *Newsweek* (April 9, 1984):91–92.

Shavlik, D. "A Time for Change." *Higher Education and National Affairs* 41, no. 10 (May 18, 1992):5.

"SSSS Sees Meese Commission as Having Dire Effect on Future Sex Research." *Sexuality Today* 9, no. 36 (June 23, 1986): 2–3.

Tanzman, E. S. "Unwanted Sexual Activity: The Prevalence in College Women." *Journal of American College Health* 406, no. 4 (January 1992):167–71.

Tennov, D. *Love and Limerence.* Chelsea, Mich.: Scarborough House, 1989, pp. 45–50.

Thornton, J. S. "Sexual Activity and Athletic Performance: Is There A Relationship? *The Physician and Sportsmedicine* 18, no. 2 (March 1990):148–54.

Ward, S. K.; Chapman, K.; Cohn, E.; White, S.; and Williams, K. "Acquaintance Rape and the College Social Scene." *Family Relations* 40 (January 1991):65–71.

Williams, L. S. "The Classic Rape: When Do Victims Report?" *Social Problems* 31, no. 4 (April 1984):459–67.

Zilbergeld, B., and Ellison, C. R. "Desire Discrepancies and Arousal Problems in Sex Therapy." In *Principles and Practice of Sex Therapy.* Ed. R. Lieblum and L. A. Pervin. New York: Guilford, 1980.

Additional Readings

Craig, M. E. "Coercive Sexuality in Dating Relationships: A Situational Model." *Clinical Psychology Review* 10 (1990):395–423. Provides a literature review related to coercive sexual behavior and presents a situational model to help explain coercive sexual behavior during dating situations.

Donnerstein, E. "Pornography: Reserach and Policy in a Free Society." *Contemporary Psychology* 36, no. 2 (1991):160–61. Provides an overview of research on pornography.

Friedman, J. "The Impact of Homophobia on Male Sexual Development." *SIECUS Report* 17, no. 5 (May/June 1989):8–9. The author points out that homophobia makes the passage of young males from childhood into adulthood very traumatic. He describes an ideal atmosphere for transition that would benefit everyone.

Herbert, T. B.; Silver, R. C.; and Ellard, J. H. "Coping With An Abusive Relationship: How and Why Do Women Stay?" *Journal of Marriage and the Family* 53, no. 2 (May 1991):311–25. Presents information about ways women cope with physical and emotional abuse while remaining with their abusive partners. This information helps develop an understanding of why women stay.

CHAPTER 8

Conception and Birth and Their Control

One of the most crucial life-cycle phases is the childbearing years. Any decision about heterosexual intercourse almost always involves questions about having children. Among the most critical consumer health decisions made are whether to have children and when, whether to use contraception and if so what type, and what should be done if an unwanted pregnancy occurs.

Conception: An Overview

Conception is the fertilization of a female's egg by a male's sperm, which results in pregnancy. Two conditions are necessary for conception to take place: (1) a mature egg must be in a position to be fertilized and (2) the sperm must reach the egg.

Conception and Birth Health Assessment

The first assessment is for females and the second assessment is for males regarding premenstrual syndrome (PMS). The third assessment is for committed couples who have had children, are currently expecting a child, or want to have children.

Female Assessment

Section A

Females, please check those items you feel or experience just prior to your menstrual period.

_____ I feel as though I am out of breath.

_____ My nose bleeds for no reason.

_____ My abdomen feels bloated.

_____ My breasts are sore.

_____ I get mouth sores or my mouth gets dry.

_____ I develop cold sores.

_____ My legs hurt or have cramps.

_____ I feel dizzy or have fainting spells.

_____ I feel like I am shaking inside.

_____ I get sharp pains.

_____ My skin itches and burns.

_____ My joints hurt, swell, or feel stiff.

_____ I get diarrhea or constipation.

_____ I get bad headaches.

_____ I get food cravings.

_____ I get backaches.

_____ Noise or light bothers me.

_____ I get clumsy and drop or bump into things.

_____ I feel fat or ugly.

_____ I feel all alone in the world.

_____ I cry for no reason.

_____ Nothing can cheer me up.

_____ I am really crabby.

_____ I feel like committing suicide.

_____ I get really angry.

_____ I feel I am a failure.

_____ I think I am going crazy.

_____ I'm tired and have no energy.

_____ People are out to get me.

_____ I am extremely afraid.

_____ I am out of control.

_____ I can't get anything done.

_____ I just can't laugh.

_____ I just want to be alone.

_____ No one listens to me.

_____ I can't concentrate.

Section B

Females, mark those items that apply to you.

_____ I rarely eat sweets or chocolate.

_____ I do not drink coffee, tea, caffeinated beverages, or take over-the-counter stimulants.

_____ I do not drink alcohol.

_____ I usually get seven to eight hours of sleep at night.

_____ I exercise thirty minutes or more, three to four times a week or more.

_____ I get plenty of vitamins through natural sources or take vitamin supplements (particularly B-6).

_____ I avoid excessive stress (check results of stress assessment in stress management chapter).

_____ I eat four to six small, well-balanced meals daily.

Interpretation

Section A is a symptom checklist for PMS. If you checked any of the symptoms because you are not as functional as normal and, in severe cases, very debilitated, then you may suffer from PMS.

Section B is a list of things that you can do to lessen the impact of PMS. If there are any items you have not checked, you may want to adopt that habit to see if the discomfort can be lessened.

Male Assessment

Read the list of symptoms in section A and note whether anyone you know demonstrates any of those symptoms just prior to her period. Respond to the following assessment items in reference to that person. Check all of the following items that apply to you.

_____ I feel sorry for someone who experiences some of those symptoms.

_____ I try to be more understanding during the time just before and during her period.

_____ Because I know that hormones are affecting her, I can deal with her problem and not let it bother me.

_____ I try to avoid fights and do not discuss important decisions or resolve arguments during this time in her life.

_____ I know that she really doesn't mean some of the things she says while she is feeling bad so I don't let it bother me.

Interpretation

If you did not think of anyone who experienced any symptoms, then there are no results to be given. If you did think of someone, then it is important for you to consider the items you did not check. It is extremely important that you understand, have compassion, easily forgive, and help the person you know through this time that males have difficulty understanding. If you did not check all items, then you are lacking in your ability to help and cope with PMS as a support person.

Committed Couples Assessment

If you have had children, are currently expecting a child, or want to have children, respond to the following checklist. Mark all items that apply to you.

1. If as a couple you have tried to become pregnant and can't, check all of the following that apply. If you do not know or haven't tried, skip to item 2.

    ____ We have had complete physicals and know the cause of our problems (if you have not checked this item, then skip to item 2).

    ____ We have considered adopting children.

    ____ We have considered artificial insemination.

    ____ We have considered foster children.

    ____ We have received professional counseling on this matter.

2. If you ever plan to have children or are pregnant, check all that apply.

    ____ We have considered a Lamaze delivery.

    ____ We have considered a Leboyer delivery.

    ____ We have selected a physician or midwife with whom we are comfortable.

    ____ We have decided that the male will accompany the female during delivery.

    ____ We have chosen a hospital or home delivery that has the options we want (rooming-in, birthing rooms, and so on).

    ____ We have talked as a couple about the pros and cons of breast-feeding versus bottle feeding.

    ____ We have reviewed our family histories for any genetic diseases (e.g., diabetes) for which we might be carriers or know we have.

    ____ We have received genetic counseling (only if you have a history of a genetic disease).

3. Which of the following apply to you as a couple if you have children or want to have children someday.

    ____ The female partner smokes.

    ____ The male partner smokes.

    ____ The female drinks alcohol.

    ____ The female takes drugs.

    ____ The male takes drugs.

    ____ The female eats a well-balanced diet with plenty of iron and calcium (see nutrition chapter for details).

Interpretation

Item 1 is a checklist for couples who desire to get pregnant but can't. If any of the items are blank, then you may want to consider acting on that item.

Item 2 is a checklist for couples to discuss prior to having children or during pregnancy. If you have not talked about any of the items, then perhaps you should do so.

Item 3 is an important list of behaviors that increase the risk of birth defects or other problems. If you are performing any of the behaviors, then your risk of having problems is increased. If you have multiple factors, then the risk greatly increases with each item and with dosages or lack of good nutrition.

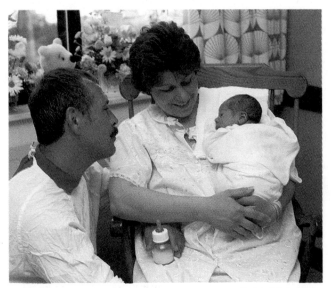

Many health decisions relate to pregnancy and childbirth.

The Menstrual Cycle

Sometime during puberty, a girl reaches **menarche;** that is, she begins to *menstruate*. **Menstruation** is the periodic discharge of blood from the **uterus** through the **vagina.** There are many myths about menstruation, including that a permanent wave will not take during menstruation, sexual intercourse should not occur during menstruation, women should not swim or exercise during menstruation, and women cannot carry on usual work activity during the menstrual period. None of these statements is true.

The **menstrual cycle** lasts approximately twenty-eight days, although cycles vary in length from woman to woman and even for the same woman at different times. Figure 8.1 illustrates the phases of this cycle. No matter how many days the cycle lasts, the first day of menstrual flow (which usually lasts about five days) is counted as the first day of the cycle. During the flow, hormonal (chemical) action that affects the upcoming cycle begins. The pituitary gland secretes **follicle-stimulating hormone (FSH),**

Contraceptive Behavior Assessment

Perhaps the most important aspect of this chapter is your sense of values and what you believe is right or wrong, particularly as it relates to sexual behavior, responsibility, human life, and when you feel life begins. Here you consider some very important questions that may help you to be in control and responsible and live in accordance with your sense of values.

1. Which of the following best describes you? (Mark all that apply.)
   a. single, never married
   b. married
   c. divorced
   d. widowed
   e. separated
2. Which of the following best describes your feelings about sexual intercourse? (Select one response.)
   a. It's okay to have sexual intercourse with anyone you would like to if both partners think it's okay.
   b. It's only okay to have sexual intercourse with someone after you know him or her well and really love the person.
   c. It's only okay to have sexual intercourse with someone after you have married him or her.
3. When do you think life begins? (Pick the closest time.)
   a. before fertilization (egg and sperm separate)
   b. when the egg is fertilized
   c. when the egg implants in the uterus
   d. when the heart begins to beat
   e. sometime between when the heart begins to beat and birth
   f. at birth
   g. after birth (systems stable)
4. Which of the following best describes your feelings? (Mark all that apply.)
   a. If I make a mistake, then I am responsible for the consequences.
   b. If I make a mistake, then I'll try not to do it again, but I'm really not responsible for the consequences.
   c. When I believe something is right, then I'll do it no matter what.
5. Which of the following best describes your behavior?
   a. I am sexually active. (When sexual opportunities come along, I will have intercourse with someone under the right conditions.)
   b. I have never had sexual intercourse, or I have in the past but I no longer have sexual intercourse.
6. Which of the following methods of birth control do you feel are wrong?
   a. Methods that are natural (abstinence, rhythm).
   b. Methods that act before fertilization (spermicides, condoms, birth-control pills, and so on).
   c. Operations that act before fertilization (tubal ligation or vasectomy).
   d. methods that act after fertilization (IUD, morning-after pill).
   e. Methods that work after implantation and growth begins (abortion techniques).

Evaluation

The method of evaluation for this assessment is somewhat different than assessment tools in other chapters. This evaluation deals with value-behavioral congruence. When your values and behaviors are congruent (what you believe is what you do), then you avoid negative emotions and guilt. Look at the assessment tool and see if you have any of the listed incongruencies.

First compare your answers to numbers 3 and 6. If you believe life begins at fertilization, for example, any method of contraception that acts after fertilization or abortion should be avoided because your belief system would imply that you are taking a life. On the other hand, if you believe that life begins at birth, then any contraceptive or abortive method is within your value system. Check for congruencies by making sure that the contraceptive or abortive methods you use (if you use them) are within your values limitations.

Check numbers 1 and 2 together and then check number 5. If you are single, for example, and checked number 2c, and if number 5 is marked a, then there is value-behavioral incongruence.

Check number 4 and number 5 together. If you checked number 4a, which indicates responsibility, and number 5a indicating sexual activity, and then checked number 6b, c, and d, then maybe you should consider abstinence unless you are able to face consequences.

You can check other areas for incongruence. There are many potential areas. The point of this evaluation is to align your values and behaviors so that you are guilt free, do not make errors forcing you into responsibilities that you do not want, and are happy.

---

which travels through the bloodstream and stimulates one of the **follicles,** the small sacs that contain a developing egg cell, in a female's ovary to grow. As the stimulated follicle grows in size, the egg inside of it begins to mature. There are actually thousands of follicles in a female's **ovary** (all of which are present at birth), so clearly most eggs never come to maturity (and a woman will never run out of eggs).

About the time the flow ends, the follicle stimulated by FSH begins to secrete the second **hormone** of the cycle, **estrogen.** As the estrogen level increases, it signals the lining of the uterus to thicken and become a hospitable place for a possible fertilized egg. The rising level of estrogen in the bloodstream also stimulates the pituitary gland to secrete a third hormone, **luteinizing hormone (LH),** into the bloodstream. The increased level of LH in the

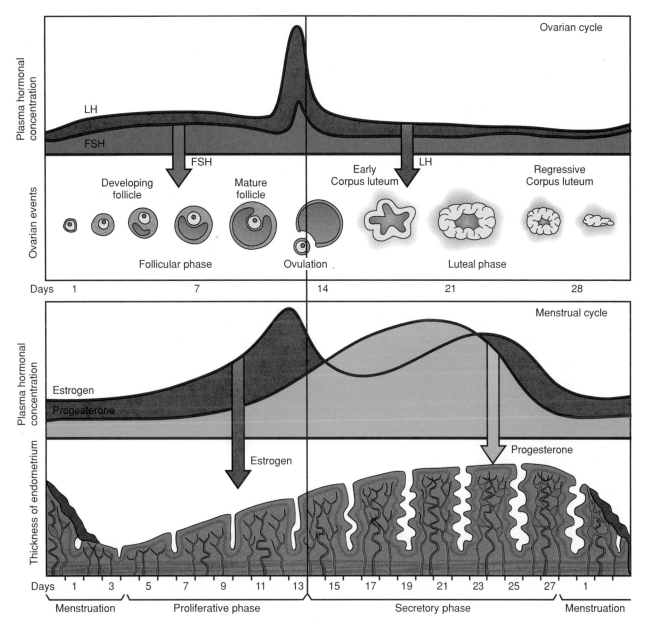

Figure 8.1

Major events in the female ovarian and menstrual cycles.

From John W. Hole, Jr., *Human Anatomy and Physiology,* 5th ed. Copyright © 1990 Wm. C. Brown Publishers, Dubuque, Iowa. All Rights Reserved. Reprinted by permission.

blood then causes the follicle to release the mature egg. This process of egg release is called **ovulation.**

Many individuals assume that ovulation occurs in the middle of the cycle. Most experts believe that ovulation actually occurs about fourteen days before the onset of menstruation. So it is impossible to tell exactly when ovulation occurred until fourteen days after the event! This makes calculations of fertile times difficult. There is no problem if a woman has a twenty-eight-day cycle; she simply figures fourteen days forward or backward from the onset of menstruation. But if a woman has a longer cycle, say thirty-three days, then ovulation occurs not in the "middle" of her cycle but closer to the end.

The average egg lives about thirty-six hours. In the example, the woman with the longer cycle would begin to ovulate on perhaps the nineteenth day of her cycle, and the egg would remain alive until sometime on the twentieth day. The maximum life of a male sperm, however, is about seventy-two hours; so the sixteenth through the twentieth day of the cycle would be the prime fertilization time in this case. Remember, however, that cycles vary tremendously, and the onset of menstruation varies for each woman within her cycle, so the time of potential fertilization is actually much longer than this. Even dietary changes can influence menstruation ("Diet Affects Menstrual Cycle" 1992/93).

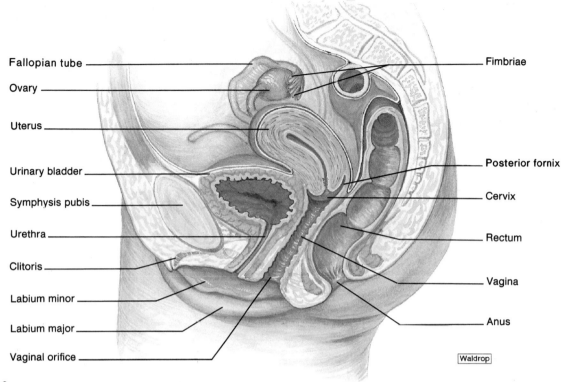

Figure 8.2

Cross section of the female reproductive system.

After ovulation, the egg is sucked into the opening of the **oviduct,** or **fallopian tube** (figs. 8.2 and 8.3). The follicle continues to produce estrogen, and the level of LH also increases. Because of the high level of LH, the tissue of the follicle changes color and begins to produce the fourth hormone of the cycle, **progesterone.** At this point, the follicle is called the corpus luteum.

The combined secretions of estrogen and progesterone continue to cause the **endometrium,** or lining of the uterus, to thicken. In addition, the presence of hormones prevents the release of another egg, which prevents women from conceiving a second time within a few days of the first fertilization. If a woman becomes pregnant, these hormones remain present at a relatively high level; if she does not, the levels of estrogen and progesterone fall. This decrease in hormonal level brings about the menstrual flow (the total flow amounts to only around four tablespoons), and the entire process starts over. An unfertilized egg is simply removed from the body by the menstrual flow.

The Course of the Sperm

Just as women are born with far more eggs than will ever come to maturity, men are provided with the capacity to produce millions of sperm each day, only an infinitesimal number of which are used. **Sperm** are produced in the **seminiferous tubules** in the **testes.** These seminiferous

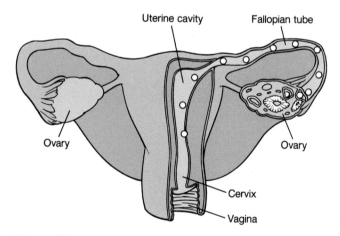

Figure 8.3

Female internal reproductive organs.

tubules produce sperm through the combined hormonal action of follicle-stimulating hormone (FSH) and **testosterone.** Mature sperm are stored in the **epididymis** before traveling through the **vas deferens** in preparation for **ejaculation.** Figures 8.4 and 8.5 show the location of these organs.

As the sperm pass through the vas deferens, they are joined by fluid secretions from the **seminal vesicles.** This fluid consists mainly of fructose, a simple sugar that

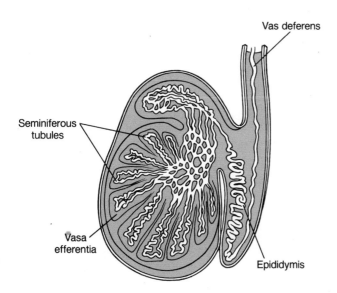

Figure 8.4
Cross section of testis.

provides nutrition for sperm. As the sperm and fluid continue their journey towards ejaculation, the **prostate gland** adds several chemical substances that help neutralize the acid in the vagina as well as possibly assist the sperm if they attempt to fertilize an egg.

The fluid mixture still needs one more secretion before it is completely prepared for ejaculation. The final fluid comes from the **bulbourethral glands,** also called **Cowper's glands.** This fluid lubricates and chemically neutralizes the **urethra** before sperm pass through. This is necessary because urination acidifies the urethra and the sperm need a neutralized passageway to survive the voyage.

Assuming the sperm are ejaculated into a vagina and no contraceptive measures are used, they set out in search of an egg to fertilize. Most of the millions of sperm

ejaculated do not survive the expedition. A few dozen probably reach the egg, if one is ready. Scientists believe that the first sperm to penetrate the egg may create a chemical change that shuts out all other surviving sperm. The head of this sperm proceeds to the center of the egg, where **chromosomes,** that part of cells containing hereditary factors, from the egg and the sperm become knitted together within a few hours. At this time, all inherited traits of the baby are determined, and the egg is now fertilized.

The union of a sperm and an egg produces a single cell called the **zygote.** The zygote begins to divide about thirty hours after fertilization. It splits into two cells, and then these two cells split into four cells, eight cells, and so on. The unborn child is called an **embryo** from approximately one to eight weeks after fertilization and a **fetus** thereafter.

Infertility

Just as many couples want to prevent conception, others wish to enhance their chances. For those who want children, **infertility**—the inability to reproduce—can be distressing. Infertility affects 15 percent to 20 percent of married couples in the United States, and its incidence is increasing (Higgins 1990).

Causes of Infertility

The cause of infertility can be psychological. For example, anxiety related to intercourse may result in sexual dysfunction in males or in muscular spasms that obstruct the fallopian tubes in females. Infertility can also be caused by physical barriers separating sperm from an **ovum** (the female egg), the failure of successful implantation of the fertilized egg in the uterus, or problems in the normal development of the embryo.

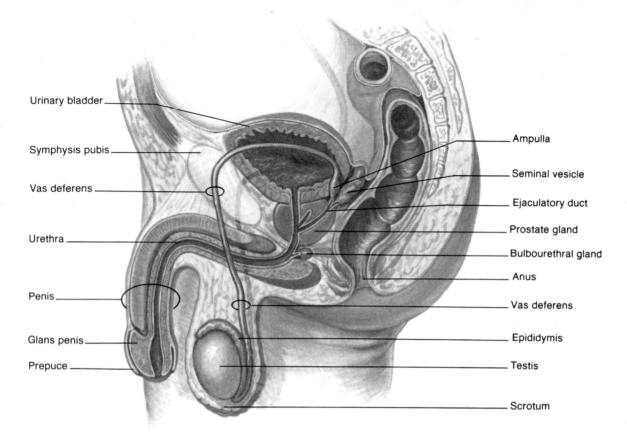

Figure 8.5

Cross section of the male reproductive system.

From John W. Hole, Jr., *Human Anatomy and Physiology*, 5th ed. Copyright © 1990 Wm. C. Brown Publishers, Dubuque, Iowa. All Rights Reserved. Reprinted by permission.

If a male's ejaculate contains fewer than twenty million sperm cells (a condition called **oligospermia,** or low sperm count), the chances of conception are not good. In addition, if the sperm does not effectively neutralize acid in the urethra or vagina, conception may be impossible. Blocked fallopian tubes, dysfunctional ovaries, an improperly functioning uterus, or inappropriate hormonal functioning, which can even be caused by drastic changes in body weight ("Infertility as a Function of Body Weight" 1992), in the woman can also lead to infertility.

Infertility can cause personal problems and problems in relationships. In addition, the loss of sexual pleasure can occur along with grief, anger, guilt, and depression (Higgins 1990).

Treatment of Infertility

If there is difficulty conceiving, it is wise to get a medical examination to determine the cause of the infertility. The male's medical examination focuses on sperm production and delivery. The female's medical examination assesses regularity of ovulation, the condition of the cervical mucus (e.g., the mucus could contain antibodies against a

male's sperm or could form a plug that blocks the passage of sperm), and the possible presence of infections or scar tissue.

If the cause of infertility is medical and identifiable, procedures involving hormonal, chemical, nutritional, or surgical therapy are available to correct the situation. As an example of medical capabilities in this area, consider the 1978 birth of the first "test-tube baby." In this instance, the mother's fallopian tubes were blocked, preventing sperm from reaching and fertilizing an ovum; therefore, an egg was surgically removed from the mother and fertilized by sperm from the father outside their bodies. The fertilized egg was then implanted in the mother's uterus for development and eventual birth.

A procedure sometimes used by infertile couples is **artificial insemination.** In cases where a male's sperm count is not high enough or he cannot complete coitus, an unknown male donor can provide sperm, which is introduced via a syringe into the woman's vagina. If a male's sperm count is consistently low, or if for some other reason the sperm cannot fertilize an egg through sexual intercourse, another remedy is to collect samples of sperm over the course of several days and then instill the whole

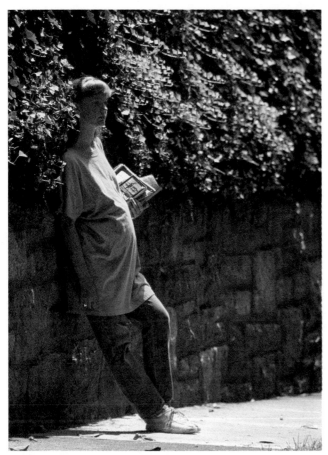

Teenage pregnancy is more common in the United States than in other Western countries.

amount at the cervical opening. This is done in a physician's office as close to ovulation as possible.

If a donor is used, he is screened for health, intelligence, and physical resemblance to the father. A potential hazard of using donor sperm is the transmission of viral illness, including AIDS. Semen can be screened, like blood, however, for the presence of AIDS antibodies.

Many couples unable to become pregnant have happily sought artificial insemination using an unknown donor. Assuming that the female's reproductive system is functioning properly, these couples can experience a pregnancy together and know that the child carries at least the genes of the mother. Some people, however, feel that artificial insemination is immoral and inappropriately meddles with human nature. Do you think artificial insemination should be used?

In some cases, drugs, commonly called "fertility drugs," can be used to stimulate ovulation. These drugs can be helpful, but they also seem to cause more multiple births. For example, from the early 1970s until 1989, multiple births increased by 113 percent (from 29 to 62 per 100,000 live births) in white mothers and 25 percent (from 32 to 40 per 100,000 live births) in black mothers. These increases are thought to be a direct result of fertility drugs (Kiely 1992).

Psychological causes of infertility should be treated with professional psychosexual counseling. Great advances in such counseling have been made in recent years.

Pregnancy

Parents can and do take an active role in both their own health and that of their unborn child because of increased knowledge about factors influencing a healthy pregnancy and available options in delivery methods. Pregnancy-related decisions that years ago were not even considered are now quite necessary, as well as quite complex. More and more women are waiting until they are in their thirties—or even later—to have a baby, and there is good news for them. There is no evidence that these older women have an increased risk of having a preterm delivery, a smaller infant or one with developmental problems, or an infant who dies during pregnancy. Because of medical advances, the few pregnancy-related problems that might occur in older women are readily manageable. Given sound counseling and appropriate prenatal care, the increasing number of older women having babies can look forward to normal deliveries and healthy babies (Berkowitz et al. 1990; Resnik 1990).

While it is possible for teenagers to have healthy babies, there are a number of problems associated with teen pregnancy. Teenage pregnancy in the United States is far more common than in other Western countries—even though girls in the United States do not engage in sexual intercourse earlier or more frequently than girls in other countries. If the present rates continue, four in ten girls who are fourteen years old will become pregnant before they are twenty. Every thirty seconds a teenage girl becomes pregnant in the United States (Sroka 1991). The teenage pregnancy rate stayed relatively constant throughout the 1980s—110 pregnancies per 1,000 girls (Portnes 1992).

Teen mothers face reduced employment opportunities, unstable marriages (if they occur at all), low incomes, and increased health and developmental risks to their children. Sustained poverty, frustration, and hopelessness are often the long-term outcomes. The national costs of health and social service programs for families started by teenagers amount to more than $19 billion a year (Wattleton 1989).

There are other tragic consequences associated with teenage pregnancy. Teenage mothers usually drop out of school and are unable to find jobs to support their children, unmarried teenage fathers rarely contribute financially to their children's support, and teenage marriages are at high risk for divorce. In addition, teenage mothers are more likely to have birth complications and are less likely to receive adequate prenatal care. Low birth weights and premature births, which can lead to problems such as childhood illnesses, neurological defects, and mental retardation, are common with teenage mothers (Stark 1986; "March of Dimes Fact Sheet" 1991).

Reducing Teen Pregnancies

It is clear that too many teenage girls are getting pregnant. U.S. teenagers have one of the highest pregnancy rates in the world—twice as high as in England, Wales, France, and Canada; three times as high as in Sweden; and seven times as high as in the Netherlands ("Teenage Sexual and Reproductive Behavior" 1991). The best way to reduce teen pregnancies is to be more open about them. There should be more open discussions and better access to accurate information. This includes information about contraception and free access to contraceptives. Only when it becomes more acceptable for teenagers to use reliable contraceptives will we reduce the teen pregnancy problem.

- **Pro:** This is the only rational approach. No matter what is done, a significant number of teenagers will participate in sexual intercourse. Regardless of how we feel about this, the problem of pregnancy must be faced. Open access to reliable contraceptives for teenagers would reduce teen pregnancies.

- **Con:** Open access to contraceptives for teenagers implies that it is acceptable for them to participate in intercourse. It would be better to emphasize why they should not participate and the problems associated with teen pregnancy. If teenagers better understood these problems, there would not be so many teen pregnancies.

How should teen pregnancies be reduced?

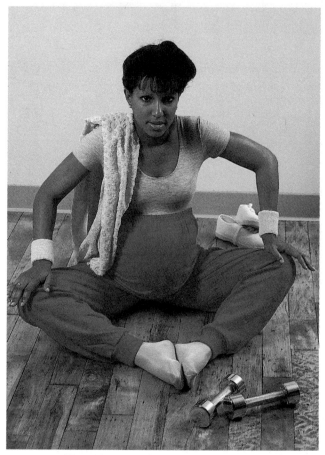

Good prenatal care is important for both mother and child.

Determination of Pregnancy

Pregnancy begins when an egg is fertilized by a sperm and is successfully implanted in the endometrium, or uterine wall, to be nourished. Pregnancy can be determined by several means. The most frequently used technique is to test the urine for the presence of **human chorionic gonadotropin (HCG),** a hormone produced by the placenta once implantation has occurred. Although pregnancy can be chemically determined as early as ten days after conception, most pregnancy tests are conducted about six to eight weeks after the last menstrual flow. When conducted and analyzed by a physician or laboratory technician, these tests are very reliable.

Pregnancy self-tests are increasingly available. These tests, which can be purchased at drugstores, are not recommended: the kits are difficult to use properly, and their negative findings are unreliable. In controlled tests, the accuracy of the kits ranged from 45.7 percent to 89.1 percent, depending on how early after a missed period the tests were performed (Doshi 1986).

Physicians have sophisticated equipment and tests that can detect pregnancy very early. One of these, sonography, which gives an image of uterine and other changes associated with pregnancy, detects pregnancy within just a few weeks of conception ("Transvaginal Sonography Detects Early Pregnancy" 1992).

Environmental and Genetic Influences: Prenatal Care

The first three months of pregnancy are the most important in the embryo's development. For this reason, if a woman suspects she is pregnant, she must act as though she is and seek **prenatal care.** Many factors can influence the health of the mother and the child. Even stress can produce major problems, such as premature delivery and low birth weight ("Stress during Pregnancy Linked to Premature Delivery" 1985).

Today, more prevention-oriented activities, such as positive health practices for a woman and her developing baby, are encouraged. More and more the emphasis is placed on the quality of behavior and care and not just on the importance of a certain number of visits to the doctor. In fact, the American College of Obstetricians and Gynecologists recommends a reduction in the thirteen traditional visits to seven for healthy women who have previously had babies and nine for healthy women experiencing their first pregnancy (Young 1990).

About 1 percent to 1.68 percent of pregnancies are **ectopic pregnancies**—implantation occurs outside the uterus. The embryo may attach itself to an ovary, one of the abdominal organs, or, most commonly, inside one of the fallopian tubes. Ectopic pregnancy should be suspected when a sexually active woman's period is a week late and she experiences abdominal pain. Other possible symptoms include absence of menstruation, vaginal bleeding, nausea, vomiting, and dizziness.

The incidence of ectopic pregnancy has quadrupled since 1970. Now there is one for every sixty-five to seventy normal pregnancies. Risk factors for ectopic pregnancy include previous ectopic pregnancy, current intrauterine device use, prior fallopian tube surgery, previous pelvic inflammatory disease, and a prior history of infertility—particularly if there has been surgery to correct blocked fallopian tubes. All of these conditions can damage the lining of the fallopian tube so the egg and sperm can't be transported to the uterus. Ectopic pregnancies are now the leading cause of maternal death.

Sources: "Ectopic Pregnancies Now Leading Cause of Death" in *Sexuality Today* 24:4, September 1984; and Richard E. Leach and Steven J. Ory, "Management of Ectopic Pregnancy" in *American Family Physician* 41(4): 1215–1218, April 1990.

Environmental Teratogens

Many factors in the mother's environment are suspected **teratogens,** which are substances that may cause birth defects or diseases in infants. There is a limit to what pregnant women can do to protect themselves from teratogens, but they can refuse chest or abdominal X rays during pregnancy, wear a lead apron during dental X rays, avoid raw meat, stay away from areas where pesticides are sprayed, avoid the use of aerosol containers, and have someone else clean the cat litter box (to avoid catching a defect-causing disease from the droppings).

Rh Incompatibility

Prepregnancy counseling is valuable for many reasons, one of which relates to **Rh incompatibility.** While the likelihood of this causing problems today has been greatly reduced, couples are still wise to reduce any possible risk. Rh incompatibility refers to a situation where the mother's blood is Rh negative (i.e., without an inherited protein substance) and the child's is Rh positive (i.e., with an inherited protein substance). Statistically, this combination is highly unlikely, but a woman with Rh-negative blood must be aware of the possibility. In response to the child's positive Rh factor, the mother's blood develops antibodies that could be harmful to a child's blood in future pregnancies. To remedy this situation, an injection (called Rhogam) that destroys the antibodies is given to an Rh-negative mother within seventy-two hours after delivery. This is done so that the next time she becomes pregnant the antibodies will not develop to a high enough level to do any damage.

Nutrition

Diet during pregnancy is extremely important. If a woman's diet is healthful, she has a much improved chance of remaining healthy during pregnancy and bearing a healthy child. Just because she is eating for two, however, does not mean she should eat twice as much. Only about three hundred extra calories per day are needed.

In general, necessary vitamins are usually provided by a balanced diet that includes milk, bread, and fresh fruits and vegetables. It is particularly important that a pregnant woman get enough protein (for building new tissues), folic acid (for growth), iron (for the blood), and calcium (for growth of the fetal skeleton and tooth buds).

Poor maternal nutrition can lead to slower fetal growth, premature delivery, and low birth weight babies. Prematurity and low birth weight cause higher infant death rates, and malnourished babies with low birth weights may have brain damage and retardation. Pregnant women must remember that they are responsible for the health and nutritional needs of two individuals.

Tobacco, Alcohol, and Other Drugs

About twice as many premature and improperly developed babies are born to women who smoke as compared with women who do not smoke during pregnancy. The exact reason for this is unknown, but one theory holds that smoking during pregnancy prohibits an adequate oxygen supply from reaching the fetus.

Moderate alcohol use can be harmful to the developing fetus, but heavier alcohol use can cause great damage. **Fetal alcohol syndrome (FAS)** includes growth deficiencies before and after birth, damage to the brain and nervous system, and facial abnormalities. Mental retardation is also sometimes found in the children of alcoholic mothers (see also chapter 10 on alcohol).

Almost every drug used by a pregnant woman crosses the placenta and enters the developing baby's circulation. Because it is not always clear which drugs affect the embryo or fetus, even drugs that seem safe should be restricted. Aspirin should be avoided because it can cause fetal bleeding, and tranquilizers can cause fetal malformations.

Pregnant women addicted to drugs such as heroin, barbiturates, cocaine, crack, designer drugs, and amphetamines expose the fetus to many problems. Low birth weight and prematurity can occur, and the baby also becomes addicted, so the first days of life are a difficult time with withdrawal symptoms.

The effects of marijuana smoking on fetal development are unclear. The active chemical ingredients are known to cross the placental barrier, but there is insufficient research to predict the exact effects on the developing fetus. Some research, however, indicates that marijuana may be more damaging to a fetus than alcohol—especially if the mother's overall life-style is unhealthy. Women whose life-styles combine smoking, drinking, marijuana use, and poor eating habits give birth to more infants with characteristics of fetal alcohol syndrome than women who are just heavy drinkers. It is difficult to isolate any single detrimental factor because individuals seldom use or abuse only one substance.

As you can see, many chemical substances can cause great harm during pregnancy, and even decisions about whether to take prescription drugs should be based on current research evidence. It is sensible to avoid any prescription drug unless it is prescribed by a physician aware of the pregnancy.

Physical Activity

Most healthy women can continue their regular physical activity patterns during pregnancy. Traditionally, women were often told to refrain from sports and sexual stimulation during the later stages of pregnancy and for six to eight weeks following delivery. In most cases, however, there is no reason to refrain from general physical exercise or sexual stimulation at any time during a healthy pregnancy. In fact, many researchers recommend regular physical activity, and it has been found that maternal exercise doesn't affect fetal development ("Exercise Through Third Trimester?" 1985). If extreme pain or spotting occurs, a physician should be consulted, but these symptoms are rare.

Many women do find sexual activity in the last weeks of pregnancy to be awkward, and some experience diminished sexual desire towards the end of pregnancy (Bogren 1991). Researchers who studied over fifty-six thousand pregnancies, however, have concluded that sexual activity during pregnancy is safe ("Sex Safe During Pregnancy" 1984). After birth, three factors determine how quickly a female can return to sexually stimulating activities: (1) when she feels like it, (2) when any surgical incision is fully healed, and (3) when all vaginal bleeding or spotting has ceased. Masters and Johnson (1966) found that these three criteria were usually met by the third week following delivery.

Potential Complications

In spite of all precautions, complications may arise for the fetus during pregnancy. One means of detecting fetal abnormalities is by testing the amniotic fluid that surrounds the developing child. The process of extracting the fluid is called **amniocentesis** (*amniotic tap*), but it is not a routine procedure (fig. 8.6). The fluid can be analyzed to detect various diseases, the sex of the child, and the exact age of the child. Amniocentesis is routinely recommended for women in their mid-thirties or older expecting a first or even third or fourth child. In the past, amniocentesis could not be done until the sixteenth week of pregnancy, but now it can be done as early as the eleventh week ("Amniocentesis Now Available in the First Trimester" 1992).

Another technique, **fetoscopy,** allows direct examination of the fetus. Using fetoscopy, physicians can actually see the fetus in the uterus and spot certain physical defects. They can even take blood and tissue from the fetus. After making a small incision in the abdomen, a very thin tube containing a scope with the ability to transmit light enables physicians to see tiny areas of the fetus.

Another means of detecting fetal abnormalities is **chorionic villi sampling (CVS).** Pieces of the villi (thin tissue) protruding from the chorion (outer layer of the amniotic sac) are removed and analyzed for birth defects. One advantage of this technique over amniocentesis is that it can be done eight to nine weeks after conception. One disadvantage is that the risk of spontaneous abortion following amniocentesis is believed to be about 0.5 percent and following CVS it is about 4.4 percent ("CVS Tops Amniocentesis?" 1985).

Ultrasound examinations are also useful during pregnancy. No radiation is used, so ultrasound is believed to be safer than X rays. The test can be used to estimate the fetal age, exclude the possibility of an ectopic pregnancy, guide the needle during amniocentesis, evaluate uterine growth that is not as expected, check for multiple fetuses, evaluate bleeding, check on fetuses at risk for birth defects, and evaluate complications during pregnancy to make sure the fetus is alive ("Ultrasound" 1985).

Finally, to help identify certain birth defects early in pregnancy, screening programs based on a test for **alpha-fetoprotein (AFP)** in the mother's blood are becoming more common. The main object of testing pregnant women for AFP is early detection of neural tube defects. If the neural tube does not form properly, the result can be improper development of the brain and skull, or spina bifida ("split spine"). An abnormal result indicates that more elaborate tests, such as amniocentesis or ultrasound, should be considered ("A New Prenatal Screening Program" 1987).

It is wise for potential parents to also pay attention to hereditary characteristics that can influence the health of a baby. According to the March of Dimes Birth Defects Foundation, 20 percent of birth defects are inherited, 20 percent are environmentally caused, and 60 percent appear to result from an interaction between the two. While it is not routinely done, prospective parents can utilize **genetic counseling** to better understand the hereditary potential of a birth defect (fig. 8.7).

Fortunately, most pregnancies result in the delivery of a healthy baby approximately nine months after conception. As with health in general, making preventive decisions before health problems occur greatly increases the likelihood of a healthy pregnancy.

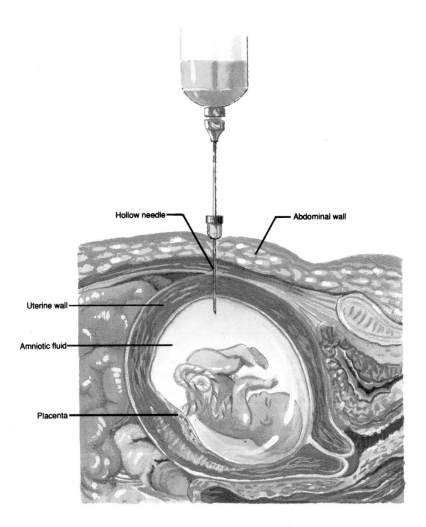

Figure 8.6

Amniocentesis. Usually the fetus is first located by sonography—bouncing high-frequency sounds off it and recording the echoes. Then, about ten milliliters of amniotic fluid, containing fetal cells, is withdrawn by a hypodermic needle inserted directly through the abdominal wall. The cells obtained by this method are grown in culture and then subjected to biochemical and chromosomal analysis.

From Stuart Ira Fox, *Human Physiology,* 3d ed. Copyright © 1990 Wm. C. Brown Publishers, Dubuque, Iowa. All Rights Reserved. Reprinted by permission.

Birth

It is important to understand the stages of labor. Then decisions related to the birth need consideration.

The Stages of Labor

In delivering a child (or children), a woman goes through three stages of **labor,** as shown in figure 8.8. The first stage lasts an average of 10.5 hours for the first pregnancy and 6.5 hours for later pregnancies. During this stage, the neck of the cervix should dilate wide enough (four inches) for the fetus to exit.

The second stage of labor, lasting approximately one hour, results in the delivery of the fetus. An involuntary contraction and pushing of the abdominal muscles aids this process. To prevent tearing of the vaginal tissue, most women choose (with their physicians) to have an incision called an **episiotomy,** made in the vaginal opening right before delivery. There is both good and bad news about episiotomies. The good news is that they do reduce the number of minor vaginal tears during childbirth. The bad news is that the number of major tears increases ("Birthing Procedure Hurts Mother More Than It Helps" 1991). Some experts argue that nature should be allowed to take its course—which means not doing an episiotomy (Edell 1990b). The final stage of labor delivers the **placenta** (afterbirth.)

Upon the baby's delivery, the **umbilical cord**—the cord linking the mother to the fetus and providing it with

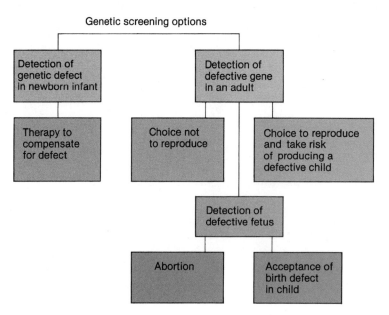

Genetic screening options

Detection of genetic defect in newborn infant

Therapy to compensate for defect

Detection of defective gene in an adult

Choice not to reproduce

Choice to reproduce and take risk of producing a defective child

Detection of defective fetus

Abortion

Acceptance of birth defect in child

Figure 8.7

Flowchart describing genetic screening options.

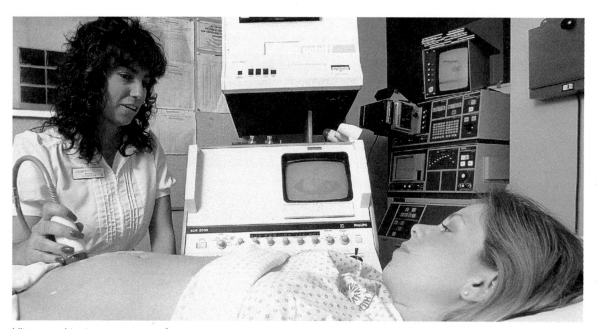

Ultrasound tests are common for pregnant women.

nourishment—is clamped and cut; the baby is checked for vital functions; and drops of silver nitrate are deposited in the baby's eyes to prevent blindness from a possible gonorrheal infection in the mother.

Generally, the head of the fetus is the first body part to come out of the mother, but sometimes the fetus is posi-

tioned in the uterus with its buttocks set to come out first. A delivery in this position is termed a **breech birth** (about 4 percent of all births) and calls for specific physician involvement to maneuver the fetus for birth. In other cases, the pressure on the head of the fetus may be so great as to decrease its oxygen supply; in these and other

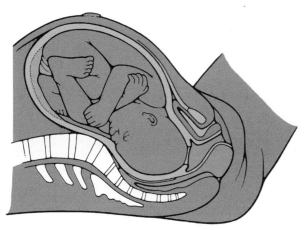

Stage 1

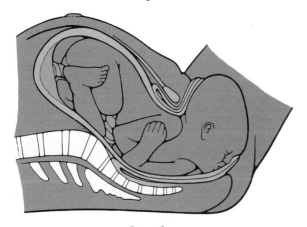

Stage 2

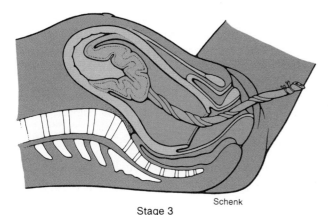

Stage 3

Schenk

Figure 8.8

The stages of childbirth, including discharge of the placenta (stage 3).

From Kent M. Van De Graaff and Stuart Ira Fox, *Concepts of Human Anatomy and Physiology,* 2d ed. Copyright © 1989 Wm. C. Brown Publishers, Dubuque, Iowa. All Rights Reserved. Reprinted by permission.

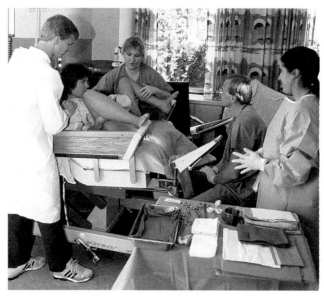

Decisions related to delivery should be considered well in advance.

situations where the mother or baby would be endangered by vaginal delivery, the best procedure for birth may be through a **cesarean section** (an incision in the woman's abdomen). Cesarean sections have become more common and now represent from 24 percent to 28 percent of deliveries in the United States. It was thought that once a woman had a cesarean she also had to have one for future deliveries. It has been found, however, that from 40 percent to 80 percent of women could successfully avoid a repeat cesarean. This greatly reduces length of hospital stay, recovery time, and costs related to delivery ("C-Section Rates Remain High, But Postcesarean Vaginal Births Are Rising" 1990).

While there may be good reasons for cesarean deliveries, the decision of whether or not to have one should be carefully considered. Some feel there are too many cesareans done unnecessarily. For example, 30 percent of emergency cesarean sections performed at a British teaching hospital were judged later to have been unnecessary. There is also a high degree of disagreement among evaluators regarding the need for many cesareans ("Evaluating the Cesarean Decision" 1990).

Decisions About the Birth

Because anesthetics to decrease the mother's pain during childbirth actually remain in the newborn long after birth, more and more women are choosing drugless births, or **natural childbirth.** One of the more popular methods of natural childbirth, the **Lamaze method,** is named after its developer, Fernand Lamaze. The Lamaze method is a program of formal class instruction to teach women how to relax through breathing exercises and how to bear down (using abdominal muscular contractions to help position the baby for birth) during the second stage of labor. Women are taught to consider labor as a time of work and concentration. They become active participants in the birth process, confident that they can help control their deliveries. Further, the father (or another person who serves as a partner) is taught how to coach the woman during childbirth—reminding her to relax, monitoring her breathing, telling her about her progress, and providing moral support.

Decisions About Where to Deliver

Although hospital delivery is still the predominant choice, more and more women choose home births. The advantages of home delivery include the familiar and comfortable setting, the potentially enlarged role of the father, faster recovery than from hospital births, and the opportunity to have the baby be an immediate part of the family and the family an immediate part of the birth. Since medical resources available at hospitals are unavailable in homes, however, home births are recommended only when the risk of complications appears low. The mother should be twenty to thirty years of age and have no potential medical problems; she should also have been well nourished during the pregnancy and had one to three full-term births without any complication. In any case, home birth should include the services of a qualified nurse-midwife or physician.

In some parts of the country, an alternative, called a **birthing center,** exists. A birthing center is usually connected with a hospital, although some are not. The center is designed to simulate the home environment, and the couple, along with their obstetrician and pediatrician, draw up a plan—based on their desires and potential medical needs—to guide the birthing center staff.

The homelike atmosphere of the birthing center facilitates relaxation with friends, family, and siblings. During labor, the mother may walk around and be near her loved ones. Usually no unexpected visitors, including hospital staff, are allowed inside unless an emergency occurs. If an emergency should arise, medical personnel and equipment are readily available.

Treatment of the Newborn

Another issue to consider is how to treat the newborn immediately after birth. There seemed to be little question about this matter until the ideas and practices of a French obstetrician, Frederick Leboyer, were publicized. Leboyer (1975) believes that entry into the world is a traumatic event for the infant and everything possible should be done to make this transition gradual. He advises that newborns be delivered in dimly lit, quiet, warm rooms. Further, he argues that rather than being held by their feet and spanked on their rears to induce breathing, babies should be placed on the mother's abdomen, where they can hear the heartbeat and begin breathing gradually. Finally, he advises that babies be placed in water at body temperature and bathed and rocked gently. Leboyer feels that babies born in this manner are psychologically better off throughout the life cycle.

Rooming-in

A mother who gives birth in a hospital must also consider if the baby will be kept in a nursery or in her room. Some feel that a mother who "rooms-in" with her first child tends to feel more competent and confident in her ability to mother than women whose babies are kept in hospital nurseries. Rooming-in, however, does not allow the mother as much rest and time to recover from childbirth.

Breast-Feeding

Lactogenesis is the initiation of milk production after delivery; **lactation** is the breast-feeding (nursing) experience. If a woman decides to breast-feed, she must remember that what she eats or drinks eventually reaches her baby. Doctors recommend against taking birth-control pills while breast-feeding because the hormones in the pills can end up in breast milk (Edell 1990c). A woman must also realize that sexual stimulation from breast-feeding is common and should cause no concern. Lastly, she should understand that she will probably have delayed onset of menstruation following delivery; however, this is not a reliable means of contraception. If another pregnancy is not desired, usual means of pregnancy prevention should be used after consulting with a physician.

Some argue for breast-feeding because a mother's milk gives the child the best nutrition available and provides antibodies that protect against disease. In addition, it can provide closeness between the mother and child, it saves money, and it does not require bottles and other equipment. Others argue that it is inconvenient, messy, and time-consuming and that adequate nutrition can be obtained from commercially available milk.

To Circumcise or Not to Circumcise

Circumcision, the surgical removal of the foreskin of a male's penis, is the most commonly performed surgical procedure in the United States. (Although circumcision of the female has flourished in many parts of the world for centuries, we will confine this discussion to male circumcision because female circumcision is rarely seen in the United States.) Circumcision has been widely practiced throughout the world for religious, ritual, and hygienic reasons.

Particularly during the past twenty to twenty-five years, circumcision has been a controversial procedure in the United States. Some feel there is no absolute medical indication for routine circumcision of the newborn. They feel potential benefits should be balanced against the surgical risk, the discomfort to the infant, and the use of medical and economic resources (Siwek 1990). Others feel routine circumcision of newborn males has many potential advantages: the procedure helps prevent urinary tract infections, penile cancer, and sexually transmitted diseases (including AIDS). The risk of complications is low, it is more economical to perform the procedure early in life, and no evidence shows that penile hygiene alone is as beneficial as circumcision (Wiswell 1990).

Even a middle-of-the-road point of view exists on this issue. Some feel that although the risks of routine circumcision performed at birth are small, the benefits are uncertain. Therefore, it should be performed at the discretion of the parents and not as a part of routine medical care (Poland 1990). What do you think?

Contraception

Contraceptive decisions are sometimes controversial. Understanding arguments for and against contraception, as well as options, is essential when making decisions about contraception.

Arguments for Contraception

Many individuals use **contraceptives** to space pregnancies, limit family size, delay childbearing, or avoid pregnancy altogether. Contraception allows us to decide when we will have any children desired. Because children conceived under such circumstances are planned for, we can avoid bringing unwanted children into the world. For some women, a pregnancy may be medically dangerous, and contraception can protect the health of the mother or let her avoid conceiving children with birth defects.

Contraception also provides a means for individuals to participate in sexual intercourse without much fear of pregnancy. Many women experience more freedom and self-actualization when they use contraception. This is particularly true for women who wish to pursue careers or other activities where unplanned pregnancies would be difficult. Lastly, contraception can also control population growth.

Arguments Against Contraception

Among the reasons commonly given for not using contraceptives are health risks and moral arguments. Some fear their bodies will be harmed by using birth-control pills or other methods, and others feel it is against the will of God to "artificially" interfere with a pregnancy. These individuals might consider abstinence or some other "natural" avoidance of pregnancy to be acceptable but not any method that involves an artificial device or chemical. Some individuals also find that certain contraceptive methods create a loss of spontaneity in sexual relationships. Finally, some minority group social leaders have argued that government advocacy of contraceptive use for their group is meant to reduce their number and eventually exterminate them.

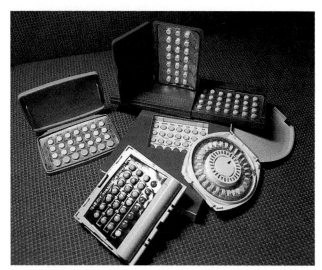

Many choices exist if the pill is the contraceptive method chosen.

Forms of Contraception

Deciding on the best contraceptive should involve consultation with a physician or appropriate persons who are trained to deal with contraceptive decisions and possess the latest information. Two of the current preferred methods (the **oral contraceptive,** or pill, and the diaphragm) require a physician's prescription. Sterilization requires a surgeon's help, and use of an *injectable* requires visits to a physician. But all other methods considered here require at most a trip to a store that carries contraceptives.

Oral Contraceptives (the Pill)

The most effective method of contraception control today—short of abstinence or a surgical procedure—is the pill. Even though the term *the pill* is frequently used, there are actually several variations of oral contraceptives. The type of oral contraceptive used since the early 1960s contains both estrogen and progestin (synthetic progesterone) and is called the **combination pill.** A variation of the combination pill is called the **multiphasic pill.** This newer version varies the amount of estrogen and progesterone throughout the menstrual cycle to match the amounts of these hormones naturally occurring in the female more closely.

The combination pill is almost 100 percent effective if taken properly. A woman must take it regularly for twenty-one days or use supplementary contraception. The chemical reactions sparked by combination or multiphasic pills can be quite complicated. Simply described, the hormones trick the body into thinking it is pregnant; these hormones, estrogen and progesterone, work exactly as they do in the usual menstrual cycle. Recall that after ovulation, elevated levels of estrogen and progesterone prevent the release of another egg during the menstrual cycle. The pill elevates the levels of these hormones and suspends ovulation altogether. The menstrual cycle continues as usual for all practical purposes, but no egg is released and conception cannot occur.

A third type of oral contraceptive contains no estrogen and is called the progestin-only pill, or **minipill.** This pill is ingested daily throughout the menstrual cycle, but it often does not suspend ovulation. The progestin inhibits implantation and causes the cervical mucus to become thicker, making it more difficult for the sperm to get through. Since the minipill contains only progesterone, it generally does not cause the side effects commonly associated with the combination pill. Researchers have concluded that it is a suitable and equally effective alternative to the combination pill in all age groups ("Minipill May Have Broader Appeal" 1991).

Research shows that taking the pill presents fewer risks than going through a pregnancy. As with any medication, however, women who take the pill risk complications and side effects. A physician and client must decide if benefits are worth the risk. The negative side effects of the pill are of two types: nuisance effects and medically serious effects. Fluid retention, weight gain, irritability, and change in sex drive fall into the nuisance category, while a tendency toward blood clots, hypertension, or gallbladder disease are medically more serious. In most cases, women's bodies adjust to the nuisance side effects after several menstrual cycles. If adjustment does not occur, however, a woman may decide that this method is unacceptable. There is no reliable evidence that birth-control pills cause cancer—even after being used for fifteen years or longer (*Better Health* 1987). It is generally recommended that women over forty, women who smoke, or women with liver function problems, hypertension, circulatory problems, sickle-cell disease, asthma, varicose veins, epilepsy, or migraine headaches should not take the pill. This does not mean that the pill causes any of these things—rather it is wise to be cautious if any of these conditions already exist. Better screening of potential pill users and lower hormone dosages have resulted in fewer reports of adverse side effects than twenty to twenty-five years ago.

Increasing evidence has shown that the pill has positive side effects. For example, it has been estimated that fifty thousand hospitalizations are prevented each year by use of the pill. The pill has a direct positive effect on the following diseases: benign breast disease, ovarian and endometrial cancers, ovarian cysts, iron-deficiency anemia, **pelvic inflammatory disease (PID),** and ectopic pregnancy. In some cases, such as benign breast disease and PID, the protective effect increases the longer the pill is used (Hatcher et al. 1986; Edell 1990d).

What happens when a female stops taking the pill? There is no strong evidence that the pill subsequently affects a woman's ability to become pregnant, increases her tendency to have multiple births, or in any other way alters her general health.

Other contraceptive techniques that also work by suspending ovulation are in various stages of experimentation and implementation. These include a capsule implant that

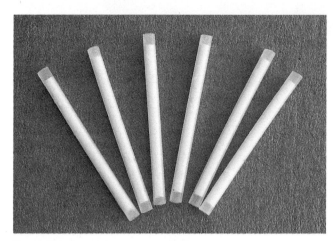
Norplant is becoming more popular.

is injected under the skin and releases hormones over a long period of time, an injection that works in essentially the same way, and a once-a-month (or other time interval) pill.

Long-acting injectable contraceptives, known as **injectables,** have been available for over a decade. The three-month DepoProvera injectable is approved for use in over ninety countries and the two- to three-month Noristerat in more than forty. Late in 1992, DepoProvera was approved by the FDA. It became available on a limited basis early in 1993. While the status of long-acting injectables is subject to change, it is safe to say that in the United States, they are in limited use.

In December 1990, the FDA approved the marketing of Norplant, a contraceptive implant system. Six capsules, thirty-four millimeters long, inserted beneath the skin of a woman's upper arm release a steady, low dose of levonorgestrel (a synthetic progestin) for up to five years. The United States was the seventeenth country to approve this method for marketing. It is already thought to be the most effective reversible contraceptive method available, with a first-year use-failure rate of 0.2 pregnancies per 100 ("FDA OKs Hormonal Implant" 1990).

Injectables are about 99 percent effective, but some users report changes in menstrual patterns, some develop amenorrhea (absence of menstruation), and some report a delayed return to fertility after stopping use of the injectable. Injectables also have beneficial health effects. They often increase blood iron levels and protect against PID and ovarian and endometrial cancers ("Hormonal Contraception" 1987).

While some nuisance side effects (such as weight changes, headaches, and mood changes) have been reported among some Norplant users, no serious side effects have been reported. Researchers have concluded that Norplant is highly acceptable to most women seeking a convenient, effective, temporary method of contraception ("Hormonal Implants Prove to be Highly Acceptable" 1990). The only downside to using Norplant seems to be abnormal menstrual flow. About 70 percent of users have

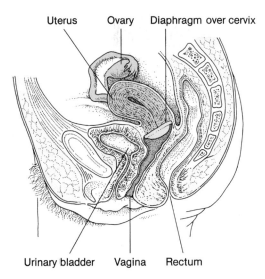

Figure 8.9

Cross section of the female pelvis showing a diaphragm in position. Generally used in conjunction with a spermicidal jelly or cream, the diaphragm blocks sperm from entry into the uterus and thus prevents conception.

a flow that is unpredictable in amount, duration, and frequency ("Pros and Cons of Norplant" 1992).

The morning-after pill, which contains an estrogen-like substance called **diethylstilbestrol (DES),** must be taken within seventy-two hours after sexual intercourse to prevent pregnancy. It does not prevent conception but it makes the lining of the uterus unacceptable for implantation of a possible fertilized egg. Unfortunately, it also tends to make some women ill for a short time. Because of this and because the side effects of repeated high dosages of DES are not yet fully known, this pill should only be considered an emergency and temporary measure.

Diaphragm

The **diaphragm** is a dome-shaped, latex device that a woman places next to the cervix to block the opening to the uterus, thereby preventing sperm from entering (fig. 8.9). Used in combination with a spermicidal jelly or foam, the diaphragm was probably the most effective birth-control method (about 85 percent to 90 percent) before the advent of pills and injectables. It is important to use the diaphragm in combination with a spermicidal jelly, which lubricates the diaphragm for insertion and, more important, greatly increases its potential effectiveness. It is also important to leave the diaphragm in place for at least six hours after intercourse.

Use of the diaphragm introduces a factor not present with either pills or injectables: the user must insert the diaphragm before actual sexual intercourse, which some individuals find undesirable. There are no adverse side effects with the diaphragm, however, as there may be with pills and injectables. Women must consult their

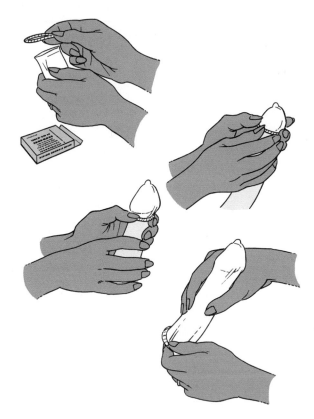

Figure 8.10

Most condoms, lubricated and plain, come packaged in foil and rolled, ready for easy use. The condom is placed over the head of the penis, with a space left at the tip to hold the semen when ejaculated. Either partner can unroll the condom down over the glans and shaft of the penis to the base of the scrotum. The condom should be in place before any vaginal contact and removed immediately after ejaculation and withdrawal.

physicians to get a diaphragm that fits correctly and to learn proper insertion and removal techniques. Never borrow another woman's diaphragm, because women are different sizes internally, just as they are externally. Also, after a pregnancy and after a body weight change of six pounds or more, a woman should be refitted for a new diaphragm.

Condom

Sometimes called *rubbers,* **condoms** cover the erect penis and prevent sperm from entering the vagina. Leading the list of nonprescriptive contraceptives, condoms can be quite effective (90 percent to 97 percent) if used properly (fig. 8.10). Correct use involves following U.S. Centers for Disease Control recommendations found in the accompanying box. There are no side effects or dangers associated with condom use. Some individuals object to condoms because they claim condoms dull physical sensation and tend to interrupt sexual intercourse, but users should personally evaluate these characteristics.

Ever since the Surgeon General's report on AIDS (Koop 1986), there has been a renewed interest in condoms. While not a guaranteed barrier, condoms do seem to be helpful in reducing the likelihood of spreading sexually transmitted diseases—including AIDS. (Animal skin condoms, however, are not as effective for this purpose as latex condoms.)

There is also a female condom in limited use, which was approved by the FDA in 1992. In a small Danish pilot study, a majority of men and women reported the female condom was easy to use and did not interfere with sexual response. Both men and women were more likely to report problems in achieving orgasm with the male condom than with the female condom ("Users Approve of Female Condom" 1991).

Jellies, Creams, and Foams

A great variety of **jellies, creams,** and **foams** are available in any drugstore for women without a prescription. Figure 8.11 shows the application of a spermicidal foam. These products all work basically the same way—they are supposed to kill the sperm before it can complete its journey. By themselves, however, they are not nearly as effective as the methods already mentioned. For best results, they should be used in combination with a diaphragm or condom. The application method and time used before intercourse vary with the product, so it is important to read the instructions carefully. There are no known serious or adverse side effects, but some women and men report skin irritation from some products, just as might be expected from some deodorants or other products that contact the skin.

Effectiveness of a **spermicide,** that is, a sperm-killing chemical, can be as low as 70 percent to 80 percent. To be effective, it must be inserted into the vagina as close to

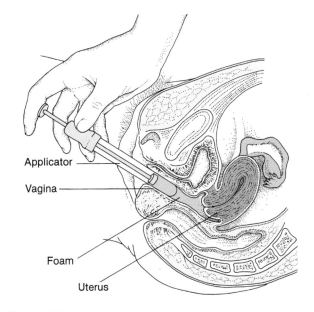

Figure 8.11
Application of spermicidal foam.

the time of intercourse as possible, but no more than an hour before. As it covers the cervix, the spermicide forms both a physical and chemical barrier to sperm. To avoid interfering with the contraceptive action, a woman should not douche for at least six hours after intercourse.

Sponge

First marketed in 1983 under the brand name of Today, the effectiveness of the spermicidal **sponge** is estimated to be 80 percent to 87 percent. The sponge is made of a special polyurethane material and contains the spermicide nonoxynol-9. After being moistened with two tablespoons

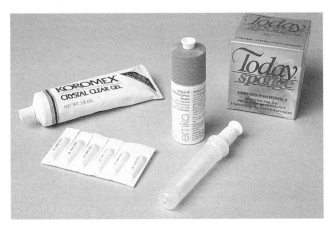

Many spermicides are available without a prescription.

of water, the sponge is inserted into the vagina to cover the cervix, forming both a physical and chemical barrier to sperm. It is believed to act in several ways: its spermicide kills the sperm, the sponge itself absorbs the ejaculate, and it acts as a mechanical barrier to block the opening to the cervix. The sponge should be left in place for at least six hours after intercourse but can be left in place and be effective for up to twenty-four hours. It should be discarded after use.

As with spermicides, a small percentage of users may experience irritations, and there are reports of difficulties removing the sponge. There have been a few cases of the rare but potentially fatal illness called toxic shock syndrome (TSS) among women using sponges. But the rate is very low—less than one TSS case per three million sponges used—and even this rate can be reduced if women carefully follow the directions on the leaflet accompanying the product.

Fertility Awareness (Rhythm Method)

A contraceptive method that requires little equipment and has been used for centuries is the **rhythm method,** also called natural family planning, the ovulation method, or **fertility awareness.** Effectiveness is highly variable, with estimates generally ranging from 53 percent to 86 percent. Avoiding pregnancy with this method requires having no intercourse during those times in the menstrual cycle when fertilization is most likely to occur.

The most common variations of this contraceptive method are the basal body temperature method, the cervical mucus method, and the calendar method. They can be used together for increased effectiveness. The **basal body temperature (BBT) method** is based on the fact that a woman's temperature drops slightly, about 0.2 degrees F, just before ovulation. A day or so after the drop, a distinct rise (about 0.6 to 0.8 degrees F) signals the beginning of ovulation. Unprotected intercourse must be avoided from the time a woman's temperature drops until her temperature has remained elevated for three consecutive days. Unfortunately, a woman's temperature can vary for other reasons, such as illness.

The **cervical mucus method** (also called vaginal mucus method) relies on the fact that cervical mucus changes from dry after menstruation to very slippery (almost like raw egg white) during ovulation to dry again after ovulation. A woman can check her cervical mucus several times a day by wiping herself with toilet paper before she urinates and observing any changes. At first, she may need help from a physician or other trained health professional to interpret her findings. Sometimes a woman may choose to combine the BBT and cervical mucus methods. When the two are used together it is termed the **symptothermal method.**

The **calendar method,** which is effective only when used with one or both of the methods just discussed, consists of keeping track of the number of days in the menstrual cycle in an attempt to pinpoint ovulation. If menstrual cycles are short, this method is highly unreliable. For best results, couples must be willing to chart ovulation carefully for a year's time and strictly adhere to a given regime. Table 8.1 shows how to calculate "safe" and "unsafe" days.

Cervical Cap

The **cervical cap** is available on a limited basis and as an investigational device in some clinics around the country. It has long been popular in Europe. It is similar to, but smaller than, the diaphragm and is made of rubber, plastic, or metal. It is more difficult to insert than a diaphragm and fits snugly around the cervix.

Like the diaphragm, the cervical cap comes in different sizes, but it can probably be left in place for days or weeks. Generally, the cap must be removed during menstruation to allow for the menstrual blood to flow from the body. There is, however, an experimental cap (the Goepp cap) that can remain in place up to a year. It has a one-way valve that allows menstrual products to flow into the vagina but doesn't allow sperm to enter the cervix. Although this method seems to hold some promise, its safety and effectiveness are still under investigation.

Intrauterine Device (IUD)

Of all methods of contraception, the **intrauterine device (IUD)** has been the most controversial. IUDs are used by millions of women around the world (fig. 8.12). In the United States, they were introduced in the early 1960s, and by 1982 they were used by over two million women (Hantula 1986). How the IUD prevents pregnancy is not known for sure, but there are several theories: (1) The presence of the IUD changes the chemical environment inside the uterus, preventing either fertilization or implantation. (2) The IUD causes the normal contractions of the uterine wall to be more violent than usual (although the woman doesn't feel them), which prevents implantation of a fertilized egg. (3) The IUD makes the egg travel more rapidly and, therefore, prevents the sperm from fertilizing it. (4) The IUD stops the sperm from getting through the uterus to the egg. (5) The IUD irritates the lining of the uterus and this prevents implantation.

As early as 1974, one IUD, the Dalkon Shield, was taken off the market by its manufacturer, the A. H. Robins Company. In 1980, the company urged physicians to remove the devices from women still using them and in 1984 said it would pay all medical costs of such removal. By the end of 1985, Robins had paid out $520 million in more than nine thousand lawsuits related to serious side effects and thousands of additional lawsuits were still pending (Hantula 1986).

The Saf-T-Coil was taken off the market by its manufacturer in 1982 and the Lippes Loop in 1985. The Copper-7, which had become by far the most popular IUD, and the Tatum-T were removed from the U.S. market in 1986 by their manufacturer, G. D. Searle and Company. It is interesting that this series of events was mainly a result of legal expenses and not medical complications.

In 1987, a copper IUD (the Copper-T 380, or TCu 380) was again put on the market, and expectations were that it would be widely used. In 1991, a slimline version of the TCu 380 became available. While it might be helpful for women with small cervical canals, there seem to be no other advantages of the newer model ("A Slimmer Copper T" 1991).

A five-year evaluation of a low-dose, levonorgestrel-releasing (the same synthetic chemical in Norplant) IUD showed the device to be as effective as the TCu 380—an advanced form of the Copper-7 IUD. Each day it releases about one-third as much hormone as the Progestasert, which was the only hormonal IUD approved in the United States as of 1993. Effectiveness rates are about the same as the TCu 380 (between 1.1 and 1.4 pregnancies per 100 users) ("The Low-Dose IUD" 1990).

TABLE 8.1

The Rhythm Method of Contraception—How to Calculate the "Safe" and "Unsafe" Days for Coitus

Length of Shortest Cycle (days)	First "Unsafe" Day After Start of Any Menstrual Period	Length of Longest Cycle (days)	Last "Unsafe" Day After Start of Any Menstrual Period
20	2nd	20	9th
21	3rd	21	10th
22	4th	22	11th
23	5th	23	12th
24	6th	24	13th
25	7th	25	14th
26	8th	26	15th
27	9th	27	16th
28	10th	28	17th
29	11th	29	18th
30	12th	30	19th
31	13th	31	20th
32	14th	32	21st
33	15th	33	22nd
34	16th	34	23rd
35	17th	35	24th
36	18th	36	25th
37	19th	37	26th
38	20th	38	27th
39	21st	39	28th
40	22nd	40	29th

Some experts feel that because of all the negative publicity, some women are missing out on a good contraceptive option by not using an IUD. Ninety-eight percent of current IUD users are happy with the method, IUDs are far safer than most assume, and the original negative statistics turn out to be misleading ("IUD Underused" 1992).

IUDs are changing rapidly, and it is difficult to keep up with the most recent information about them. As you read this, what is the current status of IUD use?

Ineffective Methods

Two other methods are sometimes classified as contraceptives but are ineffective and should not be considered reliable. These are **coitus interruptus**, withdrawal of the penis from the vagina before ejaculation, and the **vaginal douche,** a stream of water or other liquid directed into the vagina for sanitary or medical reasons. The withdrawal method is common among young people because it is simple and requires no equipment. There is a real chance of pregnancy with this method, though, because sperm may seep out of the penis before actual ejaculation. These

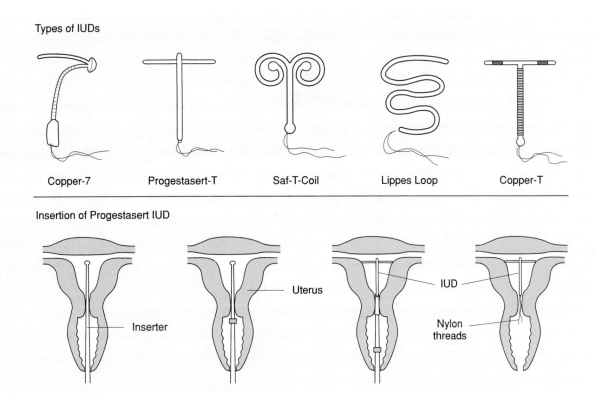

Types of IUDs

Copper-7   Progestasert-T   Saf-T-Coil   Lippes Loop   Copper-T

Insertion of Progestasert IUD

Uterus

Inserter

IUD

Nylon
threads

Figure 8.12

Intrauterine devices are made of flexible plastic, sometimes
with copper or progesterone added. Before having an IUD
inserted, a woman should discuss the pros and cons of
available models with her health-care practitioner. After being
straightened for insertion, the IUD's "memory plastic"
resumes its original shape in the uterus. Some IUDs are
designed to flex somewhat within the uterus to adjust to
changes in the shape of the uterine cavity.

sperm are just as capable of fertilizing an egg as those
ejaculated later. Sperm leaking from the penis, or deposited in a moist spot just *outside* the vagina, can swim into
the vagina and up into the uterus. These facts, combined
with the fact that the man is forced to withdraw when
that's the last thing he feels like doing (and the woman
probably isn't too happy about it either), make withdrawal
a very ineffective method of contraception. The psychological frustrations of using this method also contribute to
its undesirability.

The vaginal douche is not an effective contraceptive.
Sperm are good swimmers, and it is impossible for a
female to douche quickly or thoroughly enough to wash
out all of the sperm. Furthermore, the force of the douche
may even push some sperm further into the vagina and
make pregnancy *more* likely. Figure 8.13 gives the effectiveness rates of the methods of contraception we have
discussed.

Sterilization

Surgical **sterilization,** a procedure by which an individual
is made incapable of reproducing, has rapidly gained
popularity in the United States as a permanent way to
prevent pregnancy. It is the most popular method used
by couples over thirty. For either the man or the woman,
sterilization simply involves blocking the anatomical road-
way so that the sperm or egg can no longer make the
trip to the point of meeting. For men, this involves sever-
ing both of the vas deferens; for women, it requires sev-
ering the fallopian tubes. Some individuals believe that
sterilization alters a person's physical abilities or sexual
desires, but this is simply not true. For both men and
women, sterilization does *not* affect feelings, hormone
production, or physical function.

In both the male operation (**vasectomy**) and the
female operation (**tubal ligation**), there are a number of
ways to sever and close off the tubes. Men or women can
have this simple surgery in about fifteen to twenty minutes
as outpatients in a hospital, clinic, or physician's office.
The particular procedure and surroundings are a matter of
choice between physician and patient. Figure 8.14 shows
both a vasectomy and a tubal ligation. After the procedure,
a woman is immediately sterile. A man's system, however,
takes some time to clear out all the sperm, and men are
usually asked to bring an ejaculate sample to the doctor
several weeks after a vasectomy to be sure they are
"sperm-free."

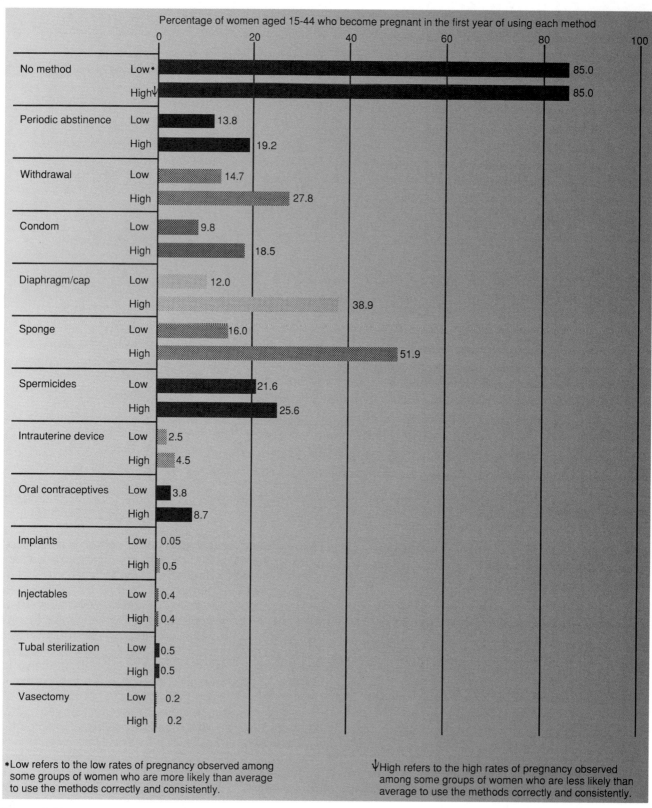

Percentage of women aged 15-44 who become pregnant in the first year of using each method

No method	Low*	85.0
	High↓	85.0
Periodic abstinence	Low	13.8
	High	19.2
Withdrawal	Low	14.7
	High	27.8
Condom	Low	9.8
	High	18.5
Diaphragm/cap	Low	12.0
	High	38.9
Sponge	Low	16.0
	High	51.9
Spermicides	Low	21.6
	High	25.6
Intrauterine device	Low	2.5
	High	4.5
Oral contraceptives	Low	3.8
	High	8.7
Implants	Low	0.05
	High	0.5
Injectables	Low	0.4
	High	0.4
Tubal sterilization	Low	0.5
	High	0.5
Vasectomy	Low	0.2
	High	0.2

*Low refers to the low rates of pregnancy observed among some groups of women who are more likely than average to use the methods correctly and consistently.

↓High refers to the high rates of pregnancy observed among some groups of women who are less likely than average to use the methods correctly and consistently.

Figure 8.13

Effectiveness of various birth-control methods. Note: Jones and Forrest (1992) have reported failure rates similar to those indicated. During the first year of use, they found 8 percent of pill users, 15 percent of condom users, 16 percent of diaphragm users, 25 percent of spermicide users, and 26 percent of those who practiced periodic abstinence became pregnant. Failure seemed to result more from improper and irregular use than from inherent limitations of the methods.

Source: Susan Harlap, Kathryn Kost, & Jacqueline D. Forrest, *Preventing Pregnancy, Protecting Health,* 1991, p. 35. © The Alan Guttmacher Institute.

Oral Contraceptive

Follow pill-taking instructions carefully and consistently. Use a backup method, such as foam or condoms, during the first month.

Intrauterine Device (IUD)

Have IUD inserted by experienced clinician.

Frequently check IUD's position during the first few months. (User should feel thread in cervical opening but not the stem of the IUD).

Use a backup method, such as foam or condoms, during the first three months and, if desired, at midcycle thereafter.

Diaphragm and Jelly

Use with every act of intercourse and leave in place for at least six hours after intercourse. Ask for thorough instruction with initial fitting and have fit checked annually by an experienced clinician.

Inspect regularly for defects or holes.

Avoid use of Vaseline or perfumed powders, as they can damage the latex. Always use ample amounts of spermicidal jelly or cream; add as necessary.

Check position after insertion: front rim must be behind pubic bone, and dome must cover cervix.

Condom

Use with every act of intercourse. Put condom on penis before *any* penis-vagina contact, leave space in tip of condom for semen, and remove carefully to avoid spillage. Avoid damage to condom; handle carefully, and avoid heat and use of Vaseline.

Buy a good brand and do not use condom that is more than two years old.

Use foam along with condom.

Vaginal Spermicides

Use ample amounts with every act of intercourse.

Follow instructions regarding time limits of effectiveness.

When using foam, shake it *vigorously* before use.

Use condoms along with spermicide.

Rhythm (Fertility Awareness)

Combine calendar, temperature, and mucus methods.

It is generally accepted that sterilization has no long-term effects on women. While some individuals express concern about the effect of sterilization on the menstrual cycle, sterilized women are unlikely to experience substantial changes in the duration of menstrual flow, their cycle length, or midcycle bleeding ("Sterilization Is Unlikely to Alter Most Women's Menstrual Symptoms" 1990).

Some individuals suspect that vasectomies might make men more susceptible to later cardiovascular problems. Even men with vasectomies for longer than ten years are no more prone to heart attacks, strokes, or other atherosclerotic problems than nonvasectomized men their age.

Male sterilization is usually preferable to female sterilization for a variety of reasons. It is safer, just as effective, and less expensive and there are fewer complications. In addition, regret is two-thirds again as high among women who have had a tubal ligation as compared to men who have had a vasectomy ("Vasectomy Proves to Be Preferable to Female Sterilization" 1989). Why do you think women feel this way?

As is expected with any surgical procedure, complications occasionally accompany sterilization. Most sterilizations, however, are performed without complications or reported regrets, and for those who know they want no more children, it is an ideal way to prevent pregnancy. Because the chances of reversing the operation at a later time are poor, it should be considered a permanent procedure. Research is underway, however, to find a means of easily reversing the procedure; the installation of valves, the use of silicone plugs, and the perfection of surgical techniques hold promise for successful reversal in the future.

Contraceptive Decisions

If there were a perfect contraceptive, it would be 100 percent effective, be very inexpensive or free, have no side effects, be reversible, involve no action, be convenient and not messy, prevent sexually transmitted diseases, be accepted religiously and morally, and not interrupt sexual intercourse. None of the methods discussed and none on the horizon meet all these criteria. Individual feelings also determine whether or not a particular method is acceptable. Contraceptive decisions are influenced by safety, reliability, convenience, religion or sociocultural considerations, aesthetics, and whether a temporary or permanent method is desired.

The use of effective contraception by college men and women is primarily associated with partner support of contraception. Effective contraceptive use tends to begin only when the relationship reaches a stage at which intercourse becomes relatively predictable and when the partner is supportive of contraceptive use. Also, less frequent intercourse is associated with condom use, and more frequent intercourse is associated with use of the pill (Whitley 1990).

What do these facts mean in relation to your contraceptive decisions? What you do about your reproductive life may be one of the most important health decisions made during your lifetime.

Contraception and the Future

As researchers try to improve further various contraceptive methods and devices, it is impossible to keep current with technological advances. Those who practice fertility awareness, as well as those who have had difficulty conceiving, could be helped by a device that is available but

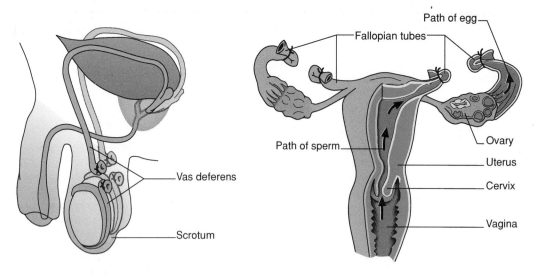

Figure 8.14

Vasectomy and tubal ligation compared. A vasectomy (*left*) is a comparatively simple surgical procedure. By comparison, tubal ligation (*right*) is somewhat more complex.

From John W. Hole, Jr., *Human Anatomy and Physiology,* 4th ed. Copyright © 1987 Wm. C. Brown Publishers, Dubuque, Iowa. All Rights Reserved. Reprinted by permission.

not widely used. A small device consisting of an oral thermometer and a computer chip gives repeated electronic beeps to remind the wearer that it is time to take her temperature. By using this device, called Bioself, the woman knows within two minutes if she is in a fertile phase of her cycle ("New Device to Aid Natural Family Planning" 1982).

Researchers have developed a contraceptive device that immobilizes sperm by generating a weak current across the lining of the cervical canal. This is the gynecological equivalent of an electric fence. The device might be combined with a specially modified diaphragm or cervical cap or attached to an intracervical implant and left in on a long-term basis ("Intracervical 'Electric Fence' Keeps Out Sperm" 1987).

Some researchers estimate that women will soon have five new methods from which to choose—all modifications of the injectables already discussed. To varying degrees, all change or disrupt menstrual patterns. Biodegradable implants, placed under the skin, are expected to prevent pregnancy for twelve to eighteen months. Injectable microcapsules prevent pregnancy for one to six months, and new monthly injectables are being developed as well. Finally, a vaginal ring can be placed by the woman in her vagina, where it gradually releases hormones and is effective for three months ("Hormonal Contraception" 1987).

A "missed-period pill" containing **mifepristone** (also called **RU486**) seems to block hormonal action necessary for a pregnancy to begin. This method, which might actually be considered a very early abortion, can be used with-

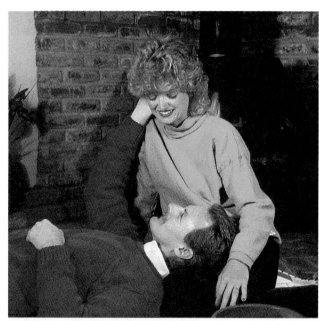

It is important to communicate effectively in an intimate relationship.

in ten days of the first missed period and is thought to be very effective ("The Missed-Period Pill" 1987).

Early French studies, in which women used mifepristone up to three weeks beyond the missed period, show an effectiveness rate of 96 percent. The administration of mifepristone seems to be a safe and effective method for

Conversing About Controlling Conception

You have heard people say that a birth of a baby was "an accident." Since you know about the male and female reproductive systems, how conception occurs, and how births can be controlled, there should be no "accidents." Having a baby and raising a child can be a wonderful experience, but it is also serious business. Babies should only be created by those who want them and are ready to be parents. To prevent "accidents," we need to communicate effectively in intimate situations and realize the consequences of our actions.

Being comfortable with conversations about sexuality can help prevent "accidents." Many of us, however, have difficulty talking with someone we care deeply about when it comes to sexuality. To help prevent "accidents" and reduce stress, try the following as they pertain to body, mind, soul, and interdependence.

Mind

Consider your sexual feelings and how they relate to other parts of your life.

Body

Think about physical responses you have to sexual stimulation (this might be responses to pictures, movies, music, physical closeness, etc.). Consider what the effects of these responses might be on effective communication with another person.

Soul

Think about your values. What are your goals for this year, the next few years, and for the long term? What effects might your sexual behavior have on these goals?

Interdependence

If you have someone with whom you have an intimate relationship, discuss the possible impact of the three preceding items on your desires and behavior. For example, what do they have to do with sexual thoughts and behavior? What do they have to do with choices about controlling births? If you are not in an intimate relationship, find several classmates who do not mind sharing some of their thoughts on this subject (you and they might not be comfortable sharing all of your thoughts).

Many "accidents" happen because individuals do not plan their behavior, consider their goals and values, or learn to communicate effectively in intimate situations. Taking these health actions can help prevent "accidents."

---

the early termination of pregnancy (Segal 1990; Silvestre et al. 1990). Because of its apparent safety and effectiveness, in 1991 the American Association for the Advancement of Science encouraged the FDA to clear the way so RU486 could be brought to the United States (Phillips, April 1991b).

Developing a male birth-control pill seems to be more difficult than developing one for the female, but research continues in several directions. One of these is research on the compound gossypol, which seems to inhibit enzyme activity necessary for sperm production. It decreases sperm production while not decreasing testosterone levels, but sperm production does not always return to normal when men stop taking it. It also seems to have potential negative effects on liver functions, gastrointestinal functions, and cardiac patterns and efficiency (Sang 1985).

Other chemicals thought to have potential as a male contraceptive have been tried on animals. So far, none of these totally prevent sperm production. Those that are most effective also have unacceptable side effects, such as decreased sex drive, decreased testosterone levels, and an inability to achieve an erection. Interestingly, weekly injections of testosterone seem to have promise as a safe and effective way to suppress sperm production ("A Male Contraceptive" 1991).

Contraceptive vaccines are also being explored. It makes sense that a vaccine in a female would prevent fertilization more effectively than a method that works after conception. Similarly, in the male there are attempts to develop a vaccine that will inhibit sperm production (Philips, March 1991a).

Some experts believe there will be fewer contraceptive methods at the end of the twentieth century than there were at the beginning. This is because of the prohibitive costs of liability insurance, the costs of developing new products, the amount of time before the FDA grants approval, and the costs involved in getting such approval ("Special Report on Contraception" 1986; Jenks 1990).

Since the introduction over three decades ago of the pill and the IUD, no fundamentally new contraceptive method has been introduced in the United States except Norplant. Many feel that new methods could become available if there were more support for their development (Mastroianni, Donaldson, and Kane 1990).

Abortion

Abortion is premature expulsion from the uterus of a fertilized egg, embryo, or nonviable fetus. It can occur naturally (usually termed a **miscarriage** or **spontaneous abortion**) or be induced. Abortion differs from most contraceptive methods in that fertilization has already occurred before intentional or spontaneous action prevents the birth.

Abortion is one of the controversial issues of our day. In 1973, it became illegal for states to prohibit abortion in the early months of pregnancy, and many considered abortion a female right. In 1989, the U.S. Supreme Court shifted the focus of the abortion controversy back to the states. This occurred because the Court again showed a willingness to intervene in state abortion policies. This had not been done since 1973 (Fulton 1990).

Many legal questions are still being considered as a result of the 1989 Supreme Court decision and the influence of the Clinton administration. For example, when does the life of a human being begin? Do unborn children (if they can even be called children) have rights? Can public funds be used for abortions? Whose permission is needed before an abortion can be performed? We will probably see the abortion controversy in the news for a long time to come. The United States, however, continues to have one of the higher abortion rates among developed countries ("Abortion in the United States" 1991). The number of abortions in the United States has leveled off at around 1.6 million per year. Women who have abortions are predominantly young (25 percent under twenty years of age and 33 percent from twenty to twenty-four), unmarried (63 percent), and of poor to modest financial means. The national abortion rate is about 27.3 per 1,000 pregnancies ("Today's News" 1992).

Major Methods of Abortion

Whether you believe abortion is acceptable or not, you should understand a little about the process. Traditionally, the most common method of abortion has been **dilation and curettage (D and C),** a procedure that must be carried out within the first twelve weeks of pregnancy. This method involves dilation of the cervix (by inserting graduated sizes of instruments to stretch the opening) and scraping of the uterine cavity (curettage) to remove all developing tissues.

A variation of this method is **suction curettage,** in which the contents of the uterus are sucked out as the uterine lining is scraped. Suction curettage is by far the preferred and most commonly performed abortion method today due to its relative simplicity and lack of extreme pain.

Another method of abortion is **saline induction,** a procedure that cannot usually be performed until after sixteen weeks of pregnancy. In this method, some **amniotic fluid** (fluid surrounding the fetus) is withdrawn through the abdominal wall and a saline (salt) solution is injected. The solution kills the *fetus* (unborn child from third month after conception on) and induces uterine contractions (labor) after twenty-four to forty-eight hours. The woman goes through labor to expel the dead fetus and the *placenta* (the organ that connects the fetus to the uterus through the umbilical cord). Sometimes a follow-up D and C is necessary to remove dead tissue.

> ### ISSUE
>
> ### Should Abortions Be Legal?
>
> Some of the pros and cons of abortion are listed here. Can you add any to the list?
>
> • Pro:
>
> 1. Government has no right to limit the freedom of a woman's choice.
> 2. Human life doesn't begin until a fetus is capable of living outside the mother.
> 3. Women should have the right to control their own bodies.
> 4. Unwanted children should not be brought into the world.
> 5. Women show few negative emotional reactions as a result of abortion; in fact, many show emotional benefit.
>
> • Con:
>
> 1. Government has no right to authorize destruction of a fetus or embryo.
> 2. Human life begins at the moment of conception.
> 3. Humans do not have the right to take the lives of other innocent humans.
> 4. Every human being—wanted or unwanted—receives its right to life directly from God.
> 5. Women are psychologically damaged by abortion.
>
> Should abortions be legal?

The final major method of abortion is a **hysterotomy.** In this procedure, an incision is made through the lower abdomen and the wall of the uterus, and the fetus and related tissue are removed. This is similar to what is done in a cesarean section delivery at the end of a pregnancy and involves several days of recovery in a hospital.

Some have feared that many women would have serious psychological consequences from abortions, but this does not seem to be the case. Although there may be sensations of regret, sadness, or guilt, evidence from the best scientific studies indicates a legal abortion early in pregnancy is not hazardous to most women's mental health ("Lack of Evidence for Post-Abortion Syndrome Found" 1990).

Even among teenagers, those who chose to have an abortion were more likely to stay in school, were no more likely to have psychological problems, and were economically better off after two years than those who decided to have a child. In addition, those choosing abortion were more likely to adopt a consistent contraceptive method and avoid a repeat pregnancy ("Study Finds No Negative Consequences for Teen Abortion" 1990).

Future Methods of Abortion

Extensive abortion research is being done with **prostaglandins,** fatty acid substances found naturally in the body. They can be injected into the uterus in a similar manner to the saline solution and induce labor much more quickly and simply. This method may be used between twelve and sixteen weeks of pregnancy, a time when other methods cannot be used. Prostaglandin abortions are available in the United States on a limited basis and should probably still be considered in a research stage.

The missed-period pill (RU486), already discussed as part of contraceptive research, might also be considered as a future abortion method—depending on your point of view. At any rate, since it is known that statistically an early abortion is safer than going through a pregnancy, it is likely that additional abortion research will continue.

Summary

1. For conception to occur, a mature egg must be in a position to be fertilized and the sperm must reach the egg.

2. Many myths exist about menstruation; however, it is known that cycle lengths vary from woman to woman and even for the same woman, that there are phases to the cycle that are controlled by hormones, and that it is difficult to calculate the most fertile time in the cycle.

3. There are many functions performed by the semen while keeping the sperm alive and capable of fertilizing an egg. Infertility can be caused by a number of reasons, but today there are many ways to treat infertility.

4. Many factors can influence a healthy pregnancy. Genetic counseling and the use of a variety of tests can be helpful to many couples interested in improving their chances of having a healthy baby.

5. A number of consumer decisions need to be made related to labor and delivery. These include the type of childbirth, the place for childbirth, immediate care of the baby after birth, and whether to circumcise a newborn male.

6. There are a number of arguments for and against contraception. Decisions related to birth control have many health implications.

7. The most effective contraceptive method available is probably the pill. Taking the pill is statistically safer than going through a pregnancy. In addition, the pill promotes a number of positive side effects.

8. Diaphragms and condoms can be effective barriers to sperm if care is used. Spermicides used alone are less effective than previously mentioned methods, but they can help increase the effectiveness of other methods.

9. The sponge method seems to have promise as an effective contraceptive. Fertility awareness is becoming more reliable as better ways to pinpoint ovulation are developed.

10. The cervical cap is considered experimental, and IUDs are only available on a limited basis in the United States. Ineffective contraceptive methods include coitus interruptus and use of the vaginal douche.

11. Sterilization is very safe and effective but should still be considered permanent. A great deal of contraceptive research is still being done.

12. Abortion has been controversial through the years and remains so today. Medically, it is a safe procedure that can be done using various methods.

Commitment Activities

1. If you are a female (or a male with a strong intimate relationship with a female), carefully follow your menstrual cycle for three to six months. Through the use of careful record keeping, try to determine as closely as possible the time of ovulation during each cycle. What can you conclude after you have this information?

2. Check with local hospitals to see what facilities are available for parents wishing to have their babies away from the traditional delivery room. What are the hospital policies about deliveries outside of the delivery room? Do they have any special facilities? Will the medical staff cooperate if a pregnant woman wishes to deliver her baby at home? Are there birthing centers away from the hospital? What would you decide about delivery if you (or your mate) were pregnant?

3. Population dynamics can be related to the quality of life. Too many or too few people in a given area might considerably influence the health of all. Survey your community to determine where overpopulation or underpopulation might contribute to potential health problems. Develop recommendations that could be used to help reduce these problems.

4. Think about your feelings concerning abortion. Is it always acceptable to you? Is it never acceptable? If it is acceptable, what circumstances make it so? After you have clarified your feelings, talk with others (particularly those who have strong feelings at both extremes on this issue) to be sure you understand why they feel as they do. Once you better understand where they are coming from, see if this new information has any effect on your feelings. Ask yourself the same questions again.

5. How do you feel about the need to control births and the use of contraceptives? What is appropriate in your own life? Once you have clarified your own feelings,

outline a plan for communicating your feelings to a potential partner or your present one. How will you handle it if your partner feels differently about decisions related to birth control? Is there a way to reconcile any differences?

References

"Abortion in the United States." *Facts in Brief.* New York: The Alan Guttmacher Institute, 1991.

"Amniocentesis Now Available in the First Trimester." *UAB Insight* (Winter 1992):12.

Berkowitz, G. S., et al. "Delayed Childbearing and the Outcome of Pregnancy." *New England Journal of Medicine* 322, no. 10 (March 8, 1990):659–63.

Better Health 4, no. 2 (February 1987):3.

"Birthing Procedure Hurts Mother More Than It Helps." *Edell Health Letter* 10, no. 10 (November 1991):7.

Bogren, L. Y. "Changes in Sexuality in Women and Men During Pregnancy." *Archives of Sexual Behavior* 20, no. 1 (February 1991):35–45.

"C-Section Rates Remain High, But Postcesarean Vaginal Births Are Rising." *Family Planning Perspectives* 21, no. 1 (January/February 1990):36–37.

"CVS Tops Amniocentesis? Miscarriage Rate Worrisome." *Sexuality Today* (January 14, 1985):4.

"Diet Affects Menstrual Cycle." *Edell Health Letter* 12, no. 1 (December 1992/January 1993):6–7.

Doshi, M. "Accuracy of Consumer Performed In-Home Tests for Early Pregnancy Detection." *American Journal of Public Health* 76, no. 5 (May 1986):512–14.

Edell, D. "Good News About the Pill." *Edell Health Letter* 9, no. 4 (April 1990d):4.

Edell, D. "Pasta and Potatoes Prescribed for PMS." *Edell Health Letter* 9, no. 4 (April 1990a):5.

Edell, D. "Q & A With Dr. Edell—Breast-Feeding." *Edell Health Letter* 9, no. 4 (April 1990c):8.

Edell, D. "Q & A With Dr. Edell—Episiotomies." *Edell Health Letter* 9, no. 4 (April 1990b):8.

"Evaluating the Cesarean Decision." *Family Planning Perspectives* 22, no. 6 (November/December 1990):245.

"Exercise Through Third Trimester?" *Medical World News* 11 (March 1985).

"FDA OKs Hormonal Implant." *Family Planning Perspectives* 22, no. 6 (November/December 1990):244.

Fulton, G. B. "Abortion . . . after Webster." *Our Sexuality Update.* Benjamin/Cummings Publishing, Winter 1990 pp. 7–8.

Hantula, R. "IUDs." *Spotlight on Health* 1, Macmillan Educational Co., 1986 p. 7.

Hatcher, R., et al. *Contraceptive Technology 1986–1987,* 13th ed. New York: Irvington, 1986.

Higgins, B. S. "Couple Infertility: From the Perspective of the Close-Relationship Model." *Family Relations* 39, no. 1 (January 1990):81–86.

"Hormonal Contraception: New Long-Acting Methods." *Population Reports,* Series K, 3 (March–April 1987): K57–K87.

"Hormonal Implants Prove to Be Highly Acceptable." *Family Planning Perspectives* 22, no. 5 (September/October 1990): 234–35.

"Infertility as a Function of Body Weight." *UAB Insight* (Winter 1992):12.

"Intracervical 'Electric Fence' Keeps Out Sperm." *Sexuality Today* (January 19, 1987):3.

"IUD Underused." *Edell Health Letter* 11, no. 2 (February 1992):1–2.

Jenks, S. "Contraceptive Choices in U.S. Scarce, Experts Find." *Medical World News* 31, no. 5 (March 12, 1990):37.

Jones, E. F., and Forrest, J. D. "Contraceptive Failure Rates Based on the 1988 NSFG." *Family Planning Perspectives* 24, no. 1 (January/February 1992):12–18.

Kiely, J. L.; Kleinman, J. C.; and Kiely, M. "Triplets and Higher Order Multiple Births." *American Journal of Diseases of Children* 146 (July 1992):862–68.

Koop, C. E. *Surgeon General's Report on Acquired Immune Deficiency Syndrome.* Washington, D.C.: U.S. Public Health Service, October 1986.

"Lack of Evidence for Post-Abortion Syndrome Found." *Behavior Today* 21, no. 17 (April 23, 1990):6–7.

Leboyer, F. *Birth Without Violence.* New York: Knopf, 1975.

"The Low-Dose IUD." *Family Planning Perspectives* 22, no. 6 (November/December 1990):245.

"A Male Contraceptive." *Harvard Health Letter* 16, no. 3 (January 1991):7.

"March of Dimes Fact Sheet." White Plains, N.Y.: March of Dimes Birth Defects Foundation, 1991.

Masters, W. H., and Johnson, V. E. *Human Sexual Response.* Boston: Little, Brown, 1966.

Mastroianni, L., Jr.; Donaldson, P. J.; and Kane, T. T. "Development of Contraceptives—Obstacles and Opportunities." *New England Journal of Medicine.* 322, no. 7 (February 15, 1990):482–84.

"Minipill May Have Broader Appeal." *Family Planning Perspectives* 23, no. 1 (January/February 1991):5.

"The Missed-Period Pill." *Harvard Medical School Health Letter* 12, no. 5 (March 1987):1–2.

"New Device to Aid in Natural Family Planning." *Sexuality Today* 20 (December 1982):5.

"A New Prenatal Screening Program." *Harvard Medical School Health Letter* 12, no. 40 (February 1987):6–8.

Phillips, P. "Contraceptive Vaccines Inch Nearer to Clinical Trials." *Medical World News* 32, no. 3 (March 1991):17.

Phillips, P. "Mainstream U.S. Scientists Back Controversial RU 486." *Medical World News* 32, no. 4 (April 1991):47.

Poland, R. L. "The Question of Routine Neonatal Circumcision." *New England Journal of Medicine* 322, no. 18 (May 3, 1990):1312–15.

Portnes, J. "Little Change in Teenage Programming Rate During 80's Found." *Education Week* 12, no. 2 (November 25, 1992):8.

"Pros and Cons of Norplant." *UAB Insight* (Spring 1992):13.

Resnik, R. "The 'Elderly Primigravida' In 1990." *New England Journal of Medicine.* 322, no. 10 (March 8, 1990):693–94.

Sang, G. W. "Gossypol—A Potential Contraceptive for Men?" *Internal Medicine for the Specialist* 6 (1985): 118–25.

Segal, S. J. "Mifepristone (RU486)." *New England Journal of Medicine* 322, no. 10 (March 6, 1990):691–92.

"Sex Safe During Pregnancy: Largest Study Ever." *Sexuality Today* 8, no. 7 (December 3, 1984):1, 3.

Silvestre, L., et al. "Voluntary Interruption of Pregnancy with Mifepristone (RU486) and a Prostaglandin Analogue." *New England Journal of Medicine* 322, no. 10 (March 8, 1990):645–48.

Siwek, J. "Circumcision: The Debate Continues." *American Family Physician* 41, no. 3 (March 1990):817–18.

"A Slimmer Copper T." *Family Planning Perspectives* 23, no. 1 (January/February 1991):5.

"Special Report on Contraception: Where Will We Be in the Year 2010?" *Sexuality Today* 9, no. 35 (June 16, 1986):1, 2.

Sroka, S. R. "Common Sense on Condom Education." *Education Week X,* no. 25 (March 13, 1991):39–40.

Stark, E. "Young, Innocent and Pregnant." *Psychology Today* (October 1986):32–35.

"Sterilization Is Unlikely to Alter Most Women's Menstrual Symptoms." *Family Planning Perspectives* 22, no. 1 (January/February 1990):44–45.

"Stress During Pregnancy Linked to Premature Delivery." *Sexuality Today* 28 (January 1985):4.

"Study Finds No Negative Consequences for Teen Abortion." *Behavior Today* 21, no. 8 (February 19, 1990):6–8.

"Teenage Sexual and Reproductive Behavior." *Facts In Brief.* New York: The Alan Guttmacher Institute, 1991.

"Today's News." United States Centers for Disease Control, Atlanta, Georgia, June 30, 1992.

"Transvaginal Sonography Detects Early Pregnancy." *UAB Insight* (Spring 1992):12.

"Trends in Use of Oral Contraceptives." *Family Planning Perspectives* 22, no. 4 (July/August 1990):169–70.

"Ultrasound: Revelations About An Unborn Child." *Better Health* (April 1985):5–7.

"Users Approve of Female Condom." *Family Planning Perspectives* 23, no. 1 (January/February 1991):5.

"Vasectomy Proves to Be Preferable to Female Sterilization." *Family Planning Perspectives* 21, no. 4 (July/August 1989):191.

Wattleton, F. "Teen-Age Pregnancy: The Case for National Action." *The Nation* (July 24/31, 1989):138–41.

Whitley, B. E. "College Student Contraceptive Use: A Multivariate Analysis." *Journal of Sex Research* 27, no. 2 (May 1990):305–13.

Wiswell, T. E. "Routine Neonatal Circumcision: A Reappraisal." *American Family Physician* 41, no. 3 (March 1990):859–63.

Young, D. "How Can We 'Enrich' Prenatal Care?" *Birth* 17, no. 1 (March 1990):12–13.

Additional Readings

"Gallup Survey Points to Frequent Contraceptive Switching and Apparent Disregard for STD Protection." *SIECUS Report* 18, no. 4 (April/May 1990):25. Describes patterns of contraceptive use at different points in life. Points out how health issues and practical matters influence contraceptive decisions.

Neef, N. F.; Scutchfield, D.; Elder, J.; and Bender, S. J. "Testicular Self-Examination by Young Men: An Analysis of Characteristics Associated with Practice." *Journal of American College Health* 39 (January 1991):187–90. The level of testicular self-examination awareness and practice of 404 male college students was determined. Results and characteristics associated with practice are discussed.

Trussell, J.; Warner, D.; and Hatcher, R. A. "Condom Slippage and Breakage Rates." *Family Planning Perspectives* 24, no. 1 (January/February 1992):20–23. Presents factors involved with condom slippage and breakage and related statistics.

Turner, R. J.; Grindstaff, C. F.; and Phillips, N. "Social Support and the Outcome in Teenage Pregnancy." *Journal of Health and Social Behavior* 31 (March 1990):43–57. Presents information on the significance of social support for the occurrence of health and birth problems among adolescent mothers and their babies. The significance of family support, friend support, and partner support are discussed.

Psychoneuroimmunology (PNI), the study of the interaction between the mind, the central nervous system, and the body's immunological system, shows that people with a fighting spirit, optimism, hope, and faith can actually build their immune systems. The brain has the capability to self-medicate and to release a variety of mental and physical painkillers and motivating substances (neuropeptides) when the demand is there.

The topics that have been covered in this part have included several social, psychological, moral, and biological issues associated with sexuality and relationships. When considering the issues of love, family, intimacy, communication, sexual behavior (masturbation, homosexuality, and other variations), date rape, birth control, abortion, and other topics, the feelings and emotions as they pertain to PNI are quite clear. With negative experiences in sexuality and relationships, the outcome can be guilt, loneliness, rejection, sadness, pessimism, hopelessness, and depression. All of these emotions and feelings contribute to a weaker immune system, not to mention the quality of living. On the positive side of sexuality and relationships, the resulting feelings can be warmth, love, caring, optimism, trust, happiness, security, cause, and perceived emotional support. With these positive traits, we are looking at a fortified immune system and a good life quality.

Based on this generalization, it should be clear that there are two PNI intervention approaches. The first is to relieve oneself from the negative emotions, and the second is to maximize the emotions and feelings that come from the social, psychological, moral, and biological aspects of sexuality and relationships. The following is a series of questions you may want to consider to avoid the negative outcomes of a relationship and feel the positive outcomes. Remember that the positive fortifies.

If you are already in a relationship, consider these questions that (with positive response) can fortify positive outcomes of relationships.

1. Are you living in a mind state of appreciation for what you have rather than looking for what you could possibly get?

2. Are you in the relationship with the idea of giving to it rather than seeing what you can get from it?

3. Are you avoiding a "take it for granted" mind state?

4. Are you staying within the bounds of what you and your partner consider moral behavioral conduct?

5. Have you talked about what each other considers moral behavioral conduct?

6. Do you avoid saying something you regret to your partner?

7. Are you aware of your emotional state when you are angry or are out of control?

8. Can you get over being angry soon?

9. Do you take pleasure in being close to someone and enjoying the moment as opposed to always looking to see how "far you can go"?

10. Are you spontaneous, playful, and fun in a relationship?

11. When you see your partner, do you link seeing him or her with positive emotional states?

12. Do you give what you most want in a relationship?

13. Do you try and find out those things that really make your partner feel loved? (Is it when I buy you something? Take you somewhere? Say I love you? Touch you a certain way? Play a certain way?)

If you are not in a relationship but want to be, consider some of the following questions.

1. Do you believe that you will find someone with whom you can have a good relationship?

2. Do you seek opportunities to meet people at places that will attract the types of partners that you would like to be with?

3. Are you being your natural yet best self when interacting with others as compared to putting on a phony front?

4. Are you looking for someone who has common interests, a compatible personality, and other commonalities or complementary traits as opposed to superficial characteristics like physical attractiveness?

5. Are you friendly and assertive?

If you are feeling the negative outcomes of a relationship, particularly guilt, be sure that you attempt to purge that guilt. If you have done something that makes you feel guilty, then quit doing that behavior. Seek a means to forgive yourself. If relieving your guilt involves the counsel of or confession to a religious leader, then go through those steps to purge yourself.

Maximize your relationships by enjoying the process of dating, courting, and just being friends. Those who worry about where the relationship is going, are not able to be themselves, or behave in a way to please others, generally see the stagnation of a relationship over time. When it is natural, honest, friendly, and fun, then relationships and the immune system can be fortified.

By reading and working through the activities in the last three chapters on sexual choices, you should have a good understanding of

1. human sexuality, its dimensions, its relationship to all people, and its connection to human well-being;
2. intimate relationships and communication;
3. parenting and sexuality education;
4. human sexual response;
5. variations in sexual behavior;
6. human reproduction;
7. influences on a healthy pregnancy;
8. ways to control conception;
9. issues related to conception control.

There has also been an opportunity to assess your feelings about many sexual issues. It is clear that human sexuality is a topic that often causes strong reactions and feelings. These can have a significant impact on health decisions.

Since sexuality is an important part of health, it is appropriate to consider ways to strengthen your well-being related to sexuality and prevent potential problems. The prevention model presented in chapter 1 provides the framework within which to consider the relevance of the issues presented in this section.

The following list includes some sample behaviors related to human sexuality. These are only possibilities and there may be others that are more appropriate for you.

1. Decide how you will educate your children (now or in the future) about sexuality.
2. Improve communication skills within your intimate relationships (friends, spouse, children, etc.).
3. Many people think negatively about some aspects of human sexuality. Develop a plan to reduce such negative thinking in your life so sexuality can become more of a positive aspect of your health decisions.
4. Recognize that those who have different sexual life-styles have emotional needs, self-esteem needs, and acceptance needs just like anyone else.
5. Sexually active students, as well as those who are not active at this time, can become process oriented (focusing on the enjoyment of the relationship and expressing feelings and love) rather than product oriented (focusing on sexual intercourse as the goal). If appropriate, try to focus more on the quality of the relationship instead of on specific sexual behaviors.
6. Take precautions to reduce the risk of sexual abuse. This might relate to date rape, rape in other situations, or teaching children how to avoid sexual abuse.
7. Develop a plan for a woman who might want to be pregnant so she can maximize her potential to have a healthy baby.

8. Be sensitive about comments made to couples who do not have children—especially if it is known that they wish to have children.
9. If you choose to participate in sexual intercourse, but do not wish to cause a pregnancy, develop a plan for ways to avoid a pregnancy.
10. Since sexual activity for many people is influenced by personal values, develop a contract to promote consistency between the activity and the values.
11. Think of a situation related to human sexuality that has caused disorganization or disruption in your life. Develop a plan to promote resilient adjustment (see chapter 1 for a review of these terms) in your life to prevent potential health problems related to sexuality in the future.

Life-Style Contracting Using Strength Intervention

I. Choosing the desired health behavior or skill

A. Keeping in mind the purposes in life and goals you identified in the mental health chapter, consider one or two health behaviors related to human sexuality (from the list here or of your own creation) that will help you reach your goals. To assess the likelihood of success, ask yourself questions similar to those used in previous sections, such as the following:

1. Is my purpose, cause, or goal better realized by the adoption of this behavior?
____ yes ____ no
2. Am I hardy enough to accomplish this goal? (This means I feel I can do it if I work hard, I am in control of what needs to be done, I am committed to do it, and the goal is a challenge for me.) ____ yes ____ no
3. Is this a behavior I really want to change and that I feel I can change? ____ yes ____ no
4. Do I first need to nurture a personal strength area?
____ yes ____ no
(If yes, be sure to include this as part of the plan.)
5. Do I need to free myself from a bad habit to accomplish this goal? ____ yes ____ no
(If yes, be sure to include this as part of the plan.)
6. Have I considered the results of the assessments in the three sexuality chapters?
____ yes ____ no
These results may be helpful in developing a plan.

(Yes answers to the first three questions are a must to be successful. It might be wise to consider a different behavior if you cannot honestly answer yes to these questions. Your answers to questions 4–6 ought to provide information for consideration in your plan.)

B.   Behaviors I will change (no more than two).

_____

_____

II. Life-style plan

A.   A description of the general plan of what I am going to do and how I will accomplish it. Consider apperceptive experiences (successes you have had in the past) since they may help you consider the best ways to carry out this plan.

_____

_____

_____

_____

_____

_____

B.   Barriers to accomplishment of the plan (lack of time, feelings of others, my own hang-ups, motivation, etc.).

1.   Identify barriers _____

_____

_____

_____

2.   Means to remove barriers (use problem-solving skills or creative approaches such as those described in the mental health chapter) _____

_____

_____

_____

C.   Implementation of the plan.

1.   Substitution (putting positive behaviors in place of negative ones) _____

_____

2.   Confluence (combining activities for time efficiency if possible) _____

_____

3.   Systematic enhancement (using a strength to help a weakness)_____

_____

4.   When_____

5.   Where _____

6.   Preparation_____

_____

7.   With whom_____

III. Support groups

A.   Who _____

_____

B.   Role _____

_____

C.   Organized support _____

_____

IV. Trigger responses_____

_____

V.   Starting date_____

_____

VI. Date/sequence the contract will be reevaluated _____

_____

VII. Evidence of reaching goal _____

_____

VIII. Rewards when contract is completed _____

_____

IX. Signature of client_____

_____

X.   Signature of facilitator _____

XI. Additional conditions/comments_____

_____

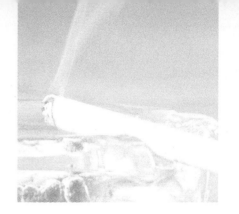

PART IV

Chemical Choices

WE ARE FACED WITH DIFFICULT CHOICES IN REGARD TO CHEMICAL SUBSTANCES WE CHOOSE TO USE. CHAPTER 10 CITES THE DANGERS, EFFECTS, AND PREVENTIVE STRATEGIES OF OVER-THE-COUNTER AND ILLEGAL DRUGS. CHAPTER 11 PROVIDES INSIGHTS INTO THE USE AND MISUSE OF ETHYL ALCOHOL FOR THOSE FACED WITH THE CHOICE OF DRINKING AFTER THEY REACH THE LEGAL DRINKING AGE. CHAPTER 12 DESCRIBES THE PHYSICAL DEVASTATION EXPERIENCED BY THOSE WHO SMOKE TOBACCO AND NONSMOKERS WHO BREATHE SIDESTREAM SMOKE. THE SOCIAL, POLITICAL, EMOTIONAL, AND MEDICAL IMPLICATIONS OF CHEMICAL USE IS PRESENTED IN ALL THREE CHAPTERS.

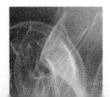

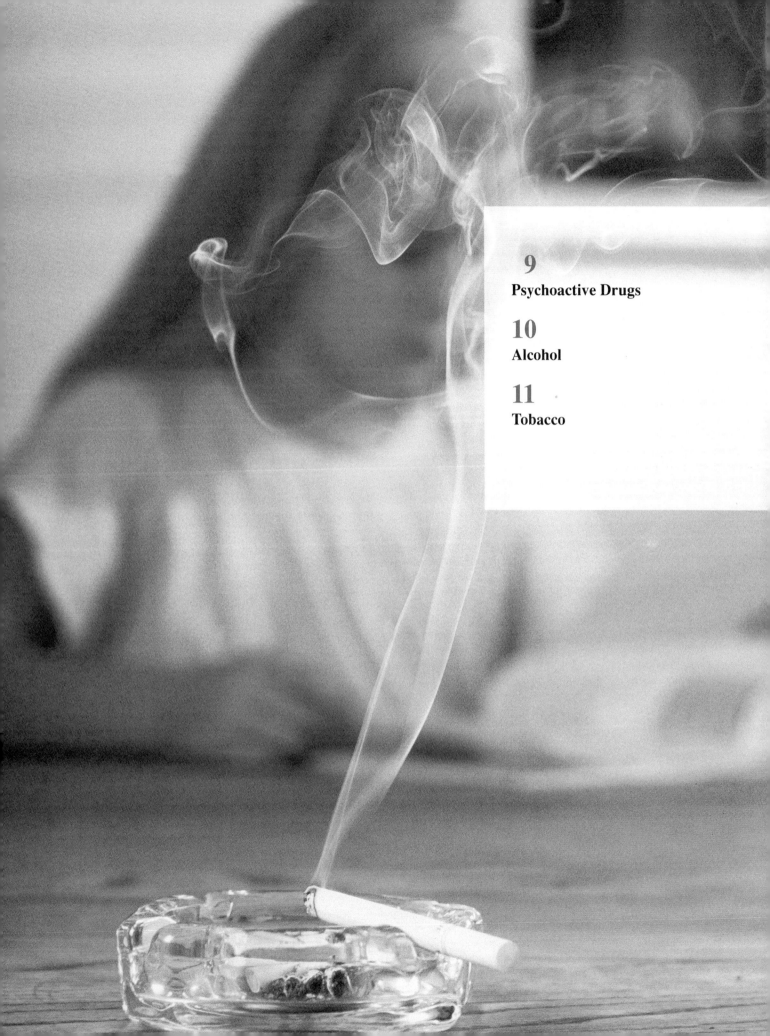

CHAPTER 9

Psychoactive Drugs

Key Questions

- What is a psychoactive drug?

- What are some reasons individuals use drugs?

- What does psychoactive substance dependence mean?

- Why are designer drugs and free-based cocaine so dangerous?

- What are the classifications of drugs?

- How does drug testing affect employees and athletes?

- What is meant by drug abuse?

- For which classification of drugs is it the most dangerous to quit suddenly after using the substance for some time?

- How can we avoid drug use or abuse?

Chapter Outline

Motivations for Drug Use
Psychoactive Substance Dependence
　　and Abuse
　　Genetic Vulnerability
　　The Addiction Cycle
Types of Psychoactive Drugs
　　Cannabis Products
　　Narcotics
　　Stimulants
　　Depressants
　　Hallucinogens
Drugs in Sports
　　Steroids and Growth Hormone
　　Drug Testing
Drug Interactions
Drug Use and AIDS
Drugs and the Law

Beginning in the mid-1980s, the United States entered an aggressive war on drugs. Not since the 1960s has the country made such efforts to educate and prevent drug use and abuse. In Harlem, angry residents painted large red Xs on crack dealers' doors and put stuffed animals in abandoned building windows as a symbolic gesture to reclaim them from drug users. In New Mexico, two children turned in their parents to police for marijuana possession, and in California, a girl turned in her cocaine-using parents. In 1986, President Reagan made several national appearances with his wife, Nancy Reagan, to stage the "war on drugs."

President Bush and his wife, Barbara Bush, continued the war into the 1990s. Although some criticized him for not doing enough in treatment and prevention, he worked intently on the international front, particularly in South America and Mexico, to crack down on the drug cartel and substitute other cash crops for drug crops. It will be interesting to see how Bill Clinton and his wife, Hillary Rodham Clinton, attack the drug problem during his administration.

Drug testing in athletics, businesses, and government positions has created much controversy. In

1986, Congress allocated hundreds of millions of dollars to prevent and treat drug use and abuse. Almost every state in the union has a governor's council on drugs to deal with drug issues particular to each state.

Why is there a renewed war on drugs? Some of the reasons are that the drugs available today are much more potent, dangerous, addicting, and available than ever before. The marijuana smoked today is twenty times more potent than marijuana smoked in 1964. Cocaine, once labeled the "rich man's" drug, is not only cheaper, but it is easily transformed (free-based) into crack, a substance that is forty times as addictive as cocaine and is sold on the streets for a relatively cheap price.

Methamphetamine (speed), which arrived here from Korea and Japan, is bad enough in its original state, but it has been refined into a rock crystalline form, intensifying the addictiveness and debilitative nature of the drug. Designer drugs, which can be mass-produced in a single laboratory, are made from readily available chemicals and are one thousand times as potent as heroin. Some botched batches have left a trail of users with symptoms such as those of Parkinson's disease and other forms of brain damage.

With all the benefits of today's technology, opportunists have gained the skills to develop drugs that can ruin lives. The knowledge exists to synthesize powerful narcotics for hundreds of dollars and make profits in the millions. Healthy individuals can be debilitated in a matter of a few days or weeks with some of the drugs produced.

This chapter will create an awareness of the new drug epidemic that has hit the United States and the world. It is hoped you will make wise decisions regarding the use of illicit, prescription, and over-the-counter drugs.

Motivations for Drug Use

Most individuals sixteen to twenty-five years old try drugs only once or twice as an experiment because they are curious or because their friends use drugs (Mannatt 1980). Some try drugs primarily for pleasure or recreation or to help them through unpleasant situations. The following list of reasons for using drugs has been suggested by experts (Schlaadt and Shannon 1986; Towers 1987):

1. to feel less afraid and more courageous;
2. to find out more about oneself;
3. to have a religious experience or come closer to God;
4. to satisfy a strong craving or compulsion;
5. to relieve boredom;
6. to find altered states and increase the intensity of moods;
7. to relieve tension or nervousness;
8. to shut things out of their minds;
9. to recreate and have fun;
10. to escape from boredom;
11. to experience a different kind of awareness;
12. to make it easier to be more social, begin conversations, and promote camaraderie;
13. to find stimulating and sensational experiences;
14. to feel less depressed or sad;
15. to demonstrate rebellion to parents and social norms by using drugs illegally;
16. because of peer pressure;
17. to escape life stressors and pain;
18. to feel capable and wanted (overcome a lack of self-worth);
19. to perform better in school, athletics, or work;
20. to follow family modeling or deal with family inconsistencies.

You must decide if these reasons for using drugs are worth the consequences of addiction, illness, emotional disruption, failed relationships, and even death.

Psychoactive Substance Dependence and Abuse

According to the American Psychiatric Association, problem use of drugs is termed either *psychoactive substance dependence* or *abuse.* Dependence has both physiological and psychological components.

Physiological dependence is characterized by tolerance and withdrawal symptoms. Tolerance, explained in more detail in the chapter on alcohol, is a condition in which it takes increasingly larger amounts of a drug to produce the same effects previously felt at lower dosages. Withdrawal refers to the physical disturbance or cluster of symptoms that occurs when the drug is taken away or becomes unavailable. Withdrawal symptoms are an indication that the body has adapted to the presence of the drug, that the drug is required for the individual to function normally, and that the development of physical dependence has occurred. "Psychological dependence is a condition in which the drug produces a feeling of satisfaction and a psychological drive that requires periodic or continuous drug use to produce pleasure or avoid discomfort" (Jensen 1987). The American Psychiatric Association (1987) suggests that any three of the following criteria are indicators of psychoactive substance dependence:

1. substance often taken in larger amounts or over a longer period than the person intended;
2. persistent desire or one or more unsuccessful efforts to cut down or control substance use;
3. a great deal of time spent in activities necessary to get the substance (e.g., theft), taking the substance (e.g., chain-smoking), or recovering from its effects;
4. frequent intoxication or withdrawal symptoms when expected to fulfill major role obligations at work, school, or home (e.g., does not go to work because hung over, goes to school or work "high," intoxicated while taking care of his or her children) or

The following assessment tools include a risk assessment for nonusers of drugs, an early detection tool, and a step to drug abuse assessment tool. The drugs referred to in this questionnaire refer to prescription or illegal drugs that can be abused (i.e., cocaine, marijuana, speed, downers, heroin, Valium, and so on).

Drug Risk Assessment

This questionnaire is designed for those who are not currently using drugs. If you currently use drugs, then this does not apply to you.

Directions: Use the a, b, and c codes to respond to the following list of characteristics or situations.

a = This definitely applies to me or applied to me.

b = This somewhat applies or applied to me.

c = This does not apply or never did apply to me.

1. My parents (guardians) and I have a good relationship.　　a　b　c
2. My parents (guardians) and I share our feelings openly and comfortably.　　a　b　c
3. I place a lot of importance on achievement.　　a　b　c
4. I am very sensitive to criticism by my friends.　　a　b　c
5. It is not important for me to do things that are socially acceptable.　　a　b　c
6. I am very religious.　　a　b　c
7. I get very good grades.　　a　b　c
8. Some of my friends use drugs.　　a　b　c
9. I feel depressed quite frequently.　　a　b　c
10. I grew up with only one parent in my home.　　a　b　c
11. The people I live with now use drugs.　　a　b　c
12. I have a rebellious nature.　　a　b　c
13. I skip class frequently.　　a　b　c
14. I have a low opinion of myself.　　a　b　c
15. My parents (guardians) use(d) drugs.　　a　b　c
16. I have experimented with drugs.　　a　b　c
17. My home is chaotic and disorganized.　　a　b　c
18. I often feel guilty.　　a　b　c
19. I have feelings of insecurity.　　a　b　c
20. I have often wanted to try a drug just to see what it was like.　　a　b　c

Scoring/Interpretation

For questions 1, 2, 3, 6, and 7, score as follows:

a = 3 points

b = 2 points

c = 1 point

For all other questions, score as follows:

a = 1 point

b = 2 points

c = 3 points

Total your score for all twenty items.

This is a risk assessment tool, which means that numerous studies have shown that there is a higher risk for some individuals to become drug abusers over others. These risk factors do not mean that someone will become a drug abuser, but it does mean that those with a particular background have become drug abusers more frequently than those who do not have these characteristics. Your total points can be interpreted as follows:

20–33 high risk

34–46 moderate risk

47–60 low risk

Detection of Drug Use Checklist

This tool is designed to aid you in helping others who might be starting to use drugs. As a roommate, sibling, or friend, it may be your opportunity to help someone who is just starting out with drugs. Picture someone in your life who you care about and want to keep off drugs, and apply this questionnaire to them.

Directions: Mark a check by any of the symptoms that might apply to a person to whom you are close.

_____ 1. Recent trend toward self-centeredness

_____ 2. Motivation to achieve life goals weakens

_____ 3. Dress becomes noticeably more bizarre

_____ 4. Whites of the eyes are often bloodshot

_____ 5. Seems to be more sensitive to light

_____ 6. Friends seem to change to a less desirable group

_____ 7. Vague about social activities

_____ 8. Capacity to think is impaired and has a poor short-term memory

_____ 9. Emotions seem to be flattened

_____ 10. Tend to react to frustration with increased irritability or anger

_____ 11. Bottles of eye drops are found

_____ 12. Has frequent infections, runny nose, chronic cough

_____ 13. Use of gum or mints to cover breath

_____ 14. Change in sleeping patterns (i.e., can't sleep until late and sleeps a lot during the day)

_____ 15. Goes directly to own room and shuts door without interaction

_____ 16. Loses appetite

_____ 17. Blames others for problems

_____ 18. Speech may be slurred or has difficulty speaking

_____ 19. Does not answer when spoken to

_____ 20. Frequently lies and maintains lie when truth is discovered

_____ 21. Missing money or items from the home/room/apartment

_____ 22. Frequent use of incense in room

_____23. Seems to be more secretive

_____24. Needle marks or bruises on body

_____25. Less attention to cleanliness

_____26. Increased physical problems such as nausea, stomach problems, fatigue, sweats, trembling

_____27. Evidences of drug use such as rolling papers, seeds, razor blades, mirrors, miniature spoons, miniature tubes, miniature bottles, or other drug paraphernalia

Scoring/Interpretation

Score one point for each item checked, except for items 24 and 27.

If item 24 or 27 is checked, then there is a strong likelihood that the person is at least experimenting with drugs.

For other items, note that something is going on that is prompting a behavior change. If you care about this person, investigation through effective communication and paying attention to other potential cues may help you to help this person before dependence or addiction takes place. These symptoms may not represent drug use but could represent relationship, academic, or other types of problems.

Steps to Drug Abuse Assessment

This tool is designed to assess where you are in the steps that can lead to potential drug abuse. All of you are at least on step 1, but consider other steps.

Directions: Mark all that apply.

_____ 1. I do not take drugs and have no idea how to get them.

_____ 2. I do not take drugs but could get them if I wanted them.

_____ 3. I do not take drugs but would like to try sometime.

_____ 4. I have tried some drugs (e.g., marijuana) but no longer use them.

_____ 5. I use some soft drugs occasionally and socially.

_____ 6. I use some soft drugs regularly.

_____ 7. I have experimented with harder drugs (cocaine, crack, heroin, speed, barbiturates) but no longer use them.

_____ 8. I use a variety of drugs socially but regularly.

_____ 9. I take drugs regularly even when alone.

_____10. I need to take hard drugs regularly.

Interpretation

Look at the highest number you have marked. If there are any marks above number 2 you are at risk of abusing drugs. If you have checked number 5 or above, then you have a one in eight chance of becoming seriously addicted. If you have checked number 7 or above, then you have a one in three chance of becoming seriously addicted. If you have checked number 8 or above, you may already be seriously addicted. If you marked number 9 or 10, then you will need help immediately to recover from your drug abuse problem.

---

when substance use is physically hazardous (e.g., drives when intoxicated);

5. important social, occupational, or recreational activities given up or reduced because of substance use;

6. continued substance use despite knowledge of a persistent or recurrent social, psychological, or physical problem that is caused or made worse by the use of the substance (e.g., keeps using heroin despite family arguments about it, cocaine-induced depression, or having an ulcer made worse by drinking);

7. marked tolerance—need for markedly increased amounts of the substance (i.e., at least a 50 percent increase) to achieve intoxication or desired effect or markedly diminished effect with continued use of the same amount.

Note: The following items may not apply to cannabis, hallucinogens, or phencyclidine (PCP):

8. characteristic withdrawal symptoms (see specific withdrawal syndromes under "Psychoactive Substance-induced Organic Mental Disorders," American Psychiatric Association 1987);

9. substance often taken to relieve or avoid withdrawal symptoms;

10. some symptoms of the disturbance have persisted for at least one month or have occurred repeatedly over a longer period of time.

Psychoactive substance abuse may be indicated by a college student who "binges on cocaine every few weekends. These periods are followed by a day or two of missing school because of crashing. There are no other symptoms" (American Psychiatric Association 1987). Other examples are when a student repeatedly drives under the influence of a drug or keeps using a drug even when it irritates an ulcer and medical advice is to quit using the drug. Any of the following list of symptoms help identify the criteria for abuse (American Psychiatric Association 1987):

1. continued use despite knowledge of a persistent or recurrent social, occupational, psychological, or physical problem that is caused or exacerbated by use of the psychoactive substance;

2. recurrent use in situations in which use is physically hazardous (e.g., driving while intoxicated);

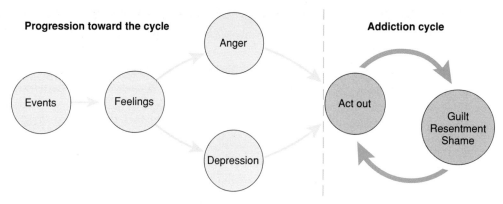

Figure 9.1
Progression toward the addiction cycle.

3. some symptoms of the disturbance have persisted for at least one month or have occurred repeatedly over a longer period of time;
4. never met the criteria for psychoactive substance dependence for this substance.

Genetic Vulnerability

One frightening fact to consider is the way that people generally begin to use drugs, that is, through the influence of someone who has had some drug experience. The assumption is that one person's reaction to a drug will be the same as the person who influences him or her. There is substantial evidence that genetic vulnerability to drugs is a significant factor in becoming addicted (Pickens and Svikis 1988). Someone using a drug may report a minimal effect, but the person to whom the user is recommending the drug may become addicted immediately. Although everyone can become addicted through repeated use, some, because of the variability among individuals, become drug addicts after one or two doses. The only safe course of action, particularly for those who are genetically vulnerable, is never to try drugs.

The Addiction Cycle

Stress reduction is a significant factor in using drugs. Life is so pressing for some individuals that they choose to escape from their problems temporarily or get an extra boost to cope through drug use. A common progression to drug abuse follows a series of events and feelings. First, it is likely that the individual experiences negative events (romantic breakup, death of a close person, academic problems, financial worries, etc.). The resultant feelings are likely hurt, inadequacy, feeling put down, rejection, abandonment, or fear. These feelings soon turn to anger and depression. Some may then act out their feelings by using drugs (or a variety of other addictions like gambling, eating, sex, shopping, etc.). After acting out, they feel self-defeated, guilty, resentment, and shame, so they act out some more. Thus, the cycle between negative feelings and acting out continues, which is the addiction cycle (fig. 9.1).

Types of Psychoactive Drugs

Many different psychoactive drugs are used, each with a different physiological and psychological effect. In the remainder of this chapter, the uses and effects of the major types of psychoactive drugs are presented. Because of the frequency of use, cannabis products are presented first, followed by the two categories that have been the major reason for the renewed war on drugs, the narcotics and stimulants. Within these two classifications, the new "ice," designer drugs, and crack have emerged. The other classifications of drugs, each with their own potential dangers, are the hallucinogens and depressants.

Cannabis Products

Aside from alcohol and tobacco, marijuana is the drug most used for nonmedical purposes in the United States. More than twenty-two million Americans use marijuana regularly. Marijuana and its sister drug, hashish, come from the Indian hemp plant Cannabis sativa, which grows wild throughout most of the tropical and temperate regions of the world. Marijuana is the dried leaves and flowering tops of the plant, while hashish is the processed resin. The solid form is dried resin, compressed into balls, cakes, or cookielike sheets. The liquid form, called hashish oil, is produced by a process of repeated extraction of the plant materials. Since marijuana is much more commonly used in the United States than hashish, most of this discussion centers on it.

Composition

Chemists have identified over 350 chemicals in marijuana and hashish, more than 50 of which are cannabinoids, that is, chemicals found only in cannabis products. Many of the effects of these chemicals are only partially understood, but we do know that the major psychoactive drug found in marijuana is **delta-9-tetrahydrocannabinol (THC).** The THC content of marijuana (and thus its effect on users) can vary greatly, from less than 1 percent to as much as 5 percent, depending on where the plants were grown and what part of the plant is used. The marijuana smoked today can be twenty to one hundred times more potent than in 1965 (Dusek and Girdano 1987).

The marijuana of today's generation is grown by hi-tech **hydroponics,** which means it is grown in nutrient solutions, with or without dirt as a base. As a result, the plant is drastically more potent and expensive than what was smoked in the late sixties. Rather than an average of 1 percent to 4 percent THC as in the late sixties, today's **sinsemilla,** the plant grown under these hi-tech conditions, produces 17 percent and higher THC concentrations. Instead of a buzz, the results are **hallucinations** (visual or imaginary perceptions), heavier withdrawal symptoms, more depressions, mood swings, and anxiety (Meacham 1990).

Marijuana and hashish work by entering the bloodstream and acting on the brain and nervous system. They can be either smoked or eaten but are about three times more potent when smoked. A single drop of hashish oil on a cigarette has the same effect as one marijuana joint; the effects are felt within minutes, reach their peak in ten to thirty minutes, and may linger for two to four hours. Effects depend partly on the amount of THC but may also vary according to the expectations and past experience of the user.

There are numerous acute effects of marijuana use on the body. Low doses can induce mood changes involving euphoria, a feeling of restlessness, a sense of well-being, relaxation, laughter, hunger, or sleepiness. Larger doses can cause confusion and disorientation to the environment, which users call "getting stoned." There may be changes in sensory perception, including more vivid senses of sight, smell, touch, and taste. Marijuana effects are based largely on the expectations of the user and the setting.

Stronger doses of marijuana also produce other physiological reactions. There is a 30 percent to 60 percent increase in heart rate, depending on the dosage, which is not very significant in a healthy person but potentially dangerous in a person with heart problems. Bronchodilation, an increase in the diameter of the air passages of the lungs, occurs. If inhaled deeply, the smoke may irritate these air passages.

Stronger doses may also produce changes in mental performance. Memory is impaired and time sense altered, so performance on various tasks is impaired. High doses may also result in image distortions, a loss of sense of personal identity, fantasies, relaxed inhibitions, and hallucinations. There is definite impairment of driving skills, even after ordinary social use of the drug (Liska 1981).

Heavy and prolonged use may also impair lung function (Liska 1981). When tobacco and marijuana are inhaled together, there is a synergistic effect more intense than the effect of either alone. It appears that marijuana may be more pathogenic than tobacco, due to the greater irritant effect, a greater degree of upper-airway involvement, and deeper smoking technique. Though lung cancer has not yet been seen, this may be because the latent period for lung cancer extends over decades.

Extensive government research has also suggested that daily use of substantial amounts of marijuana may adversely impair aspects of reproduction. It may (1) decrease the levels of sex hormones in males and females; (2) lower the level of testosterone in males, the major masculinizing hormone; (3) reduce sperm count and the sperm's ability to move, as well as increasing the incidence of abnormal sperm; (4) cause sexual dysfunction and impotence; (5) disrupt gonadal function; and (6) impair ovulation, cause defective menstrual cycles, and increase testosterone levels in females. It is not known if this last possibility can lead to problems with fertility or lactation or to cancer of the reproductive organs, but any drug that affects normal menstrual cycles may adversely affect fertility and reproductive health in later life. Researchers are also exploring the possible effects of marijuana use on chromosomes (Meacham 1990).

Since 1975, marijuana users have also had to worry about marijuana contaminated with **paraquat.** The U.S. and Mexican governments have tried to stop marijuana growing in Mexico by spraying the fields with this defoliant (plant killer). If the sprayed crop is harvested immediately, however, it can still be sold; thus, much Mexican marijuana is contaminated by high levels of paraquat. Smoking paraquat-contaminated marijuana can cause irreversible lung damage ("Pot and Paraquat" 1978).

People still grow marijuana, either for personal use or for sale, in forests, on government land, or in their own homes. The U.S. Forest Service has established hotlines in an effort to stop the illegal cultivation of marijuana in national forests (Howe 1992). A typical plant produces up to one and a half pounds of marijuana, enough to generate $6,000 on the market. Home-grown sinsemilla, the high-potent marijuana, is available through mail-order seed catalogues. Home-grown sinsemilla was Oregon's highest cash crop (Meacham 1990) and may be the nation's. On one day in Tucson and West Los Angeles, the highest pollen count causing allergy problems was from the illegally grown flowering marijuana plant (Wise 1989).

Abuse Potential

Psychological dependence on marijuana depends on the frequency of use, ranging from little or no dependence by intermittent users to compulsive behavior by very heavy users. Individuals apparently do not become **physically dependent** when marijuana is taken in relatively small amounts, but there is a possibility of dependence among very heavy users. **Withdrawal** symptoms from very high doses begin six to eight hours after the last dose and include restlessness, irritability, tremors, nausea, vomiting, diarrhea, and sleep disturbances (Meacham 1990).

Marijuana and the Law

The Marijuana Tax Act of 1937 regulated marijuana use until it was repealed by the more lenient Comprehensive Drug Abuse Prevention and Control Act of 1970. Possession of a small amount is usually considered a misdemeanor punishable by a fine. Often the misdemeanor does not become part of the person's criminal record.

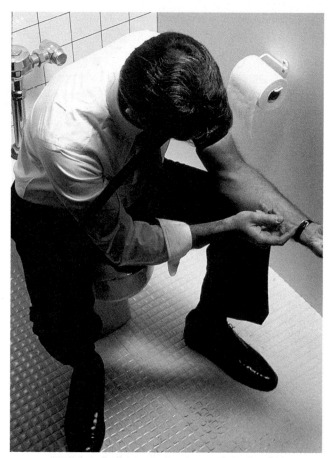

Illicit drugs have infiltrated all segments of society.

The initial effects of narcotic use may be extremely unpleasant, ranging from drowsiness, apathy, and constipation to nausea, vomiting, and depression of the respiratory system. These effects, however, are usually followed by a state of euphoria.

Repeated use of a narcotic tends to increase tolerance, forcing the user to obtain larger and larger doses to get the same effects and prevent withdrawal symptoms from occurring. Withdrawal symptoms are directly related to the amount of narcotic used daily. If the narcotic is withheld, symptoms appear before the next scheduled dose, and withdrawal peaks about thirty-six to seventy-two hours afterward. Initial symptoms include watery eyes, running nose, yawning, and perspiration. These are followed by restlessness, irritability, loss of appetite, insomnia, tremors, and severe sneezing. After forty-eight hours, the user is weak and nauseous and may also experience stomach cramps and diarrhea. Pain and muscle spasms occur. The person often becomes suicidal. Without treatment, the symptoms will probably disappear in seven to ten days, but the psychological need remains for several weeks.

Laws vary from state to state, but most still provide stiff penalties for possession or sale of a large quantity of marijuana and possession of hashish. Such acts may be considered felonies punishable by jail terms (Liska 1981).

Narcotics

Narcotics, the major drug problem of the 1960s, appear to be making a major comeback in the wake of the cocaine problem. Drug users are now mixing heroin and cocaine, resulting in a mix of emotional highs and lows and death in some cases.

The term **narcotics** refers to opium and opium derivatives, such as **morphine, heroin,** and **codeine** and to synthetic opiates, such as hydromorphione (**Dilaudid**) and **methadone.** Narcotics are indispensable in the practice of medicine because of their ability to relieve pain; however, this same ability accounts for a large portion of their abuse.

Under medical supervision, narcotics are used not only to relieve pain but also to suppress coughs and relieve diarrhea. They are administered orally or injected into a muscle. As drugs of abuse, however, they are sniffed, smoked, or injected under the skin (skin popping). Most abusers inject narcotics into a vein, which is called mainlining.

Narcotics of Natural Origin

The opium poppy is the main source of nonsynthetic narcotics. The milky fluid of the dried plant is extracted and transported in liquid, solid, or powder form. There were no legal restrictions on the use of opium until the early 1900s, but today there are state, federal, and international laws governing the production and distribution of narcotic substances such as opium, and there is little abuse of opium in the United States.

Twenty-five alkaloids can be extracted from opium and used to produce other narcotics. One group of alkaloids, the phenanthrene alkaloids (such as morphine and codeine), are used as **analgesics,** which are medicines that relieve pain, and cough suppressants. Another group, the isoquinoline alkaloids, have no significant influence on the central nervous system, so they are not drugs of choice on the illicit market. A small amount of opium is also used to make antidiarrheal preparations such as paregoric.

Morphine, the principal constituent of opium, is one of the most effective drugs known for relieving pain. It is used medically, usually for postoperative pain or pain associated with terminal illness. Abusers inject the drug intravenously, with tolerance and dependence developing rapidly. Most codeine is produced from morphine. Compared with morphine, it produces less sedation and analgesia; thus, it is used for the relief of moderate pain and in combination with other products such as aspirin. It is by far the most widely used naturally occurring narcotic in medical treatment.

Heroin was medically used to reduce pain from 1898 until 1914, when it was shown to be highly habit forming. Since then, it has become strictly a street drug. Pure heroin is a white powder with a bitter taste; it is rarely sold in unadulterated form on the street.

In the 1960s and early 1970s, a **bag,** a single dose of heroin, was about 4 percent to 7 percent heroin. Today it is about 40 percent pure. With the increased purity, the addiction rates are much higher. With the high demand in the U.S. market, heroin produced in Afghanistan, Iran, Burma, Laos, Thailand, Mexico, and other places is pouring into the country ("The Return of a Deadly Drug Called Horse" 1989).

Heroin is usually some shade of brown in color, depending upon the impurities left from the manufacturing process and/or the presence of additives. A fix of heroin is usually injected directly into a vein. Because dependency becomes extreme, the user can rapidly go from using twenty to thirty milligrams a day to four hundred milligrams or more.

Heroin may enslave users so completely that they spend every waking hour determining how to get the next fix. Withdrawal symptoms begin eight to twelve hours after each fix, so the user is continually on a physical and emotional roller coaster. It is difficult for users to hold a regular job, not only because of the constant need for the drug but also because of the large income needed to support the habit. Many heroin users turn to crime to pay for the habit they have acquired.

Synthetic Narcotics

Synthetic narcotics have been developed to help drug addicts become productive members of society, but at the same time the technology has created a new threat in the form of "new heroin." Synthetic narcotics such as hydromorphione and methadone have been derived by modifying the chemicals found in opium. Hydromorphone (Dilaudid) abuse does not necessarily follow the same pattern as heroin, but the end result is the same dependency. Hospitals and pharmacies have administered it as a painkiller for more than fifteen years, and heroin addicts now are turning to it when they are unable to get heroin. It is marketed in both tablet and injectable form. Its effects last for a shorter period, and it is more sedative than morphine, but its potency is much greater; thus, it is a highly abusable drug.

Methadone has the same general properties as morphine. It is a highly effective analgesic agent but more recently has been used for the treatment of narcotic dependence. Though methadone itself creates a dependency, the withdrawal symptoms appear more slowly and are of lesser intensity than those of heroin (Gerald 1981).

In 1979, a dealer unveiled a drug that looked like heroin. It was cut with milk sugar, and the dealer called it Asian White, the street name for the finest Southeast Asian heroin. The dealer charged a comparable price. He shortly lost two of his customers. One was found comatose in a motel room, and the other died in a bathroom. Both had the obvious heroin paraphernalia—needle, syringe, and white powder. Forensic scientists examined the bodies, and they found no trace of heroin. Since that time, numerous chemicals have surfaced, each with a slight variation, and have become known as synthetic narcotics, or **designer drugs** (Gallager 1986).

These drugs originally were legal because they were not considered a controlled substance. When researchers found out that the chief ingredient of the drugs was **fentanyl,** they became controlled substances and illegal. The drug-producing chemists then created a new drug that was similar to fentanyl but with a slight molecular variation that resulted in a legal, or uncontrolled, substance. The frustrating thing was that hundreds of variations of fentanyl were created and the designer drugs, now called China white or new heroin, use any number of the variations and in many cases are legal.

The base drug, fentanyl, is one hundred times as strong as morphine and twenty to forty times as strong as heroin. The analogs such as sufentanyl and lofentanyl are respectively two thousand and six thousand times as strong as morphine. It is, under controlled situations, an effective anesthetic and in the illicit markets, results in a very fast "rush" and an extraordinary high. On a comparative basis, it may take a couple of years to get addicted to alcohol, a couple of months for cocaine (not crack), and one dose for fentanyl. Because of the potency, the drugs have varied and bizarre effects. They have been called the drug version of Chernobyl, that is, a problem that was never imagined twenty years ago. Reports indicate that students are smoking cocaine cut with the fentanyl, which has been called "juice."

Every abusable drug can be synthesized in a laboratory. In California, 20 percent of the heroin abusers use fentanyl instead of the more expensive heroin, and in some counties, as many as 90 percent of the heroin abusers use fentanyl. These problems do not only occur on the coast but throughout the United States. For example, a county in Pennsylvania recently reported sixteen overdose drug deaths due to fentanyl ("An Outbreak of Designer Drug-Related Deaths" 1991). Some of these criminal chemists have botched batches and sold the drugs anyway. MPTP is a contaminant that was discovered in new heroin. After its distribution, MPTP left users suffering from the devastating symptoms of Parkinson's disease, in many cases after one dose. The brain uses MPTP to produce the toxin that causes Parkinson's disease (Shafer 1985).

MDMA (outlawed in July 1985), better known as **ecstasy,** is a type of synthetic cocaine. Ecstasy is a drug hybrid, a cross between the hallucinogen mescaline and the stimulant amphetamine ("New Data Intensify the Agony over Ecstasy" 1988). Labeled the LSD of the 1980s and 1990s, MDMA appears to stimulate the emotions and cognitive functions. Before it was outlawed it was used by psychiatrists to speed psychotherapy (Gallager 1986). As with most drugs, there seemed to be some positive effects in therapy, but in the streets, it was abused and resulted in hospitalizations and dependency.

Treatment of Narcotics Abuse

Treatment programs for narcotic abuse usually involve three stages: (1) crisis intervention, (2) detoxification, and (3) aftercare. Crisis intervention relieves whatever problem brought the user to the treatment center. If the user decides to continue in the treatment program, **detoxification,** the process of eliminating the drug from the user's system, must be started. This usually entails controlling the withdrawal symptoms so that the user experiences as few ill effects as possible. The initial concern is to determine polydrug use, to identify the drugs used, and to assess the degree of dependency of each drug. For example, barbiturate/alcohol withdrawal is treated first with mild barbiturates to withdraw the individual gradually. Methadone would likely be used for opiate users.

After the process of detoxification, the long, hard job of rehabilitation begins. There are several aftercare approaches currently available to those who choose to kick their habits. There are two basic, and opposing, philosophies of rehabilitative treatment for heroin abuse. In general, the maintenance programs (such as the British system and methadone maintenance) do not try to break the user's drug dependence. Rather, their goal is to make the users' criminal or antisocial acts unnecessary by providing them with a monitored legal supply of narcotics. By contrast, the goal of abstinence programs is to help users become functioning members of society again by breaking the drug habit for good.

Stimulants

Drugs known as stimulants, or "uppers," speed up the central nervous system. There are probably as many legal stimulants on the market as there are illicit drugs in this category. The chief legal stimulant that is widely used and abused is caffeine. The two most dangerous and popular illicit drugs are cocaine, with its free-based derivative **crack** and methamphetamine (speed or **crank** and its more potent crystalline form, **ice**).

Physiological Reactions to Major Stimulants

Stimulants mimic the action of the sympathetic nervous system; that is, at proper dose levels, they increase system activity to respond to the need for improved mental and physical performance when fatigue impairs them. The physiological reactions to stimulants include increased heart rate and strength of contraction, elevated blood pressure, increased muscle tension, stimulation of adrenal glands to produce adrenaline, constriction of blood vessels, dilation of the bronchi in the lungs, relaxation of intestinal muscle, and increased blood sugar. These reactions combine to produce alertness, wakefulness, and attentiveness; thus, the drugs seem to make their users feel stronger, more decisive, and more self-confident. They can also act as appetite suppressants.

Stimulants are quickly absorbed from the alimentary tract (digestive system) or from sites of injection. The effects are greatly intensified if stimulants are injected intravenously rather than taken orally or inhaled. Injection produces a sudden sensation known as a "rush," often described as orgasmic in nature, which probably results from the intense stimulation of the sympathetic nervous system. A period of euphoria occurs, which is usually followed by a period of depression (Carroll 1989). To remain "high," abusers must increase the dose level, which often leads to psychological dependence.

Caffeine

Most Americans take a legal stimulant, caffeine, each morning. It is fairly easy to ingest over 500 milligrams of caffeine in one day, which can be harmful. Table 9.1 shows the amount of caffeine in commonly used substances. Caffeine is a stimulant: it speeds the heart rate, temporarily elevates the blood pressure, interferes with sleep, and increases the fatty acid levels in the blood.

Caffeinism refers to the acute or chronic overuse of caffeine and caffeine poisoning. The symptoms of caffeinism include anxiety, mood changes, sleep disturbances, and other psychophysical complaints. Caffeine intoxication is characterized by the described traits and an excess consumption of 250 milligrams. Caffeine withdrawal results in headache, irritability, lethargy, mood changes, sleep disturbance, and mild physiological arousal.

Cocaine and Crack

Cocaine use has rocketed over the last decade: twenty-two million Americans have tried it, and 15.2 percent of graduating high school students have tried the drug. One out of every eighteen young people have used crack, and six million people use cocaine regularly (Clouet, Asghar, and Brown

TABLE 9.1

Caffeine in Selected Substances (in milligrams)

Coffee (5 oz)		Diet Pepsi	36
Brewed, drip method	60–180	RC Cola	36
Brewed, percolator	40–170	Cherry RC	36
Instant	30–120	Canada Dry Jamaica Cola	30
Decaffeinated, brewed	2–5	Canada Dry Diet Cola	1.5
Decaffeinated, instant	1–5	*Prescription Drugs*	
Tea (5 oz)		Cafergot (for migraine headache)	100
Brewed, major U. S. brands	20–90	Darvon compound (for pain relief)	32.4
Brewed, imported brands	25–110	*Nonprescription Drugs*	
Iced (12 oz)	67–76	No-Dōz (alertness tablets)	100
Instant	25–50	Vivarin (alertness tablets)	200
Soft Drinks (12 oz)		Aqua-Ban (diuretic)	100
Sugar Free Mr. PIBB	58	Aqua-Ban Plus	200
Mountain Dew	54	Anacin	32
Mellow Yellow	52	Excedrin	65
TAB	46	Midol	32.4
Coca-Cola (classic and new)	46	Vanquish	33
Diet Coke	46	Duradyne	15
Shasta Cola	44	Coryban-D capsules	30
Shasta Cherry Cola	44	Triaminicin tablets	30
Shasta Diet Cola	44	*Other*	
Mr. PIBB	40.8	Cocoa (5 oz)	2–20
Dr. Pepper	40.8	Chocolate milk (8 oz)	2–7
Diet Dr. Pepper	40.8	Milk chocolate (1 oz)	1–15
Pepsi-Cola	38.4	Semi-sweet chocolate (1 oz)	5–35
Big Red	38	Chocolate flavored syrup (1 oz)	4

Denise Grady/© 1986 Discover Magazine.

1988). Just a few years ago, cocaine was not considered addictive, but now it is recognized as a powerful addictive drug. Even after treatment and months of abstinence, many people cannot resist its lure. The national cocaine hotline receives 1,200 calls per day, most from users of crack or concerned family and friends of crack users. Other callers are users of powder cocaine (Holtzman 1986).

Cocaine is the most powerful stimulant of natural origin. In its pure form before being cut, it is a white crystalline powder that looks much like sugar. Cocaine is also found in the rock form or flake form (like shavings from a bar of soap). It is either snorted, liquified and then injected, or free-based and smoked. It is extracted from the leaves of the coca plant, which has been cultivated in South America since prehistoric times. In South America, as much as 90 percent of the adult male population living at high altitudes chews the leaves of the plant for refreshment and relief from fatigue.

The following statements are descriptive of the nature and effect of cocaine (Holtzman 1986):

1. general psychological stimulant that mimics the stress response by increasing heart rate, respiratory rate, body temperature, blood pressure, constriction of the blood vessels, and dilation of the pupils;

2. reduces hunger and fatigue—the more fatigued a user, the more powerful the effect;

3. temporarily increases reaction time and muscular strength, but then there is a letdown;

4. acts as a local anesthetic;

5. if snorted, it reaches the brain in three to five minutes; if injected, it reaches the brain in fifteen seconds; and if smoked, it reaches the brain in five to seven seconds;

6. psychological effects include anxiety, hallucinations, impotence, and insomnia;

7. large doses may cause multisensory (visual, tactile, and auditory) hallucinations, paranoid delusions, quick changes in perception, impaired judgment, aggressions, panic reactions, agitated depression, and a perception of power, which may make a person potentially antisocial and dangerous;

8. death from overdose is due to respiratory failure on a lethal dose of about 1.2 grams at one time.

Free-basing cocaine has become very popular because the intensity of the cocaine high is dramatically more powerful and intense. It is comparable to methamphetamine in intensity. Free-basing, up until 1985, was a dangerous process. Cocaine, purchased on the street in its adulterated form, was refined using water and ether or ammonia. The procedure removes most of the sugars and other substances and leaves an intensive form of cocaine. The use of ether is extremely dangerous and has resulted in fires and explosions. After about 1985, free-basing was accomplished with common baking soda. Suddenly, crack, or rock, emerged as a cheap (about $5 to $10 a hit) and powerful drug, and it has swept America. Crack is generally sold as slivers or pellets (like soap shavings) in a vial, folding papers, or aluminum foil. According to experts, crack is many times more powerful and more addictive than cocaine, and addiction occurs sometimes after a few uses. It is so intense that it can cause instant death, particularly for a small percentage of the U.S. population who can't metabolize its enzymes ("The War on Drugs" 1991). Cocaine and crack have been responsible for many instant deaths in normally healthy people. Many of these deaths have received a great deal of attention, as in the case of athletes and Hollywood figures. Crack joins the designer drugs, methamphetamine (crank), and ice as the most potent, quick addicting, and dangerous street drugs of our times.

Cocaine powder is usually sniffed, or "snorted," through the nasal passages, but free-basing, vaporizing the cocaine and inhaling the smoke, has recently become popular among some heavy users. Within twenty minutes, the drug enters the bloodstream and is carried to the brain, where it serves as a central nervous system stimulant. The effects of cocaine, which last from one to two hours, have been described as extremely pleasurable; users say the drug makes them feel happier, more energetic, more seductive, and more exciting.

Cocaine overuse can damage the mucous membranes of the nose. The drug acts as a **vasoconstrictor,** that is, it narrows blood vessels and reduces the oxygen supply. The lining of the nose eventually deteriorates, and the septum (cartilage that separates the nostrils) crumbles. Some chronic users have so abused this drug that they have "sniffed" holes in their noses, which require surgical repair.

With chronic use, new symptoms can develop from the constant stimulation and lack of rest. As tolerance increases, larger doses are required at shorter intervals, until the user's life is largely committed to the habit. Tactile hallucinations can seem so real that some chronic users injure themselves attempting to remove imaginary insects from under their skin. Excessive doses can even cause seizures and death from respiratory failure or heart attack (Carroll 1989). Many dramatic cases are reported in the media, such as the case of the athlete Len Bias.

A major problem is the increasing number of cocaine babies born to cocaine-abusing mothers. Cocaine babies begin life in the agonizing state of withdrawal and may go

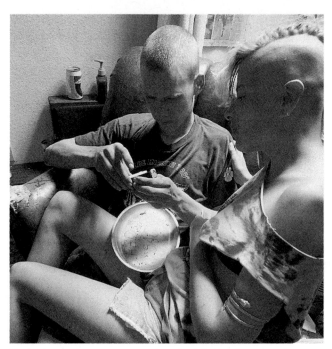

Crack is much more powerful and addictive than cocaine, with addiction sometimes occurring after a few uses.

through life with severe physical (motor development) and emotional (learning disabilities) problems (Carroll 1989).

To help yourself or others, call the toll-free Cocaine Hotline at 1-800-COCAINE, or see your college/university counseling or drug services. Many community services are also available through county or city agencies.

Amphetamines

Amphetamine abusers usually follow one of two patterns. Some compulsively take low-dose oral amphetamines daily to maintain a fast pace, reinforce an outgoing personality, keep their mood elevated, and postpone the inevitable depression that follows discontinued use. They alternate stimulants and depressants, taking "uppers" in the morning and "downers," such as barbiturates or alcohol, at night.

The other pattern of amphetamine abuse involves the intravenous use of high-dose methamphetamine (speed or crank). In this pattern, the abuser goes on "runs," episodes lasting from several hours to a few days, during which he or she remains "up" with continued injections. Within minutes after the initial injection, the user experiences an intense tingling sensation (a "buzz"), which is followed by more intense tingling sensations, muscle contractions, and a feeling of extreme pleasure. During a run, the user typically does not eat and thus loses weight and may experience other symptoms of malnutrition. The longer the run persists, the more problems occur, including a mood change from pleasant optimism and euphoria to hyperactive aggression. Even though tolerance develops, overdoses of amphetamines are uncommon and rarely fatal (Dusek and Girdano 1987).

Ice

One of the latest hi-tech forms of methamphetamine to arrive in the United States is a crystalline rock form called ice ("An Invitation to Sudden Death" 1991). The drug originated in Japan and Korea and gradually spread to Hawaii, where it has become a major problem (Cho 1990). It has arrived on the West Coast and is reaching major cities inland (Lerner 1989). Women seem particularly attracted to it, and it is hypothesized by some as a weight-reduction drug. The sense of euphoria of ice lasts for up to fourteen hours.

Ice can cause vitamin and mineral deficiencies, rapid loss of weight, and lower resistance to disease. Prolonged use may cause lung, liver, and kidney damage. Side effects are somewhat puzzling but include anorexia, brittle bones, and wounds that won't heal (Culhane 1990). In Hawaii, case studies indicate addiction after a single use. Users take the drug for up to four days and then crash, just as with speed or crank.

Illicit amphetamine use closely parallels that of cocaine in the range of its short-term and long-term effects. Despite the risks, undercover laboratories continue to produce vast amounts of amphetamines, especially methamphetamine, for distribution on the illicit drug market.

Unfortunately, amphetamines are often prescribed as diet pills, such as phenmetrazine hydrochloride (Preludin), dexedrine, and methamphetamine. Many states have already passed legislation that virtually bans the use of amphetamines for the treatment of obesity. Similar legislation is pending in several other states.

The FDA continues to approve the use of amphetamines in the treatment of narcolepsy and hyperactivity in children. Dextroamphetamine and methylphenidate (Ritalin) are the most effective drugs for the acute management of hyperactivity, with about two-thirds of the children taking the drugs being helped. The drugs seem to reduce aggressive and impulsive behavior in children, as well as improving goal orientation and attention span. Unlike the activating effects observed in adults, these drugs do not produce euphoria or overstimulation in hyperkinetic children nor do they slow the children down or suppress their initiative. The medical reason for this is not well understood, but the calming effect does improve academic performance (Gerald 1981).

The treatment of cocaine and other stimulant abuse involves absolute abstaining from all drugs, teaching consequences of drug stimulation and alternative forms of stimulation, and involving family members in the treatment when possible.

Depressants

Depressants are drugs designed to slow the functioning of the central nervous system. There are two classifications of depressants: sedative hypnotics and antianxiety drugs. Sedative hypnotics can calm the individual and thereby relieve anxiety and tension by inducing a state resembling natural sleep. The sedative hypnotics include **barbiturates,** such as phenobarbital and secobarbital, and nonbarbiturates, such as methaqualone (Quaalude) and glutethimide (Doriden). Tranquilizers also calm the individual and relieve anxiety and tension but do so without inducing a hypnotic state.

If you suspect or know that you have become dependent on a particular drug(s), whether legally or illegally obtained, draw up a decision tree about your choices concerning future use of this drug. You may wish to include the physical, psychological, social, and professional consequences of continuing or discontinuing use. As you consider the choices, locate a drug counselor who can assist you in making your decision.

Physicians often prescribe depressants to reduce tension and anxiety and counteract insomnia. Taken in excessive amounts, however, depressants produce a state of intoxication similar to drunkenness. These effects can vary not only from person to person but also from time to time in the same individual; invariably, however, excessive use of depressants results at least in impaired judgment, slurred speech, and loss of motor coordination. Users rapidly develop tolerance to the intoxicating effects, which can lead to overdosing.

Depressants vary in their potential for overdose, but users who have severe depressant poisoning can fall into a coma, have a weak and rapid pulse, or evidence slow and shallow respiration. Users can even die from an overdose, generally respiratory failure, if they do not receive medical attention.

Treatment for Withdrawal from Depressants

The treatment for withdrawal from depressants requires intensive care that should be given in a medical setting. Signs and symptoms of withdrawal first appear within eight hours after the user discontinues the drug and become severe during the next eight hours; they become even more severe after twenty-four hours and, if untreated, will likely develop into **grand mal** (major) **convulsions** between thirty and forty-eight hours. After the first forty-eight hours, there may be recurrences of insomnia, culminating in delirium, hallucinations, and marked tremors. This stage lasts about five days, ending in a long sleep. Treatment, or detoxification, consists of administering short-acting barbiturates to relieve the first symptoms and then tapering off with either the same drug or decreasing doses of a long-acting drug. Along with this treatment for the physical withdrawal from the drug, users need psychological help to prevent a relapse into drug use. Death is a real danger in uncontrolled, untreated withdrawal (Dusek and Girdano 1987).

Chloral Hydrate

Chloral hydrate, first synthesized in the 1860s, is the oldest of the hypnotic drugs. Its popularity declined with the advent of barbiturates, but it is still considered an effective sedative and hypnotic that is unlikely to induce tolerance (although it may be habit forming). Chloral hydrate disturbs rapid eye movement (REM) sleep less and depresses respiration less than the barbiturates, but it does show some drug interactions. When used with alcohol, it is known as a "Mickey Finn," or knockout drops. These drugs in combination react synergistically, that is, they cause each one to be more powerful than when consumed alone. Chloral hydrate is not a street drug of choice (Liska 1981).

Barbiturates

Some 2,500 derivatives of barbituric acid have been synthesized, but only about 15 remain in medical use. Doctors prescribe barbiturates in small therapeutic doses to calm nervous conditions and in large doses to induce sleep. These drugs are classified as ultrashort (pentathol), short-intermediate (seconal or amytal), and long acting (luminal).

Because the ultrashort-acting drugs produce anesthesia within seconds and because their duration is also short, drug abusers do not seek them out; instead, they seek out the short- and intermediate-acting barbiturates with durations up to six hours. Long-acting barbiturates are not marketable as illicit drugs because of the length of time needed for onset. One of the most dangerous aspects of all barbiturate use is the high risk of both physiological and psychological dependence.

Glutethimide (Doriden) and Methaqualone (Quaalude)

When it was introduced in 1954, glutethimide (Doriden) was thought to be a safe barbiturate substitute, but experience has shown that it has no particular advantage over the barbiturates and several disadvantages. The sedative effects are similar to those of the intermediate-acting barbiturates, but because this drug's effects are of long duration (six hours), it is difficult to reverse overdoses, and overdoses of this drug often result in death (Carroll 1989). The mortality rate is four times higher than is generally observed in barbiturate overdose (Gerald 1981).

Methaqualone (Quaalude), also a synthetic sedative, has been widely abused because users mistakenly thought it was nonaddictive. Users often take Quaaludes to heighten a feeling of excitement. They say that they feel more in control than with other drugs and don't have to worry about hangovers, alcohol on the breath, or "bad trips," but the drug can impair reflexes and judgment. Large doses cause coma, sometimes accompanied by convulsions. Users rapidly develop dependence, and some say that it is easier to become dependent on this drug than on narcotics. The amount of methaqualone needed to overdose does not increase with a user's tolerance, so heavy users can overdose before the drug has even made them feel high. This drug also has a synergistic effect in combination with alcohol.

Tranquilizers

Tranquilizers are divided into two groups: major and minor. The major tranquilizers such as Thorazine and Reserpine are prescription drugs most often used in mental hospitals for the treatment of psychoses. They are not street drugs of abuse. The minor tranquilizers are used to relieve anxiety, tension, and muscle spasms, to produce sedation, and to prevent convulsions.

Meprobamate, synthesized in 1950, introduced the era of minor tranquilizers. It is also sold as Miltown, Equanil, Kesso-Bamate, and SK-Bamate. In onset and duration of action, meprobamate is similar to the intermediate-acting barbiturates, but it does not produce sleep and is less toxic. Excessive use, however, can result in psychological and physical dependence. Minor tranquilizers of the benzodiazepine family include Librium and Valium. The **benzodiazepines,** namely **Valium** and **Librium,** are the most widely prescribed medicine in the United States. The FDA cites evidence that Valium is overprescribed and abused, and that it can cause psychological and physical dependence. Over 90 percent of the physicians in the United States prescribe Valium for anxiety, muscle spasms, ulcers, and other anxiety-related psychosomatic disorders. Women users outnumber men 2.5 to 1. Valium is also a popular street drug.

Librium (Chlordiazepoxide) is also habit forming and overprescribed. Users commonly experience clumsiness, drowsiness, and dizziness. Valium and Librium used as tranquilizers cause drowsiness, respiratory depression, and a decrease in memory and motor functions. Side effects include skin rashes, lethargy, menstrual irregularities, conjunctivitis, overexcitement, constipation, stammering, slurred speech, hypertension, and thirst. Valium and Librium, like most drugs, are dangerous to pregnant women, particularly during the first trimester. Valium in combination with alcohol is **synergistic,** that is, it has a multiplying effect, and it may result in coma or death.

Valium dependence can occur with a dosage as low as thirty milligrams a day over time. Withdrawal from Valium can be as dangerous as barbiturate withdrawal, which is characterized by violent shaking and possibly seizures.

Hallucinogens

The hallucinogenic drugs discussed in this section, LSD, peyote and mescaline, psilocybin and psilocyn, and PCP, have much more powerful effects than marijuana or hashish. They bring about greater excitation of the central nervous system, characterized by alterations of mood. These moods are usually **euphoric,** that is, characterized by a feeling of extreme well-being, but may also be so severely depressive that suicide is possible.

When individuals use hallucinogens, their pupils dilate, their body temperatures rise, and their blood pressures elevate. Senses of direction, distance, and time are distorted. These drugs produce **delusions** (false beliefs) and visual hallucinations, such as the intensification of color, the apparent motion of a fixed object, or the confusion of one object with another. The most common danger is impaired judgment, which can lead to accidents and rash decisions. Long after hallucinogens are eliminated from the body, users may experience spontaneous **flashbacks,** which are recurrences of the hallucinatory effects.

Lysergic Acid Diethylamide (LSD)

Lysergic acid diethylamide (LSD) is produced from lysergic acid, a substance derived from the ergot fungus that grows on rye, or from lysergic acid amide, a chemical found in seeds of the morning glory flower. The LSD user gets his or her drug in a tablet or other consumable form. Because the usual dosage (one hundred or two hundred micrograms) is too small a quantity to weigh out, the drug is always found diluted in some other substance (Liska 1981).

Just how LSD acts to produce hallucinations is unknown. Successful treatment of a bad LSD trip can often be accomplished by friends who talk the user down in familiar surroundings. Minor tranquilizers have also proved useful.

LSD remains high on the list of drugs to be controlled. Because of the belief that the original laws were not stringent enough, legislators have passed even stiffer laws, and today the maximum federal penalty for first-time unlawful possession is a $5,000 fine and one year in jail (Liska 1981). LSD is now marketed as little drops on the back of postage stamps. There has been some resurgence of LSD use, particularly among teenagers.

Peyote and Mescaline

Mescaline is the primary active ingredient of the fleshy parts, or buttons, of the **peyote** cactus. It can also be synthetically produced. It is legal in the United States to use peyote as a part of the religious rites of the native American church; outside this church community, the drug is used illegally.

Peyote or mescaline intoxication first brings on a feeling of contentment and hypersensitivity, which is followed by a period of nervous calm during which visual hallucinations often occur. A 350 to 500 milligram dose of mescaline produces delusions and hallucinations lasting five to twelve hours. As used in religious ritual, four to twelve peyote buttons are ingested, followed by a period of meditation during which visual aberrations, nausea, or vomiting may occur.

Peyote buttons can be found on the illegal drug market, but it is rare to find mescaline; only about two in every one hundred street samples offered as mescaline actually turn out to be the drug. Like LSD, no physical dependence seems to occur, but it is possible that some psychological dependence may develop. Tolerance to the drug develops very quickly.

Psilocybin and Psilocyn

Psilocybe mushrooms have also been used for centuries in traditional Mexican Indian religious services to produce visions and hallucinations. When these mushrooms are eaten, they affect moods in the same way that mescaline and LSD do. Their active ingredients, psilocybin and psilocyn, are chemically related to LSD. The hallucinatory experience is roughly comparable to that produced by LSD, except that the trip lasts about half as long. Dangers involved stem not from physical harm but from the potential for inducing psychotic states that remain long after the expected end of the experience. Tolerance to these mushrooms develops quickly, and a period of five days must elapse before the user can get high again. Psilocybin and psilocyn head the list of the most misrepresented drugs on the street; most mushrooms sold on the street are the grocery store variety spiked with LSD (Liska 1981).

Phencyclidine (PCP), or Angel Dust

Phencyclidine is sold under at least fifty names, including **angel dust,** animal tranquilizer, crystal, supergrass, and killer weed. In its pure form, PCP is a crystalline powder that readily dissolves in water; however, most illicit PCP contains contaminants that cause the color to range from tan to brown and the consistency to range from a powder to a gummy mass. It is most often applied to a leafy material such as parsley, mint, oregano, tobacco, or marijuana and smoked. The bizarre and volatile effects of this drug include numbness, slurred speech, loss of coordination, rapid or involuntary eye movements, and image distortions like those seen in a funhouse mirror. Severe mood disorders, sometimes violent or psychotic, may also occur. Because of the catatonic (trancelike) state produced, evidenced by the inability to speak or walk, PCP effects are often indistinguishable from the effects of schizophrenia.

At one time, PCP was tested as a human anesthetic but was abandoned because of its bizarre aftereffects. Until 1979, it was used as a tranquilizer on large animals. PCP has perhaps the highest potential for bad experiences of any hallucinogen. Even emergency room professionals are not quite sure what to do for a "PCP freakout." Persons who are badly affected by this drug should be kept in a dark, quiet room because of their tendency to become hyperactive on high doses, and medical attention is definitely needed. Another problem is that PCP is often used to adulterate other drugs. Some drug samples alleged to be cocaine, for example, are partly or wholly PCP; the opposite problem can also occur when a user believes that the drug is PCP when it is something else. This can cause a particular problem for a doctor trying to treat a drug overdose.

In the spring of 1978, PCP was added to the Comprehensive Drug Abuse Prevention and Control Act of 1970, which made much harsher penalties for possessing the drug. There are no legal manufacturers of PCP in the United States today.

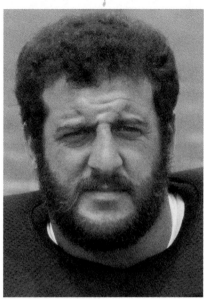

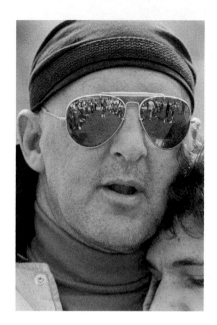

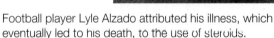
Football player Lyle Alzado attributed his illness, which eventually led to his death, to the use of steroids.

Drugs in Sports

The National Collegiate Athletic Association (NCAA) approved mandatory drug testing on January 13, 1986, and since that time there has been increased public awareness regarding drugs and athletes. This has been facilitated by national media coverage of the cocaine-related deaths of several athletes as well as exclusion of some athletes from postseason bowl games related to anabolic steroid use. Mandatory drug testing has been the first strategy to curtail widespread use of drugs in athletics. Athletes realize that they can lose their eligibility to compete in athletics if they have a positive test. New ways to get the edge in sports are through more natural means such as self-hypnosis, meditation, and imagery rather than steroids and cocaine. Professional sports have also adopted drug testing.

Steroids and Growth Hormone

Anabolic steroids are derived from the male hormone testosterone and are available in pill form or injectable solution. During World War II, anabolic steroids were used effectively to increase aggressiveness in German soldiers and restore vitality to nitrogen-depleted prisoners of war. They soon became available to weight lifters and other athletes. In the 1970s and early 1980s, there was widespread abuse among NCAA members and professional athletes until drug testing began. Physicians have dramatically reduced the number of steroids they prescribe, but the black market supply of steroids has increased. Steroids are used to increase levels of workout intensity and duration, in addition to speeding up the recovery from the workouts. Although the side effects studies are antidotal, athletes who use steroids, attribute death and illness to steroid use. Table 9.2 lists the effects of steroids.

Another hormone that some athletes use in a dangerous attempt to get the edge in sports is **human growth hormone (HGH)**. HGH is the natural hormone (a polypeptide with 191 amino acids) that is released from the pituitary gland and promotes general body growth. Until recently, HGH could only be obtained in an expensive retrieval process from cadavers. Now HGH can be manufactured synthetically and is available from physicians by prescription but also illegally (White et al. 1989).

HGH is used therapeutically in children who can't produce their own HGH and would have been victims of disabling dwarfism. Athletes' indiscriminate use of growth hormone may cause the medical condition acromegaly. Acromegaly is associated with heart problems, arthritis, impotence, and bony enlargement of the forehead, jaw, hands, and feet (White et al. 1989). HGH should be avoided by athletes as well as anyone who thinks it would benefit them physically.

Drug Testing

In recent years, testing for drugs in athletes, federal workers, transportation service personnel, and a variety of other workers has become an important issue. Beginning with Utah in 1987, many states are considering or have implemented mandatory drug testing of employees.

Drug tests are conducted by giving an employee about a one-hour notice to provide a urine specimen (which is witnessed by an observer) to be analyzed for any abused drugs. Two specimens are sent to the lab. One for an initial screening, and a second test for confirmation of a positive test. Two forms of analysis include the **immunoassays** and **gas chromography/mass spectrometry (GC/MS)** tests. Immunoassays work by allowing selected antibodies to come in contact with drugs in the specimen. Antibodies are proteins that have sites where specific drugs will bind. An

ISSUE

Drug Testing

"It was impossible to get high any more, or to stop," stated a thirty-one-year-old former narcotics addict who at the time was in the last stages of his disease. He needed eight to ten shots a day and when he woke up, he was either overdosing or he was detoxing. "My world was hopeless, and I was helpless. I had no more relationships, and I had accepted the fact that I was doomed to die alone, in fear."

This sounds like the confession of a street "junkie," but this confession ends with "By that point, I was either on the street scoring, or in the hospital working as an emergency room physician." He was spending the $1,500 per week he was earning in the emergency room for either heroin or designer drugs after he was suspected, rightly so, of diverting drugs from the hospital pharmacy. Unfortunately, this physician's story is not uncommon among many respected professionals. It is frightening to know that this physician worked for four years practicing medicine in his condition. To try to deal with this problem, drug testing has become mandatory in some professions and businesses.

• **Pro:** It is imperative that drug testing be done. What kind of harm could this physician have done? What harm could a police officer, pilot, bus driver, or nuclear power plant operator do under the influence of drugs? It must be done.

• **Con:** Drug testing is an invasion of privacy. If people want to kill themselves with drugs, it is their option to do so. It can result in lost jobs for false positive tests.

What will you do if asked to take a drug test?

Source: *Discover,* August 1986.

analysis of what drugs have bonded to the antibodies provides a positive test. Some errors have occurred, and, in unfortunate instances, employees have lost their jobs because of occasional false positive tests. GC/MS is a gas chromatograph that breaks down all substances in a specimen and spreads each test on a printout. This test is 99.9 percent accurate and has not had any reported errors. The only errors with GC/MS are human handling errors.

Students must realize that a condition of current or future employment may be a drug test. If found positive, the prospective employee will not be hired in many cases. Drug testing is being challenged in courts by those who refuse to be tested on the grounds of invasion of privacy. In some cases, the court has ruled in favor of the person refusing to take a test.

Costs for drug tests in 1988 ranged from $25 to $30 for drugs of abuse and $100 for drugs of abuse and anabolic steroids. Table 9.3 lists some of the drugs that can be detected through drug testing and how long they can be detected after use (Hawks and Chiang 1986). This list is only for a sample of drugs. For example, there are over three thousand brand-name drugs that contain a substance banned by the NCAA (NCAA 1986).

Drug Interactions

When two or more drugs are used together, the possibility arises that they will adversely interact in a person's body. **Drug interactions** are of several types; perhaps the most serious occurs when the drugs multiply each other's effects, termed *synergism.* For example, barbiturates and alcohol each depress the central nervous system when taken alone, but when taken together, they increase the depressant effects and result in a "superdepressant." Alcohol potentiates the effects of tranquilizers, antihistamines, and sedatives. Other kinds of potentiation occur when one drug inhibits the metabolism of another, displaces another from its plasma-binding site (thus allowing a greater amount to reach its receptor site, such as the

TABLE 9.3

NCAA Banned Substances

Substance	Intensity	Positive Test with GC/MS After Use
Marijuana (THC)	Chronic user (daily)	Up to 1 month
Marijuana (THC)	Two times/week	1–3 days
Cocaine/crack	Single dose	48 hours
Methamphetamine	Single dose	23 hours
Methamphetamine	Chronic user	48 hours
Opiates	Light to heavy	1–3 days
PCP	Light to heavy	7 days
LSD	Light to heavy	2 days
Quaaludes	Light to heavy	1 week
Barbiturates	Depending if short or long acting	30–76 hours
Valium/Librium	Chronic	Weeks to months

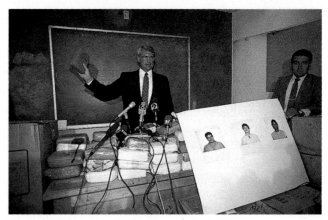

Drug law enforcement is only one aspect of the "war on drugs."

brain), or alters elimination so that the drug is not passed from the body as quickly as it would be if taken alone.

A second type of interaction occurs when one drug acts as a therapeutic antagonist to another, thereby reducing or nullifying its effect. For example, caffeine nullifies the effect of sedatives, barbiturates reduce the effectiveness of major tranquilizers, alcohol reduces the effect of minor tranquilizers, and nicotine decreases the effectiveness of certain analgesics (Liska 1981).

Cross tolerance of one drug with another is also dangerous. For example, a person who abuses alcohol and has built up a tolerance to its effects would have the same tolerance for barbiturates. Cross tolerance also occurs between a number of the hallucinogens.

The possibilities of dangerous interactions are almost endless. Certainly, the safest action is to assume that the potential for a dangerous reaction exists whenever two drugs are taken at or near the same time.

Drug Use and AIDS

A detailed discussion of the HIV virus and AIDS is provided in the chapter on communicable diseases, but it is worth noting that AIDS is a disease that has no cure. Those who get AIDS will have a significantly shortened life. One of the common ways of spreading AIDS is through the sharing of needles among drug users. Many professionals are looking to methadone maintenance programs as one way to curb AIDS, because even though the addict continues to receive a drug, at least conditions are sterile and an option exists to intravenous drug use. Some larger cities have even made sterile syringes available for drug abusers to avoid the sharing of needles.

Drugs and the Law

Laws are made in an effort to safeguard the members of our society. The drug laws now in force are a combination of federal, state, and local laws that have accumulated since the passage of the Harrison Act of 1914. The most current federal law for the control of illicit drugs is the Comprehensive Drug Abuse Prevention and Control Act of 1970, Title II. Better known as the Controlled Substances Act, this law was designed to control the distribution of all depressant and stimulant drugs as well as others with abuse potential.

Under the act, persons cannot lawfully manufacture, distribute or dispense, or possess with intent to distribute any of the drugs mentioned. The penalties vary depending on the drug. The act also covers illegal possession (obtained without a doctor's prescription) of controlled drugs and assesses penalties for violation, with possible one-year probation for a first-time offender caught in simple possession. Stiff penalties may be administered for adults who break the law by distributing a controlled substance to a person under the age of twenty-one.

Federal laws are enforceable throughout the United States, but individual states have their own laws, as do cities and counties. Though it is important to be aware of these penalties, it is more important that we know the statutes of the state in which we live, because the laws vary from state to state.

Decriminalization of drug use has resurfaced as a hot political topic in Washington, D.C. Some legislators and health professionals are in favor of removing the laws on drug use. The billions of dollars spent trying to stop the importation of drugs and keep citizens from growing or manufacturing their own are not working. The legal, political, agricultural, health, advertising, emotional, and psychological implications of such a debate are mind boggling. The most important implication of this whole drug issue is your own personal behavior and choices. Knowing the negative consequences of participating in any dimension of over-the-counter, prescription, or illicit drug use, it is hoped you will make healthy choices.

Psychoactive Drugs

Drugs are a predominant part of our society. The good that drugs do in medicine to relieve pain and to speed recovery leave us all grateful. It is unfortunate that drugs have been abused and now represent a major threat to our society. It is not healthy to use drugs to fortify the body, quicken the mind, or strengthen the soul. You can achieve similar outcomes if you use natural means to accomplish the maximization of mind, body, and soul and their interdependence. Consider the following health actions. These skills work without the negative aftereffects of drugs.

Mind

Use the mental skills described in chapter 2 to acquire desired mental states. Rather than using drugs to be creative, use imagery, psychological pairing, or creative personal problem solving to project yourself into a desired mental state. If you feel the urge to take a drug to relax or to sleep, try the relaxation skills described in chapter 2 and experience the power of the mind to create a relaxed state.

Body

During a week, reflect upon those times that your body feels best. Perhaps it is after exercise, after a good night's sleep, after eating nutritiously without eating too much, or after a shower. Once you have identified those activities or times that you feel best, practice those habits to create a physical high. Take that shower, get adequate sleep, or exercise to reach a peak physical state.

Soul

In chapter 2 is a description of psychological pairing. You can control your emotional state. If you want to be happy, then think of a time when you were extremely happy in the past. Remember the feeling, then try and feel the same emotions.

Interdependence

Find a trigger from your environment or from someone around you that will spark your desired emotional state. Triggers such as a musical theme from a favorite movie, music in general, some photographs, or a keepsake of some sort can trigger the right emotions for you. Reminiscing with a loved one or friend, asking for support, or visiting with a person who may represent your desired state (a religious leader to acquire a spiritual state) can help. You do not need drugs to reach an emotional high—just your own mind.

Summary

1. State-of-the-art chemical technology has produced some devastating new drugs, such as designer drugs and crack, that have quick addicting, debilitating, and death risks.

2. Individuals use drugs for a variety of reasons, including recreation, experimentation, coping, sensation seeking, and escape.

3. Psychoactive substance dependence involves both psychological and physiological factors.

4. Cannabis products are more potent than twenty years ago and are some of the most widely used illicit drugs.

5. Natural and synthetic narcotics are still abused in society, with the fentanyl designer drugs beginning to dominate the narcotic abuse scene.

6. Stimulants include the amphetamines, caffeine, and cocaine (also free-based cocaine), which are some of the strongest addictive drugs in America.

7. Depressants are extremely dangerous, particularly when they are mixed with alcohol, because of the synergistic effect of the drugs.

8. Hallucinogens include LSD, PCP, mescaline, psilocybin, and other drugs that create illusions and hallucinations.

9. Polydrug use can result in effects that are synergistic, are antagonistic, or show cross tolerance.

10. Drug laws in our society are designed to prevent manufacturing, distributing, or possessing controlled substances.

Commitment Activities

1. If you know of someone who may have trouble with cocaine or crack, you can call the Cocaine Hotline by dialing toll-free 1–800–COCAINE. They will identify the local Cocaine Anonymous chapter and provide other information for you.

2. Determine what your community has done to counteract the problem of narcotic abuse. You may want to visit a halfway house and talk to those recovering from narcotic abuse. Ask them for help in developing a prevention program for young people in your community.

3. Interview a member of the police department whose responsibility lies in drug enforcement. Discuss the types of persons who take drugs and other problems

specific to drug abusers, including drugs of choice in your community, legal aspects, and rehabilitation facilities.

References

American Psychiatric Association. *Diagnostic and Statistical Manual of Mental Disorders DSM III.* Washington, D.C. 1987.

Carroll, C. R. *Drugs in Modern Society,* 2d ed. Dubuque, Iowa: Wm. C. Brown, 1989.

Cho, A. K. "Ice: A New Dosage Form of an Old Drug." *Science* 249 (August 10, 1990):631.

Clouet, D.; Asghar, K.; and Brown, R. "Mechanisms of Cocaine Abuse and Toxicity." NIDA Research Monograph 88. U.S. Department of Health and Human Services, Public Health Services, p. ix.

Culhane, C. " 'Ice' Spreads to West Coast Area." *U.S. Journal of Drug and Alcohol Dependence* 14, 1 (1990):16.

Dusek, D. E., and Girdano, D. A. *Drugs: A Factual Account,* 4th ed. New York: Random House, 1987.

Egan, T. "Life, Liberty, and Maybe Marijuana: Choosing Sides in Alaska." *New York Times* (February 5, 1991):B1, A6.

Gallager, W. "The Looming Menace of Designer Drugs." *Discover* (August 1986):24–35.

Gerald, M. *Pharmacology: An Introduction to Drugs.* Englewood Cliffs, N.J.: Prentice-Hall, 1981.

Hawks, R. L., and Chiang, C. N. *Urine Testing for Drugs of Abuse,* National Institutes of Abuse Research Monograph 73 (1986).

Holtzman, D. "Crack Shatters the Cocaine Myth." *Insight* 23 (June 1986).

Howe, S. "Looking for Grass in the Forests." *Backpacker* 20, no. 1 (February 1992): 9.

"An Invitation to Sudden Death." *USA Today.* (February 1991): 5.

Jensen, M. A. "Understanding Addictive Behaviors: Implications for Health Promotion Programming." *American Journal of Health Promotion* 1, no. 3 (1987):48–57.

Lerner, M. A. "The Fire of Ice." *Newsweek* (November 27, 1989):37.

Liska, K. *Drugs and the Human Body.* New York: Macmillan, 1981.

Mannatt, M. *Parents, Peers, and Pot.* DHS pub. no. 80. Washington, D.C. 1980, p. 812.

Meacham, A. "Potent Pot Causes More Health Problems." *U.S. Journal of Drug and Alcohol Dependence* 14, no. 1 (1990):13.

National Collegiate Athletic Association. *NCAA Banned Drugs Reference List,* 1986.

"New Data Intensify the Agony over Ecstasy." *Science* 239 (February 1988):864–66.

"An Outbreak of Designer Drug-Related Deaths in Pennsylvania." *Journal of the American Medical Association* 265, no. 8 (February 28, 1991):10–12.

Pickens, R. W., and Svikis, D. S. "Genetic Vulnerability to Drug Abuse." *Biological Vulnerability to Drug Abuse,* NIDA Research Monograph 89, U.S. Department of Health and Human Services, Public Health Service, 1988, pp. 1–7.

"Pot and Paraquat." *Current Health* (November 1978): 26–29.

"The Return of a Deadly Drug Called Horse." *U.S. News and World Report* (August 14, 1989):31–32.

Schafer, J. "Designer Drugs." *Science* (March 1985):60–67.

Schlaadt, R. G., and Shannon, T. T. *Drugs of Choice: Current Perspective of Drug Use.* Englewood Cliffs, N.J.: Prentice-Hall, 1986.

Towers, R. L. *Student Drug and Alcohol Abuse.* Washington, D.C.: National Education Association, 1987.

"The War on Drugs (Continued)." *U.S. News and World Report* (December 30, 1991):viii, 21.

White, G. W., et al. "Preventing Growth Hormone Abuse: An Emerging Concern." *Health Education* 22, no. 4 (1989):4–8.

Wise, T. "Weed It and Reap: Domestic Marijuana Production Soars with Drug War." *Dollars and Sense* (March 1989):12–15.

Additional Readings

Carroll, C. R. *Drugs in Modern Society,* 2d ed. Dubuque, Iowa: Wm. C. Brown, 1989. This comprehensive textbook discusses in depth the causes, effects, descriptions, and problems associated with drug use and abuse.

Gallager, W. "The Looming Menace of Designer Drugs." *Discover* (August 1986):24–35. This article gives an excellent overview of designer drugs, how they surfaced, and their destruction.

Jensen, M. A. "Understanding Addictive Behaviors: Implications for Health Promotion Programming." *American Journal of Health Promotion* 1, no. 3 (1987):48–57. This is an excellent article that provides a psychological and physiological explanation of addiction.

CHAPTER 10

Alcohol

 Japanese proverb says: "First the man takes a drink, then the drink takes a drink, then the drink takes the man."

Alcohol abuse and dependence (i.e., alcoholism) are serious problems that affect about 10 percent to 20 percent of adult Americans. About three out of every one hundred deaths in the United States can be attributed to alcohol-related causes (U.S. Department of Health and Human Services 1990). Alcohol, because of its widespread use, causes more problems nationwide and internationally than any other drug (Villalbi et al. 1991). According to the National Institutes of Drug Abuse, there are ten to eighteen million problem drinkers and alcoholics in the United States today. Unfortunately, only one out of thirty-five will effectively recover from alcoholism, and those who do will need to abstain from any alcohol for the rest of their lives. The families of those alcoholics are often emotionally, socially, and spiritually devastated, and, in some cases, physically abused. Alcohol is responsible for crime, it is a precursor to suicide, it is responsible for over half of all traffic accidents, and it causes disease and death in many Americans. Yet the social grace, "Would you like a drink?" is still prevalent in society.

Directions: Mark all responses that apply to you.

1. If you still live with your parents or when you lived with your parents, it is (was) with
   a. both parents.
   b. mother only.
   c. mother and stepfather.
   d. father only.
   e. father and stepmother.
   f. neither.

2. Your parents are
   a. married.
   b. divorced.
   c. separated.
   d. widowed.

3. Mark any of the following situations that apply to you.
   a. I live at home with parent(s) who drink regularly.
   b. I socialize with friends or roommates who drink regularly.
   c. I live at or am a member of a sorority or fraternity that has alcoholic drinks at socials.
   d. I live with a spouse who drinks regularly.

4. When you have problems, who among the following can you reach quickly and talk with freely?
   a. father/stepfather
   b. mother/stepmother
   c. friend
   d. girlfriend/boyfriend
   e. spouse
   f. no one really

5. Which of the following statements apply to you? (Mark all that apply.)
   a. I really enjoy the academic part of school.
   b. I am content with the grades I earn.
   c. I like school, but my grades are probably not as good as they could be.
   d. I don't like school.
   e. I am not getting grades I am happy with.
   f. I put a lot of pressure on myself to get good grades.
   g. My family puts a lot of pressure on me to get good grades.
   h. Someone else (i.e., coach, advisor, and so on) puts a lot of pressure on me to get good grades.

6. Mark all of the following that describe your family life (closeness and relationships) now and growing up.
   a. It was great growing up, but poor now.
   b. It was poor growing up, but good now.
   c. We did (do) lots of things as a family (vacations, outings, played games, and so on).
   d. We didn't (don't) do much as a family.

7. If you drink, indicate which of the following types of beverages you generally drink. (Leave blank if you do not drink.)
   a. beer
   b. wine
   c. wine coolers
   d. liquor (Scotch, gin, bourbon, vodka, and so on)

8. Which of the following best describes the drinking patterns of your best friends?
   a. They do not drink.
   b. They drink socially with no more than one or two drinks.
   c. They drink regularly, but not more than one or two drinks per time.
   d. They drink socially and occasionally get drunk.
   e. They drink regularly and get drunk often.

9. Which of the following best describes the drinking patterns of your immediate family (parents, siblings, grandparents). Think of the family member(s) that drink(s) the most.
   a. They do not drink.
   b. They drink socially with no more than one or two drinks.
   c. They drink regularly but not more than one or two drinks per time.
   d. They drink socially and occasionally get drunk.
   e. They drink regularly and get drunk often.

10. Are any of your family members alcoholic or seriously abusing alcohol?
    a. father/stepfather
    b. mother/stepmother
    c. brother/sister
    d. one grandparent
    e. more than one grandparent
    f. no one in my family

11. Which statements best describe how you feel about yourself? (Mark all that apply.)
    a. I feel good about how I am.
    b. I wish I was the way I used to be.
    c. I don't like the way I am.
    d. I like my life-style and how I turned out.
    e. I want to be just like my mother (if female) or father (male).

12. Which best describe how you feel about religion? (Mark all that apply.)
    a. In my religion, it does not really matter whether you drink or not to be in good standing.
    b. My religion is not important to me.
    c. I am not religious.
    d. My personal religious beliefs are that drinking alcohol is okay.
    e. My personal religious beliefs are that drinking is wrong.

13. Which of the following apply to you? (Mark all that apply.)
    a. I am influenced by beer and wine cooler commercials on television.
    b. I sometimes drink to escape my problems.
    c. I feel like I want to run away from my problems.
    d. I am sad a lot of the time.
    e. I am a happy person most of the time.

14. The following statements may describe your situation. (Mark all that apply.)
    a. People consider me rebellious.
    b. I do what I want to do no matter what others think.
    c. I have a lot of problems that are difficult to deal with.
    d. I can handle just about every stress that is thrown at me.
    e. I am currently experiencing a lot of stress.

15. Which of the following best describes your drinking habits?
    a. I do not drink alcohol.
    b. I drink socially with no more than one or two drinks.
    c. I drink regularly, but not more than one or two drinks per time.
    d. I drink socially and occasionally get drunk.
    e. I drink regularly and get drunk often.

Scoring/Interpretation

Total the points you received based on the following key.

1. a = 0   b = 4   c = 1   d = 4   e = 1   f = 4
2. a = 0   b = 4   c = 4   d = 2
3. a = 5   b = 5   c = 5   d = 5
4. f = 5, for a-e if you were only able to mark one response give yourself 1, for two or more responses give yourself 0
5. a = 0   b = 0   c = 1   d = 2   e = 2   f = 2   g = 2   h = 2
6. a = 4   b = 4   c = 0   d = 2
7. a = 1   b = 3   c = 2   d = 7
8. a = 0   b = 3   c = 3   d = 5   e = 7
9. a = 0   b = 3   c = 3   d = 5   e = 7
10. a = 7   b = 7   c = 6   d = 4   e = 6   f = 0
11. a = 0   b = 2   c = 3   d = 0   e = 0
12. a = 2   b = 2   c = 2   d = 2   e = 0
13. a = 3   b = 3   c = 3   d = 3   e = 0
14. a = 3   b = 0   c = 3   d = 0   e = 3
15. See interpretation that follows.

1. For moderate to high risk based on question 15:

   If you indicated response a, then refer to number 3 following to see what your risk is.

   If you selected response b or c, then you are already at a moderate risk. One out of ten social drinkers becomes an alcoholic.

   If you selected response d or e, you may already have a serious drinking problem.

2. You are low risk if you did all of the following:

   left question 3 blank

   selected two or more responses other than f on question 4

   selected 8 a, 9 a, 10 f, 11 a, 12 e, and 15 a.

3. From the total score for questions 1 through 14, interpret your risk of alcohol abuse as follows:

   Low risk = See number 2 previously or a score of less than forty

   Moderate risk = 41–89

   High risk = See number 1 previously or a score of 90 or higher

Directions: If you have a close relationship with someone who, in your opinion, has an alcohol problem, then respond to the following statements.

Indicate by circling the appropriate response as to the degree the statements apply to your actions when you are with the person.

		Never	*Sometimes*	*Frequently*
1.	I confront the person with his or her drinking problem.	2	1	0
2.	I have to hide my real feelings around this person.	0	1	2
3.	I know in advance of being with this person whether I will be loved or abused.	2	1	0
4.	I feel like I am the cause of this person's drinking problem.	0	1	2
5.	I cover for this person when he or she is drinking.	0	1	2

Scoring/Interpretation

Total the number of points circled.

0–1 points	You are probably not in a dysfunctional relationship with this person.
2–4 points	You are likely having some problems in this relationship as it pertains to his or her drinking. Read the section on enabling and codependency in this chapter, and you may need to seek some professional help.
5 or more	You are likely in a dysfunctional relationship with this person, either through enabling or as a codependent. You should seek counseling to help you in this relationship.

The purpose of this chapter is not necessarily to suggest that you stop drinking (although this is the safest action) but to suggest responsible habits if you do choose to drink. Because any drinker has at least a one in ten chance of becoming an alcoholic, extreme caution and awareness should accompany any drinking habits. For nondrinkers, this chapter should encourage continued abstention based on the logic that if someone never drinks, he or she will never become an alcoholic. This chapter also helps the nondrinker to consider the relationship he or she has with someone who drinks and help determine whether or not that person has a drinking problem and if that problem is negatively affecting the nondrinker.

Alcohol is something most of us have tried (estimates are up to 92 percent of college freshman) and remains an accepted part of life on many campuses. Alcohol abuse remains a major problem on most campuses. Some campuses have banned alcohol from all college or university activities in an attempt to avoid the problem of alcohol (e.g., private institutions such as Baylor University and Brigham Young University). Others have alcohol programs, campus chapters of Students Against Driving Drunk (SADD), and other innovative educational and preventive programs to reduce the negative effects of alcohol. National campaigns and educational programs appear to have had some effect. Alcohol consumption began to drop in the 1980s and has continued to do so to the present time.

The most important aspect of using alcohol is for the drinker and the nondrinker to understand the effects of alcohol, the potency of alcohol in different drinks, how many drinks can be consumed before irresponsibility ensues, and how to be a responsible host and drinker. It is appropriate to begin with the understanding of the nature of alcohol, the drug.

Nature of Alcoholic Beverages

The intoxicating ingredient in alcoholic beverages is **ethyl alcohol** (C_2H_5OH), which is a colorless liquid with a sharp, burning taste. There are other types of alcohols found in nature but not used in drinks. Isopropyl alcohol is rubbing alcohol used to cleanse and disinfect. Methyl alcohol is wood alcohol and is extremely poisonous. Methyl alcohol is used in many industrial products such as antifreeze.

Each of the major alcoholic beverages, beer and ale, wine, and liquor, contains a different percentage of ethyl alcohol and is made differently. Beer and ale are made by controlled fermentation of cereal grains plus malt. Hops may be added for a distinctive flavor. Wine is made by the fermentation of grapes and other fruit. Wine is sometimes fortified with the addition of more alcohol after the fermentation process is complete, such as in dessert wines (port and sherry). Liquor is made by distilling an already fermented brew from grain, fruit, or molasses.

TABLE 10.1

Percentages of Alcohol in Selected Drinks

Drink	Alcohol (%)
Beer	3–6[a]
Ale	6–8
Wine coolers	3.2–6
Hard cider	5–10
Champagne	12
Regular wines (red, white, rosé, sparkling)	10–16
Dessert wines	17–20
Whiskey	42–52
Brandy	40–50
Gin	27–45
Vodka	37
Cognac	45
Scotch	45

[a]Depending on the state and brand.

From Dorothy Dusek and Daniel A. Girdano, *Drugs: A Factual Account,* 4th edition. Copyright © 1987 McGraw-Hill Book Company, New York, NY. Reprinted by permission of McGraw-Hill Inc.

In this chapter, reference is made to a number of drinks. Although there is some variability in the amount of alcohol in each drink, as shown in table 10.1, a drink refers to twelve ounces of beer (4.1 percent alcohol), four ounces of regular wine (12.5 percent alcohol), two to four ounces of sherry or port (20 percent alcohol), or one ounce of liquor (50 percent alcohol).

Proof

The **proof** of a beverage is a measure of its alcohol content. Proof is given as roughly twice the value of the percentage of alcohol. For example, a beverage that is 50 percent alcohol would be given a value of 100 proof. This designation is helpful in controlling drinking. It is not a matter of which drink is consumed (beer, gin, or wine) but the proof of the beverage that helps you know how much alcohol you drink. For example, beer ranges from 6 proof (3 percent alcohol) to 12 proof (6 percent alcohol). Interestingly, the term *proof* came from an early test of the quality of whiskey. Mixed with gun powder, a drink was lighted with a match. If it did not light, then the alcohol content was low; if it flamed orange, then the alcohol content was too high; if it lit with a cool blue flame, then it was "proof" of a good whiskey (Dusek and Girdano 1987).

Absorption and Metabolism

When you swallow alcohol, it passes down the esophagus and into the stomach; no digestion is required for it to have its effects. A small amount is absorbed directly into

TABLE 10.2

Blood Alcohol Concentration: Effects on Behavior

Blood Alcohol Concentration (BAC) (%)	Number of Drinks	Behavioral Response
0.02	1	Pleasant feeling; sense of warmth and well-being; minor impairment of judgment and memory
0.03	1½	Doesn't worry; time passes quickly; feeling of superiority
0.04	2	Motor skills may be impaired; slight trembling of hands
0.06	3	Decreased reaction time; coordination affected; may become aggressive or amorous
0.10	5	Vision, speech, balance affected; staggering; judgment and memory affected
0.16	8	Further effect on ability to stand and walk
0.20	10	Has trouble standing; needs help walking; gross distortion of motor and sensory capacities
0.40	20	Loss of consciousness
0.50	25	Coma; death

Note: Blood alcohol concentration is expressed in percentages: a BAC of 0.05 percent means an alcohol content of 5 ml for every 10,000 ml of blood.

W. Wayne Worick/Warren E. Schaller, *Alcohol, Tobacco, and Drugs: Their Use and Abuse,* © 1977, p. 45. Adapted by permission of Prentice Hall, Inc., Englewood Cliffs, New Jersey.

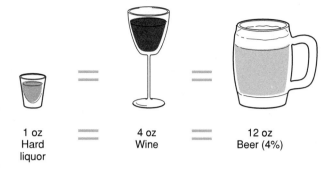

Figure 10.1

These three drinks have the same alcohol content.

1 oz Hard liquor = 4 oz Wine = 12 oz Beer (4%)

per hour results in little, if any, alcohol in the blood, but if an individual drinks faster than that, the alcohol begins to accumulate, resulting in a higher and higher blood alcohol concentration in the body.

Blood Alcohol Concentration (BAC)

Although the safest approach to alcohol is to avoid it, if you choose to use this potentially devastating drug, you should learn about **blood alcohol concentration (BAC).** The amount of alcohol in the blood has clear psychophysiological effects, as shown in table 10.2.

To be a responsible drinker, you should know how much you can drink and still be functional. The standard rule of one drink per hour may not be a good rule for everyone. Anyone can calculate his or her own BAC for different drinks and different time frames to determine the approximate concentration of alcohol in his or her own system. BAC is a function of body weight, the number of drinks, and the time it takes to drink the number of drinks. The definition of one drink is twelve ounces of beer, four ounces of wine, or one ounce of 100 proof distilled spirits (fig. 10.1).

To determine your BAC, first convert your weight to kilograms by dividing your weight in pounds by 2.2. If you weigh 140 pounds, your weight in kilograms would be 63.63 kilograms. The formula* for BAC is

$$BAC = c/BV - (H \times .015)$$

Where:

    c = the number of drinks on one occasion multiplied by 14

  BV = the body weight multiplied by 8

    H = the number of hours it takes to drink the number of drinks you have on this one occasion

*Note: Formula developed by Dr. Wayne Wiley, Director, Alcohol Abuse Prevention Project, Texas A&M University.

the bloodstream from the stomach, but the major portion passes into the small intestine, where it is absorbed directly into the bloodstream and carried rapidly to the brain.

The blood vessels carry alcohol to the various parts of the body. The liver is the organ most significantly involved in the metabolism, or breaking down, of alcohol. Approximately 90 percent of the alcohol is eliminated as a function of the liver, and 10 percent is eliminated by perspiration, exhalation, and urination. Enzyme action in the liver eventually converts alcohol into energy, carbon dioxide, and water. The process of metabolizing excessive amounts of alcohol over long periods of time has several debilitating effects on the liver, which are presented later.

Alcohol is metabolized in the body at a fairly constant rate in any individual, although the rate varies from person to person. The average 150-pound person metabolizes approximately one-half an ounce of absolute (100 percent) alcohol per hour. At that metabolic rate, taking one drink

For example, if you weigh 140 pounds and had three drinks at a party between 8:00 P.M. and 10:00 P.M., what would your BAC be at 10:00 P.M.? (See the Health Actions box on page 230 for a chart on BAC.)

$$140/2.2 = 63.63 \text{ (140 lb converted to kg)}$$
$$c = 3 \text{ drinks} \times 14 = 42$$
$$BV = 63.63 \text{ kg} \times 8 = 509$$
$$H = 10:00 - 8:00 = 2 \text{ hours}$$
$$BAC = (42/509) - (2 \times .015) = .052$$

Effects of Alcohol on the Body

Medically, alcohol is a depressant, a drug that slows the activity of the central nervous system, especially the brain and the spinal cord. In small doses, alcohol may psychologically seem to act as a stimulant, a drug that speeds up the bodily processes. As more alcohol is consumed, however, the activity of the central nervous system declines.

As individuals absorb their first drinks, they are likely to feel better, gaining a sense of warmth and well-being. At the same time, the ability to think clearly begins to deteriorate. As they drink more and more, mental ability further deteriorates and physical coordination declines. Physical symptoms include staggering, slurred speech, and diminished sensitivity to glare and to certain colors and sounds. Alcohol can reduce our sense of fear, which accounts in part for the fights that break out among drinkers. Even though inhibitions are lowered by alcohol, sexual performance is actually often decreased.

Different blood alcohol concentrations have different effects on motor skills and body functions, but again, individuals vary in their responses. Alcohol also affects other body organs. Minor amounts of alcohol in the small intestine increase the flow of digestive juices, which may be mistaken for hunger pangs. With the ingestion of larger amounts, the throat, gullet, and lining of the intestine and stomach may be irritated. Alcohol also increases the urinary activity of the kidneys.

In the long term, alcohol can permanently affect several systems of the body. Chronic alcoholism can cause brain damage or brain disorders. Many studies suggest that at least 50 percent of those who have drunk heavily for years will develop some sort of brain disorder by the time they are forty (Schlaadt and Shannon 1986). Brain atrophy may be as high as 50 percent to 100 percent in alcoholics.

The liver is the primary site of alcohol metabolism and is susceptible to alcohol abuse. Repeated use of alcohol causes the liver to swell and become tender. As alcohol abuse continues, liver function deteriorates into one of the three main types of disease: (1) fatty liver, (2) alcoholic hepatitis, which may be reversible with abstinence, and (3) cirrhosis of the liver, which is not reversible. According to a National Geographic feature, "When alcohol is present in the liver, it preempts the breakdown of fats, which accumulate within liver cells. As fatty cells enlarge they can rupture or grow into cysts that replace normal cells. After years of heavy drinking, fibrous scar tissue, or cirrhosis, impedes the normal flow of arterial and venous blood through the organ" (Gibbons 1992). **Cirrhosis,** the ninth leading cause of death in the United States (U.S. Department of Health and Human Services 1990), is characterized by diffuse scarring of the liver, which is a common complication of alcoholism. Those who have alcoholic cirrhosis and continue heavy drinking often die from **hepatic failure** (liver failure).

Excessive alcohol consumption can also cause diseases of the heart and circulatory system. The most common of these is congestive heart failure, with symptoms including an enlarged heart, elevated diastolic blood pressure, and edema (retention of fluid in body tissues). In the National Geographic feature previously mentioned, a Finnish alcoholic's heart was compared to a normal heart. The alcoholic heart was nearly twice the size. The growth was induced by ethanol-induced high blood pressure and the scar tissue left (about one-third of the entire heart) by massive doses of vodka (Gibbons 1992). Mild drinking (i.e., a drink a day) does not seem to affect the heart adversely, though it does cause the blood vessels to relax and dilate, and blood pressure falls slightly.

In the gastrointestinal tract, regular alcohol consumption can cause inflammation of the esophagus and irritate peptic ulcers. Alcoholic beverages are also known to contain cancer-producing compounds. Tobacco users who also drink alcohol are at even higher risk of cancer. Though the mechanism of how tobacco combined with alcohol increases the risk is unclear, one theory suggests that alcohol is a solvent for cancer-producing compounds and enhances their penetration into susceptible areas.

Negative effects to many organs of the body occur largely due to poor nutrition. Alcohol in the gut impairs the intestinal absorption of many nutrients, notably folate and vitamin B-12. It also represents empty calories substituting for more beneficial foods. In addition, alcohol or one of the substances it changes into during metabolism is a toxic poison. A high level of acetaldehyde has been one of the chief substances implicated in injury to the liver, heart, and other organs (Robbins and Kumar 1987).

Why People React Differently to Alcohol

Some individuals can drink alcoholic beverages all evening without any effects, while others are affected after a few sips of wine. Why do these variations occur? Five main factors appear to be involved: rate of consumption, stomach contents, type of beverage, body weight, and body chemistry (Miles 1974). Keeping these factors in mind may help you decide how much to drink, what to drink, and how fast you should drink.

Rate of Consumption

If you sip a drink slowly enough to last for an hour, you should have no significant rise in blood alcohol concentration. The body burns the alcohol at the same rate at which it is absorbed in the bloodstream. If you gulp the drink, however, its effects are felt immediately and take about an hour to wear off.

Stomach Contents

If you eat while you drink, or just before, food in the stomach slows the rate at which the alcohol is absorbed, and thus the alcohol reaches the brain at a slower rate. Foods that have fat and protein content are best (cheese, low-salt crackers, Swedish meatballs, cold cuts, and so on). Fruits are less effective in slowing down absorption.

Type of Beverage

Beer and wine affect the central nervous system more slowly than does liquor. Beer and wine contain certain nutrients and other substances that slow the absorption of alcohol, resulting in a lower alcohol concentration in the blood. Carbonated substances added to alcoholic beverages speed the rate of absorption because carbon dioxide relaxes the pyloric sphincter (the valve opening from the stomach to the small intestine) and allows alcohol to pass more readily into the small intestine. Sparkling burgundy and champagne have high carbon dioxide content and are absorbed faster than other beverages.

Body Weight

Someone who weighs 180 pounds has more blood and other fluids in his or her body than does a person weighing 120 pounds. The same amount of alcohol is more diluted in the bloodstream and thus does not show its effects as soon.

Body Chemistry

For an unexplained reason, some individuals have an internal body chemistry that keeps them from getting intoxicated as quickly as others. This allows them to drink a great deal and remain sober, whereas another person may react to even the smallest amounts of alcohol. If a person has already developed a tolerance to alcohol, then the effect is lowered.

Tolerance

Tolerance is the condition in which it takes larger and larger amounts of alcohol to produce the same effects felt previously at lower levels of alcohol consumption. An understanding of tolerance is critical to controlling alcohol consumption. You may find that you soon can "hold your liquor" better, that is, drink more and not feel the effects as much. For example, if you find that it takes two drinks instead of one to relax you, then you are developing tolerance. This means that the body is adapting to alcohol on the cellular level. This adaptation is the first step toward serious physiological addiction, even though an individual may already be psychologically addicted.

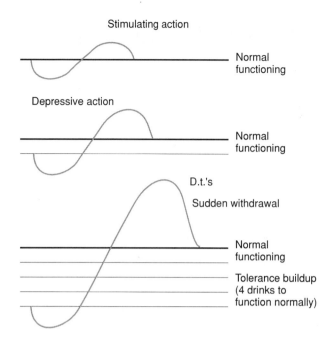

Figure 10.2
Alcohol and tolerance.

Figure 10.2 represents how the effect of alcohol and tolerance work. Initially, alcohol acts as a depressant. As with all drugs, after the depressing effect, there is a stimulating effect that is part of the cause of a hangover. In the figure, the horizontal line in the first drawing represents normal bodily functioning. With one drink, there is a depressive action that, after the alcoholic effect wears off, is followed by a stimulating effect. Over time, as the body develops tolerance, it adapts to the alcohol and the normal functioning line drops some because the body begins to need alcohol to function optimally. With continued use, the normal functioning lines drop more and more as tolerance increases. With problem drinking, when a person needs four or five drinks to have the same effect as one drink used to have, then that person must have three or four drinks in his or her system to function normally.

When an individual who may need several drinks to function optimally is suddenly deprived of alcohol, problems can occur. The withdrawal effect of the drug is felt at the low-tolerance normal functioning line (bottom), but for complete withdrawal, the person experiences the peak of the balancing stimulating effect as well. The stimulation is so severe it is manifested by trembling and convulsions, called the **delirium tremens (D.T.s)**. D.T.s indicate a serious state of withdrawal that, without medical help, can result in death. Medical intervention generally includes mild injections of a depressant to reduce the peaking effects of withdrawal.

Alcohol Dependence

Almost all social drinkers have experienced the immediate physical and psychological effects of overindulgence at one time or another, but they rarely drink to excess. Some

Psychologists have tried for years to understand the psychological reasons why people drink and become alcoholics. Although there are many theories, here are four basic theories from which most stem (Blane and Leonard 1987).

1. Tension Reduction Theory: People may drink to reduce stress and tension. If the drinking is successful in relieving the tension or problems, then the drinking is reinforced, and after some time the person continues to drink to relieve tension.

2. Personality Theory: There are certain personality types that are more prone to drinking than others. If, through inheritance or learning, people find themselves with a certain personality type, then they will be more prone to drink. Personality characteristics associated with drinking include nonconformity, negative self-esteem, and certain negative cognitive styles.

3. Social Learning Theory: This theory assumes that all drinking that progresses from incidental social use to alcoholism and abuse is governed by learning from others, cognition, and reinforcement from peers or effects of the alcohol.

4. Interactional Theory: This theory suggests that drinking is a function of the interaction between the person, his or her environment, and behavioral factors.

individuals, however, develop a dependence on alcohol that leads to problem drinking and eventually to alcoholism. In alcohol dependency, a person experiences a craving or uncontrollable desire for alcohol. At first, the dependence is psychological as the drinker builds up a certain level of alcohol tolerance; eventually, physical dependence can develop.

Psychological dependence is the compulsive need for alcohol to relieve emotional discomfort. Alcohol-dependent individuals feel the need to escape from the tension and pressures confronting them in the real world, and they often find the social atmosphere of a bar more accepting of their behavior. Once involved, they need the sense of belonging given to them by the group.

Physiological dependence does not occur as quickly as psychological dependence. Generally, it takes from three to fifteen years of heavy alcohol consumption, although young drinkers may develop a dependency after one or two years of heavy drinking. Someone physically dependent on alcohol experiences withdrawal symptoms (hangovers or the delirium tremens) when drinking is stopped or decreased.

Why People Drink

People drink for many reasons. Some drink out of habit or family tradition, while others drink to celebrate a religious, cultural, or social event, such as the champagne toast to a bride and groom. For some, drinking is a way to show sophistication—drinking is thought to go hand in hand with elegance, as evidenced by the fine wine served with a good meal. The cocktail hour has become a great American pastime, with restaurants and bars promoting "happy hours" by serving drinks and appetizers at reduced rates for several hours in the early evening.

There is no question that alcohol advertising has a great deal of influence on the decision to drink. Alcohol is portrayed as feminine, macho, fun-loving, sophisticated, cool, and every other positive image imaginable to appeal to the broadest audience as possible.

Some young people drink as a way of rebelling against their parents. Children of **teetotalers** (complete abstainers), for example, may drink excessively as a form of self-assertion against their parents, even while feeling guilty for doing so. Others drink to be accepted by their peers, to relax, to forget their problems, to relieve boredom, or simply because they enjoy doing so.

Still others drink because they like the feeling that intoxication gives them. **Intoxication** is the direct result of alcohol depressing the central nervous system. Drinkers tend to become talkative, sociable, and relaxed. For some, this is the way to loosen up in a social situation, regardless of possible alcohol dependence.

It is interesting to note that in the elementary years, attitudes against drinking are high. Young children do not think that people should drink often or to excess and that drinking and driving are dangerous. After young people become drinkers, the attitudes change to acceptance and tolerance of drinking, excessive drinking, drinking and driving, and use of alcohol to cope with life crises (Carver, Kittleson, and Andrews 1991).

Responsible Drinking

Responsible drinking of alcohol is a function of the drinker, the drinker's friends and family, social hosts, and servers of alcoholic beverages. Responsible drinking means making provisions to be taken home if you plan to drink, understanding limits through the calculation of blood alcohol concentration, and recognizing when enough alcohol has been consumed. Responsible drinking is realizing that the toughest problem you may have is not whether to drink but rather how to live with the decision to be a drinker and the potential outcomes of drinking.

Social Impact of Alcohol

In the Fifth Special Report to the U.S. Congress (1984), it was noted that there are several social consequences that result from citizens' use of alcohol. The following is a list of those consequences.

1. Traffic accidents. One study showed that in one-third of the traffic fatalities, drivers had BAC of over .10 and that with other victims 50 percent to 60 percent of all traffic fatalities were influenced by alcohol. Drivers with BACs over .10 are three to fifteen times as likely to have a fatal crash.

2. Pedestrian accidents. Of the 8,000 pedestrians killed and 100,000 injured in 1984, 35 percent to 75 percent had measurable BACs.

3. Airplane accidents. In one study of 678 fatal plane crashes, alcohol impairment was identified in thirty pilots.

4. Occupational accidents. This area is not as well studied, but one study showed only 2 percent of employees drinking on the job, while another study showed that in job-related accidents 79 percent had measurable BACs.

5. Home and recreational accidents. In home accidents, one-third come from falls and another 20 percent come from burns and injuries from fire. In recreational activities, accidents come from drownings, falls, and other recreational activities. Studies involving alcohol-related accidents showed a range of 20 percent to 45 percent measurable BACs.

6. Homicide. There are approximately 9.8 homicides per 100,000 people in the United States. Studies have differed but show that alcohol was involved in from 25 percent to 85 percent of the homicides.

7. Rape. There are approximately thirty-six forcible rapes per 100,000 people. Studies have shown that the rapist had been drinking alcohol prior to the rape in from 50 percent to 81 percent of the cases.

8. Marital problems. Forty percent of family court problems involve alcoholism in some way, and it is estimated that 33 percent to 40 percent of intact alcoholic couples have poor marital relationships.

9. Family violence. The abuse of children by their parents and the abuse of spouses by their marital partners, although difficult to study, have yielded evidence that alcohol is involved in 11 percent to 17 percent of child abuse cases and from 29 percent to 71 percent of spouse abuse cases.

10. Suicide. Between 15 percent and 64 percent of suicide attempts and up to 80 percent of completed suicides have been associated with drinking alcohol at the time of the attempt.

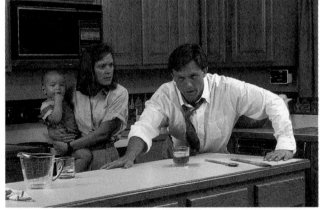

The conflict, marital problems, and family violence often caused by alcoholism can make growing up in an alcoholic home confusing and challenging.

Personal Decisions and Society

The social life of most students is very important and is a significant motivator in their lives. When important social groups or individuals offer you a drink, it may be difficult to say no when you prefer not to drink or have had more to drink than you would like. A fraternity or sorority party or nightclubs often revolve around drinking. Ordering a nonalcoholic drink at a club may be met with criticism.

In spite of the possible social stigma, more students are finding the courage to say no when they have had enough to drink or even say no to any drink. They handle the situation by being very open about being a nondrinker or by covertly ordering a look-alike soft drink or ordering a drink but not drinking it. The question you must ask yourself is, What are my standards and limits to be responsible? Once your standards and limits are established, then planning how to implement and abide by them should ensue. If you choose to drink, even moderately, it is important to continue to assess and reassess your drinking patterns and attitudes to pick up any problems early. Cohen (1985) has suggested the following questions that the social drinker should continually ask himself or herself. Any positive response to any question may necessitate a period of abstinence.

1. Do I get drunk when I intended to stay sober?
2. When things get rough do I need a drink or two to quiet my nerves?
3. Do other people say I'm drinking too much?
4. Have I gotten into trouble with the law, my family, or my business associates in connection with drinking?

5. Is it not possible for me to stop drinking for a week or more?

6. Do I sometimes not remember what happened during a drinking episode?

7. Has a doctor ever said that my drinking was impairing my health?

8. Do I take a few drinks before going to a social gathering just in case there won't be much to drink?

9. Am I impatient while waiting for my drink to be served?

10. Have I tried to cut down, but failed?

11. Can I hold my liquor better than other people?

12. Have many members of my family been alcoholics?

Available Help

Because alcohol may impair judgment, it is important as roommates, family members, sorority sisters, fraternity brothers, and friends to look for early problems in loved ones. Asking loved ones, when they are sober, about potentially problem drinking is awkward but important.

Many groups are available to help and educate people about how to avoid the problems associated with drinking alcohol. MADD (Mothers Against Drunk Driving) was started by a woman whose child was killed by a drunk driver, and chapters exist all over the country to help prevent alcohol abuse and treat and prosecute drunk drivers. Students Against Driving Drunk (SADD) and Removing Intoxicated Drivers (RID) groups have formed around the country and on college campuses. These organizations try to reduce the number of drunk drivers on the road through education, by providing rides, and with awareness functions.

Responsible Hosting

Responsible hosting used to be an ethical issue. As a host, you showed your concern and care for guests and made sure that if they became intoxicated, they got home safely. Now, responsible hosting has become a legal issue as well. For example, on January 11, 1980, Donald Gwinnell drove away from the home of Joseph and Catherine Zak after consuming reportedly thirteen drinks of Scotch. Minutes later, while attempting to pass another car on a curve, he hit another car and injured Marie Kelly, who suffered a broken ankle and lost six teeth. Gwinnell was legally intoxicated. Kelly sued Gwinnell and later included the Zaks in her suit. In 1984, the New Jersey Supreme Court ruled that "where the social host directly serves the guest and continues to do so even after the guest is visibly intoxicated, knowing that the guest will soon be driving home, the social host may be liable for the consequences of the resulting drunken driving." Several months later in court, the Kelly case was settled, with the Zaks paying $72,000 and Gwinnell paying $100,000. At

least twelve states now include a provision in the law for action against social hosts for injuries caused by their intoxicated guests (Prugh 1986).

Whether an ethical or legal issue, it is important to watch guests carefully who are drinking. There are several things that you can do to be a responsible host (National Clearinghouse for Alcohol Information, Rockville, Md.):

1. Do your best to establish and maintain a tension-free atmosphere. Guests should not have to drink in order to relax.

2. Have food available before and during alcohol service, but avoid salty foods that promote thirst. High-protein foods—meatballs or chicken, for example—are best at slowing the absorption of alcohol.

3. Do not have an open bar. De-emphasize alcohol by putting the bar someplace out of the way. Serve your guests yourself or hire someone to do it. In either case, measure the alcohol carefully and use light doses. Have an attractive variety of nonalcoholic beverages on hand, and make them at least as easily and prominently accessible as the alcoholic drinks. If you are serving mixed drinks, be aware that noncarbonated mixers retard the absorption of alcohol into the bloodstream while carbonated mixers speed it up.

Liability Lawsuits: Prevention Steps for Colleges and Universities

University and college groups can do several things to reduce liability and damages associated with university functions where alcohol is served. The responsible hosting techniques described in this chapter should be practiced in addition to and with special emphasis on the following:

- Assure that nonalcoholic drinks are displayed with more or equal prominence as alcoholic drinks at an event.
- Make sure that plenty of food is available where alcohol is served, especially protein-rich items such as cheese, crackers, and pizza, which slow the rate of alcohol absorption into the bloodstream.
- Develop alcohol-free events, such as dance marathons, dorm campouts, casino nights, sports competitions, and "mocktail" parties to take the place of traditionally alcohol-related activities.

- Eliminate "happy hours," discount prices, keg parties, and other practices that encourage the consumption of alcohol.
- Stop the service of alcohol an hour prior to the expected conclusion of any event.
- Establish an alcohol-problem awareness group on campus to educate students on responsible drinking.
- Restrict to appropriate levels the amount and kinds of alcohol served, according to the type of event, participants, and duration of the activity.
- Post notices stating the legal drinking age at the entrance and in beverage serving areas of campus functions where alcohol is served.
- Avoid open bars by requiring all campus alcohol service events to be attended by a responsible server at all times.

- Establish a designated-driver program, allowing the driver for a group to drink nonalcoholic beverages free of charge in order to eliminate the risk of drunk-driving incidents.
- Take steps to ensure that the campus health services, the counseling center, and the disciplinary systems are sensitive to alcohol-related problems and are prepared to inform and intervene.
- Maintain adequate liquor-liability insurance.
- Provide due warning to the campus community on the health and safety hazards of alcohol abuse through educational and informational activities such as health fairs, panel discussions, demonstrations, film festivals, and a dedicated alcohol-problem awareness day or week.

Source: National Clearinghouse for Alcohol Information, Rockville, Md.

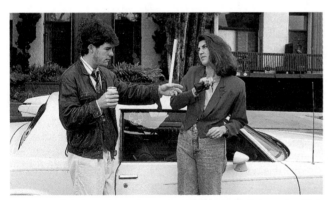

A responsible host can take several steps to help guests drink responsibly, but when one of them overindulges, the host should ensure that the guest does not drive home drunk.

4. If the event is a dinner-and-drinks affair, keep the drinking period short and have hors d'oeuvres available throughout.
5. Don't push drinks. Respect your guests' right to refuse drinks. Make sure that nonalcoholic beverages are available during dinner as well as before.

6. Never serve alcohol, or allow it to be served, to a guest who seems to be intoxicated.
7. Stop serving alcohol at least an hour before the party is over.

If, despite these precautions, a guest drinks to the point of impairment (not necessarily drunkenness) and you are not certain he or she will be driven home by a sober companion, then drive the guest home yourself, arrange for a taxi, or put him or her up in your home for the night. *Never let a guest drive away intoxicated.*

As a guest, support and cooperate with your host's efforts to make the event safe and pleasant for all (National Clearinghouse for Alcohol Information, Rockville, Md.):

1. Do not hesitate to exercise your right to refuse drinks or to avoid alcoholic beverages altogether.
2. If you choose to drink, moderate your intake. If you arrive with a group, arrange for one member to take responsibility for doing the driving. That person should not drink alcohol on that occasion.
3. Be aware that, while most people can metabolize about one standard drink every hour (a standard drink is twelve ounces of beer, four ounces of wine,

or one ounce of spirits), metabolic rates vary. In general, women are more readily affected by alcohol than men are, because of lower average body weight, different tissue composition, and other factors.

4. If a woman is pregnant or nursing, the safest decision for her and her baby is not to drink.

5. Party goers taking medication should be aware that many drugs—both prescription and over-the-counter—can interact with alcohol to produce unpleasant or even dangerous side effects. If in doubt, consult your physician or pharmacist.

Responsible Service

Legal and ethical issues are associated with serving alcoholic drinks from commercial establishments. Successful lawsuits have been filed against bartenders and drinking establishments. Consequently, server intervention programs around the country train bartenders to spot potential drunk drivers, call them a cab, and quit serving them before legal drunkenness occurs.

Problem Drinking

When alcohol begins to control a person's life, create accidents, cause arguments, and take the person away from activities he or she should be doing, that person may be considered a problem drinker. **Problem drinking** is the repeated use of alcohol that causes physical, psychological, or social harm to the drinker or to others. The drinker is unable to cope or function normally without alcohol. The actual amount, frequency, or pattern of alcohol use is not particularly important; what is important is the person's consistent reliance on alcohol.

In the Health Assessment at the beginning of this chapter, a list of items indicating that alcohol is becoming a problem were noted. Those signs represent early symptoms of serious problems. Becoming seriously addicted is a subtle process, and people generally do no realize they are sinking into alcoholic addiction and serious problems.

Pathway to Problem Drinking

The steps to alcoholism occur differently for every individual, but some common steps in the gradual decline might include the following (Strug 1986):

Step 1: The occasional drink.
A drink at social gatherings, a drink at dinner as a cultural tradition, and an occasional drink for pleasure.

Step 2: Initial use as a "crutch" or "escape."
A drink for the purpose of calming nerves, to relax after a difficult day.

Step 3: Frequent use of alcohol as a "crutch" or an "escape."

When regular use of alcohol is the means to control stress.

Step 4: Physical symptoms and overt symptoms.
When the psychological use of alcohol as a coping mechanism or escape is routine, and it is accompanied by occasional blackouts (not passing out, but not remembering events while drinking). Some preoccupation with alcohol, gulping first drinks, and drinking alone. Increasing tolerance.

Step 5: Alcohol becomes central to life-style.
Job, home life, appearance, possessions, and significant others become second to alcohol. Cannot stop at one drink. Interpersonal conflicts, resentment, and self-pity dominate.

Step 6: Continuous drinking.
Drinking starts in the morning and may continue, daily routine of drinking everywhere he or she goes, danger of withdrawal and the D.T.s if alcohol is not in the system at all times. Generally malnourished and has the "shakes."

Step 7: Medical intervention or death.

Alcoholism

Alcoholism is an old problem. Today, however, alcoholism is one of America's top health problems: at least one in every ten adults—about ten to eighteen million Americans—are alcoholics!

Alcoholism is a condition in which individuals have so lost control over their drinking that they are consistently unable to refrain from or stop drinking before becoming intoxicated (Miles 1974). Alcoholism differs from problem drinking in that the alcoholic not only suffers problems due to drinking but also suffers a loss of control.

Alcoholism is recognized by professional organizations as a disease. The disease process is a downward progression from social drinking to debilitating alcoholism. Individuals who need help in overcoming alcoholism include both those who have the powerful genetic predisposition to alcohol addiction and those who have become addicted by using alcohol as a coping mechanism. Professional intervention is generally the only way to curb the downward spiral to addiction and begin the process of recovery.

Alcoholism creates problems for individuals, their families, and the community. Alcoholics lose self-respect. Their health, ability to relate with people, happiness, and safety are affected, and this leads to ruined lives. Three of every four alcoholics are reasonably well-accepted members of their communities, not "skid row bums," as is often thought. An alcoholic affects an average of at least four

TABLE 10.3

Stages of Alcoholism

Early Stage	Middle Stage	Final Stage
Frequent drinking	Conceals drinking	Loneliness and isolation
Increased tolerance	Drinks alone, in morning	Lives to drink
Promises to quit but doesn't	Work affected	Extreme personality changes
Changes in personality	Feels bad regardless of amount consumed	Health definitely affected

Source: Alton L. Blakeslee, "Alcoholism: A Sickness That Can Be Beaten" in New York Public Affairs Pamphlet No. 118A, pp. 8–9, 1976.

The middle stages of alcoholism are characterized by a lack of control after taking the first drink. Drinking becomes a daily necessity, at any time of the day. The drinker is unable to abstain, even though the effects of drinking are pronounced. Definite physical, mental, and social changes occur in the alcohol-dependent individual, including severe guilt feelings, efforts to deny or conceal drinking, and general deterioration of normal social relationships within the family and the profession.

After a number of years of drinking, the alcoholic reaches the final stage—drinking to live and living to drink. The person's entire life revolves around obtaining and consuming alcohol. The alcoholic is usually isolated from family, friends, and co-workers; alcohol comes first. Health problems begin to appear: tremors, hallucinations, and malnutrition (because the alcoholic drinks rather than eats). Unless the alcoholic realizes there is a severe problem, he or she will likely lose everything—family, job, friends—and may eventually die from the health complications.

others by his or her behavior. Loss of income and respect can lead to divorce, delinquency, crime, and even suicide.

Alcoholism can cause a huge drain on the economy within the community. There is money lost from lost productivity, vehicular accidents, health and social service costs, and violent crimes. Some $55 billion is lost through alcoholism, including money spent on recovery from the disease (Galizio and Maisto 1985).

Alcoholism attacks humans without regard to social standing, occupation, intelligence, education, national origin, religion, or race. In fact, typical alcoholics include bright, middle-management executives in their thirties, married and living in middle-class neighborhoods. There are also middle-aged homemakers who no longer have children at home and who have found little to occupy their lives other than drinking from a "hidden bottle." There are even twelve- to fifteen-year-old alcoholics who go to school every Monday morning with a hangover. There are many theories about the causes of alcoholism, but no one has presented conclusive evidence that pinpoints a definitive cause.

Stages of Alcoholism

Alcoholics have different drinking patterns, but all these patterns usually fall into similar stages. The **stages of alcoholism** are outlined in table 10.3. After a period of apparently normal drinking, the alcoholic begins a period of heavy social drinking—the early stages of alcoholism. The individual drinks more frequently, usually to relieve tensions, and develops an increased tolerance to the effects of alcohol. The person may experience blackouts and not remember the drinking episode. Other personality changes, including increased irritability and forgetfulness, are also likely to occur. The person promises to quit but promptly breaks the promise to cope with social stress. During this stage, which may last as long as ten years, the person invents occasions for drinking if none exist.

Treatment and Rehabilitation

The only "cure" for alcoholism is **abstinence,** or never drinking again. An alcoholism treatment study designed to help alcoholics become social drinkers (rather than abstainers) through behavior modification techniques has been discredited ("Alcoholics as Social Drinkers" 1982). Records show that of the twenty subjects enrolled in the program, only one has become a successful social drinker. Alcoholics are unable to stop drinking if they have even one sip of alcohol. To achieve abstinence, the alcoholic must admit there is a problem, sincerely desire to recover, and be willing to accept and stick with some form of treatment, whether self-imposed or institutional.

Most alcoholism treatment programs begin in a medical facility and include physical and psychological components. The first step in treatment is physical **withdrawal** from alcohol, a period in which the body adapts to functioning without alcohol. During withdrawal, hallucination and convulsive seizures known as delirium tremens (D.T.s) occur, and without drug assistance, these can be very painful and dangerous experiences. Sedation may be needed to help the person through this period. Vitamin injections may be given, because most alcoholics suffer from nutritional deficiencies. Tranquilizers may also be used to control anxiety temporarily but they must be used with great care because of the danger of transferring dependence. Sometimes, Antabuse therapy is used. **Antabuse** is a drug that prevents drinking because its intake with alcohol causes nausea, dizziness, and heart palpitations.

The psychological component of the treatment program, psychotherapy, is provided to help the alcoholic face the problems that have caused and resulted from drinking. Group and individual therapy are available, depending on personal preference. The family of the alcoholic is often included in the therapy program to create a more supportive home environment for **rehabilitation.** A

Alcohol

Alcohol is a legally approved drug for those who have reached drinking age (age dependent upon the state law). Yet, alcohol is a factor in over half of traffic deaths and homicides and in many dysfunctional families and relationships. The decision to drink is yours, but it is also your responsibility to control it and use alcohol wisely. To contribute to better control and responsibility, consider the health actions of mind, body, and soul and their interdependence that follow.

Mind

Whether you are a drinker or a nondrinker, calculate several BACs for different situations. See what your BAC would be for two drinks an hour, three drinks an hour, or four drinks in two hours. Determine the maximum number of drinks that you could have for different times to keep below a .04 BAC.

For a general picture of the relationship between body weight, number of drinks, and time, the blood alcohol concentration chart provides an overview. Blood alcohol concentration can be obtained by testing blood samples, breath, urine, saliva, or even spinal fluid. If alcohol is found in these samples, the corresponding amount of blood alcohol can be calculated.

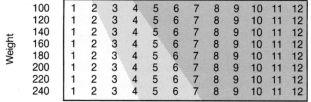

Number of drinks in a two-hour period

BAC =
0.00 to 0.05
Be careful

BAC =
0.05 to 0.09
Driving impaired

BAC=
0.10 and over
Do NOT drive

Blood alcohol concentration chart.
Source: U.S. Department of Transportation.

Body

If you drink, consider how you feel the morning after drinking. Were you responsible enough not to have a hangover or are you going to pay the price for irresponsibility? Treat your body with care. To avoid liver and heart problems, headaches, and other problems of the body, do not drink more than a drink per hour.

Soul

If you have an alcohol problem, consider the Twelve Steps of Alcoholics Anonymous in dealing with it:

1. We admitted we were powerless over alcohol—that our lives had become unmanageable.
2. Came to believe that a Power greater than ourselves could restore us to sanity.
3. Made a decision to turn our will and our lives over to the care of God as we understood Him.
4. Made a searching and fearless moral inventory of ourselves.
5. Admitted to God, to ourselves, and to another human being the exact nature of our wrongs.
6. Were entirely ready to have God remove all these defects of character.
7. Humbly asked Him to remove our shortcomings.
8. Made a list of all persons we had harmed and became willing to make amends to them all.
9. Made direct amends to such people wherever possible, except when to do so would injure them or others.
10. Continued to take personal inventory and when we were wrong promptly admitted it.
11. Sought through prayer and meditation to improve our conscious contact with God, as we understood Him, praying only for knowledge of His will for us and the power to carry that out.
12. Having had a spiritual awakening as the result of these steps, we tried to carry this message to alcoholics and to practice these principles in all our affairs.

(Source: *44 Questions and Answers about the AA Program of Recovery.* Alcoholics Anonymous, New York, 1952.)

Although the AA program is considered to be one of the most successful, many people have questioned the first step, which suggests that people are powerless over alcohol. Some think that the first step should state that we believe we *are* capable of overcoming the effects of alcohol and only *we* are going to make the difference.

Interdependence

Alcohol alters attitudes and behaviors and can powerfully affect others. Many families are destroyed by alcohol-related irresponsible actions and words and accidents affecting other nondrinkers. If you are going to drink, drink responsibly, if not for yourself, then for those you care about.

number of excellent organizations assist in the rehabilitation of alcoholics. There are private counseling services, councils on alcoholism, and the Veterans Administration (VA), but perhaps the largest and most successful program is Alcoholics Anonymous (AA). Alcoholics Anonymous is a worldwide self-help organization with only one qualification for membership: the person must want to stop drinking. A person joins simply by attending a meeting, and members assist each other in maintaining sobriety. The AA program recognizes that the only cure is abstinence, which can be maintained through personal commitment, humility, a day-by-day plan for not drinking, and the "Twelve Steps" for personal recovery (see the Health Actions box above).

Each state has its own statutes regulating the use, purchase, and sale of alcoholic beverages. Many of these laws, however, particularly those prohibiting public intoxication and habitual drunkenness, have been found unconstitutional in Supreme Court decisions prohibiting the punishment of persons for public intoxication except as a misdemeanor. In various states, laws prohibit the following:

1. *Public intoxication.* Courts have interpreted a public place to include virtually every place but the home. The criminal aspect of this has been eliminated in approximately fifteen states.
2. *Drinking in public.* Some states prohibit this. Legal action could occur under statutes that prohibit loitering and disorderly conduct.
3. *Drunk and disorderly.* In some states, this is an offense.
4. *Sale to minors.* All states prohibit the sale of alcoholic beverages to "minors."

ISSUE

Drunk Driving: Losing Your License

Every state has the power to rescind drivers' licenses in cases where the drivers are convicted of driving while intoxicated. With the massive plea bargaining that occurs in some courts, however, very few drivers ever lose their licenses.

- **Pro:** Intoxicated drivers should lose their licenses because these drivers will do it again and the next time may kill someone.
- **Con:** These drivers are not criminals in the same way that a robber or rapist is, and in most cases they need their cars to support a family.

  Should problem drinkers (convicted more than once) and social drinkers (first-time offenders) be treated the same? Should mandatory treatment programs be required for either or both groups?

If you could make the law, what would it be?

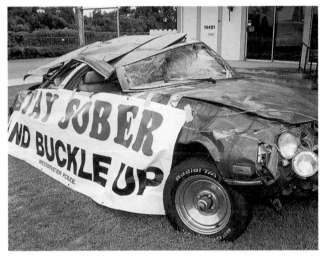

The message is clear: if you drink, don't drive.

Drinking and Driving

"If you drink, don't drive." Unfortunately, many persons disregard this message, and today alcohol is a leading factor in more than half of all fatal automobile accidents. Regardless of our own drinking behavior, it is important to understand the dangers presented by drinking drivers.

All fifty states have laws and varying penalties against driving under the influence of alcohol. Most states base "driving under the influence" on a person's blood alcohol concentration (BAC), as determined by a **breathalyzer** (breath tester) or direct analysis of the blood. In Utah, California, and Idaho, a BAC of 0.08 percent or higher is classified as "drunk driving"; all other states and the District of Columbia use a BAC of 0.10 percent as the criterion. Current evidence indicates that compulsive drinkers with consistently high BAC levels are involved in a disproportionate number of fatal crashes, even though they may be skillful drivers when sober (Galizio and Maisto 1985).

The average person arrested for driving while intoxicated has a BAC of 0.20 percent, which means that the person has probably had close to ten drinks and that motor and sensory capacity are severely distorted. Such drivers are abusers of alcohol, not mainstream social drinkers. Within the last several years, organizations such as MADD (Mothers Against Drunk Driving) and RID (Remove Intoxicated Drivers) have formed throughout the United States. These organizations attempt to ensure that drunk drivers, especially those who have been involved in fatal accidents, are brought to trial and prevented from driving as long as possible. Early in 1982, President Reagan decided that drunken driving had become such a mammoth problem that he appointed a special commission to look into possible solutions. In 1984, he signed a law requiring all states to establish their legal drinking age at twenty-one or lose federal highway funds.

Fetal Alcohol Syndrome

A pregnant women who drinks can cause her baby irreversible damage. Fetal exposure to alcohol is one of the leading known causes of mental retardation in the Western

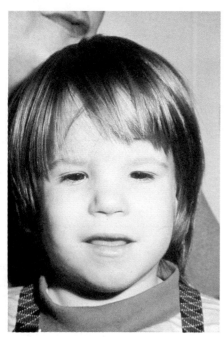

Fetal alcohol syndrome can result when pregnant women drink alcohol.

world, and treatment costs one-third of a billion dollars per year (U.S. Department of Health and Human Services 1990). Scientists still do not understand just how alcohol damages unborn children. They do know, however, that the ingestion of alcohol interferes with normal pregnancy, that the effects on the fetus are permanent, and that whether or not damage occurs depends on the basic metabolism of both the expectant mother and the fetus.

Fetal alcohol syndrome (FAS) is a pattern of physical, mental, and behavioral abnormalities often found among newborns whose mothers drank heavily during pregnancy. Anatomical defects that may be signs of FAS include small head circumference, low nasal bridge, underdeveloped groove in the center of the upper lip between the nose and lip edge, thin reddish upper lip, short nose, and small mid-face. Potential effects of fetal alcohol syndrome are brain injury, mental retardation, and behavioral problems. In addition, children born to alcoholic mothers are born dependent on alcohol; they go through withdrawal symptoms that begin during the first twenty-four hours after birth and last anywhere from one week to six months (Furey 1982).

Fetal alcohol effect (FAE) is a group of less obvious and more subtle abnormalities that often go undetected in children (Steinmetz 1992). Mild retardation or moderate behavioral problems often are undetected because these children seem to be talkative and outgoing. These children may have impaired memory, brief attention spans, poor judgment, and a decreased capacity to learn from experience.

Not all women who drink alcohol during pregnancy have babies with FAS or FAE. Genetic factors and other life-style variables may account for differences in outcome and may explain why some infants are spared the negative effects. Animal studies indicate that peak blood alcohol concentration levels rather than drinking large amounts of alcohol over time is one critical variable. Researchers are working to identify women at greater risk of having babies with FAS. Risk factors such as length of drinking history, reported tolerance to alcohol, and history of alcohol-related illnesses are some of these factors being used to help to identify those at highest risk (U.S. Department of Health and Human Services 1990).

To recommend a safe level of alcohol consumption to avoid FAS would be foolish. Genetic variability, bodily makeup, and psychological characteristics vary too much for such a recommendation. The only safe way to avoid FAS is to not drink during pregnancy.

There is an epidemic of addicted babies born to addicted mothers. The expense of dealing with FAS, the task of helping these babies recover from alcoholism, and the likelihood that these babies will be abandoned by their mothers are major problems in the United States.

Problems of Those Close to Alcoholics

You may not be a drinker yourself but come from an alcoholic family or have an alcoholic partner. There are potential problems that may surface in those types of relationships.

Codependency

In an attempt to help someone who is experiencing drinking problems, caring support people sometimes are affected by the alcohol problem. **Codependency** occurs when individuals are so entrapped by love and concern for the alcohol abuser that they themselves lose their identities in the process of trying to help. They essentially become addicted to the addict's behavior. Codependents are forced to hide their feelings, and the mental and emotional disruption is as destructive to the codependent as alcohol is to the abuser.

For example, a child of an alcoholic mother learned to ignore her feelings and hide the secret of her mother's alcoholism. She later married a man who abused alcohol and drugs: "He filled my needs as a codependent—I needed to be needed and he needed me." Even after her husband got off drugs, she continued her codependent behavior until she went into therapy ("Codependency" 1989).

The process of becoming codependent, according to Gary Jorgensen (1990), starts when someone becomes a victim of a problem drinker. In an alcoholic family or relationship, a child or partner becomes a victim when physically or emotionally abused and experiences assaults to his or her sense of self-worth. The victim then forms some core beliefs, thinking, "I must have done something to have caused my parents/partner to drink." A filtering process then occurs through conscious and unconscious thought, which is a product of family, genetics, temperament, and culture. The codependent emerges after the filtering process thinking, "Anger is not okay." He or she subsequently withdraws and is not directly angry with the person but may "act out" in other ways. The victim becomes anxious and forms the belief that if he or she just shows love, then the alcoholic will be okay. Operational beliefs are: "I feel secure when I don't confront him or her. If I pray hard enough, God will deal with it." The final stage of codependency is when the person becomes an enabler, or thinks, "I will dance all around the behavior but never deal with it." Figure 10.3 illustrates this process. The person becomes trapped in a situation that, without confrontation and disruption, will not be solved, and life is miserable. Groups to help codependents are available through Codependents Anonymous in Phoenix, Arizona, at (602) 944–0141.

Enabling

Enabling can be positive or negative. In the positive sense, support or skills can enable or help a person to succeed. In a negative sense, enabling means to help a person to continue to abuse alcohol. "Enabling systems consist of that constellation of ideas, feelings, attitudes, and behaviors that unwittingly allow and/or encourage alcohol problems to continue or worsen by preventing the alcohol abuser from experiencing the consequences of his or her condition" (Anderson 1988). The enabler covers for the person by making excuses for him or her for not attending parties, school, or work. The enabler does not confront the person directly about the problem and thinks that in some way the problem will go away. Reflecting on the prevention model discussed in chapter 1, recall that growth occurs through the process of experiencing disruption or adversity, becoming disorganized, and after the experience acquiring more coping and protective skills than before the disruption. Enabling overprotects the addict from disruptions and confrontations, which stagnates growth and facilitates the continuation of problem drinking.

The only way to help a person whom you care about to deal with alcoholism is for them to receive help. As a codependent or an enabler, you do not help the person. Confrontation and not allowing the behavior to continue is an important stand. The result is disruptive but is likely to be the only real way to help.

Children of Alcoholics

When children live with one or more alcoholics, they find themselves living in a chaotic household. Rules are never stable, they hide from parents who are episodically abusive and loving, they ride with drunk drivers, and they have no one to talk to about the horrid situation. These children are sometimes forced to run households in these dysfunctional families. One comment from a child of an alcoholic

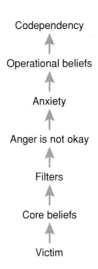

Figure 10.3
The process of becoming codependent.

(COA) who was essentially robbed of his childhood was, "I grew up in a little Vietnam. I didn't know why I was there, and I didn't know who the enemy was" ("Alcohol and the Family" 1988). Children of alcoholics learn to trust no one and do not learn how to experience joy.

As children grow up, these adult children of alcoholics (ACOA) tend to have the following characteristics (Woititz 1988):

1. guess what normal behavior is;
2. have difficulty following a project from beginning to end;
3. lie when it would be just as easy to tell the truth;
4. have difficulty having fun;
5. overreact to changes over which they have no control;
6. constantly seek approval and affirmation;
7. feel that they are different from other people;
8. are super-responsible or super-irresponsible;
9. are extremely loyal even in the face of evidence that the loyalty is undeserved;
10. tend to lock themselves into a course of action without giving consideration to consequences;
11. judge themselves without mercy;
12. have difficulty with intimate relationships;
13. take themselves very seriously.

The chances of an ACOA becoming an alcoholic is 40 percent to 60 percent. Many ACOAs function extremely well and are resilient in spite of their upbringing. Those who do survive are aware of their heritage and ensure that they do not have the problem, often by never drinking alcohol. If you need help you may contact Adult Children of Alcoholics in Torrence, California, by calling (213) 534–1815.

Summary

1. There are ten to eighteen million alcoholics in the United States.

2. Drinking has declined slightly in the United States through the efforts of numerous groups and organizations.

3. Ethyl alcohol is a depressant.

4. Alcohol is metabolized mostly by the liver at the rate of one drink per hour.

5. A knowledge of how many drinks it takes to become an irresponsible drinker is determined by estimating blood alcohol concentration.

6. Negative physiological effects of excessive alcohol intake include brain disorders, cirrhosis, heart failure, and malnutrition.

7. Alcohol can cause both psychological and physiological dependence.

8. Tolerance is a condition in which it takes increasingly larger amounts of alcohol to produce the same effects previously felt at lower levels of alcohol intake.

9. Responsible drinking incudes personal commitment and monitoring, helping others, responsible hosting, and responsible serving.

10. Problem drinking is repeated use of alcohol that causes physical, psychological, or social harm to the drinker or to others.

11. Alcoholism is a treatable disease that can be described as a condition in which people have so lost control over their drinking that they are consistently unable to refrain from or stop drinking before becoming intoxicated.

12. Enabling helps a person to continue or worsen an alcohol problem by preventing the alcohol abuser from experiencing the consequences of his or her condition.

13. Codependency is when people are so entrapped by love and concern they have for the abuser that they themselves lose their identities in the process of trying to help.

Commitment Activities

1. Alcohol use and social activities tend to go hand in hand. List your suggestions for dealing with irresponsible drinking at a university social function (if drinking is allowed at your university functions).

2. Discuss with classmates ways to help the university community become more aware of the warning signs of potential problem drinking.

3. Visit an open meeting of Alcoholics Anonymous, Al-anon, or Ala-teen to hear a firsthand account of the problems associated with alcoholism.

References

Alcoholics Anonymous. *44 Questions and Answers About the AA Program of Recovery.* New York: Alcoholics Anonymous 1952.

"Alcohol and the Family." *Newsweek* (January 18, 1988):62–68.

"Alcoholics as Social Drinkers: Benchmark Study Attacked as Fraud." *Science News* 122 (1982):20.

Anderson, G. L. *Enabling in the School Setting.* Minneapolis, Minn.: The Johnson Institute, 1988.

Blane, H. T., and Leonard, K. E. *Psychological Theories of Drinking and Alcoholism.* New York: Guilford Press, 1987.

Carver, V. C.; Kittleson, M. J.; and Andrews, V. J. "Assessing Alcohol Consumption Attitudes of Adolescent Drinkers: Implications for Alcohol Education Programs." *Health Values* 15, no. 1 (1991):32–36.

"Codependency." *U.S. News and World Report* (September 11, 1989).

Cohen, S. *The Substance Abuse Problems,* vol. II. New York: The Haworth Press, 1985.

Dusek, D. E., and Girdano, D. A. *Drugs: A Factual Account,* 4th ed. New York: Random House, 1987.

Fifth Special Report to the U.S. Congress. "Adverse Social Consequences of Alcohol Use and Alcoholism." *Alcohol and Health.* Washington, D.C., 1984.

Furey, E. M. "The Effects of Alcohol on the Fetus." *Exceptional Children* 49 (1982):30–34.

Galizio, M., and Maisto, S. A. eds. *Detriments of Substance Abuse.* New York: Plenum Press, 1985.

Gibbons, B. "Alcohol: The Legal Drug." *National Geographic* (February 1992):3–35.

Jorgensen, G. Q. "Building Prevention Skills." Presentation made at the 39th School on Alcoholism and Other Drug Dependencies. University of Utah, Salt Lake City, Utah, June 1990.

Miles, S. ed. *Learning About Alcohol.* Washington, D.C.: American Alliance for Health, Physical Education, and Recreation, 1974.

Prugh, T. "Social Host Liability: Kelly versus Gwinnell." *Alcohol, Health and Research World* (Summer 1986):32–35.

Robbins, S., and Kumar, V. *Basic Pathology.* Philadelphia: W. B. Saunders, 1987.

Schlaadt, R. G., and Shannon, T. T. *Drugs of Choice: Current Perspectives on Drug Use.* Englewood Cliffs, N.J.: Prentice Hall, 1986.

Steinmetz, G. "Fetal Alcohol Syndrome: The Preventable Tragedy." *National Geographic* (February 1992): 37–39.

Strug, D. L.; Priyadarsini, S.; and Hyman, M. M. *Alcohol Interventions.* New York: Haworth Press, 1986

U.S. Department of Health and Human Services. *Alcohol and Health,* Seventh Special Report to the U.S. Congress from the Secretary of Health and Human Services, NIAAA, Rockville, Md., 1990.

Villalbi, J. R.; Comin, E.; Mebot, M.; and Murillo, C. "Prevalence and Determinants of Alcohol Consumption Among School Children in Barcelona, Spain." *Journal of School Health* 61, no. 3 (1991):23–26.

Woititz, J. G. "Adult Children of Alcoholics." Referenced in "Alcohol and the Family." *Newsweek* (January 18, 1988):62–68.

Additional Readings

Blane, H. T., and Leonard, K. E. *Psychological Theories of Drinking and Alcoholism.* New York: Guilford Press, 1987. This book describes the many theories of alcohol abuse, with a chapter on each theory.

Gibbons, B. "Alcohol: The Legal Drug." *National Geographic* (February 1992):3–35. This issue has a special section on alcohol and discusses its history, social effects, physical effects, and emotional effects.

Miller, J. *Addictive Relationships: Reclaiming Your Boundaries.* Deerfield Beach, Fl.: Health Communications, 1989. A short book that describes the characteristics of destructive relationships and co-dependency and suggests approaches to confronting the problem. Suggestions on finding comfortable boundaries, degrees of involvement, and monitoring progress are provided.

CHAPTER 11

Tobacco

Key Questions

- What are the physiological effects of tobacco?

- Why do people decide to smoke?

- What health hazards result from smoking?

- How can you quit smoking or help someone else quit?

- What consumer rights do and can nonsmokers have?

- Why is it so difficult for tobacco users to quit?

- What are the health hazards associated with passive smoke?

- What are the health hazards associated with smokeless tobacco?

- What can we do to improve our quality of life as it relates to tobacco?

Chapter Outline

The Nature of the Tobacco Problem
Physiological Aspects of Smoking
    Chemistry of Smoking
    Diseases of the Heart and Blood
        Vessels
    Cancer
    Respiratory Disease
    Digestive Disease
Mothers and Smoking
Pipe and Cigar Smoking
Smokeless Tobacco
Psychological and Social Aspects of
    Smoking
Involuntary Smoking
Fighting Tobacco and Nicotine
    Addiction
Kicking the Smoking Habit
    Nicotine Substitution Approaches to
        Smoking Cessation
    Behavioral Approaches to Smoking
        Cessation

I f a new drug suddenly were to be proposed by a company for acceptance by the Food and Drug Administration, and that drug was shown to contain some three thousand toxic chemicals, double the risk of a fatal heart attack, make the risk of death from chronic obstructive lung disease six times greater among users, and make the risk for dying from lung cancer ten times greater among users, and it was known that this new drug contributed to over 300,000 deaths a year in the United States, there is little question that the drug would not be approved for consumer use. Yet, those devastating effects are clearly established for tobacco smokers today. With the common knowledge of the serious detrimental effect, it is difficult to understand why tobacco (behind caffeine and alcohol consumption) is one of the most widely used drugs in America.

The Nature of the Tobacco Problem

It is difficult to understand why people start smoking. Beginning smokers must actually learn how to smoke, because smoke inhalation by itself is not particularly pleasurable; to some, it is even nauseating. With practice, however, smokers learn to adjust the depth of inhalation and the frequency of puffs so that inhaled air and tobacco smoke are drawn into the lungs in a tolerable way. Through this "learning," a smoker's craving for nicotine soon becomes the chemical motivation for smoking. Nicotine is a very deadly poison if taken in sufficient concentration, but with normal smoking levels, it acts as a powerful reward, or "hooker." Smokers seem to develop a level of daily nicotine consumption that they find satisfying. If they switch to a brand of cigarettes with less nicotine, they're likely to compensate by inhaling more deeply, smoking more cigarettes, or both.

The strong evidence of the detrimental effects of smoking and the difficulty in learning how to smoke might make us think that smoking would not persist in our society, yet many Americans continue to smoke. The incidence of smoking among men peaked at 54 percent in the mid-1950s and declined to 32 percent in 1987. The highest rate of smoking in women of 34 percent occurred in 1966 and declined to 27 percent in 1987. Although fewer women than men smoke, the fastest growing segment of smokers is women under the age of twenty-three. More than 80 percent of smokers start before the age of twenty-one. Although percentages of smokers among black males (32 percent) and females (25 percent) compare closely to white males (29 percent) and females (24 percent), other cultural groups are much higher. About 40 percent of Hispanic men smoke, although their female counterparts are less likely to smoke (24 percent). Among youth, smoking prevalence among high school seniors declined from 28 percent in 1977 to 19 percent in 1987. Now, more adolescent females than males smoke (Kellie 1989).

In the United States, cigarettes were responsible for approximately 390,000 premature deaths in 1985 by causing coronary heart disease (115,000), chronic obstructive pulmonary disease (57,000), cerebrovascular disease (27,500), other vascular and pulmonary diseases (45,000), lung cancer (106,000), other cancers (31,600), infant and neonatal deaths (2,500), lung cancers in nonsmokers (3,800), and deaths from fires caused by cigarettes (1,700) (Slade 1989).

C. Everett Koop, the former U.S. Surgeon General, stated: "There is no serious debate about the hazards of cigarette smoking. It is the chief avoidable cause of death in this country. It is a 'disease' which each year is costing us billions of dollars in economic loss as well as much human suffering" (Koop 1986).

Cigarettes have become a major international problem, fueled by American advertising. An estimated one billion people smoked five trillion cigarettes in 1986, resulting in 2.5 million deaths attributed to smoking. By the year 2000, the number of deaths are expected to rise to 4 million annually. While smoking rates are declining in industrialized countries at a rate of 1.5 percent per year, the rates are increasing at 2 percent per year in developing countries (Connolly 1989).

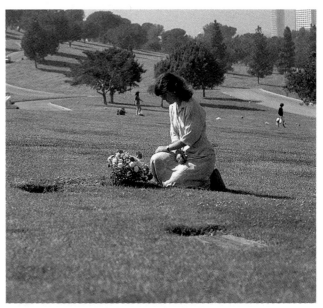

Smoking, the leading cause of preventable death, causes great suffering for both smokers and their loved ones.

Physiological Aspects of Smoking

The negative physiological aspects of smoking are conclusive after thirty-five years and over fifty-five thousand studies from eighty countries. Scientists now understand, for the most part, why smokers have three times the risk of sudden heart attack, 85 percent more lung cancer, and, for pregnant women who smoke, an increased risk of having premature babies, spontaneous abortions, stillbirths, and babies that live only a few hours or days (McGinnis 1987).

Chemistry of Smoking

The smoke from a lighted cigarette consists of a mixture of more than three thousand chemical substances that are dangerous to body tissue. These substances include tars, nicotine, and gases such as carbon monoxide, hydrogen cyanide, and nitrogen oxide that produce undesirable effects on health. The toxic effect of these gases and compounds with the nicotine is responsible for many cigarette-related deaths each year.

Tobacco products contain hundreds, if not thousands, of chemical additives used as flavors and fillers. No federal agency has any authority to require that these additives be disclosed or even removed if found to be harmful. Many of the additives used in tobacco products are suspected of being carcinogenic (cancer-causing).

Tobacco **tar** is made up of hundreds of chemicals that together account for most of the known cancer-causing agents in cigarettes. Research has shown these tars to be carcinogenic and other chemicals in the tar to be carcinogens, that is, substances that, while they do not directly cause cancer, can stimulate the development of cancers while in combination with other chemicals.

Health Assessment for Smokers (nonsmokers proceed to questionnaire for you)

Current Health Status as It Relates to Tobacco Use

1. Keep a diary for one week. Record each cigarette smoked, or each time you chew, dip, or snuff tobacco (number). Also indicate when you used it (time), where you were when you used it (place), what you were doing (activity), and what or who triggered the use of tobacco (prompt). A copy of the chart that follows can be wrapped around the cigarette pack or smokeless tobacco container with a rubber band to remind you to keep the record. A new chart can be attached to the pack or container each day.

Daily Tobacco Use Chart

Number	Time	Where	Activity	Prompt

Directions: Please consider carefully and answer honestly.

	Usually	Sometimes	Rarely	Never
2. Smoking (using smokeless tobacco) helps to pick me up.	4	3	2	1
3. I like the feel of having something in my hand.	4	3	2	1
4. I only smoke (use tobacco) when others smoke (or use it).	4	3	2	1
5. I associate smoking (using tobacco) with pleasant or relaxing experiences.	4	3	2	1
6. When I run out of cigarettes (smokeless tobacco), I feel an urgent need to get some more.	4	3	2	1
7. I smoke or use tobacco more when under stress.	4	3	2	1
8. Sometimes I reach for a cigarette or smokeless tobacco when I already have a cigarette lit or am already using tobacco.	4	3	2	1
9. I really like smoking (using tobacco products).	4	3	2	1
10. Smoking (using tobacco products) really keeps me going.	4	3	2	1
11. Unpacking, lighting, watching exhaled smoke (or the process of using smokeless tobacco) is part of the enjoyment of using tobacco.	4	3	2	1
12. If my friends and family didn't smoke or use tobacco products, I probably wouldn't smoke or use tobacco products.	4	3	2	1
13. I don't think I can go very long without smoking or using tobacco.	4	3	2	1
14. When angry or emotionally down, I generally smoke or use tobacco.	4	3	2	1
15. I often find myself smoking or using tobacco products and don't remember reaching for the tobacco or lighting the cigarette.	4	3	2	1

Likelihood of Being Able to Quit Using Tobacco Products

Directions: Circle all answers that apply except where noted.

16. Which of the following statements best describe your feelings about quitting smoking or using smokeless tobacco?
    a. I do not want to quit smoking or using smokeless tobacco.
    b. Someday I would like to quit smoking or using smokeless tobacco, but not now.
    c. I would like to quit smoking or using smokeless tobacco now.
    d. I am very motivated to quit smoking or using smokeless tobacco now.

17. If you decided to quit smoking or using smokeless tobacco, who would be willing to support and help you quit? (Check all that apply.)
    a. all family members
    b. some family members
    c. roommates
    d. good friends
    e. other co-workers or students
    f. spiritual or religious leader
    g. other

18. People who are heroes or someone I want to be like are:
    a. smokers or users of smokeless tobacco.
    b. nonsmokers or do not use smokeless tobacco.
    c. I don't know.

19. My usual level of stress is (refer to chapter 2 on stress for a complete psychological stressor assessment)
    a. very high.
    b. high.
    c. moderate.
    d. low.

20. Which of the following statements describes your feelings?
    a. I don't think smoking/using tobacco has any negative effects on me.
    b. I tried to quit and failed so I don't think I can quit again.
    c. I know why I smoke or use smokeless tobacco.
    d. I feel better about myself when I smoke/or use tobacco.
    e. Because I can't stop using tobacco or smoking, I don't feel good about myself.
    f. I have been able to quit for short periods of time in the past.
    g. I feel more confident when smoking or using tobacco.

21. Which of the following statements best describes your feelings?
    a. I control whether I smoke (or use smokeless tobacco) or not.
    b. The only thing that prevents me from quitting is me.
    c. For me to quit, I just have to make up my mind.
    d. Whether I smoke (or use smokeless tobacco) or not depends a lot on other people.
    e. My smoking (use of smokeless tobacco) is beyond my control.
    f. The way I was raised determined that I would be a smoker or a tobacco user.

Interpretation

Amount Smoked or Tobacco Used (from question 1)
For cigarettes: Calculate the average number of cigarettes per day for the week.

  25 or more cigarettes per day = heavy smoker
  10–24 cigarettes per day = moderate smoker
  0–9 cigarettes per day = light smoker

This information may not be new to you, but the chart you have completed will be helpful in quitting, as you will learn by reading this chapter.

For smokeless tobacco: Calculate the number of chews or dips you have per day for the week.

  10 or more per day = heavy user
  5–9 per day = moderate user
  0–4 per day = light user

Why Do You Smoke or Use Tobacco? (questions 2–15)
Each of the following pairs of questions represents a reason for smoking or using tobacco. Total the scores for the two questions (range of 2 to 8). If you scored 7–8, then it is a strong reason why you smoke or use tobacco. If you score 5–6, then it may be a reason why you smoke. If you scored 4 or below on the two questions, it is probably not a reason for smoking or using tobacco.

Questions	Reason for Smoking/Using Tobacco
2, 10	Stimulation
3, 11	Need to handle things
4, 12	Need to fit in/social
5, 9	Pleasure/enjoyment
6, 13	Addicted
7, 14	Coping
8, 15	Habit

Likelihood of Your Being Able to Quit
Score yourself on questions 17 through 20 as follows:

17. a = 1, b = 2, c = 3, d = 4
18. Give yourself 2 points for each answer you respond to for a maximum of 6 points.
19. a = 1, b = 2, c = 3, d = 4
20. If a, then 1 point, if not selected give 3 points
    If b, then 1 point, if not selected give 3 points
    If c, then 3 points, if not selected give 1 point
    If d, then 1 point, if not selected give 3 points
    If e, then 1 point, if not selected give 3 points
    If f, then 3 points, if not selected give 1 point
    If g, then 1 point, if not selected give 3 points
21. If a = 3
    If b = 3
    If c = 3
    If d = 1
    If e = 1
    If f = 1

Total your points for questions 17 through 20. The following scoring system applies:

  38 to 44 = strong likelihood to be able to quit
  30 to 37 = good chance to quit, will need to work on attitude or support system
  Below 30 = fair chance, will need to make some attitudinal changes or improve relationships to be successful

Health Assessment for Nonsmokers

Current Health Status for Nonsmokers

1. Identify those situations indoors where you associate with people who smoke in your presence.
   a. where I live
   b. at work
   c. at parties, social events, and clubs
   d. at school
   e. at my social or service organization meetings
   f. other indoor activities
   g. no situations

2. Indicate any of the following that describes you.
   a. I used to smoke but quit over a year ago.
   b. I never smoked.
   c. I used to smoke but quit less than a year ago.
   d. My grades recently had a sudden decline.
   e. I recently went through a divorce or my parents recently went through a divorce.
   f. I have recently seen an increase in the amount of stress in my life.

For questions 3 through 5, a, b, c, d, e, and f are characterized by the following reactions.
   a. Allow them to smoke, even though I didn't want them to.
   b. Allow them to smoke, because I don't mind.
   c. Ask them politely not to smoke, but not insist if they persist.
   d. Ask them politely not to smoke and if they persisted, I would insist that they not smoke.
   e. I would demand that they not smoke.
   f. If a person persisted in smoking I would leave or move.

Indicate which of the reactions you would have in the following situations:

3. A friend or family member asks if he or she can smoke in my house/room or car.
   a   b   c   d   e   f

4. A person I do not know too well asks if they can smoke in my room/house or car.
   a   b   c   d   e   f

5. In a nonsmoking section of a public place such as a restaurant or airplane, a person begins smoking.
   a   b   c   d   e   f

Risk of Beginning Smoking (circle the response that agrees with your feelings)

	Strongly Agree	Agree	Not Sure	Disagree	Strongly Disagree
6. The thought of smoking appeals to me.	5	4	3	2	1
7. My friends/family want me to start smoking.	5	4	3	2	1
8. The thought of dipping or chewing tobacco appeals to me.	5	4	3	2	1
9. My friends or family want me to start dipping or chewing tobacco.	5	4	3	2	1
10. I think smoking or using tobacco would help me cope better with my problems.	5	4	3	2	1
11. I want to start smoking but don't dare.	5	4	3	2	1
12. Smoke makes me nauseated.	1	2	3	4	5
13. Dipping or chewing tobacco is disgusting.	1	2	3	4	5
14. I like to chew or suck on things.	5	4	3	2	1
15. Smoking really doesn't hurt people.	5	4	3	2	1

Interpretation

Likelihood of Involuntary Smoking

Question 1   If a, b, or d, give three points for each response
               If c, e, or f, give one point for each response
               If g, give zero points

Questions 3, 4,   If d, e, or f, give zero points
and 5   If c, give one point
                    If a or b, give three points for each

If total points is ten or more, then you are likely being exposed to chronic sidestream smoke. If total points is less than three, then you are probably free of chronic excessive sidestream smoke.

Attitudes About Smoking

Scoring for questions 6–15.
After totaling points

   44 or higher = unfavorable attitude about smoking
   23 to 44   = neither favorable nor unfavorable attitude
   22 or less = favorable attitude against smoking

Scoring high on this scale means that you should be careful to use healthy approaches to coping with life's stressors.

Read chapter 2 carefully. Nurture your personal strengths, and get support from family and friends.

Risk of Your Starting to Smoke
The following suggests your risk of starting (or returning) to smoke. For high or moderate risk, you should be extremely strong in resisting smoking opportunities.

High risk: If on question 2 you selected c in combination with d, e, or f and scored forty or higher on the attitude score.

Moderate risk: If on question 2 you selected a in combination with d, e, or f and scored forty or higher on the attitude scale.

Low risk: If on question 2 you selected b in combination with d, e, or f and scored forty or higher on the attitude scale.

Note: Over 90 percent of those who become regular smokers do so by the time they are twenty years of age. If you have never smoked, then you have likely learned to cope in other ways and are not likely to begin smoking, although 10 percent do. Please don't start and become one of the unfortunate 10 percent.

Cigarette Labeling

The Federal Comprehensive Smoking Education Act is an attempt to counteract the effects of cigarette advertising. The law requires that cigarette companies rotate one of the following four health warnings on cigarette packages and in their advertising (Koop 1986):

Surgeon General's Warning: smoking causes lung cancer, heart disease, emphysema, and may complicate pregnancy.

Surgeon General's Warning: quitting smoking now greatly reduces serious health risks.

Surgeon General's Warning: pregnant women who smoke risk fetal injury and premature birth.

Surgeon General's Warning: cigarette smoking contains carbon monoxide.

Nicotine, an alkaloid poison, is the addictive element in tobacco. According to Slade (1989), "Nicotine addiction is the most medically serious drug problem in the United States today with social, behavioral, physiologic, and pharmacologic aspects. . . . Nicotine regularly causes a true drug addiction in a high proportion of regular tobacco users." The addiction to nicotine is clear as evidenced by the failure of nicotine-free products in the marketplace.

Drug addiction is evidenced by tolerance, physical dependence, continued use despite harmful effects, pleasant (euphoric) effects, stereotypic patterns of drug use, relapses following drug abstinence, and recurrent drug cravings. The major nicotine effects on the body are respiratory stimulation and gastrointestinal hyperactivity, which are manifested in increased heart rate, blood pressure, cardiac output, oxygen consumption, irregular heart rhythms, and coronary blood flow. Nicotine, tars, and carbon monoxide are inhaled through cigarette smoking, while nicotine in smokeless tobacco is absorbed through the cheek and mouth membranes.

It is estimated that approximately 90 percent of the nicotine found in cigarettes is actually inhaled and absorbed into the bloodstream. The body readily absorbs smoke, and some of the nicotine goes directly to the brain (Schlaadt and Shannon 1986). Nicotine affects not only the respiratory and gastrointestinal systems but also the brain, spinal cord, and peripheral nervous system. It can stimulate, then depress, production of saliva, constrict the bronchi (the air passage tubes to the lungs), increase amounts of free fatty acids in the bloodstream, and cause other effects as shown in figure 11.1.

Carbon monoxide (CO) is a deadly gas that is a by-product of burning tobacco. It is the same deadly gas in the automobile exhaust that pollutes the air. The reasons this gas is deadly rests in its powerful affinity or bonding potential to hemoglobin. **Hemoglobin** is an iron-containing compound in red blood cells that carries oxygen to the cells of the body. There are four sites where oxygen can attach to a red blood cell for the journey through the circulatory system to the cells. The fight for these sites between oxygen and CO is generally won by CO, since the CO chemical bond is two hundred times stronger than the oxygen chemical bond. The result is that the body's cells that rely on oxygen to function are deprived. Figure 11.2 demonstrates this process at the site of the oxygen exchange.

Red blood cells returning from the circulatory system to the tissues of the body have carbon dioxide (a by-product of metabolism) attached and are still carrying carbon monoxide (from the previous inhalation of smoke before the journey). At the oxygen exchange site in the lungs, the carbon dioxide and some of the carbon

Carbon monoxide
(reduces oxygen carrying
capacity of the blood)

Tars
(carcinogens)

Nitrous oxide
(reduces the number of
white blood cells)

Additives
(suspected carcinogens)

Hydrogen cyanide
(increases nerve poison
and reduces cilia
function of lungs)

Nicotine affects the CNS
Heart rate ↑
Blood pressure ↑
Vasoconstriction ↑
Skin temperature ↓
Epinephrine release ↑
Adrenalin release ↑
Gastrointestinal tract activity ↑
Fatty acids in blood ↑
DNA synthesis of lymphocytes ↑
Physical dependence ↑
Psychological dependence ↑
Withdrawal symptoms ↑

Figure 11.1

Chemical elements and effects of tobacco smoke.

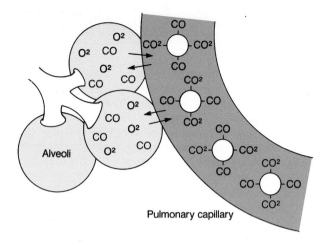

Figure 11.2

Exchange of oxygen and carbon monoxide.

monoxide detach themselves from the red blood cell to be expired via the lungs. The detachments and expiration open some carrying sites on the red blood cells, and the fight between oxygen from the air and carbon monoxide from the smoke again wages.

The result of this reduced supply of oxygen to the brain is impaired judgment—reducing the performance of a driver, a student on an exam, or an athlete in competition. This gas may also lead to disturbances in rhythmic activity of the heart and promote atherosclerosis. When smoking is stopped, oxygen uptake improves soon after. Energy levels return after a few months.

CO is particularly devastating to the unborn fetus of pregnant mothers. The CO is supplied to the fetus from the mother's blood, which travels through the umbilical cord and is internalized in the fetus's circulatory system. The result can be lower birth weight, premature delivery, and a greater risk of sudden infant death syndrome (crib death).

Diseases of the Heart and Blood Vessels

Coronary heart disease, a disease of the arteries nourishing the heart muscle, is the chief contributor to excess deaths in the cigarette-smoking population. Smokers have severe and extensive narrowing of the coronary arteries, higher LDL cholesterol ("bad" cholesterol), and hypertension, which can lead to heart attack. Smoking is not only one of the three major risk factors of heart attack, but it is also a major risk factor for cardiovascular diseases affecting the peripheral blood vessels, the vessels that constitute the circulatory system (Schlaadt and Shannon 1986).

Smoking also increases the possibility of a recurrent heart attack and tends to lower the threshold for the onset of **angina**, the chest pain associated with heart disease. Women who smoke and use oral contraceptives increase their risk of heart attack, blood clots, and brain hemorrhaging (fig. 11.3).

Cancer

The risk of developing lung cancer is ten times greater for cigarette smokers than for nonsmokers. Lung cancer risks for both sexes increase proportionately to the number of cigarettes smoked, the length of time the individuals have smoked, the age at which they started, and the amount they inhale (depth of inhalation). The tar and nicotine content of the cigarette smoked also affects lung cancer risk. Other types of cancer caused by cigarette smoking include cancers of the larynx, esophagus, bladder, kidney, pancreas, and mouth.

Respiratory Disease

Cigarette smoking slows down the action of the cilia in the lungs. The **cilia** are the hairlike projections that help clean the lungs. When these cilia are immobilized, dust and dirt particles can cause lung inflammation and disease, even early in life; so children of parents who smoke are more likely to contract bronchitis and pneumonia during infancy and childhood.

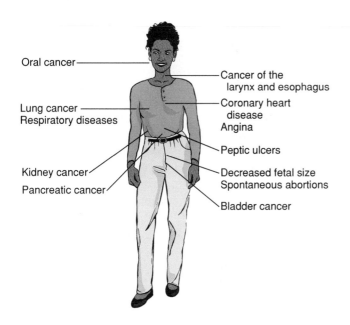

Oral cancer

Cancer of the larynx and esophagus

Coronary heart disease
Angina

Lung cancer
Respiratory diseases

Peptic ulcers

Kidney cancer

Decreased fetal size
Spontaneous abortions

Pancreatic cancer

Bladder cancer

Figure 11.3
Diseases and disorders closely associated with tobacco use.

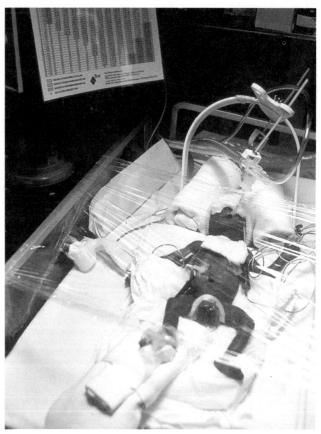

Smoking during pregnancy has adverse effects on the developing fetus and can lead to premature birth and complications during birth.

Cigarette smokers also have more chronic coughs, phlegm production, wheezing, and other respiratory symptoms. Both men and women smokers tend to report more acute and chronic **bronchitis** (inflammation of the bronchi), **sinusitis** (inflammation of the sinus), and **emphysema.** Chronic smoking also leads to tissue changes in the respiratory tract. People with allergies, especially asthma, are more sensitive to cigarette smoke than others (*Smoking and Health* 1979).

Digestive Disease

Cigarette smoking is also associated with the incidence of **peptic** (stomach) **ulcer** and increased risk of dying from this disease; smoking also tends to slow down the healing of peptic ulcers (Schlaadt and Shannon 1986).

Mothers and Smoking

Smoking during pregnancy has an adverse effect on the well-being of the developing fetus. Smoking can reduce the size of the newborn; in fact, babies born to smoking mothers are on the average two hundred grams (approximately seven ounces) lighter than those born to nonsmoking mothers. Smoking mothers are also more likely to have a premature baby (who would also weigh much less than a full-term baby).

Smoking mothers have more complications than non-smoking mothers during pregnancy: they have more spon-taneous abortions, and the death of the unborn child is more likely. The mothers themselves also have more complications, including hemorrhaging and improperly developed placentas.

The more a woman smokes, the greater the risk to both her and her child. Children of smoking mothers tend to have deficiencies after birth as well: physical growth, intellectual development, and emotional development may be affected for several years (Dusek and Girdano 1986).

Pipe and Cigar Smoking

Although the risk of lung cancer is less with pipe and cigar smokers, there is still a significant risk of other problems. There is less risk with pipe and cigar smoke because the smoke is not inhaled into the lungs. The increased health risks, however, do include cancer of the lip, oral cancer, cancer of the larynx, and cancer of the esophagus. Since some of the tars are swallowed, there is also an increased risk of stomach cancer and urinary bladder cancer.

Smoking and Medical Cost Responsibility

Smoking costs business $26 billion a year in lost productivity and $8 billion in smoking-related medical costs ($200 to $500 per smoking employee per year). The companies must pay for the medical bills, and to do so, they have to raise the price of their products. Smokers and nonsmokers alike must pay for the higher-priced goods. That is the main reason companies are implementing smoking cessation programs for their employees (Glasgow et al. 1991). The federal government spends about $26 billion a year for medical care coverage for illnesses that result from cigarette smoking. Smokers and nonsmokers must then pay the higher taxes to cover those costs. The issue is why nonsmokers should have to pay for the increased costs that smokers cause.

- **Pro:** Most illnesses have a number of causative factors in addition to smoking. To label a disease clearly as a direct cause of smoking is impossible in many cases but possible in others. If the program resulted in different rates of taxes or insurance premiums, how do you determine a smoker from a nonsmoker? Is a person who quit twenty years ago a smoker? How about someone who quit a year ago or a week ago? We all just need to pay. Otherwise, it would be a discriminatory subjective practice.

- **Con:** Some insurance companies give premium reductions to nonsmokers. A similar system could be worked in light of taxes. For example, if 10 percent of the gross national product is spent on health care and a significant percentage is associated with tobacco, then nonsmokers could have a reduction in taxes by that percentage. The country would be healthier.

What do you think the best system would be to pay for medical expenses resulting from tobacco use?

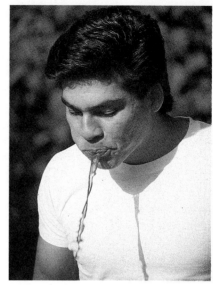

All the advertising in the world can't change the reality that the use of smokeless tobacco is a dirty and disgusting habit.

Smokeless Tobacco

Smokeless tobacco is sold in three forms—snuff, loose leaf, and plug forms. Chewing tobacco may be packaged as loose-leaf tobacco, which is sold in a pouch. The user places the tobacco between the cheek and gum, and tobacco juice and saliva are expectorated (spit). Chewing tobacco also can be found as plug tobacco, which is a solid brick form of tobacco. The user cuts off a piece with a knife and chews it. **Snuff** is a finely ground tobacco sold in circular cans that is usually placed between the cheek and gum, also called dipping, or placed on the back of the hand and sniffed through the nose. Television and magazine advertisements have made smokeless tobacco appear to be a healthy alternative to the smoking of tobacco. The advertisements also present a macho image of tobacco-chewing cowboys and athletes. Advertisements have made headway into social acceptance of smokeless tobacco in some settings where at one time it was considered to be a dirty, disgusting habit. The advertising success has resulted in an increase of 52 percent in sales of smokeless tobacco since 1978. Most estimates are that seven to eleven million Americans use smokeless tobacco, though some estimates go as high as twenty-two million.

The reality is that chewing tobacco is a dirty habit, necessitating frequent expectorating of the mixture of tobacco juice and saliva. It is also an unhealthy practice. Although users of smokeless tobacco do not experience the effects of carbon monoxide, tar, and other gases associated with cigarette smoking, the following is a list of harmful effects or results of smokeless tobacco generally agreed upon by the American Cancer Society (1989) and researchers (Marty et al. 1986; McDermott and Marty 1986; Brubaker and Loftin 1987):

1. There is damage to the soft and hard oral (mouth) tissue.
2. There are excessive abrasions of tooth surfaces caused by abrasive grits in tobacco.
3. Smokeless tobacco contains nitrosonornicotine, a known cancer-producing agent.
4. There is an increase in heart rate and blood pressure.
5. Nicotine is absorbed in the body through the buccal mucosa (inner lining of the cheek) of snuff dippers and can produce cancers.
6. Dipping and chewing tobacco are also associated with the development of leukoplakia, which is a disease manifested by thick, white irregular patches

on the cheek, tongue, and other parts of the mouth in regular users. Leukoplakia often evolves into squamous cell carcinomas (malignant skin tumors).

7. Smokeless tobacco has been linked to suppressed immunological responses, which reduce the ability to ward off disease.

8. Use increases the number of dental caries.

9. Use is associated with gingival (gums) inflammation.

10. It has been shown to decrease birth size in infants whose mothers used smokeless tobacco during pregnancy.

11. It is associated with cancers of the pharynx, esophagus, urinary bladder, and pancreas.

12. Use causes the teeth to darken and results in bad breath.

Regular use may result in psychological addiction to smokeless tobacco. Many people seek professional help in an attempt to quit using it. Addicted users claim it helps them cope with problems, perform better, and gives them a lift, which is characteristic of nicotine that they absorb with each use. Stopping use results in cravings and restlessness that many have described as more difficult than quitting cigarette smoking.

Psychological and Social Aspects of Smoking

More and more people acknowledge the dangers and risks attributed to smoking and yet do not change their behavior. Even though almost all adolescents today know the dangers, approximately 19 percent of them smoke. Psychological influences seem to account for this early experimentation. Young people start because of rebellion, curiosity, peer pressure, and the belief that smoking makes you grown up. It is interesting that the most common age to start smoking is age ten (fifth grade) and to start using smokeless tobacco is seventh grade, but the most intensive tobacco use prevention and education programs in the schools are in the tenth grade (Chen et al. 1991).

Family patterns influence teenagers' smoking behavior. Fewer smokers come from "intact" homes (where both a father and mother are members of the household) than from homes where one or both parents are not present. Smoking practices of other family members, both parents and older siblings, heavily influence teenagers. If both a parent and an older sibling smoke, that teenager is much more likely to smoke (Schlaadt and Shannon 1986).

Peer relationships and educational aspirations are also important. Adolescents who smoke have friends who smoke, those who do not smoke seem to associate with nonsmokers, and those who plan to go to college have lower smoking rates than those who do not (Green 1979).

Until recently, more boys than girls smoked, but now more girls than boys smoke. This may be due to how advertisers depict the changing sex roles in our society. For example, the slogan, "You've come a long way, baby" is used in tobacco advertising to emphasize to women the liberation—sexual and otherwise—with which smoking is associated.

Regardless of why smokers start, they tend to continue to smoke because they are accustomed to smoking in many situations and during many activities. The smoking habit becomes part of the daily routine. Watch the "chain reaction" that takes place when several smokers sit around a table and one person starts to smoke. Also, watch the way a smoker lights up: practically every movement is ritualistic. Learning these habits results in the constant desire for a cigarette—during relaxing times, during boring times, and during stressful times. It is particularly difficult for longtime smokers to quit, even though they understand the risks to their health.

If you are going to smoke during your lifetime, you most likely will be smoking by the time you are twenty years old. Many start experimenting around the age of twelve for various reasons. These children try to look older, they copy their parents, they are persuaded by their peers, the cigarettes feel good in their mouths (oral gratification reduces tension), or they have a quick addiction.

Involuntary Smoking

Involuntary smoking (sometimes called passive smoking) occurs when a nonsmoker breathes the air that has been partially saturated by **sidestream smoke.** Sidestream smoke is the smoke that comes directly from the lit cigarette. Numerous reports from 1986 to 1993 confirm the dangers and risk of involuntary smoking.

According to the Surgeon General, as many as five thousand nonsmokers die each year of diseases caused by inhaling smoke released into the air by tobacco products. The 1986 Surgeon General's report contained the following conclusions:

1. Involuntary smoking is a cause of disease, including cancer, in healthy nonsmokers.

2. Children of parents who smoke, compared with the children of nonsmoking parents, have an increased frequency of respiratory symptoms and slightly smaller rates of increase in lung function as the lung matures.

Studies also confirm that nonsmokers living with smokers have a higher risk of heart disease (Steenland 1992), and children living with smokers have a higher rate of asthma (Fackelmann 1992).

The reason the Surgeon General has reached these conclusions is that one cigarette has been shown to release seventy milligrams of cancer-producing **particulate**

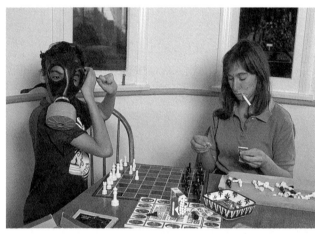

In addition to causing their own health problems, smokers also endanger the health of all those who are present when they smoke.

matter in the air and twenty-five milligrams of carbon monoxide. A smoke-filled room reaches eighty parts per million of smoke, which is considered hazardous to health by the Environmental Protection Agency (Dusek and Girdano 1986). McGinnis (1987) noted that sidestream smoke contains two and one-half times the amount of carbon monoxide as direct smoke and 70 percent more tar.

Because sidestream smoke is dangerous and many are allergic to cigarette smoke, nonsmokers' demands have resulted in nonsmoking sections in public restaurants and airlines and nonsmoking rooms in hotels. New legislation also designates nonsmoking in public buildings and worksites. The National Interagency Council on Smoking and Health has suggested a Nonsmokers' Bill of Rights (see the accompanying box).

Fighting Tobacco and Nicotine Addiction

A very difficult part of the drug war is fighting nicotine addiction. Many states rely on tobacco as a cash agricultural product, and many jobs are at stake in the growing, processing, manufacturing, and advertising aspects of the

ISSUE

Advertising Smoking

Cigarette companies have spent billions of dollars linking cigarettes with the values and trends of the times. Young-looking models in the ads represent what every teenager wants to become. The subliminal, magical message of the ads is: "If you smoke, you'll be popular, handsome/beautiful, and alive with pleasure." The companies even sponsor tennis tournaments, auto races, bowling championships, jazz festivals, and horse races. They spend even more money on advertising and promoting cigarettes than they were before radio and television cigarette advertising was banned in 1971.

- **Pro:** Any company should have the right to advertise its product provided it is not illegal to sell the product. It is not the government's right to interfere with this aspect of free enterprise. Individuals must decide for themselves whether to take any notice of the advertisements. We should not attempt to legislate good sense.

- **Con:** Each day more evidence is brought forward demonstrating that cigarette smoking is dangerous to our health. More and more people are attempting to give up smoking. There is no provable benefit observed from the habit of smoking. Tobacco companies should not be permitted to persuade people, particularly young people, to do something that is bad for their health just so the company can make a profit.

Should all types of cigarette advertising be banned?

tobacco industry. This legal drug creates more medical problems than any other drug in the drug war. The tobacco companies wield a great deal of power, but there are strategies for fighting the drug battle.

Tobacco advertising is a $2.6 billion a year industry that focuses on specific populations, particularly youth, women, and cultural groups and internationally in developing

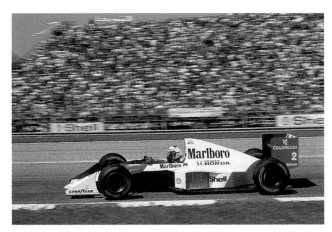

In spite of bans on radio and television advertising of tobacco products, tobacco companies continue to target specific groups in other advertising, promotions, and sponsorship throughout our culture.

countries. Since cigarette advertising on radio and television is banned, advertising is even more subtle. Philip Morris paid $350,000 to have Lark cigarettes prominently featured in *License to Kill,* a James Bond movie, and $42,500 for Lois Lane to smoke Marlboro cigarettes in *Superman II.* Cigarette advertisements still show up on television, with cigarette companies as sponsors of sports events (e.g., Virginia Slims tournaments) or with cigarette brands on billboards at sporting events or written on cars in racing events.

The cigarette companies have employed a variety of tactics to promote sales of cigarettes in light of restrictive advertising laws. One ploy is to own several other companies with more acceptable products as a cover. For example, Philip Morris produces Marlboro, Merit, Benson & Hedges, Players, Virginia Slims, and Parliament, but it also owns the Seven-Up Company, General Foods (Post cereals), Kool-Aid, Jello products, Oscar Meyer meats, Country Time, Good Seasons dressings, Minute Rice, Birds Eye, Tang, Log Cabin syrups, and others. The R.J. Reynolds Tobacco Company, which produces Camel, Winston, Salem, Sterling, Bright, Doral, Winchester, and nine other brands of cigarettes, also owns Kentucky Fried Chicken, Canada Dry, Hawaiian Punch, Nabisco Brands, Life Savers, Planters Nuts, Blue Bonnet margarine, and many others. Other tobacco companies, such as Brown & Williamson Tobacco, Liggett Group, Lorillard, American Tobacco Company, U.S. Tobacco Company, and Culbro, Inc., also own food, beverage, and insurance companies, department stores, restaurants, and other companies ("Tobacco Industry Conglomerates" 1986).

In 1991, Philip Morris spent some $60 million promoting a fifty-two-city nationwide tour of the historic document the Bill of Rights. The implication was that smoking is a constitutionally protected right. A positive association was made among heightened patriotism following the Persian Gulf War, rights of the people, and Philip Morris cigarettes. Local coalitions against smoking protested the tour.

Another ploy is to project an image of really caring about people. Although companies manufacture a product, they market freedom of choice, freedoms of nonsmokers, and their hope that children will not smoke. People continue to smoke, and they think the company is a good company at the same time they experience the chemicals and the addiction. And, children watch older people smoke as role models of being grown up.

Boycotting tobacco company products is one way to fight tobacco companies. Also effective are demanding local legislation through boards of health to restrict accessibility to tobacco products through limited licensing of vendors, eliminating vending machines, eliminating advertising by local stores, and keeping cigarettes behind the counters. Tobacco liability suits may ultimately be successful. The argument by tobacco companies continues to be that the warning labels on cigarettes meet the tenure of the law. Still, several lawsuits have been brought in recent years by individuals who have developed major complications from smoking, such as lung cancer. Litigation has a number of benefits for the overall effort to control the nicotine addiction epidemic. Liability suits typically claim that the plaintiff was addicted to tobacco before the age of consent and before the legal age of sale. Although the plaintiff accepts some responsibility for smoking, the claim is that the responsibility should be shared with the tobacco company because of nicotine addiction, the inherently dangerous characteristics of the product, and the company's behavior (Slade 1989).

Obviously, the best way to fight the tobacco industry is to reduce the demand for tobacco products by not using them. Smoking cessation and smokeless tobacco cessation programs are somewhat effective (15 percent to 40 percent rates for permanently quitting).

Nearly two-thirds of the American population report that they find it annoying to be near a person who is smoking. They believe that nonsmokers have the right to breathe air free of cigarette smoke. Federal agencies control the regulation of smoking on buses, trains, and airplanes, and some progress toward healthier air has been made in this respect. Smoking on intercontinental airline flights is now prohibited. The Interstate Commerce Commission permits smoking only in the rear 30 percent of seats on interstate buses. In trains, smoking is permitted only in designated cars. Enforcement of these regulations is not easy. If someone smokes in the nonsmoking section of the carrier, it is up to other passengers to ask the smoker to quit; if the smoker refuses to comply, the other passengers often must endure the smoke for the entire trip. The passengers may then lodge a formal complaint, but this action does not eliminate the probability that the person will smoke illegally in a similar situation.

Action on Smoking and Health (ASH), a nonprofit organization in Washington, D.C., was organized in the mid-sixties to focus on the legal aspects of smoking. ASH was instrumental in removing cigarette advertisements from television, getting nonsmoking sections in commercial airlines, and working with states on clean air legislation. Other projects include action on the dangers of smoking, the dangers of smoke to nonsmokers, and economic loss from smoking (health and life insurance issues).

The legal recommendations given from the health community to the president and Congress were as follows (Blakeman 1989):

1. Tobacco advertising and marketing must be severely restricted to eliminate its influence on our nation's children.

2. Excise taxes and user fees on tobacco products should be increased to raise revenues and discourage use by children.

3. The financial umbilical cord tying the federal government to the tobacco industry—Tobacco Price Support Program—should be severed to reduce tobacco's undue political influence on the federal decision-making process.

4. The federal government must eliminate the cynical inconsistency between its domestic health policy and the way in which it exercises its international trade leverage to open up tobacco marketing in other nations thereby enabling American tobacco manufacturers to increase overall tobacco use in those countries.

Kicking the Smoking Habit

The key to kicking the smoking habit is personal. Those who highly value health usually have the easiest time quitting. Many adults quit primarily to set a good example for their children, because children of smoking parents tend to smoke. Others quit because they are disturbed by the unpleasant aspects of smoking—the smell of stale smoke in their clothing, bad breath, and stains on fingers and teeth. Perhaps a list of positive aesthetic benefits of kicking the habit would help motivate this type of person to quit. Finally, some individuals like to excel in different situations, and perhaps awareness of this challenge to self-control is sufficient incentive for them to begin kicking the habit. Table 11.1 lists some activities that may help kick the smoking habit.

Nicotine Substitution Approaches to Smoking Cessation

One of the better approaches to smoking cessation is the use of federally approved prescriptions for **nicotine gum** (Nicorette). This approach involves dealing first with the behavioral aspects of smoking, which are the purchasing of cigarettes, social aspects of smoking, etc., but not dealing with the addiction to nicotine. Instead, nicotine is supplied in the nicotine gum (about two milligrams of nicotine per piece). Nicotine addicts chew about ten to twelve pieces per day, with a maximum of thirty pieces per day. After the behavioral aspects of smoking are overcome, then the smoker can suddenly or gradually reduce the consumption of nicotine gum. The advantage is that the smoker immediately stops the intake of carbon monoxide, tars, and other irritants. Smoking cessation rates vary dramatically, depending upon the individual and the program, but 17 percent to 65 percent smoking cessation rates have been reported. Many of those who quit smoking are still addicted to nicotine.

A similar approach uses the **nicotine skin or arm patch.** The smoker places a patch with nicotine on the arm over a twenty-four-hour period and about twenty to twenty-four milligrams (about one milligram/hour) of nicotine are absorbed by the skin. The patch is changed each day. Side effects include mild to sometimes severe skin irritations (Higgins 1990). The FDA regulates nicotine when it is sold as a drug, such as in Nicorette brand gum or skin patches.

Behavioral Approaches to Smoking Cessation

The twelve-step recovery approach, which has been successful with other kinds of chemical addiction, is also effective with nicotine addiction (Thanepohn 1990). The behavior component of smoking cessation is the most critical to quitting tobacco use. Group therapy programs are usually sponsored by local voluntary health agencies. Volunteers—including physicians and psychologists, as well as ex-smokers—are trained to assist. Those attempting to quit are supported with **positive reinforcement,** which accentuates the positive aspects of quitting and rewards positive moves toward quitting, and group interaction, in which individuals share their experiences in the quitting process.

Several profit-making corporations have entered the field of group therapy smoking-cessation programs in the last several years. One such corporation, SmokEnders, has chapters in more than thirty cities around the country. Participants attend nine weekly meetings, and reunions are organized after the final meeting for added reinforcement. SmokEnders also contacts participants periodically for a year after the completion of the program. The fee is high for this type of profit-making program.

Schick Laboratories operates more than twenty smoking-cessation centers around the country that conduct individual therapy sessions for one hour on five consecutive days. The centers use behavior modification techniques and **aversion therapy,** which is negative reinforcement for smoking. After participants complete the initial program, they are reinforced for eight weeks in weekly one-hour group sessions. This type of program is quite expensive, but the fee includes one year of free service for anyone who has difficulty controlling the urge to smoke or who has resumed smoking.

TABLE 11.1

Activities to Help Break the Smoking Habit

Type of Smoker	Reasons for Smoking	Activities to Substitute
Stimulation	You smoke to keep from slowing down. You smoke to stimulate yourself. You smoke to give yourself a "lift."	Take a short walk instead of smoking. Try moderate exercise. Take a mildly stimulating drink, such as tea or coffee.
Handling	Handling a cigarette adds to the enjoyment of smoking. Lighting a cigarette adds to the enjoyment. Watching the exhaled smoke adds to the enjoyment.	Play with a pencil, coin, paper clip, or any small object. Keep the hands busy by knitting, cooking, or engaging in another hobby.
Relaxation	Smoking is pleasant and relaxing. The best time for a cigarette is when you are comfortable and relaxed.	Rewards help; use nonfattening foods such as diet drinks, fruits, carrots, or celery. Start a new hobby or social activity. Change your behavior pattern or activity after meals.
Crutch	You smoke when you feel angry about something. You smoke when you are upset. You smoke when you want to take your mind off something.	Consciously do something else when you feel tense. Try deep breathing. Make up a phrase to say to yourself when you want to smoke. Practice it so it is almost automatic. Try sugarless gum or mints as a substitute. Splash cold water on your face. Practice conscious relaxation.
Habit	You smoke cigarettes automatically without even being aware of it. You sometimes light a cigarette with one already burning. You sometimes find a cigarette in your mouth without realizing you put it there.	Leave cigarettes in a different place; don't carry them. Wrap the package in paper and rubber band; make it difficult to get a cigarette. Designate nonsmoking areas of your home and workplace. Don't carry matches.

Source: *Stop Smoking and How to Go About It.* Scottish Health Education Unit, Edinburgh, Scotland, 1979.

Accurate success rates for these programs are unavailable because there have been few scientific follow-up surveys. Those who run commercial smoking-cessation programs are often unaware of their failures, because individuals who don't stop smoking feel guilty and don't come back. Moreover, the high costs of many commercial programs are beyond the reach of many smokers.

Several companies suggest that their cigarette filters, which reduce the tar and nicotine in cigarettes, serve as a route to kicking the habit. Unfortunately, smokers who use these filters seem unable to get past the last filter to become smoke-free.

Other methods of smoking cessation include **hypnosis** and **acupuncture.** Hypnosis has been used in various ways, but most often the individual is taught self-hypnosis as a way to stop smoking. Because the use of acupuncture to help smokers quit is a relatively recent development in this country, there are few studies on its use. Auricular (earlobe) acupuncture, however, has been used for cessation purposes, with participants who did quit reporting that cigarettes became distasteful. While the success reported for each of these methods alone is not particularly high, acupuncture in combination with psychotherapy or another therapy has shown noteworthy success rates.

Seventh-Day Adventist's "Five-Day Plan"

The five-day plan of the Seventh-Day Adventist Church is a successful withdrawal clinic that meets for two hours a day for five days straight. The clients are expected to quit smoking upon entering the program. At the end of five days, they will be over the physical withdrawal symptoms and receive instruction to deal with the psychological aspects of withdrawal. The program substitutes exercise and nutrition for cigarettes. At the same time, the client is purged of other stimulants, such as coffee, tea, colas, and also the depressant alcohol. Clients are shown visuals of lungs with cancer and emphysema to reinforce the need to stop smoking. They are urged to seek help from their

Smoking Cessation Using Strength Intervention (Individualized Program)

The only outcome used in strength intervention is to quit cold turkey (i.e., for the client to select a day to quit smoking and not smoke after that day). If some of the methods such as brand switching or gradual reduction of the number of cigarettes smoked are desired, then those activities occur before the selected quitting day. For strength intervention to be effective, three screening factors must be considered. The first is the issue of readiness. If you do not feel that you really want to quit, then some readiness issues must first be resolved. The readiness scale at the beginning of the chapter should be considered. If you scored in the ready range, then you should proceed. If not, then you should engage in a readiness program. For example, a readiness program might include the following:

1. Read this chapter carefully, particularly those concepts that deal with diseases that result from smoking. You may also want to read additional material available from the American Cancer Society and American Lung or Heart associations.

2. It is likely that someone you know or socialize with is a nonsmoker. Talk with him or her about smoking, and seek his or her encouragement and support.

3. Do some imagery. The following scenarios can be used anytime, but they are particularly effective when you are smoking.

Scenario 1: When you are smoking, close your eyes and imagine that you are able to see with Superman's X-ray vision. As you smoke, imagine that you see yourself in the mirror and, with X-ray vision, can see the smoke you are inhaling go into your lungs. Picture the black tar making your lungs blacker and blacker. With each puff the healthy pink dims with the onslaught of the gray and black smoke. Picture your heart, straining as it beats faster than it wants to under the influence of the smoke. Continue to watch the lungs deteriorate with each puff.

Scenario 2: Close your eyes and concentrate on how good you feel. Do not smoke at this time. Either sit or lie down and relax, taking several deep breaths, enjoying this relaxed state. Now imagine that you begin to smoke and feel a nauseating churning in your stomach. Concentrate on how you feel with a bad stomach flu and you are in pain. When you stop smoking, the ache goes away. When you imagine smoking, the nausea returns.

Scenario 3: Picture yourself as a nonsmoker. You no longer have a desire to smoke; you do not need to buy any more cigarettes. You are in control. Go through a typical day in your life, with people inviting you to smoke and you saying, "No thank you," and you feeling the power of controlling the cigarette, rather than it controlling you. Sense how good you feel, how fresh you smell, and how your teeth are brighter.

A second consideration prior to the initiation of a smoking-cessation program is the problem of barriers. If there are obstacles that make smoking cessation impossible or very difficult in your environment, then some action must be taken to deal with those elements. For example, if school or job pressures are excessive, high stress results (see chapter 2), or if significant others smoke or are not supportive of your quitting, then some work must be done to remove those barriers. Do stress management, encourage family members or good friends to quit with you, or use other strategies necessary to quit smoking successfully.

The third prerequisite to quitting smoking is the nurturing of strength areas and soliciting support. Be sure that the activities you do or people you are with provide the strength, comfort, support, or happiness that they are capable of providing. You will want to use those areas of strength to overcome the smoking challenge.

If you are ready, have removed potential barriers, and have an adequate resource of personal strengths, then you can begin this program. The first step is to complete a life-style contract.

---

spiritual source of strength during withdrawal. For further information, contact any Seventh-Day Adventist Church or medical facility.

American Cancer Society's Stop Smoking Program

The American Cancer Society's Stop Smoking Program consists of eight 2-hour sessions, two days a week for a four-week period. Specific guidelines for the program are contained in the *Stop Smoking Program Guide* published by the American Cancer Society, California division. Generally, the eight sessions consist of general emphases: sessions one through four are for insight development; sessions five through eight are for resource development and to try going the first forty-eight hours without cigarettes; and sessions nine and ten follow the program and are used as support in the form of the I.Q. (I quit) club.

The strength intervention approach for life-style contracting used in this text can also be used for smoking cessation. Consider the recommendations in the accompanying box.

Tobacco

The best health action to take is to avoid smoke in any form. If you smoke, then you need to quit smoking. If you do not smoke, then you need to avoid sidestream smoke. The following health actions of mind, body, and soul and their interdependence will help to facilitate this avoidance of tobacco smoke.

Mind

Use the skills of self-counseling or creative personal problem solving to resolve any problems you may have with tobacco. If you are a nonsmoker but are exposed to sidestream smoke, come up with some creative ways to solve the problem. For smokers, figure out the best way for you to quit smoking or chewing tobacco and then implement your plan. For nonsmokers, figure a way to avoid sidestream smoke.

Body

For smokers, it may be time to consider one of the smoking-cessation programs described in this chapter to quit smoking. Your body needs time to recover from the damage that smoking may already have inflicted. The sooner you quit, the sooner the recovery process can begin.

For nonsmokers, think of those times that your body and clothes have smelled after being around tobacco smoke. Perhaps you can recall a mildly irritated throat or runny nose following exposure to smoke. Resolve to protect your body from smoke to avoid the immediate negatives as well as the long-range dangers of being in the presence of tobacco smoke.

Soul

Get in touch with your emotions and spiritual feelings as they pertain to tobacco exposure. How do you really feel about exposure to tobacco? Once established, emotionally ready yourself to take action to avoid tobacco exposure to be in line with your true feelings. Use the psychological pairing technique described in chapter 2 to reinforce and anchor these feelings.

Interdependence

In light of the reconfirmation that passive smoke can cause heart disease, cancer, and respiratory problems, interdependence on the part of the smoker and the nonsmoker is clear. Nonsmokers should practice assertiveness and communication skills as described in the stress management and mental-health chapters to ensure that they are not exposed to sidestream smoke unnecessarily. Be assertive to avoid passive smoking in buses, meeting rooms, restaurants, and other locations. Smokers, even with their freedom to smoke if they so desire, should no longer ask nonsmokers if it is okay to smoke in their homes or cars or in other places. Instead, interdependent courtesy and caring for the welfare of others dictates that you smoke only where others are not affected.

Summary

1. Smoking would not likely be an accepted new drug if it was not already firmly established in the economic structure and personal lives of Americans.

2. Smoking tobacco is the chief avoidable cause of death in this country.

3. A cigarette contains three thousand chemical substances, such as tars, nicotine, carbon monoxide, hydrogen cyanide, and nitrogen oxide.

4. Smoking increases the risks of heart disease, cancer, respiratory disease, digestive diseases, and complications in pregnancy.

5. Pipe smoking and cigar smoking also result in significant health risks.

6. Smokeless tobacco increases the incidence of cancers of the mouth, throat, and stomach, and it is extremely difficult to quit using smokeless tobacco after being addicted.

7. People begin to smoke for numerous reasons, generally before reaching the age of twenty.

8. Those who do not smoke should avoid sidestream smoke because of the high amounts of gases and carcinogens in the smoke.

9. Health-care providers, voluntary agencies, and personal approaches to quitting are available to those who want to kick the smoking habit.

Commitment Activities

1. The federal government no longer allows tobacco advertising or antismoking messages on television. Determine whether this regulation has created any problems for young people in our country. You might want to have the class debate the pros and cons of cigarette advertising and antismoking messages on television.

2. Each cigarette package and cigarette advertisement must contain a warning about the health hazards of smoking. Using the examples given in his chapter and other information about smoking, rewrite the warning label to be a more effective deterrent to smoking.

3. Plan to have a smoke-free day at the university where all agree to quit for a day. Call the American Cancer Society and be a part of their "Great America Smoke-Out" or use their guidelines for your university smoke-free day.

References

American Cancer Society. *Cancer Facts,* 1989.

Blakeman, E. M., ed. *Introduction: Final Report and Recommendations From the Health Community to the 101st Congress of the Bush Administration from the Tobacco Use in America Conference.* Houston, Texas. Washington, D.C.: American Medical Association, 1989.

Brubaker, R. G., and Loftin, T. L. "Smokeless Tobacco Use by Middle School Males: A Preliminary Test of the Reasoned Action Theory." *Journal of School Health* 57, no. 2 (1987):64–71.

Chen, M. S.; Schroeder, K. L.; Glover, E. D.; Bonaguro, J.; and Capwell, E. M. "Tobacco Use Prevention In the National School Curricula: Implications of a Stratified Random Sample." *Health Values* 15, no. 2 (1991):3–9.

Connolly, G. N. "The International Marketing of Tobacco." In *Introduction: Final Report and Recommendations From the Health Community to the 101st Congress of the Bush Administration from the Tobacco Use in America Conference,* ed. E. M. Blakeman. Houston, Texas. Washington, D.C.: American Medical Association, 1989.

Dusek, D. E., and Girdano, D. A. *Drugs: A Factual Account,* 4th ed. New York: Random House, 1986.

Fackelmann, K. A. "Passive Smoking Risk Proves a Family Affair" *Science News* 141, no. 4 (January 25, 1992):54.

Glasgow, R. E.; Hollis, J. F.; Pettigrew, L.; Foster, L.; Givi, M. J.; and Morrisette, G. "Implementing a Year-Long Worksite-Based Incentive Program for Smoking Cessation." *American Journal of Health Promotion* 5, no. 3 (1991):192–99.

Green, D. E. *Teenage Smoking: Immediate and Long Term Patterns.* Washington, D.C.: Government Printing Office, 1979.

Higgins, L. C. "Arm Patch May Help Kick the Butt." *Medical World News* 31, no. 11 (1990): 29.

Kellie, S. E. "Tobacco Use: Women, Children, and Minorities." In *Introduction: Final Report and Recommendations From the Health Community to the 101st Congress of the Bush Administration from the Tobacco Use in America Conference,* ed. E. M. Blakeman. Houston, Texas. Washington, D.C.: American Medical Association, 1989.

Koop, C. E. "The Quest for a Smoke-Free Young America by the Year 2000." *Journal of School Health* 56, no. 1 (1986):8–9.

McDermott, R. J., and Marty, P. J. "Dipping and Chewing Behavior among University Students: Prevalence and Patterns of Use." *Journal of School Health* 56, no. 5 (1986): 175–77.

McGinnis, J. M. Distinguished Scholar Lecture, University of Utah, Salt Lake City, May 7, 1987.

Marty, P. J., et al. "Prevalence and Psychosocial Correlates of Dipping and Chewing Behavior in a Group of Rural High School Students." *Health Education* 17, no. 2 (1986).

Schlaadt, R. G., and Shannon, T. T. *Drugs of Choice: Current Perspectives of Drug Use.* Englewood Cliffs, N.J.: Prentice Hall, 1986.

Slade, J. "Nicotine Addiction." In *Introduction: Final Report and Recommendations From the Health Community to the 101st Congress of the Bush Administration from the Tobacco Use in America Conference,* ed. E. M. Blakeman. Houston, Texas. Washington, D.C.: American Medical Association, 1989.

Smoking and Health: A Report of the Surgeon General. Washington, D.C., 1979.

Steenland, K. "Passive Smoking and the Risk of Heart Disease." *Journal of the American Medical Association* 267, no. 1 (January 1, 1992):94.

Thanepohn, S. G. "How to Kick the Butts." *U.S. Journal of Drug and Alcohol Dependence* 14, no. 1 (1990):1, 10.

"Tobacco Industry Conglomerates: Status Report on Diversification in the Tobacco Industry." *Smoking and Health Reporter* 3, no. 4 (1986):7.

Additional Readings

Blakeman, E. M., ed. *Introduction: Final Report and Recommendations From the Health Community to the 101st Congress of the Bush Administration from the Tobacco Use in America Conference,* Houston, Texas. Washington, D.C.: American Medical Association, 1989.

This report, available from the American Medical Association, Public Affairs Group, 1101 Vermont Avenue, N.W., Washington, D.C. 20005, is the best comprehensive and up-to-date report on the effect of nicotine addiction on society. The booklet includes discussions by the top people in the country on (1) tobacco use: women, children, and minorities, (2) nicotine addiction, and (3) federal regulation of tobacco products, cigarette excise tax, protecting nonsmokers, tobacco marketing and promotion, U.S. agricultural policy on tobacco, the international marketing of tobacco, and grassroots lobbying.

Danaher, B. G., and Lichtenstein, E. *Become an Ex-smoker.* Englewood Cliffs, N.J.: Prentice Hall, 1978. Provides information needed to quit smoking.

Iverson, D. C. "Smoking Control Programs: Premises and Promises." *American Journal of Health Promotion* 1, no. 3 (1987). This is an excellent overview of smoking patterns, health implications of smoking, stages of smoking, and smoking cessation. Methods of controlling smoking in worksites, schools, and communities through physician, policy, and economic intervention are discussed.

Psychoneuroimmunology (PNI) is the study of the interaction of the mind, the central nervous system, and the body's immunological system. It has been shown that people with a fighting spirit, optimism, hope, and faith can actually build their immune systems. The brain has the capability to self-medicate and to release a variety of mental and physical painkillers and motivating substances (neuropeptides) when the demand is there.

We have learned that alcohol, tobacco, and drugs artificially influence our mood states. Alcohol initially has a stimulating effect but this is followed by the hangover, or depressing effect. Tobacco is a stimulant followed by a depressing withdrawal effect. Tobacco also wears down the immune system. Other drugs and substances also artificially send your body into painkilling, stimulating, depressing, and hallucinogenic effects without the body having voluntary control. The result is that the use of drugs (most often marijuana) can inhibit optimal functioning of the immune system and leave the person at higher risk of disease (Friedman, Klein, and Specter 1991). When the body is not forced to help itself, it may tend to lose its effectiveness when called upon to do so.

The obvious resolve is to fortify the immune system by not using chemical substances, including tobacco, alcohol, or recreational drugs, and perhaps, over-the-counter drugs. This challenge is easier said than done, but suggestions are included in the chapters. As it pertains to PNI, the challenge is to fortify yourself with alternatives to drugs. The essentials to relieving yourself from stress and fortifying yourself are the same throughout the PNI sections.

1. People use drugs to escape, forget, get high, or just out of habit. PNI suggests that these mood states should be created naturally rather than by chemical substances. One way to create a mood state is through anchoring. Obtain or create any mood you want by anchoring. That is, when you naturally reach a happy, high, or emotional state, mentally anchor it to music, an action, a photograph, a piece of clothing. During the experience, repeat the anchoring over and over. The next time that you want to acquire the same mental state, play the music, wear the clothing, or bring out the photograph, and acquire that same mental state.

2. One key to a resilient, happy, and drug-free life (consequently a fortified mind and body) is through four basic actions or understandings that you can do. Most of the information you need to implement these concepts is contained within the chapters in this text.

   a. Experience varied, repeated, and successful new experiences. You do not need the thrill or habit of chemical substances if you are looking forward to new experiences. Nor do you need artificially induced highs when you can get a high by doing something that you do repeatedly, which generally means that you will do it well. The thrill of accomplishment, the self-esteem that results, and the focus can well substitute for alcohol, tobacco, and other drugs.

   b. Create a cause and purpose in life. Substances tend to get in the way when you have a true cause. Recognize that the cause keeps you going and fortifies your immune system and makes you feel better.

      The difference between a cause and a goal is clear. A cause is when you are trying to benefit someone or something else besides yourself or, at least, in addition to yourself. A cause is made up of many goals, generally one after the other. A goal is usually personal and brings self-gratification. Examples of causes include civil rights, caring for a family, contributing to the welfare of a family, providing service for the homeless, making the life of people in hospitals or rest homes happier, preserving the environment, and making a club or organization the best.

3. Understand yourself. There are generally reasons for using chemical substances, and these generally deal with something that you have not resolved, something that may be subconsciously bothering you, or a need that is not being met. Self-understanding can occur by taking personality tests and, if you are using substances, seeking professional help to resolve those needs or unresolved issues. Unresolved issues or needs result in the negative emotions that trigger weaker minds and bodies.

4. There are many mental health skills that have been endorsed in this text. Learning assertiveness, self-esteem, or creative personal problem solving; promoting a cause and purpose; communication; and numerous other skills help you to be fortified in body and mind.

Reference

Friedman, H.; Klein, T.; and Specter, S. "Immunosuppression by Marijuana and Components" in *Psychoneuroimmunology,* 2d ed. Ed. R. Ader, D. L. Felton, and N. Cohen. San Diego: Academic Press, 1991.

After reading and pondering the last three chapters on chemical substances and choices, you should have a good understanding of:

1. the nature and devastating effect of alcohol, tobacco, and other types of substance use in human beings;
2. how dependence on these substances may disrupt your life-style;
3. how substance use and abuse affects loved ones by potentially making them codependent and enablers;
4. the genetic variance between people, which leaves them either programmed to addiction with use or resistant to addiction of any substance;
5. substance abuse as merely "acting out" a function of negative feelings such as hurt, fear, and rejection.

You have been provided an opportunity to assess your health status as it relates to chemical substance nonuse, use, or abuse. Based on these assessments, the information you have read reflecting life-style implications, the importance of chemical substance behavior, and in light of codependency issues, the following list includes some suggested behaviors that you could employ to enhance your health as it pertains to chemical substance use and to complete a life-style contract.

1. Stop using tobacco, reduce drinking, or stop using illicit drugs—if you need to, seek professional help.
2. Drive with extreme caution, using defensive skills, when people might be abusing substances (especially after athletic events, New Year's Eve, graduations, etc.).
3. When hosting socials where substances are used, assure that all guests have a means of returning home safely.
4. When hosting socials, do not provide chemical substances or allow them, and provide low-salt foods and soft drinks.
5. Help someone else shake an addiction, and do not enable their behavior—this may mean confrontation and conflict.
6. Improve your refusal skills and increase your own self-confidence, self-esteem, social problem solving, and purpose in life focus.
7. If your social group participates in substance use, then you may want to gradually change social groups (e.g., start attending church or spiritual meetings, change Greek organizations, join a different service or interest club, etc.).
8. Spend more time around those who give you uplifts and exemplify how you want to be.
9. Do some personal imagery to rehearse mentally saying no in a socially acceptable way or acquiring coping skills.
10. When seeking employment, choose a job that provides a drug-free and smoke-free workplace.
11. Be careful not to begin to rely on over-the-counter or prescription medications unless encouraged to do so by a physician.
12. Read more about chemical substances, and keep current and aware of the changing drug scene.
13. Enhance your spiritual health.

Life-Style Contracting Using Strength Intervention

I. Choosing the desired health behavior or skill

A. Keeping in mind the purposes in life and goals you identified in the mental-health chapter, consider one or two health behaviors related to substance abuse (from the list here or your own creation) that will help you reach your goals. To assess the likelihood of success, ask yourself questions similar to those used in previous sections, such as:

1. Is my purpose, cause, or goal better realized by adoption of this behavior?
____ yes ____ no
2. Am I hardy enough to accomplish this goal? (This means I feel I can do it if I work hard, am committed to do it, am challenged by it, and see myself in control enough to make it happen.) ____ yes ____ no
3. Is this a behavior I really want to change and that I feel I can change? ____ yes ____ no
4. Do I first need to nurture a personal strength area? ____ yes ____ no (If yes, be sure to include this as a part of the plan.)
5. Do I need to free myself from the negative effects of a behavior (break a bad habit)? ____ yes ____ no (If yes, be sure to include this as a part of the plan.)
6. Have I considered the results of the assessments in the three previous chapters? ____ yes ____ no

(Yes answers to the first three questions are a must to be successful. It might be wise to consider a different behavior if you cannot honestly answer yes to these questions. Your answers to questions 4–6 ought to provide insights for your consideration in making your plan.)

B. Behaviors I will change (no more than two)

_____

_____

II. Life-style plan

   A. A description of the general plan of what I am going to do and how I will accomplish it. Consider apperceptive experiences—successes you have had in the past—since they may help you consider the best ways to carry out this plan.

     _____

     _____

     _____

     _____

     _____

     _____

     _____

     _____

   B. Barriers to the accomplishment of the plan (lack of help, overcoming the addiction, etc.).

     1. Identify the barriers _____

       _____

     2. Means to remove the barriers (use problem-solving skills or creative approaches such as those described in the mental-health chapter). _____

       _____

       _____

       _____

   C. Implementation of the plan.

     1. Substitution (putting positive behaviors in place of negative ones)_____

       _____

       _____

     2. Confluence (combining a mental and a physical activity for time efficiency if possible)

       _____

       _____

     3. Systematic enhancement (using a strength to help a weakness) _____

     4. When_____

     5. Where _____

     6. Preparation_____

       _____

     7. With whom _____

       _____

       _____

III. Support groups

   A. Who _____

     _____

     _____

   B. Role_____

     _____

     _____

   C. Organized support _____

     _____

IV. Trigger responses _____

   _____

   _____

V. Starting date _____

VI. Date/sequence the contract will be reevaluated _____

   _____

VII. Evidence(s) of reaching the goal _____

   _____

   _____

   _____

VIII. Reward(s) when contract is completed _____

   _____

   _____

IX. Signature of student _____

X. Signature of facilitator _____

XI. Additional conditions/comments _____

   _____

   _____

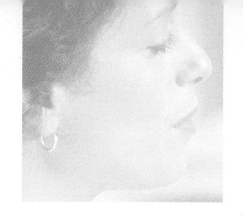

PART **V**

Choices and Disease

OUR HEALTH CHOICES IN-VOLVE UNDERSTANDING DIS-EASE IN A WAY THAT HELPS US DETECT SYMPTOMS OF DISEASE EARLY, MODIFY RISK FACTORS, TAKE PREVENTIVE ACTION, AND ADOPT HEALTHY LIFE-STYLES. HEALTHY LIFE-STYLE IMPLICATIONS HELP FORTIFY US AND KEEP US AS FAR AWAY FROM DISEASES AS POSSIBLE. CHAPTER 12 WILL DISCUSS COMMUNICABLE DISEASE, WHICH INCLUDES CHILDHOOD DISEASES, SEXUALLY TRANSMITTED DISEASES, AND AIDS. CHAPTER 13 WILL DEAL WITH CHRON-IC DISEASE, WHICH INCLUDES CARDIO-VASCULAR DISEASE, CANCER, AND OTHER DISEASES.

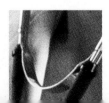

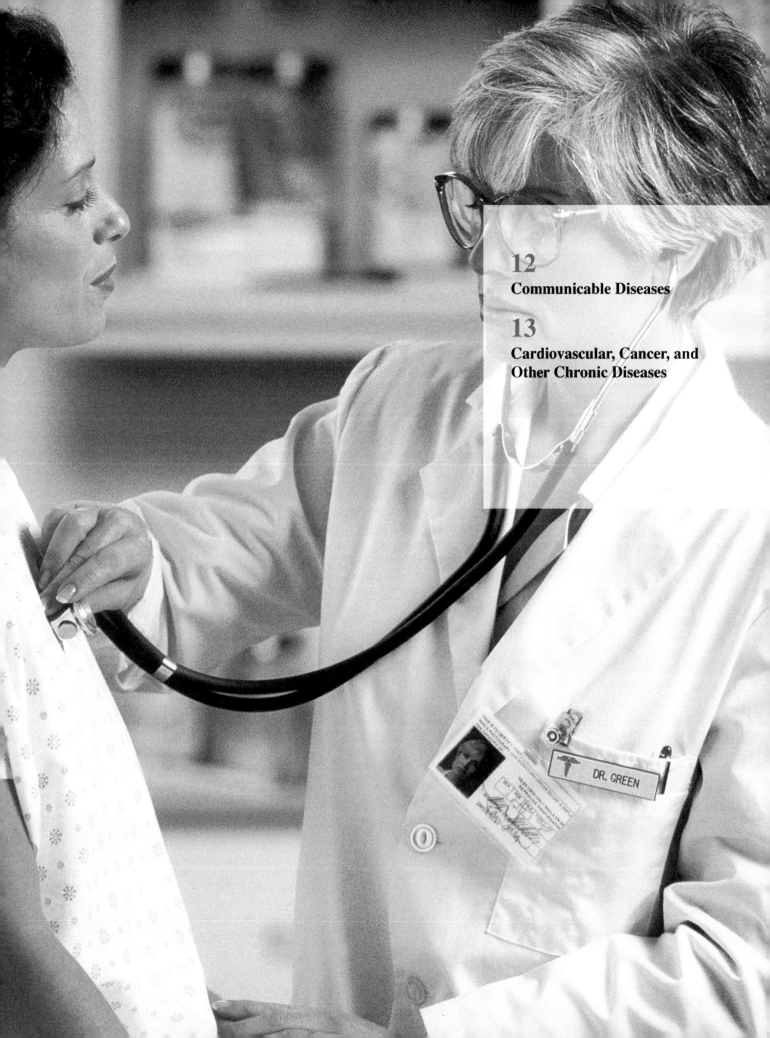

CHAPTER 12

Communicable Diseases

Key Questions

- What are some general principles for avoiding communicable diseases?

- What are some of the most common communicable diseases?

- What are the agents that cause infections?

- Which diseases can be prevented through immunizations?

- How can you be safe from AIDS?

- What life-style changes can you make to reduce the chances of getting a communicable disease?

Chapter Outline

In America, there has emerged a renewed concern over communicable diseases. With the eradication of smallpox from the earth, many Americans believed that communicable diseases were no longer serious threats to life. A minority of people died each year from complications of influenza and pneumonia, but for most people, even a sexually transmitted disease (STD) could be cured by an injection of penicillin. This state of denial and apathy is shown by some people who do not even immunize their children against preventable diseases such as polio.

Today, there is a fear of contracting a new incurable disease, acquired immunodeficiency syndrome (AIDS). There is also a fear of getting other incurable STDs. This chapter presents the principles of communicable diseases, the most common of these diseases, and, most important, what can be done to avoid or control these diseases.

Principles of Communicable Diseases

Throughout the life cycle, we are subject to **communicable diseases,** which are contagious diseases that can be passed from one person to

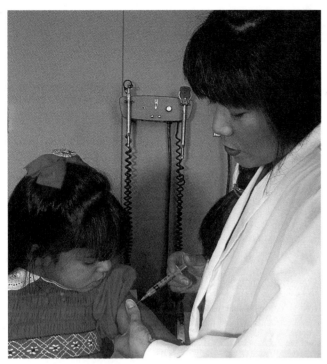

Why do childhood diseases such as rubella and polio still exist when immunizations could prevent them?

another. Some of these diseases, including chicken pox, mumps, diphtheria, polio, German measles (rubella), measles (rubeola), and pertussis (whooping cough), usually occur during childhood. Most of these diseases are now fully preventable. **Vaccines** have been developed to prevent them from occurring. Unfortunately, there are other communicable diseases for which no adequate preventive vaccine exists. These include tuberculosis, typhoid fever, leprosy, syphilis, gonorrhea, encephalitis, typhus, ringworm, AIDS, and the common cold.

We should all be aware of which communicable diseases we may have had during our lives. Some of these diseases can only be contracted once, while others can be contracted many times; therefore, by providing a brief communicable disease history, we can help our physicians understand our susceptibility to particular diseases.

Even early in this century, communicable diseases were by far the major cause of death in the United States. With progressive improvements in sanitation and nutrition, the introduction of numerous vaccines, and the discovery of penicillin and other antibiotics, a marked decrease occurred in the frequency of fatal communicable diseases among the U.S. population.

Today, the leading reported communicable diseases (diseases that physicians must report to public health officials) in our country, such as AIDS, chlamydia, gonorrhea, and herpes, are sexually transmitted. Even though the common cold is not a reportable disease, we know that the cold and other upper respiratory ailments are also common. These diseases account for the majority of lost hours in both industry and school. With the exception of the influenza vaccine, scientists have been unsuccessful

so far in developing a vaccine that prevents any of today's leading communicable diseases.

A fight occurs constantly in the body between invading microbes—microorganisms that are one-celled animals or plants that cause disease—and body defenses. Whether a communicable disease occurs depends on three factors: (1) the ability of the infecting microbes to invade the body and produce disease; (2) the number and virulence of microbes entering the body; and (3) the resistance put forth by the body's defenses, both natural and acquired (Boyd and Sheldon 1980).

The development of a communicable disease follows a regular pattern. First, the microbes enter the body through a natural body opening, such as a break in the skin or mucous membrane, or through the nose, lung, or intestine. The microbes attach themselves to cell surfaces and multiply to form a primary **lesion,** or abnormal change in the organ. At that time, the microbes begin to spread locally. Eventually, they spread through the body via the bloodstream and form lesions in other tissues, called secondary lesions. The body's ability to provide resistance to fight off the invasion is the immune response.

Agents of Infection

Communicable diseases are transmitted from human to human or from animal to human through several different agents of infection. These agents are bacteria, viruses, rickettsia, parasites, and fungi.

Bacteria

Bacteria are tiny cells similar to, but more primitive than, the cells that make up higher organisms. Like all living things, bacteria require food as a source of energy and a favorable environment in which to grow. Each species has its own nutritional needs and a set of preferences concerning body temperature, oxygen level, and acid-alkaline balance. When bacteria invade the body, one of three things may happen: (1) the bacteria may die; (2) they may survive without causing disease; or (3) they may survive and produce disease.

The diagnosis of an illness believed to be of bacterial origin is made by taking an appropriate specimen—for example, sputum, feces, urine, or a throat swab—and sending it to a laboratory. The specimen is allowed to grow in a controlled atmosphere until colonies of bacteria are formed. These colonies have different characteristics, depending on the microbe (type of bacteria) that is the causative agent. When the particular microbe is distinguished, treatment can start.

For an active bacterial infection, antibiotics are usually the physician's treatment of choice. Since antibiotics are widely used, many strains of bacteria have become resistant to certain antibiotics; the best known is probably a penicillin-resistant strain of gonorrhea.

If bacterial infection does occur, the body's immune defenses come into play. **Antibodies** are produced by

A. *Immunization Checklist:* For all of the immunizations listed, indicate which applies to you according to the following scale.

a. Yes, I have had the immunization and I know the year.

b. Yes, I have had the immunization, but I don't know when.

c. I don't know if I have had the immunization or not.

d. I have not had the immunization.

1.	Cholera	a	b	c	d
2.	Diphtheria	a	b	c	d
3.	Pertussis (whooping cough)	a	b	c	d
4.	Tetanus	a	b	c	d
5.	Influenza (flu)	a	b	c	d
6.	Measles (rubella)	a	b	c	d
7.	Mumps	a	b	c	d
8.	Plague	a	b	c	d
9.	Polio	a	b	c	d
10.	Rabies	a	b	c	d
11.	Typhoid	a	b	c	d
12.	Yellow Fever	a	b	c	d
13.	Typhus	a	b	c	d

Scoring/Interpretation

You should have checked a or b for the following to be safe:

DPT (Diphtheria, Pertussis, and Tetanus)

Mumps and Measles

Polio

You should have had most of these as a child, so if you know you have had them, then they generally have a lifelong effect. For measles, you will want to read the immunization schedule, table 12.1. If you selected c for any of the listed diseases, then contact parents or medical records to find out. If you selected d, then contact your physician or local health department and see about getting immunized.

You should have checked a for tetanus, influenza, and rabies for the following conditions:

Tetanus: If you have a wound, particularly if it was a puncture wound or caused by metal.

Rabies: If you have been bitten by an animal and cannot produce the animal for tests or verification.

Influenza: If you have respiratory problems, are fifty or older, or have another condition that is hazardous in connection with influenza. The immunization must be specific to each viral strain.

You should have marked an a for the following conditions only if you plan to travel or have traveled out of the United States:

Cholera

Typhus

Yellow Fever

Plague

Typhoid

You should be immunized within six months of travel for each of these diseases. Immunizations specific to the country you will visit may vary this need. Check your local health department for specifics if you plan to travel out of the country.

If you have marked c or d and plan to travel, then see the health department to be immunized.

B. *Behavioral Risk Factors:* Mark all that apply to you.

_____ 1. I use syringes (diabetes or drug use).

_____ 2. I have had intercourse with more than one partner.

_____ 3. I have never had intercourse with anyone.

_____ 4. I am a practicing male homosexual.

_____ 5. If I have sexual intercourse with someone, I use or ask my partner to use a condom.

_____ 6. I participate in oral sexual practices (mouth to genitalia).

_____ 7. I am married or have a permanent relationship with someone.

_____ 8. My sexual partner has never had sexual intercourse with anyone but me.

Scoring/Interpretation

If you checked any of these statements, interpret them as follows:

1. = 3
2. = 4
3. = –5
4. = 4

If you chose 2 and 4, add seven more points

5. = –1
6. = 4

If you also selected 6, add five more points

7. = –5
8. = –7

Total the values for all questions to help determine how your life-style puts you at risk for contacting serious communicable diseases. Interpret as follows:

12 or higher = high risk behavior

–3 to 11 = moderate risk

–4 or lower = low risk

C. *Symptoms Checklist:* For the following list of symptoms, indicate those that you have experienced recently.

_____ chills

_____ weakness

_____ fever

_____ headache

_____ muscular aches and pains

_____ sore throat

_____ dry cough

_____ nausea

_____ vomiting

_____ physical discomfort

_____ lack of appetite

_____ lack of energy

_____ lymph glands in the neck become swollen

_____ lymph glands in the neck become sore and tender

_____ diarrhea

_____ tenderness in the liver area

_____ jaundice (yellowing of the skin or eye tissue)

_____ skin rash over much of the surface of the body

_____ swelling of the floor of the mouth

_____ coughing

_____ runny nose

_____ shortness of breath

_____ purple blotches on skin

_____ sudden unattempted weight loss

_____ pain at the angle of the jaw

_____ skin eruptions

_____ yellowish or whitish discharge from the penis or vagina

_____ mild to intense burning when urinating

_____ cold sore or fever blisters on genitals

_____ painless sores or chancres on genitalia or oral cavity

_____ unpleasant smelling discharge from penis or vagina

_____ itching or inflammation of the genitals

_____ white curdlike discharge from the vagina

_____ warts on the genitals

Scoring/Interpretation

The fear of providing a symptoms checklist of this nature is that we often overreact and suddenly begin, by suggestion, to feel the symptoms described. But, at the same time, it is important to have any symptoms checked to assure that any serious conditions that you may have are treated, especially if you lead a risky life-style (e.g., multiple sexual partners).

You will recognize that symptoms can be indicative of a number of problems, some serious and others that pass with no harmful effects. To be safe, if you are manifesting any of the symptoms, and, particularly, if they do not pass in a couple of days, then you should see a physician, who can give you a certain diagnosis. The following are typical symptoms, some of which may or may not apply to you. The only sure diagnosis is thorough medical tests, but the

purpose of this assessment is to increase your awareness and encourage you to see a physician if any of these symptoms appear or persist.

The following are symptoms that are common with the following types of diseases.

Influenza

chills	sore throat
weakness	dry cough
fever	nausea
headaches	vomiting
muscular aches and pains	

Infectious Mononucleosis

moderate fever	lymph glands in neck
physical discomfort	become enlarged
lack of appetite and energy	and tender
white blood count	sore throat
elevates	

Hepatitis

feel miserable	tenderness in the liver
vomiting	area
diarrhea	jaundiced (yellowish
fever	skin or eyes)

Chicken pox

skin eruptions

Rubella

rash	swelling of the lymph
fever	glands

Mumps

swelling of the floor of	pain near the angle
the mouth	of the jaw
fever	

Rubeola

rash that covers most	runny nose
of the body	fever
coughing	

AIDS

cough	symptoms of
fever	pneumonia
shortness of breath	purplish blotches and
	bumps on skin

Gonorrhea

yellowish or whitish	mild to intense burning
discharge from penis or	sensation when
vagina	urinating

Nongonococcal Urethritis

    same as gonorrhea

Herpes

    cold sores on genitals   fever
       or mouth   headaches
    fever blisters on genitals   lymph nodes enlarge

Syphilis

    painless sore or chancre   rash over much of body
      on penis or oral area   (second stage)
      (first stage)   ulcer on any part of
                        the body (third stage)

Trichomoniasis

    discharge from genitals   itching and inflammation
      with unpleasant odor   of genitals

Monilia

    white curdlike discharge   intense itching
      occurs from the vagina

Genital Warts

    warts on genitals

---

specialized cells to combat the threatening microbes. These antibodies are then released into the bloodstream, where they provide immunity, or resistance, to a particular infection. We can also obtain immunity artificially. Vaccines containing weakened or killed microbes are used to induce the formation of antibodies without causing illness.

Viruses

Another type of disease-producing agent is the **virus.** Viruses are extremely small infective agents, so tiny that a special type of microscope is needed to make them visible at all. They are believed to be the simplest form of life, and they depend on living animal or vegetable cells to exist and multiply. Viruses are present in our bodies at all times, but various inner defense and immunity mechanisms usually keep them in check.

Some of the most common viral diseases include the cold, polio, hepatitis, influenza, measles, German measles, chicken pox, mumps, shingles, mononucleosis, and encephalitis. Even ordinary warts and cold sores are caused by viruses. Many types of upper respiratory infections and stomach upsets are also viral in nature. Scientists have identified about three hundred viruses that cause infections, half of which cause respiratory tract infections (Robbins and Kumar 1987). Most viral diseases, in contrast to those caused by bacteria, confer a permanent immunity on those who recover from them.

After contracting many of the communicable diseases, we are immune to having the disease again. This is called **active immunity** and occurs with diseases such as measles and chicken pox. There are important exceptions, however, such as the common cold, where repeated attacks may occur.

Medical research has produced a number of vaccines to prevent viral diseases, and we should be immunized against these diseases, including the following:

Cholera

Diphtheria (part of the DPT immunization)

Influenza

Measles

Mumps

Pertussis (whooping cough)

Plague (when traveling to selected countries)

Polio

Rabies

Rubella

Smallpox (no longer needed)

Tetanus

Typhoid (when exposed to a known carrier)

Typhus (when traveling to some areas of the world)

Yellow Fever (when traveling to specific areas of the world)

As with any infection, viral diseases are spread from one person to another in various ways, most often by breathing germs from another's coughing or sneezing or by using contaminated objects. Common-sense precautions, including avoiding unnecessary exposure to an infected person, are very important in reducing your chances of catching a viral disease.

Antibiotics, extremely successful in treating bacterial infections, are useless for treating most viral diseases. Generally, after catching a virus, a physician can only treat the symptoms until the body's natural defenses can overcome the invading virus.

Other Agents of Infection

Rickettsiae are tiny bacterialike organisms that seem to be on the borderline between bacteria and viruses. Like viruses, they demand the presence of living cells and cannot be grown in the laboratory. These organisms grow in the intestinal tract of insects called **vectors**—usually bloodsucking insects, such as lice, rat-fleas, mites, and ticks—which transmit the organisms from one host to another. Rickettsial diseases include typhus and Rocky Mountain spotted fever (Robbins and Kumar 1987).

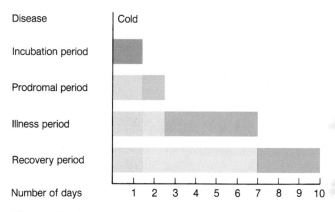

Disease	Cold									
Incubation period										
Prodromal period										
Illness period										
Recovery period										
Number of days	1	2	3	4	5	6	7	8	9	10

Figure 12.1

A typical course of the common cold.

An **animal parasite** can live in the body of another animal and may or may not produce disease in this host organism. In either case, it can spread to another host (a person), where it remains until it dies. Animal parasites belong to one of two groups, protozoa and worms. Protozoa are one-celled animals that cause diseases such as amoebic dysentery, malaria, African sleeping sickness, and trichomoniasis. They are most prevalent in human beings in tropical areas and areas with poor sanitation (Boyd and Sheldon 1980). Worms live in the intestine and can become very long (up to sixty feet) or be very small. Although there are many types of worms, two common types are tapeworms and hookworms. The tapeworm comes from infected beef or pork and is passed on to humans when the meat is poorly cooked. Hookworms, on the other hand, burrow directly into humans through bare feet walking on soil.

Fungi are parasitic organisms of simple structure that live in soil, rotting vegetation, and bird excreta. Examples of fungal diseases include candidiasis, ringworm and athlete's foot (which are contagious), histoplasmosis, and coccidioidomycosis.

Immune Response

Our bodies fight the invasion of microbes in a variety of ways. One line of defense is the activation of white blood cells, also called phagocytes, which recognize, attack, and destroy microbes or antigens (other foreign substances) upon entering the body.

Humoral immunity means that the body produces antibodies to fight a particular type of antigen. Antibodies are types of proteins that function to deactivate, rather than destroy, the antigen. They are manufactured to fit against the antigen to form an antigen-antibody complex, which becomes harmless. Once the body has triggered the production of an antibody, it remains in the bloodstream to ward off future invasions of the same antigen. Childhood diseases such as rubella produce antibodies, so we rarely get rubella more than once. **Immunization** is the process of triggering the formation of antibodies by injecting small doses of the disease in mild forms to ward off a serious attack. The immune response may also be fortified with antibiotics such as penicillin to help fight bacteria (but not viruses).

Interferon is a protein that has been shown to be effective against a variety of viral diseases. When a virus attacks a cell, interferon is produced, and although it does not protect the invaded cell, it does seem to inhibit the reproduction of the virus. The viral infection is thereby localized, and surrounding cells are protected. Interferon has great promise in treating previously incurable viral diseases.

Other mechanisms to defend against disease include the skin, tears (which wash away bacteria), cilia in the respiratory tract (small hairs that move foreign particles out of the respiratory tract), and mucous membranes lining the air passages (which catch foreign particles before they enter sensitive areas).

If a microbe enters a **susceptible host**—one who is unable to resist infection—the disease occurs. The course that the disease normally follows can be divided into four stages: (1) an incubation stage; (2) a prodromal stage; (3) an illness stage; and (4) a recovery stage. Figure 12.1 illustrates a typical course of the common cold.

The **incubation stage** is the interval between the time of entry of the microbe into the body and when symptoms first appear. During this stage, the microbes multiply until disease symptoms are produced. This stage may be as short as a few hours, as with the common cold, or as long as several months or years, as with tuberculosis, but it usually lasts from a few days to a few weeks. Diseases are highly contagious at the end of the incubation stage, just before symptoms appear.

The **prodromal stage** is the time during which non-specific symptoms appear. This stage is characterized by fever, headache, and other aches and pains, such as watery eyes and the scratchy throat that precede other cold symptoms. Many diseases are extremely contagious during this stage, which may last from a few hours to several days.

The **illness stage** occurs next. The symptoms characterizing the specific disease begin to occur, such as the sneezing and runny nose that accompany the common cold or the skin rash characteristic of chicken pox.

The **recovery stage** begins when the body's defenses start to overcome the microbes and symptoms begin to disappear. (With a cold, sneezing often subsides and other symptoms are not as pronounced.) Microbes are still present, so recovery cannot be rushed. If you resume full activity too soon, a relapse can occur.

Specific Communicable Diseases

Specific communicable diseases most common in the adult population include the common cold, influenza, infectious mononucleosis, hepatitis, AIDS, gonorrhea, chlamydia, and other sexually transmitted diseases.

The Cold

The most common of all communicable diseases is the **cold.** The cold itself is not a serious disease, but complications (such as pneumonia in rare cases) can result from improper care of a cold.

At least fifty different viruses cause symptoms of the common cold, which appear one to three days after the virus enters the body. The first clue is usually a scratchy throat. Within a few hours, a stuffy nose develops and sneezing begins. High fever is not a normal symptom of a cold. When a high fever accompanies a cold, either a secondary infection or another disease is present.

Within forty-eight hours, the cold is usually full-blown. Teary eyes, a runny nose, a husky voice, obstructed breathing, and dulled senses of taste and smell occur. A moderate headache may be present. Once a cold has fully developed, it usually continues at its peak from seven to fourteen days. Too often, complications can occur that may lead to other, more serious, chronic diseases.

No effective immunization has been developed to prevent the common cold, but you can take some common-sense precautions, including getting enough rest, washing your hands frequently, eating well-balanced meals, and avoiding unnecessary contact with people who have colds. The best treatment for the cold is quite simple (Hansen 1987): (1) rest in bed during the early stages as dictated by the severity of the symptoms; (2) drink lots of fluids or breathe humidified air (which stimulates the fluid production in the respiratory passages, easing the pain of sore throat and reducing coughing); and (3) use an appropriate cold remedy. It is important to remember that any drug can cause an allergic reaction, so follow a physician's advice if you have any questions about over-the-counter drugs.

Although there is no cure for the common cold, millions of dollars are spent on cold remedies to treat the symptoms rather than cure the cold. The following is a breakdown of functions of various cold remedies (Hansen 1987):

1. **Nasal decongestants** help to open nasal passages by constricting the dilated nasal blood vessels.
2. **Analgesics** such as aspirin and acetaminophen are appropriate painkillers to relieve musculoskeletal pains.
3. **Expectorants** help to stimulate the formation of secretions from the respiratory passages and result in an increased flow and decreased viscosity of the sputum.
4. **Antitussives** are used to suppress dry coughing.
5. Local **anesthetics** such as throat lozenges are effective local painkillers that help relieve sore throats.

It is important to remember that many cold remedies have one to ten active compounds and thus take the "shotgun" approach to treating symptoms. The FDA has cited the dangers of multiple ingredients in cold pills. It is better to recognize a particular symptom and purchase a

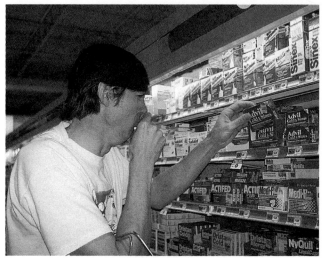

Cold remedies don't remedy; they only mask the symptoms.

medication to treat it specifically rather than "shotgun." It is unfortunate that we waste a lot of money for many over-the-counter drugs that really do not work.

It is important to follow these guidelines for the treatment of common colds. Secondary infections, such as pneumonia, can result if the body does not have the chance to build resistance to the virus. Excessive stress and lack of sleep can reduce the body's ability to ward off the virus.

Influenza

Influenza, or "flu," is another infectious disease caused by a virus. One person passes it directly to another by spreading the droplets from coughing and sneezing. It can also be indirectly spread by using common drinking glasses, towels, and other items.

Influenza often affects many individuals in a community at the same time, producing an **epidemic.** Such epidemics generally last about a month and may occur in different sections of the country at the same time. Deaths from influenza occur mainly among the elderly or those with a chronic disease.

Symptoms of all types of flu are similar, but the severity of the illness varies. An attack begins suddenly. There may be a general feeling of weakness, chills, fever, headache, muscular aches and pains, sore throat, dry cough, nausea, and vomiting. All these symptoms need not be present. As a rule, the acute stage of the illness lasts only a few days, but weakness may persist for some time, especially among older or chronically ill people. With the onset of suspected influenza symptoms, you should go to bed as soon as possible, keep warm, and eat sensibly. If symptoms persist longer than a few days, or if fever remains more than slightly elevated, consult a physician.

No known medicine cures influenza. Antibiotics have no effect, although they are used to combat certain complications that may follow. If the complications are bacterial problems, then the use of antibiotics may be prescribed by a physician. Getting well without developing any dangerous complications depends on giving the immune system every known advantage while it fights off the infection. To treat influenza, do the following:

1. Go to bed when symptoms begin.
2. Keep warm and out of drafts.
3. Eat simple and agreeable foods.
4. Drink plenty of water or other fluids.
5. Call the doctor if fever occurs.
6. Take any prescribed medication.
7. Get enough rest.

Vaccines that combine protection against the common strains of viruses, including the Asian strain, are available for high-risk groups. A single dose of vaccine is about 60 percent effective if given during the late autumn months, before the beginning of the usual influenza season. An influenza vaccine is recommended for anyone over six months of age who is at increased risk (for age or medical condition) for complications of influenza. Health-care workers and others in close contact with high-risk persons, in addition to anyone who wishes to reduce the chance of becoming infected with influenza, can be immunized (Centers for Disease Control, May 1990). A serious disease that sometimes follows influenza or other viral infections is Reye's syndrome. During recovery of the disease, there is a sudden turn for the worse, with vomiting, delirium, convulsions, and even coma. Death can occur in twenty-four to forty-eight hours. Most milder forms are reversible. In severe cases, the infection results in a fatty change in the liver and encephalopathy (brain disease). This occurs in younger people from age six months to seventeen years (Robbins and Kumar 1987).

Infectious Mononucleosis

Infectious **mononucleosis** is a viral disease of the lymphatic system—the connecting link between the blood and the cells—and is extremely common among high school and college-age students. It is called the "kissing disease" because the virus seems to be transmitted in saliva, although not necessarily through kissing.

Symptoms of the illness begin about one or two weeks after exposure. At the onset, there is usually a moderate fever, a general feeling of discomfort, and a lack of appetite and energy. Lymph glands in the neck become enlarged and sometimes tender, and a sore throat is common and often quite severe. The spleen becomes enlarged about one-third of the time. Because outward symptoms are often misleading, diagnosis is made by a very specific blood test. When the disease is present, the total white blood cell count is elevated and the percentage of mononuclear cells, or **lymphocytes,** is higher than normal.

Few people exposed to active cases of "mono" become infected themselves. Nevertheless, you should avoid exposure to known cases. There is no medication to cure mononucleosis. Bed rest is indicated when symptoms are severe. With rest, complete recovery with no aftereffects takes place after a period of one to several weeks (Robbins and Kumar 1987).

Hepatitis

Hepatitis is another disease that has been a public health problem through the ages. Its name literally means "liver inflammation," one of the symptoms of the disease. There are several types of hepatitis. The most common are hepatitis A (formerly called infectious hepatitis) caused by hepatitis A virus (HAV), and hepatitis B (formerly called serum hepatitis) caused by the hepatitis B virus (HBV). A third category is known as non-A and non-B hepatitis caused by a hepatitis C virus (HCV), which includes hepatitis that is transmitted parentally and through fecal contamination. About 28,500 cases of hepatitis A, 23,200 cases of hepatitis B, 2,500 cases of non-A and non-B hepatitis, and another 2,400 unspecified cases are reported annually, which is probably only a fraction of the actual cases (Centers for Disease Control, February 1990).

Type A, infectious hepatitis, is transmitted by direct contact with an infected person or with contaminated food or water. This type usually occurs in areas where many people live, such as a university residence hall or a military barracks. Type A may also occur when drinking water is polluted by backed-up sewers during a flood.

Type B, serum hepatitis, was previously thought to be transmitted primarily by blood transfusions or by hypodermic needles shared by illicit drug users. New evidence indicates that the virus can also be passed along by sharing a razor, manicure scissors, or anything else sharp enough to make a cut. Some people have been infected by having their ears pierced with nonsterile instruments. Type B can probably also be spread by close social contacts, including kissing, using someone else's toothbrush, or having sexual intercourse with an infected person or carrier.

Within the past several years, incidence patterns for both types of hepatitis have changed. In the past, rural areas seemed to have more cases, but today there are more cases in the cities. Although children once were the most affected group, today young adults are. This group typically contracts the type B virus.

Characteristically, those who have hepatitis feel miserable. Symptoms include vomiting, diarrhea, fever, tenderness in the liver area, and **jaundice,** a yellowing of the skin or eye tissue. If hepatitis is suspected and the illness lasts for more than two or three days, a physician should be consulted. Generally, a blood sample is sent to a laboratory to test for hepatitis. If the test is positive, the individual is usually put to bed, either at home or in a hospital, depending on the severity of the symptoms. Bed rest and inactivity may be prescribed for weeks or even months. During the acute stage, the person should be isolated, and throwaway dishes and utensils should be used to avoid contaminating others. The spread of hepatitis can be slowed by improving personal hygiene and sanitation, practicing safe sex, and if intravenous drug users avoid sharing needles.

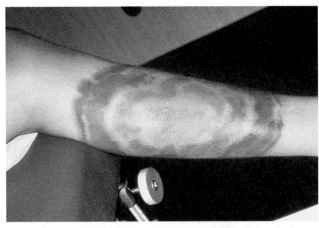

Ring-shaped sores such as these characterize the rash that appears days to weeks after a Lyme tick bite.

Lyme Disease

Lyme disease is a disorder that was first described in 1976 as an epidemic of inflammatory arthritis clustered in the northeastern United States near the town of Lyme, Connecticut. The disease has now been reported in several locales within and outside the United States, and it appears to be spreading. Experience with the disease has shown that the condition affects more than just the joints. It was renamed Lyme disease in 1979.

Lyme disease is caused by a newly identified spirochete called *Borrelia burgdorferi,* which is transmitted by a specific tick (*Ixodes dammini*). The course of the disease follows three stages if left untreated. Lyme disease is difficult to diagnose because early symptoms are much like those of other diseases and blood tests used to detect Lyme disease produce unclear results (Stroh 1992). First skin conditions surface, beginning days to weeks after a tick bite. A rash shows large, ring-shaped sores that may enlarge to several inches before fading. Then, in 10 percent to 15 percent of the cases, heart and neurological problems exist. Heart problems include pericarditis (inflammation of the membrane that surrounds the heart) and atrioventricular blocks (disruption of the transmission of nerve impulses within the heart). Neurological problems include meningitis (inflammation of the membrane that covers the brain and spinal cord), encephalitis (inflammation of the brain), and cranial neuritis (inflammation of the nerves of the skull). The third stage is an arthritic condition, generally in the knees, and is manifest in about 50 percent of the cases.

Prevention of Lyme disease includes using a repellant, avoiding uncut grasses and weeds, and inspecting the skin for bites and ticks (Hamburger 1992). Lyme disease is treatable with antibiotics, including penicillin, which are effective if used early. They prevent the secondary and tertiary symptoms of the disease. In light of the recent spread of Lyme disease, any time you are bitten by a tick, particularly when followed by a rash, you should see a physician for possible treatment with antibiotics to prevent secondary and tertiary problems.

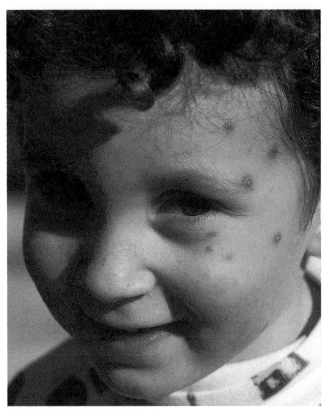

This child with chicken pox was contagious the day before this rash appeared.

Childhood Diseases

Three common childhood diseases are chicken pox, mumps, and rubella (German measles). Generally, one attack of each of these diseases confers lifelong immunity to the person, although there are exceptions. Immunizing more people, particularly children, for each of the diseases can dramatically affect the number of cases in a community (Schlenker et al. 1992). A chicken pox vaccine is being researched, and it is hoped that it will be available soon.

Chicken pox is caused by a virus called *varicella zoster.* After exposure to someone with chicken pox, it usually takes thirteen to seventeen days for symptoms to appear. Someone with chicken pox is contagious the day before the skin eruptions are present. The disease runs its course with the manifestation of a rash, skin eruptions, and fever. Itching may be severe and can be treated with antihistamines or by taking warm baths with baking soda.

Rubella, or **German measles,** is caused by the rubella virus, but its symptoms are generally mild and may go undetected until a rash appears. Additional symptoms of the disease include fever and swelling of the lymph glands. Sometimes called the three-day measles, the course of the disease may actually last only one or two days and up to four days. After exposure to someone with rubella, the manifestations of the disease occur after two to three weeks. Rubella becomes a devastating disease when pregnant women are infected because of the high risk of deformity in the unborn fetus. The incidence of measles is on the rise in most parts of the country (Centers for Disease Control 1991). If you live in an area where measles outbreaks are common or, most important, if you are three to four months away from the chance of getting pregnant, a second vaccine is recommended if there are no problems with taking the vaccine.

The symptoms and signs of **mumps** are infection of the salivary glands, swelling of the parotid gland (in the floor of the mouth), fever, and pain near the angle of the jaw. The disease is spread, as with other childhood diseases, by droplets from the respiratory passages from sneezing and coughing. Although uncomfortable, in children mumps are usually harmless and pass within a few days. The incubation period is ten to thirty-five days. The mumps virus can be localized in the testes or ovaries, causing sterility in young people, particularly in young men. It may also localize in the brain, causing brain damage (although this is very rare).

Rubeola, also called **red measles,** is very contagious and can be manifested ten to twelve days after exposure. This form of measles is more severe and may include fever, coughing, and runny nose followed by a rash that often covers the body in a couple of days. The duration of the disease is longer than rubella, in that it may take a week to ten days for recovery to begin. Rubeola is a serious disease that can lead to infections in the brain.

Table 12.1 provides information on immunization for most of the diseases we have discussed.

Sexually Transmitted Diseases

Sexually transmitted diseases (STDs) are usually spread by sexual contact. Eighty-six percent of the over twelve million cases occur in fifteen- to twenty-nine-year-olds. These diseases are spreading more rapidly than all other communicable diseases combined. According to the Centers for Disease Control and U.S. Public Health Service, the problem of STDs has reached epidemic proportions, despite the fact that modern medicine has effective ways of diagnosing and treating the majority of these diseases.

Sexually transmitted diseases are highly contagious. A single sexual contact with an infected person can transmit the disease. Sexually active people face an increased risk of infection because sexual partners can unknowingly have one or more of the STDs and infect others.

These diseases affect individuals of all races, ages, and socioeconomic levels. This section covers AIDS, gonorrhea, nonspecific urethritis, herpes genitalis, syphilis, chlamydia, and other sexually transmitted diseases.

HIV Infection and AIDS (Acquired Immunodeficiency Syndrome)

Just a few short years after eradicating smallpox, a new communicable disease emerged that is causing fear around the world. Although **AIDS (acquired immuno-**

deficiency syndrome) has existed for some time, it was first identified in the United States in 1981, when five patients in Los Angeles were diagnosed with the disease. Some researchers believe that **HIV (human immunodeficiency virus),** the virus that causes AIDS, was born when experimental research on polio vaccines was done in the Belgian Congo in 1957 and some of the vaccines were contaminated then harbored in green monkey tissues (Brownlee 1992). It should be noted that about 62.5 percent of the HIV infection cases are in Africa (Weeks 1992).

Historically, the disorders HIV (human immunodeficiency virus), AIDS (acquired immunodeficiency syndrome), and ARC (AIDS related complex) were thought to be distinct diseases. It is now believed that HIV disease (HIV positive) is a condition that ranges from no symptoms to the serious conditions of AIDS. The use of the term *ARC* is no longer current. The terms *HIV infection* and *HIV disease* refer to this continuum of disease, with AIDS suggesting the end stages of the disease (Benson and Stuart 1992).

AIDS has spread very rapidly in spite of major efforts by the government, health professionals, and other organizations to warn people. The Centers for Disease Control have shown a dramatic increase in death due to AIDS. Health researchers are desperately trying to find a treatment for AIDS or a vaccine to prevent it. To compound the problem, several cases of AIDS appeared during the summer of 1992 in individuals who had tested negative for HIV. The idea of people becoming infected by HIV and this not being detectable is a frightening thought for this deadly disease.

The number of AIDS cases has spiraled since the first cases were identified. According to the Centers for Disease Control AIDS Hotline, there were 242,146 AIDS cases in the United States at the end of 1992. Since records have been kept on AIDS (1981), some 160,372 deaths have been reported. It is also estimated that over one million people are infected with HIV, which means that one out of every one hundred males and one out of every eight hundred females carries the virus in the United States.

Just one decade after the disease was identified, the lifetime cost for treating HIV infection and AIDS for one person was about $80,000 (Lord 1989), with annual costs reaching $11 billion for all cases. Insurance companies are threatened by the social, political, and economic costs of AIDS and are concerned about increasing their premiums even more to deal with the high costs (Getz and Bentkover 1992).

AIDS Virus

AIDS is caused by the human immunodeficiency virus (HIV), which has been named by scientists as the AIDS virus, HTLV-III (human T-lymphotropic virus type III), or LAV (lymphadenopathy associated virus). The AIDS virus attacks white blood cells (T-lymphocytes) in the human blood. The attack on the white blood cells results in damage to the immune system and destroys the body's capability to ward off other microbes. When the AIDS virus

TABLE 12.1

An Immunization Checklist

Disease	Immunization Available?	When Given	Number of Doses	Booster
Chicken pox	No			
Cholera	Yes	When traveling to remote areas of some countries	2; 2–4 weeks apart	Every 6 months for maximal protection
Diphtheria (the D in DPT)	Yes[a]	2 months	3; 4–6 weeks apart	At 18 months; before entering school; repeat as needed
Influenza	Yes	To elderly, chronically ill, and others at high risk before flu season	1 per strain (type of influenza)	Yearly, as needed
Gonorrhea	No (experimental stage)			
Herpes genitalis	No (experimental stage)			
Measles (in combination with mumps, rubella)	Yes[a]	12 months	1	Possibly if high risk (see text)
Mumps (in combination with measles, rubella)	Yes[a]	12 months	1	Possibly if high risk (see text)
Pertussis (whooping cough) (the P in DPT)	Yes[a]	2 months	3; 4–6 weeks apart	At 18 months; before entering school
Plague	Yes	When traveling to certain countries, such as Vietnam	3; 4–12 weeks apart	Every 6–12 months, as needed
Polio	Yes[a]	2 months	2–3; 4–6 weeks apart	At 18 months; before entering school
Rabies	Yes	To exposed persons (animal bite)	14–21 daily injections	No
Rubella (in combination with measles, mumps)	Yes[a]	12 months	1 to 2 is now recommended	Possibly if high risk (see p. 431)
Smallpox	No longer needed			
Tetanus (the T in DPT)	Yes[a]	2 months	3; 4–6 weeks apart	At 18 months; before entering school; as needed for wound management
Typhoid	Yes	For persons exposed to known carrier	2; 4 weeks apart	Every three years
Typhus	Yes	For persons traveling to certain remote areas of world	2; four or more weeks apart	Every 6–12 months
Yellow fever	Yes	For persons traveling to specific areas of world	1; at certain designated centers	

[a]Required for entry to school

Source: Data from E. W. Hook et al., *Current Concepts of Infectious Diseases.* Copyright © 1977 John Wiley & Sons, Inc. New York, NY.

enters the bloodstream, antibodies are produced by the body, but they are ineffective in slowing the progression of the disease. Scientists do not know why these antibodies have no effect. The production of the antibodies makes detection easy. A simple blood test taken eight to twelve weeks after infection detects the antibodies that have been produced to fight the AIDS virus. Routine practice is to test to confirm the HIV infection. A positive test does not mean you have AIDS—only the virus.

Once individuals have been infected by the AIDS virus, they can either contract AIDS, HIV infection, or have no ill effects even though they may produce the antibodies. The

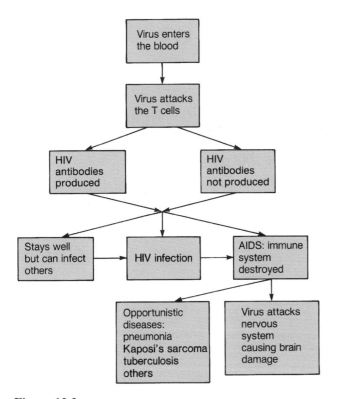

Figure 12.2
Outcomes of the AIDS virus in the blood.

incubation period for HIV infection is variable, ranging generally from two to five years, but shorter and longer time periods have been evidenced. After a person has AIDS, he or she usually lives two to five years. Some AIDS patients have lived up to nine and ten years, but the Surgeon General has stated that once a person is diagnosed as having AIDS, the fatality rate approaches 100 percent.

The range of symptoms for AIDS is varied, largely because of the breakdown of the immune system. This breakdown allows almost any opportunistic virus, bacteria, fungi, or other microbe to invade without the hindrance of an immune response from the body. Some symptoms and signs of AIDS may include a persistent cough, fever, shortness of breath, symptoms of pneumonia, or symptoms of Kaposi's sarcoma. Kaposi's sarcoma was a once obscure cancer that has gained attention as an important complication of AIDS. It generally creates skin lesions on the legs characterized by purplish blotches and bumps. The type of pneumonia that AIDS patients contract is called Pneumocystis Carinii pneumonia, named after the opportunistic protozoa whose invasion rarely affects healthy individuals but is seen in 50 percent of AIDS patients.

If individuals who test positively for HIV do not get AIDS, they may develop a less serious disease referred to as HIV infection. HIV infection is a condition in which symptoms are generally less severe than those of AIDS. Symptoms include loss of appetite, weight loss, fever, night sweats, skin rashes, diarrhea, tiredness, lack of resistance to infection, or swollen lymph nodes.

Some individuals exposed to the HIV virus form antibodies but show no ill effects even after many years; in

fact, they may never get AIDS or HIV infection (fig. 12.2). But since they have been infected by the virus, they can transmit the disease to others.

Methods of Transmission of AIDS and High-Risk Groups

The AIDS virus has been found in many body fluids, including blood, semen, and possibly vaginal secretions. Some reports suggest that the AIDS virus has also been found in tears and saliva, although no known transmission has occurred through this means. To date, the six documented methods of transmission of AIDS are as follows:

1. male homosexual or bisexual contact;
2. intravenous drug administration by contaminated needles;
3. administration of blood and blood products (although the risk of contaminated blood products has been greatly reduced since the implementation of required screening in 1985);
4. blood to blood or body fluid to body fluid contact with an HIV-infected person;
5. heterosexual contact;
6. passage of the virus from infected mothers to their newborns.

The following represents the number of AIDS deaths that have occurred from infections via these sources (Centers for Disease Control, January 1991):

1. Homosexual or bisexual males comprise by far the largest group, accounting for 59.1 percent of the reported cases.
2. Intravenous drug users with no previous history of homosexuality are about 28 percent of the total number of deaths.
3. Hemophiliacs receive large amounts of plasma concentrates (blood transfusions) and make up about 1 percent of the AIDS deaths.
4. Recipients of multiple blood transfusions comprise 3 percent of deaths.

5. Infants born to parents who are homosexual, bisexual, or intravenous drug users make up 1.2 percent of deaths.

6. Heterosexual contact accounts for 4.0 percent of deaths.

7. No identified risk results in 3.3 percent of deaths.

In May of 1991, a disturbing report was revealed through the media of the transmission of the AIDS virus through organ donation and transplant. Apparently the donating person, who had been murdered, was infected just prior to his death. Tests did not reveal the AIDS virus, so the organs were donated. Some of the organs were sterilized prior to transplant, but because of size or other reasons, several of the organs were not. Consequently, three of the patients who received the transplants died of AIDS, and eight more have tested positive for the AIDS virus.

There is concern among health workers who are exposed to the HIV-infected patient's blood, stool, and other body fluids. Although precautions against HIV infection are now mandatory and routine in hospital settings, still one study showed 3 out of 750 workers tested positive for the AIDS virus, and each of these individuals had accidentally stuck themselves with contaminated needles. More recently, some 4,500 health-care workers in the United States were reported to have AIDS (Mishu et al. 1990).

Another study observed surgical services at a reputable hospital for six months, and in 30 percent of the operations at least one blood contact (a splash to the eyelash or on the skin) was observed (Panlilio et al. 1991). The chances for continual spread among health-care workers is high, but the vast majority of infections occur as a result of life-style rather than hospital accidents.

The questions then arise: Do patients of health-care workers need to be concerned about exposure to the AIDS virus if their physicians, nurses, dentists, or other health-care practitioners are HIV positive? And should these health-care professionals be allowed to practice? One study of a surgeon revealed that while he had AIDS he operated on 1,896 patients. None of the surviving patients has AIDS, and of the 264 who died, none died of AIDS except for one. This patient was also an intravenous drug user, and it is likely that the AIDS virus was contracted by a contaminated needle. One news report in 1990 reported that the first person to contract the AIDS virus from a health-care provider contracted the disease from a dentist with AIDS. Perhaps while injecting a painkiller contact was made between a cut on the dentist's hand and a sore in the patient's mouth, but the actual mode of transmission has not been determined.

Another report tracks the increased cases of AIDS attributed to heterosexual activity (Holmes, Karon, and Kreiss 1990). From 1983 to 1988, the percentages of women who contracted AIDS from heterosexual activity went from .9 percent of reported cases to 4.0 percent. In men, during the same period, the rate rose from .1 percent to 1.4 percent. As the disease continues to infiltrate various segments of our society, the rate will likely continue to increase.

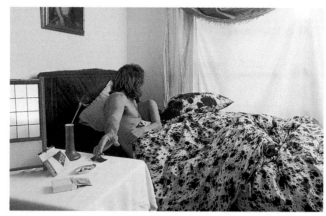

The practice of safer sex has become a fact of life for many couples.

Anyone who has sex with a prostitute or has multiple sexual partners (male or female) is at a higher risk of contracting AIDS. Anal intercourse, which is common among male homosexuals and some heterosexuals, is especially risky.

Prevention, Guidelines, and Myths

Couples who have had monogamous relationships for the last five years or longer have a low risk of getting AIDS. If both partners have never had sex with anyone else and do not fall into the categories listed previously, there is virtually no risk. It is important to know your partner well before engaging in sexual activities.

The Surgeon General's *Report on AIDS* describes some personal measures that are adequate to protect yourself from AIDS (U.S. Department of Health and Human Services 1987):

1. If people have been involved in any high-risk sexual activities (multiple sex partners, unprotected sexual contact or anal intercourse) or have injected intravenous drugs into their bodies, they should have a blood test to see if infection with the AIDS virus has occurred.

2. If a test is positive, or if people decide to engage in high-risk activities and choose not to have a test, they should tell their partners. If they jointly decide to have sex, they must protect their partners by always using a condom (rubber) during (start to finish) sexual intercourse (vaginal or rectal), and avoid oral contact with sex organs.

3. A condom (rubber) should always be used during (start to finish) sexual intercourse (vaginal or rectal). This is especially important if a person's partner has a positive blood test showing that the partner has been infected with the AIDS virus, or if the person suspects that the partner may have been exposed by previous heterosexual or homosexual behaviors, or if the person suspects that the partner might have used intravenous drugs with shared needles and syringes.

4. If a person is at high risk, avoid mouth contact with the penis, vagina, or rectum.

5. Avoid all sexual activities that could cause cuts or tears in the lining of the rectum, vagina, or penis.

6. Single teenagers have been warned that pregnancy and contracting sexually transmitted diseases can be the result of only one act of sexual intercourse. They have been taught to say no to sex. They have been taught to say no to drugs. By saying no to sex and drugs, they can avoid AIDS, which can kill them.

7. People should not have sex with prostitutes. Infected male and female prostitutes are frequently also intravenous drug abusers; therefore, they may infect clients through sexual intercourse and other intravenous drug abusers by sharing their intravenous drug equipment. Female prostitutes also can infect their unborn babies.

The implication from the report is this: the only unprotected sex that should occur is in monogamous relationships (only one permanent partner) and when both partners are sure that they are HIV negative.

Researchers all over the world are frantically trying to control AIDS. A few drugs are available, but only three, AZT, DDI, and DDC, have been approved for prescription use and have shown some promise in slowing down the progress of AIDS. Early use of AZT can delay the onset of AIDS but does not extend the life span of an HIV-infected individual (Cowley 1992). New information about this dreaded and deadly disease are evidenced each day. It is important for students to keep informed about the advances made in the fight against AIDS.

If you have questions regarding any aspects of HIV infection and AIDS, call the AIDS information line toll-free 24 hours a day, 7 days a week: 1–800–342–AIDS.

Gonorrhea

Gonorrhea has been a major health problem in this country for many years. It has surpassed syphilis in frequency in the last decade and is still common on college campuses. Caused by the bacterium *Niesseria gonorrhoeae,* it attacks the mucous membranes of the penis, eyes, vagina, rectum, or throat and can be spread by vaginal, oral, or rectal contact with individuals of either sex.

Penile gonorrhea occurs within three to seven days after contact. The disease causes a thick, whitish yellow discharge, or "drip," of pus from the penis, which is accompanied by a mild to intense burning sensation during urination. Sometimes a drip without burning, or burning without a drip, occurs, but either should be reported for medical treatment. Unfortunately, some men with penile gonorrhea have no apparent symptoms. If untreated, the disease can cause painful inflammation of the prostate gland, or scar tissue can build up inside the penis, leading to difficulty in urination or to sterility. Penile gonorrhea can also cause intense irritation and swelling of the testicles.

Women with vaginal gonorrhea usually have no symptoms, or the symptoms are so slight they go unnoticed.

Occasionally, a vaginal discharge and a burning sensation during urination may occur. Gonorrhea in women can become extremely serious, leading to **pelvic inflammatory disease (PID),** the leading cause of infertility in women. PID is an infection of the urethra (the channel for the passage of the urine from the bladder to the outside) that is evidenced by swelling and reddening. PID symptoms include difficulty or pain when urinating, bleeding between menstrual periods, and excessive vaginal discharges.

Men and women with rectal gonorrhea also may have no symptoms. When symptoms are present, however, they include a rectal mucus discharge, intense rectal irritation, a feeling of incomplete bowel movements, and burning pain during either intercourse or a bowel movement.

Symptoms of oral gonorrhea in both men and women usually go unnoticed. If symptoms are noted, they include a mild to severe sore throat, fever, and chills.

Gonorrhea is diagnosed with a smear test or a culture. For people with symptoms, gonorrhea is diagnosed with a smear test. A microscopic analysis is performed, using pus discharged from the penis or a scraping from the lining of the cervix. A culture is used to detect gonorrhea when no symptoms are present. In this test, scrapings are taken from the mucous membrane lining the suspected area and placed on a nutrient substance. The small, round bacterial colonies grow in twenty-four hours, and a positive diagnosis can be made in about forty-eight hours.

Penicillin is the drug of choice in the treatment of gonorrhea. For those who are allergic to penicillin or have a penicillin-resistant strain of the disease (rare in the United States), tetracycline or spectinomycin are used (Hook et al. 1977). Men and women with known recent exposure to gonorrhea should receive the same treatment as individuals who have actually contracted the disease, and all diagnostic tests should be repeated after treatment to be certain the person is cured. Because no immunity develops, the same individual can contract gonorrhea repeatedly; a one-time treatment does not prevent reinfection.

Gonorrhea is quickly and completely cured, without lasting damage to the body, if the disease is diagnosed and treated soon after infection. Inadequate treatment may cause symptoms to disappear, but further damage to vital organs may still occur, and the disease may be spread to others. Treatment with antibiotics left from an initial treatment is ineffective because the amount or strength of the antibiotic is improper; in fact, this type of treatment could contribute to the development of resistant strains of the bacteria.

Women with gonorrhea can infect their babies at childbirth. The attending physician or midwife at birth can put silver nitrate into the eyes of newborn infants and protect them from gonorrhea.

Chlamydia and Nongonnococcal Urethritis (NGU)

Chlamydia is a disease that symptomatically is similar to gonorrhea. It results in the infection of several pelvic areas, and if not treated, it can result in scarring of the fallopian tubes, sterility, and ectopic pregnancies. Other than the symptoms of burning when urinating, the infection does not seem to have any long-range effects in males, but a male can infect his partner.

Chlamydia trachomatis is a bacteria that acts much like a virus in that it functions inside other cells. The difference is that it has its own RNA and DNA, unlike viruses (Robbins and Kumar 1987). Its action and resulting symptoms are much like the *gonococcus* bacteria, except that the symptoms are somewhat milder.

Chlamydia is part of a group of STDs called **nongonococcal urethritis (NGU),** or **nonspecific urethritis (NSU),** because they cause the inflammation of the urethra but not by the *gonococcus* bacteria. Other than chlamydia, *ureplasma urealyticum* also causes NGU. *Chlamydia trachomatis,* in addition to causing NGU, is responsible for lymphogranuloma venereum (ulcer on the genitalia and enlargement of the lymph nodes of the groin); hyperendemic blinding trachoma (infection of the conjunctiva and cornea of the eye, which results in blindness); inclusion conjunctivitis (adult and newborn inflammation of the eye); cervicitis (inflammation of the cervix); salpingitis (inflammation of the uterine tube); proctitis (inflammation of the rectum); epididymitis (inflammation of the epididymis); and pneumonia in newborns.

NGU is the most prevalent STD in the United States today, accounting for some four million cases per year. The identification of NGU requires a smear and tissue culture. The treatment for NGU and chlamydia is tetracycline, erythromycin, or doxycycline (U.S. Department of Health and Human Services 1985).

Herpes Genitalis

Herpes, or **herpes genitalis,** is caused by the **herpes simplex virus type 2,** a virus closely related to the one that causes cold sores, fever blisters, and shingles (a nerve disorder). Exactly how that virus is transmitted is unknown, but it is thought to be spread by direct contact with an infected carrier. Blisters appear on the genitalia two to twelve days after infection. Persons infected for the first time may also experience fever, headache, and enlarged lymph nodes. These symptoms may last one to three weeks.

Recurrences of herpes are probable, since the virus is retained within the body in a dormant state and may break out again. An expectant mother may pass the virus on to her child from a new infection or an old case that becomes active. Routine practice to avoid potential exposure is to deliver the baby as a cesarean birth if the mother has an active case of herpes.

There is still no effective cure for genital herpes. Locally applied compresses and antibiotic creams (such as Acyclovir) are often prescribed to lessen pain from the blisters and ulcerations, which run their course and disappear, only to reappear at a later date. It is clear that herpes is highly contagious when blisters or lesions are present. It is suspected that herpes is contagious during the prodro-

mal period (early stage) before blisters or lesions appear. Those with an active case of herpes should refrain from sexual contact until the virus becomes inactive, that is, until all scabbing is gone from the blisters. To protect against mild or hidden cases of herpes, the male partner should use a condom.

Syphilis

Although unchecked **syphilis** can have serious consequences, the availability of penicillin and an organized control effort have almost eliminated this disease in the general population. There are still certain high-risk groups, however, including male homosexuals, migrant workers, and the poor.

Syphilis is caused by a bacteria called *Treponema pallidum,* classified as a spirochete because of its corkscrew appearance. The spirochete is an extremely delicate organism that cannot live for more than a few moments outside the human body; however, it can pass from person to person through direct physical contact.

The spirochete burrows into the soft mucous linings of the sex organs, rectum, and throat. Once the organisms pass through the mucous membranes, they are carried throughout the body in the bloodstream. The course of untreated syphilis follows a series of stages that produce characteristic symptoms.

The average incubation period for syphilis is twenty-one days but may be as short as ten days or as long as ninety. During this time, the disease is present in the body, but there are no symptoms and the disease cannot be detected. After the incubation period, the first outward symptom of syphilis, a red swelling, appears on the body at the point where the spirochetes first gained entrance. This sore, called a chancre, becomes eroded to form a small, painless ulcer with firm, hardened edges. Its surfaces produce a discharge seething with spirochetes. These spirochetes are also transported throughout the body by the lymph system and bloodstream. One to five weeks after its appearance, the chancre disappears, even without treatment.

If an infected person does not treat the initial stages of syphilis, the disease progresses into the still contagious secondary syphilis, the signs and symptoms of which appear six to twenty-four weeks after infection. The most prominent symptom is a skin rash that covers all or part of the body, especially the palms of the hands and soles of the feet. Other symptoms include the loss of large patches of hair, lesions or white blotches in the mouth, headache, chronic sore throat, joint pains, and swelling of the lymph glands. The signs may linger for only a few days or for as long as months at a time and then disappear. Relapses may occur, and new eruptions may appear over a period of a year.

If the infected person still remains untreated, the disease can progress to the latent stage, during which there are usually no outward signs or symptoms. This stage begins about two years after contact. During the latent

Communicable Disease

The number of communicable diseases we are exposed to (and whether we actually come down with the disease) is, to a great extent, determined by our actions of mind, body, and soul and their interdependence. Our inherited abilities to deal with communicable disease vary, but to maximize your individual potential, consider the following suggestions for avoiding communicable disease.

Mind

You have a great amount of control in preventing communicable disease in your life. With your powerful mind, analyze the situations in which you might be exposed to communicable disease. Think through some strategies you can use to protect yourself against exposure. Make a life-style plan to assure you implement the strategies.

Body

You are exposed to microbes daily and constantly, but whether or not the microbes are activated to cause disease depends a great deal on your physical state. If you are not getting enough sleep, if you are sedentary, and if you eat poorly, your chances of getting a communicable disease are high. To prevent disease, make sure that you exercise regularly, get adequate rest, and eat nutritiously.

Soul

Your resistance to communicable diseases is higher when you have positive emotions. From psychoneuroimmunology, we know that a fighting spirit, optimism, hope, and a good laugh periodically fortify the body against communicable disease. Reflect upon those skills described in chapter 2 and adopt them into your life-style.

Interdependence

We are exposed to most communicable diseases when we are around someone who is a carrier of the disease. Part of open, honest, and caring communication is to inform others when you are infected with a disease and then take precautions. Cover your mouth when sneezing or coughing and keep your distance from others if you are contagious. In the case of STDs, it is extremely important to practice the responsible strategies suggested in this chapter.

---

stage, the microbes multiply relentlessly and begin to destroy the body's tissue, bones, and organs. The person is no longer contagious at this stage.

From the latent stage, the disease progresses to the late stage. This process usually takes ten to twenty years. By this time, the destruction of tissue, bones, and organs is irrevocable. Any body tissue is vulnerable, but the nervous system is most often affected. Frequent results include blindness, paralysis, deafness, insanity, and heart disease.

During pregnancy, syphilis is dangerous not only to the mother but also to the unborn baby. After the eighteenth week of pregnancy, syphilis germs can cross the placenta from an infected mother to her fetus. The fetus may be stillborn or may appear uninfected, only to develop symptoms several days, weeks, or as long as two to ten years later. Early prenatal care, including a blood test for syphilis, is thus very important for pregnant women.

Penicillin remains the best and most effective treatment for syphilis; for those allergic to penicillin, tetracycline and erythromycin are the most effective substitutes.

Monilia or Candidiasis

A yeast infection called candida albicans is the most frequent cause of disease from all of the fungi. **Candidiasis,** also called **monilia,** is very common on college campuses, mostly among women. Candida albicans is present on the skin, mouth, vagina, large intestine, and rectum of many healthy people. At times, a woman's body is upset by stressful circumstances, by taking antibiotics or birth-control pills, or during the menstrual cycle. Under these conditions, organisms can flourish in large numbers, causing a yeast infection. A yeast infection is manifested by small sores on the labia. In infants, patchy sores in the mouth and diaper areas are symptoms. In men and women, infections may occur on the skin or mouth in addition to the genital areas. The infection often results in a white, curdlike discharge from the vagina, accompanied by intense vaginal and vulval itching. The infection can be spread through direct sexual contact or incidental contact from shared towels, toilet seats, and so on.

The test for monilia is done by taking a swab from the infected area, looking at it under a microscope, and making a laboratory culture. A vaginal cream or suppository is prescribed for approximately seven to ten days after diagnosis. The condition can become quite persistent and difficult to control unless prescribed treatment is followed. Over-the-counter medications are also available for monilia. Douching with clear water is recommended to relieve the itching. Both partners can help in the prevention of vaginal infections, but once an infection does occur, medical assistance should be secured (Robbins and Kumar 1987).

Trichomoniasis

Trichomoniasis is a common infection caused by the protozoa *Trichomonas.* It is usually transmitted through sexual contact; however, trichomonas can survive for several hours at room temperature on moist objects such as toilet seats, towels, and washcloths. Most infected males are carriers without symptoms who pass the organism on to women.

In women, the infection is characterized by a profuse, frothy white or yellow discharge with an unpleasant odor, which is accompanied by itching and inflammation. The disease is diagnosed by an examination of the discharge and treated with a drug called Flagyl. Both partners must receive treatment, or the organism is passed back and forth during sexual contact (Robbins and Kumar 1987).

Condylomas (Genital Warts)

Condylomas were once fairly rare, but the condition is being diagnosed more frequently on college campuses, with an estimated one million cases per year. Both men and women can develop condylomas (warts) in the anal or genital regions. Evidence suggests that these warts are caused by a virus (*human papillomavirus,* or HPV infection) similar to the one that causes warts on other areas of the body. The virus is transmitted by sexual activity and appears one to three months after infection. Genital warts are generally small skin- or pink-colored growths. Warts appear alone or form clusters. Sometimes the clusters are very large, covering several centimeters.

Prescribed treatment with Podophyllin, a brown liquid that is spread on the warts, can remove them. It is extremely difficult to rid the body totally of the warts because a part of one wart causes the continual spreading of warts. Early treatment is vital, because condylomas can spread and become more difficult to treat. Treated with Podophyllin, about 15 percent to 50 percent of the cases return. It appears that when treated with lasers and interferon, almost all cases are cured (Bauman 1992). Sexual intercourse should be avoided during the course of infection.

Pediculosis Pubis (Crabs)

Crabs, or pubic lice, are pinhead-sized insect parasites that live in the hairy parts of the body, usually around the genitals. Some people have no symptoms, while others experience intolerable itching from these parasites. Crabs can be passed by physical contact during sexual intercourse or by contact with infected bedding, clothing, or towels (DeLora, Warren, and Ellison 1977).

Treatment includes a medicated lotion prescribed by a physician. Instructions with the lotion must be followed completely to eliminate both the crabs and their eggs. Sex partners and roommates must be treated at the same time to avoid repeat infections. Bedding, towels, clothing, and other washables are also treated.

Prevention and Control of Sexually Transmitted Diseases

Prevention and control of STDs should be a primary concern in communities throughout the United States, but the intimate nature of sexual concerns presents many prob-

lems. Guilt feelings, for example, make it difficult for people to talk about STDs and to seek proper medical care.

Though condoms are rejected by some individuals as interfering with sexual activity, they can prevent the spread of some STDs. To be effective, a condom must be worn on the penis prior to and during any sexual activity. If used properly, the condom can provide complete protection against gonorrhea and NGU and good protection against syphilis, herpes, and genital warts. The most protective condoms are made of latex; viruses may be able to penetrate natural lambskin and other nonsynthetic condom materials. Female condoms may provide even greater protection because of the strength of the strong polyethylene material they are made of and their more complete coverage of the genitals. Urinating and washing the genitalia and adjacent areas with soap and water immediately following intercourse affords a little protection against STDs. Spermicides (foams) may also be useful in prevention of STDs (U.S. Department of Health and Human Services 1985).

Sexually transmitted diseases can be controlled if those exposed to them are aware of the possibility of infection and advised about proper medical care. In most communities there are STD epidemiologists, who are experts in determining the source and spread of these diseases. The epidemiologist works with each patient to alert all contacts about their exposure. In all states, minors may consent to their own confidential treatment, and in most instances, confidentiality is maintained. The essential elements for controlling STDs include public education, screening high-risk groups, treating all infected persons, and identifying and treating sexual contacts.

Ten steps to prevention are highlighted here. Some of these provide very little protection (as specified), and others provide more.

1. Be highly selective with sexual partners.
2. Wash with soap and water after coitus.
3. Have open communication with partners.
4. If a disease is contracted, avoid exposing a partner.
5. Use latex condoms.
6. Urinating and douching after coitus might help.
7. Abstain from intercourse.
8. Talk openly with your partner about the potential (sexual history) for STDs.
9. Avoid oral-genital contact.
10. Watch carefully for symptoms of any disease, and seek medical help if you have any suspicions.

Summary

1. The development of any communicable disease follows a four-stage pattern: the incubation, prodromal, illness, and recovery stages.

2. Communicable diseases may occur whenever microbes enter the body and disrupt any of the vital processes.

3. Diseases are caused by bacteria, viruses, rickettsiae, animal parasites, or fungi.

4. The common cold and influenza are two respiratory infections for which there is no cure, yet remedies are marketed.

5. Hepatitis and infectious mononucleosis, which can be passed along by sharing razors or scissors and kissing, are prevalent in the college-age population.

6. Sexually transmitted diseases are spreading rapidly, and some of the most common strains such as herpes genitalis and AIDS are incurable.

7. AIDS is an incurable disease that almost always results in death and involves both homosexual and heterosexual populations.

8. Chlamydia, nongonococcal urethritis, gonorrhea, monilia, and other STDs are irritating diseases that are extremely common among sexually active students on college campuses and require medical treatment.

9. Preventive activities include abstinence, use of condoms, washing and douching, open communication with partners, seeking medical help with any symptoms, and safer sexual practices.

Commitment Activities

1. List the ways you could provide STD information to other students at your school. What kinds of material would you use? Where would you look for current information relevant to your community? Check with the student health service or the residence hall council to see if a series of STD programs could be given at your university. How could you assist in setting up these programs?

2. List the cold remedies you have in your medicine cabinet. Decide why you use each medication. Is it for sneezing, coughing, headache, allergy, or something else? From now on, read the labels on all over-the-counter medications that you buy for respiratory infections. Analyze as well as you can the ingredients contained in each medication. Consult your physician or the student health service if you have a doubt about any of these medications.

3. There are many misconceptions about STDs. Prepare a list of facts and a list of misconceptions about STDs; then ask students at your university to judge the accuracy of each list. Report your findings to the class.

References

Bauman, N. "Interferon and Lasers May Cure Severe Condylomas." *Medical World News* 33, no. 3 (March 1992):36–37.

Benson, H., and Stuart, E. M. *The Wellness Book: A Comprehensive Guide to Maintaining Health and Treating Stress-Related Illnesses.* New York: Birch Lane Press, 1992, p. 354.

Boyd, W., and Sheldon, H. *An Introduction to the Study of Disease.* Philadelphia: Lea and Febiger, 1980.

Brownlee, S. "Origins of the Plague: Scientists Are Searching for the Beginning of the AIDS Epidemic." *U.S. News and World Report* 112 no. 12 (March 30, 1992):50–52.

Centers for Disease Control. "Increases in Rubella and Congenital Rubella." *Journal of the American Medical Association* 265, no. 9 (1991):1076–77.

Centers for Disease Control. "Mortality Attributable to HIV Infection/AIDS—United States, 1981–1990." *Morbidity and Mortality Weekly Report* 40, no. 3 (January 1991).

Centers for Disease Control. "Prevention and Control of Influenza." *Morbidity and Mortality Weekly Report* 39 (May 1990): RR-7.

Centers for Disease Control. "Protection against Viral Hepatitis." *Morbidity and Mortality Weekly Report* 39, no. S-2 (February 1990).

Cowley, G. "For Users of AZT, Sobering News." *Newsweek* 119, no. 8 (February 24, 1992):63.

DeLora, J.; Warren, C.; and Ellison, C. *Understanding Sexual Interaction.* Boston: Houghton Mifflin, 1977.

Getz, K. A., and Bentkover, J. D. "The Impact of AIDS on the Insurance Industry." *Journal of the American Society of CLU & ChFC* 46, no. 2 (March 1992):54–65.

Hamburger, M. I. "Demystifying Lyme Disease." *Newsweek* 119, no. 19 (May 11, 1992):A12.

Hansen, G. R. *Common Medicines,* 2d ed. Salt Lake City: University of Utah Press, 1987.

Holmes, K. K.; Karon, J. M.; and Kreiss, J. "The Increasing Frequency of Heterosexually Acquired AIDS in the United States, 1983–1988." *American Journal of Public Health* 80 (1990):7.

Hook, E. W., et al. *Current Concepts of Infectious Diseases.* New York: Wiley, 1977.

Lord, J. *Infection, Your Immune System and AIDS* (1990 Edition). Enterprise for Education in Association with the Massachusetts Medical Society, 1989.

Mishu, B. W.; Schaffner, T. J.; Horan, J. M.; Wood, L. H.; Hutcheson, R. H.; and McNab, P. C. "A Surgeon with AIDS." *Journal of the American Medical Association* 264, no. 12 (1990):467–70.

Panlilio, A. L., et al. "Blood Contacts during Surgical Procedures." *Journal of the American Medical Association* 265, no. 12 (1990):1533–37.

Robbins, S. L., and Kumar, V. *Basic Pathology,* 4th ed. Philadelphia: W. B. Saunders Company, 1987.

Schlenker, T. L.; Bain, C.; Baughman, A. L.; and Hadler, S. C. "Measles Herd Immunity: The Association of Attack Rates with Immunization Rates in Preschool Children." *Journal of the American Medical Association* 267, no. 6 (February 12, 1992):823–27.

Stroh, M. "Picking Out Lymes from Lemons (Misdiagnosing Lyme Disease)." *Science News* 141, no. 20 (1992):325.

U.S. Department of Health and Human Services. *1985 STD Treatment Guidelines.* Washington, D.C. 1985.

U.S. Department of Health and Human Services. *Surgeon General's Report in Acquired Immune Deficiency Syndrome.* Washington, D.C. 1987.

Weeks, D. C. "The AIDS Pandemic in Africa." *Current History* 91, no. 565 (May 1992): 208.

Additional Readings

Benson, H., and Stuart, E. M. *The Wellness Book: A Comprehensive Guide to Maintaining Health and Treating Stress-Related Illnesses.* New York: Birch Lane Press, 1992, p. 354. This contemporary book on preventing stress-related illness incorporates the principles of psychoneuroimmunology and mind, body, and soul approaches to prevention. Excellent reading.

Hansen, G. R. *Common Medicines,* 2d ed. Salt Lake City: University of Utah Press (1987). This is an excellent book that deals with immunization, cold remedies, and other treatments for common communicable diseases.

Lord, J. *Infection, Your Immune System and AIDS* (1990 Edition). Enterprise for Education in Association with the Massachusetts Medical Society, 1989. This excellent fifty-two-page booklet simply describes the immune system and how AIDS affects it. Some beautiful color photography and illustrations. Provides the reader with a broad understanding of the nature of the disease, prevention, history, and social and world impact.

U.S. Department of Health and Human Services. *1985 STD Treatment Guidelines.* Washington, D.C. 1985. This government guide provides an overview of the treatments and nature of several sexually transmitted diseases.

U.S. Department of Health and Human Services. *Surgeon General's Report in Acquired Immune Deficiency Syndrome.* Washington, D.C. 1987. This is a frank and bold declaration of the nature of AIDS, high-risk populations, and how to prevent AIDS from occurring.

CHAPTER 13

Cardiovascular, Cancer, and Other Chronic Diseases

Key Questions

- How can you prevent chronic disease?

- What is cardiovascular disease?

- What are some life-style decisions you can make to reduce your chance of developing cardiovascular disease?

- What are the different types of cardiovascular disease?

- What are some examples of risk factors associated with cardiovascular disease?

- How has medical technology advanced to treat heart disease?

- What is cancer?

- What are the warning signs of cancer?

- What are the major sites of cancer?

- How successful is treatment for different forms of cancer?

- What are the warning signs of diabetes?

- What are the warning signs of kidney disease?

- What consumer decisions can you make to help prevent diseases?

Chapter Outline

Since the beginning of the twentieth century, the overall death rate in the United States has been reduced from seventeen per one thousand persons per year to less than nine per one thousand. Much of the credit for this reduction must go to the efforts we have made in prevention, based on knowledge gained from medical research. The once-great killers—typhoid fever, smallpox, and the plague—have been eradicated due to improvements in sanitation, housing, nutrition, and immunization.

Today, the primary killers in the United States are chronic diseases. Currently, 75 percent of all deaths in this country are due to **chronic diseases**—diseases that occur over a long period of time and are usually disabling, such as cardiovascular diseases and cancer. For many, prevention of these diseases requires changes in life-style. Our ability to make life-style changes depends on our understanding of the basics of chronic disease, our understanding of the impact of health habits we acquired during childhood and young adulthood, and our sincere desire to change.

Most of us think that chronic disease, such as heart disease or cancer, is something that cannot happen to us. We are particularly vulnerable to this myth before we are thirty years old. But just as our daily decisions about nutrition and exercise affect our future life expectancies and quality of life, so we must deal daily with the issue of chronic disease if we are to lessen the risks and enhance the quality of our lives. The food we eat and the amount of exercise we get today directly influences the health of our bodies.

In this chapter, we look at disease prevention in general and then turn to the major cause of death in the United States—cardiovascular disease. We then discuss cancer and other chronic diseases.

Disease Prevention

Prevention of disease means inhibiting the development of disease and interrupting or slowing the progression of disease after it has started. Prevention can be divided into three stages: primary prevention, secondary prevention, and tertiary prevention.

If your immediate relatives have suffered from any chronic disease, you may be more predisposed to that disease. You can decide to take preventive measures now, before any disease symptoms occur. This is called **primary prevention.**

In some instances, a disease is already present but is being treated at an early stage. This is **secondary prevention**—prevention that attempts to keep the disease from worsening (such as bypass surgery or removal of a localized tumor). Unfortunately, no matter what life-style changes we make, we still may develop a major chronic disease at some stage in the life cycle. Consequently, it is important to know the signs and symptoms of cardiovascular disease, cancer, stroke, diabetes, and other diseases, because it can help us seek early diagnosis and treatment.

You or someone you know has probably had a disease and undergone rehabilitation to lessen or eliminate the sometimes serious effects. This process is known as **tertiary prevention.**

You can significantly influence your future health and increase your quality of life by developing prevention strategies, including controlling certain risk factors that increase the probability of chronic disease, disability, or premature death. There are a number of identified risk factors associated with potential cardiovascular diseases (heart attack, stroke, high blood pressure), cancers, digestive diseases, mental disorders, injury and poisoning, nervous system diseases, and sense organ diseases. Note

that these are risk factors and not causes. Risk factors that are common to many diseases (in no particular order) include the following:

1. Smoking
2. Hypercholesterolemia (high levels of cholesterol)
3. Lack of exercise
4. Poor nutrition (high-fat, high-salt, high-sugar diets)
5. Obesity
6. Stress
7. Alcohol
8. Illicit drug use
9. High blood pressure
10. Exposure to carcinogens (excessive sun, pollutants, asbestos, etc.)

Increasing evidence suggests that much of the incidence of chronic disease is generally due to the typical American life-style. Americans tend to eat foods high in saturated fat, sugar, and salt while consuming lesser amounts of whole grains, breads, vegetables, and fruits. Many Americans drink large quantities of alcohol and smoke cigarettes. When these behavior patterns are added to our sedentary way of life, the result is an awesome incidence of chronic disease. If we are to reduce the incidence of chronic disease, we must begin to value primary prevention rather than treatment and rehabilitation, as we have in the past.

Cardiovascular Diseases

Cardiovascular diseases, which are diseases of the heart and blood vessels, have been the major cause of death in the United States for more than forty years and account for over half of all deaths (Levy and Moskowitz 1982). The major types are hypertensive disease (characterized by continued elevation of blood pressure above the normal), coronary artery disease (caused by a narrowing of the blood vessels that nourish the heart), and stroke (caused by a blockage of the blood supply to some part of the brain).

Recent estimates show that more than seventy million people in the United States today have some form of cardiovascular disease (American Heart Association 1992). These diseases are responsible for close to one million deaths each year, more than the deaths from all other causes combined. There are 540,400 deaths annually in the United States just from heart attack, the result of cardiovascular disease that affects the heart muscle. Many thousands of these deaths occur not among older people but among those in the prime of their lives.

These statistics suggest that cardiovascular disease are beyond human control. Actually, of all the chronic diseases, cardiovascular diseases seem to have the most potential for primary prevention because of our knowledge of the risk factors. Studies show, for instance, that those who have heart attacks often have histories of high blood

Heart Disease Risk Assessment

Directions: Total your score adjacent to the best response to the following items.

1. Gender
   - 3 Male
   - 0 Female
2. Family history of heart disease
   - 0 I am not aware of any of my parents or grandparents having died of a heart attack before age sixty.
   - 1 One grandparent died of a heart attack before age sixty.
   - 2 Two grandparents or one parent died of a heart attack before age sixty.
   - 4 Three or more grandparents or one parent died of a heart attack before age sixty.
   - 8 Both parents or all four grandparents died of a heart attack before age sixty.
   - 10 One parent or two grandparents died of a heart attack before age forty-five.
3. Family history of high blood pressure, diabetes, or cholesterol (family in this question refers to brothers, sisters, mother, father, or grandparents)
   - 0 No one in my family has high blood pressure, diabetes, or high blood cholesterol.
   - 1 Only one member of my family has high blood pressure, diabetes, or high blood cholesterol.
   - 4 Two or three members of my family have high blood pressure, diabetes, or high blood cholesterol.
   - 6 Four or more members of my family have high blood pressure, diabetes, or high blood cholesterol.
4. Serum cholesterol
   If you have had your cholesterol levels analyzed through blood analysis, what was your total cholesterol amount? If you have not had it checked, add 2 to your score since you do not know if you are at risk or not.
   - 0 190mg/dl or below
   - 2 191–219mg/dl
   - 4 220–239mg/dl
   - 6 240–289mg/dl
   - 12 290–319mg/dl
   - 16 320mg/dl or higher
5. HDL cholesterol
   - 0 Over 50mg/dl or ratio of HDL to total cholesterol is one-fourth or better
   - 3 40–50mg/dl
   - 6 30–39mg/dl
   - 10 23–29mg/dl
   - 16 Below 23mg/dl
6. Smoking
   - 0 Never smoked
   - 1 Quit over five years ago
   - 2 Quit two to four years ago
   - 3 Quit about one year ago
   - 6 Quit during the past year
   If you still smoke, what is the number of cigarettes you now smoke?
   - 9 One-half to one pack a day
   - 12 One to two packs a day
   - 15 More than two packs a day
7. Blood pressure
   - 0 120/75 or below
   - 2 120/75 to 140/85
   - 6 140/85 to 150/90
   - 8 150/90 to 175/100
   - 10 170/100 to 190/110
   - 12 190/110 or above
8. Exercise
   - 0 Aerobic exercise four to five times a week
   - 2 Aerobic exercise two to three times a week
   - 4 Aerobic exercise on weekends
   - 6 Occasional exercise
   - 8 Rarely exercise if any
9. Weight
   - 0 Always at or near ideal weight
   - 2 Presently 10 percent overweight
   - 4 Presently 20 percent overweight
   - 6 30 percent overweight
   - 8 Have been 20 percent overweight or more for most of my life
10. Are you a diabetic?
    - 0 No
    - 5 Noninsulin dependent diabetic
    - 10 Insulin dependent diabetic
11. Alcohol consumption
    - 0 Zero to one drink per day (one oz hard liquor, four oz wine, twelve oz beer = one drink)
    - 2 Two to three drinks per day
    - 4 Four drinks per day
12. Stress
    Refer to the stress assessments in chapter 2. Add the following points according to those results.
    - 0 Low stress
    - 3 Moderate stress
    - 6 High stress

Scoring/Interpretation

0–25	= low risk
26–50	= moderate risk
51–80	= high risk
Over 80	= very high risk

Cancer Risk Assessment

Directions: Check all of the following that apply to you.

A. Indicate how many of your family members have had any of the following types of cancer. If only one member that you know of had cancer, put a 1 in the blank; if two members, put a 2 in the blank; and over two members, place a 3 in the blank. (Family members in this questionnaire refer to parents, grandparents, siblings, aunts, or uncles.)

____ 1. Colon and rectal cancer

____ 2. Breast cancer

____ 3. Prostate cancer

____ 4. Skin cancer

____ 5. Endometrial or uterine cancer

B. Which of the following statements apply to you?

____ 1. I work in conditions where I am exposed to industrial chemicals such as nickel, chromate, asbestos, vinyl chloride, and so on.

____ 2. I smoke one-half pack of cigarettes or less a day.

____ 3. I smoke one to two packs of cigarettes a day.

____ 4. I smoke two or more packs a day.

____ 5. I have been smoking for over fifteen years.

____ 6. I work around people who smoke cigarettes in smoke-filled settings.

____ 7. I use smokeless tobacco regularly.

____ 8. I work in conditions where I am exposed to industrial chemicals and I smoke two or more packs a day.

____ 9. I work with cadmium regularly.

____ 10. I work with rubber, dye, or leather regularly.

____ 11. I am fair skinned and often suntan or frequent tanning salons.

____ 12. I work around coal, tar, pitch, creosote, arsenic compounds, or radium.

____ 13. I had some severe sunburns as a child.

____ 14. I burn easily and do not tan very much.

____ 15. I burn slightly but get darker with each exposure to the sun.

____ 16. During the right weather, I try to suntan and expose myself frequently (more than thirty minutes per time and two or more times per week).

____ 17. I do not use sunblock or sunscreen (number 12 or higher).

____ 18. I am generally about 20 percent or more overweight.

____ 19. I eat processed meats (bologna, hams, bacon, and so on) more than three times a week.

____ 20. I generally include fatty foods in my diet (mayonnaise, fried foods, beef, pork, and so on).

____ 21. I drink three or more alcoholic drinks (one beer, four oz wine, or one oz liquor) when I drink.

____ 22. I really don't eat enough fiber or am not aware of what foods have a lot of fiber.

____ 23. Generally, when I have a bowel movement, the feces sink to the bottom of the commode (a floating stool is an indication of eating plenty of fiber).

____ 24. I don't eat at least four servings of green and yellow vegetables or fruits daily.

____ 25. I drink coffee daily.

C. Which of the following descriptions apply to you? (females only)

____ 1. I am taking estrogen supplements.

____ 2. I have an annual pap test or pap smear taken.

____ 3. I give myself a monthly self-breast examination.

____ 4. I have never had children nor plan on having children.

____ 5. I had my first child when I was over thirty years of age.

____ 6. I had intercourse for the first time at an early age (mid-teens).

____ 7. I have multiple sex partners.

____ 8. I have a history of infertility or failure to ovulate.

D. Do you have any of the following symptoms? (males and females)

____ 1. Persistent cough.

____ 2. Sputum streaked with blood.

____ 3. Chest pain.

____ 4. Recurring attacks of pneumonia or bronchitis.

____ 5. Bleeding from the rectum.

____ 6. Blood in the stool.

____ 7. Change in bowel habits.

____ 8. Breast changes that persist such as a lump, thickening, swelling, dimpling, distortion, retraction, or skin irritation.

____ 9. Nipple scaliness, discharge, pain, or tenderness.

____ 10. Intermenstrual or postmenopausal bleeding or unusual discharge.

____ 11. Enlarged abdomen.

____ 12. Digestive disturbances (discomfort, gas, distention) in women over forty, which are prolonged and unexplained.

____ 13. Sore that bleeds and doesn't heal.

____ 14. A lump in the mouth.

____ 15. A reddish or whitish patch that persists in the mouth.

____ 16. Difficulty in chewing, swallowing, or moving tongue or jaws.

____ 17. Weak or interrupted flow of urine.

____ 18. Frequent inability to urinate, especially at night.

____ 19. Blood in the urine.

____ 20. Urine flow that is not easily stopped.

____ 21. Painful or burning urination.

____ 22. Continuing pain in lower back, pelvis, or upper thighs.

____ 23. Any unusual skin condition.

____ 24. Change in the size, shape, or color of a mole or dark pigmented spot.

____ 25. Scaliness of the skin.

____ 26. Oozing, bleeding, or the appearance of a bump or nodule.

____ 27. The spread of pigment beyond a border.

____ 28. A change in skin itchiness, sensation, tenderness, or pain.

____ 29. Paleness.

____ 30. Fatigue.

____ 31. Undesired weight loss.

____ 32. Repeated infections.

____ 33. Easy bruising.

____ 34. Frequent nose bleeds or other hemorrhages.

E. Which of the following examinations have you had?

____ 1. Digital rectal examination.

____ 2. Stool blood test.

____ 3. Proctosigmoidoscopy examination.

____ 4. Breast cancer detection test.

____ 5. Skin cancer examination.

Scoring/Interpretation

Section A: Several cancers have been identified as running in families. If there is one member of the family who has had a particular cancer, then you are at a significant risk. If there are two or more family members who have had the same type of cancer, then you would be at high risk. The cancers of the colon/rectum, breast, prostate, skin, uterus, and endometrium have shown significant risks. It is important to have regular cancer checks if you have a family history of cancer.

Sections B, C, and D: It is difficult to score a cancer risk test into a generalized cancer risk, but this assessment does break down the various types of cancers into risks and symptoms. In the case of risk factors, it should be noted that if you check several risk factors for a particular type of cancer, then it is important for you to reduce those risk factors where appropriate. If you have any of the symptoms described, then you should see a physician to assure that the symptom is not cancer. Many of these symptoms could be symptomatic of different problems, many minor, but they also could be serious.

---

pressure, have high levels of blood cholesterol, smoke cigarettes, do not get sufficient exercise, are excessively overweight, have diabetes, and/or have a family history of heart attack in middle age. Each of these risk factors increases the chance of heart attack; in combination, they multiply the risk tremendously (fig. 13.1).

Understanding Major Risk Factors

You can prevent heart disease by understanding your risk factors, detecting any symptoms early, and modifying lifestyle habits to reduce the risks. There has been a reduction in heart disease over the last few years because people are watching their diets, exercising, quitting smoking, and monitoring their blood pressure and cholesterol levels. The following describes in more detail the risk factors of heart disease.

Family History

It appears that the tendency toward heart disease is hereditary. Individuals with close relatives who died from heart disease between the ages of forty and sixty tend to

have more heart attacks than others. This is a risk factor that cannot be controlled, so it is extremely important for high-risk individuals to monitor the health of their heart (medical examination) carefully and reduce other risks as well.

Cigarette Smoking

Cigarette smokers have higher levels of carbon monoxide in their blood than nonsmokers. This not only displaces oxygen in the blood but also tends to damage the arterial walls. Smoking makes the heart beat faster, raises the blood pressure, and narrows the blood vessels of the skin, especially in the fingers and toes. Given these facts, it is not surprising that numerous studies indicate that cigarette smokers are highly prone to heart disease.

High Blood Pressure

Blood pressure is simply the force the flowing blood exerts against the arterial walls. In any of us, blood pressure varies from moment to moment, rising when we are excited and falling when we rest. In some individuals,

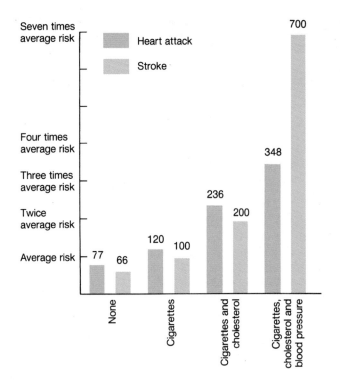

Figure 13.1

Relationship of multiple risk factors to heart attack and stroke (of a forty-five-year-old male).

however, blood pressure is always higher than normal. This condition is known as high blood pressure, or **hypertension.**

High blood pressure has been associated with an increased incidence of heart attack and stroke. When high blood pressure is not treated adequately, it can damage the heart, kidneys, and other organs of the body. Unfortunately, high blood pressure can go undetected for years because it rarely has any alarming symptoms in the early stages. With regular medical checkups, you can uncover a case of high blood pressure while it is still in an early stage.

High Blood Cholesterol

High blood cholesterol can cause a buildup on the arterial walls, narrowing the passageway through which the blood flows and leading to subsequent heart attack and stroke. The body generates its own cholesterol in addition to cholesterol that is ingested. The determination of how much cholesterol is manufactured by the body seems to be hereditary. A physician can measure the amount of cholesterol in your blood, and it is also common to see cholesterol screening programs at health departments or shopping malls. A diet low in cholesterol and saturated fat and high in fiber, particularly oat bran (Humble 1991), can help lower a blood cholesterol level that is too high. In difficult cases, hypercholesterolemia (high blood cholesterol disease) can be treated with medications.

It is difficult to make any absolute judgments about how high is too high a level of cholesterol. Robbins and Kumar (1987) state, "There is no single level of plasma cho-

lesterol that identifies those at risk, the higher the level, the greater the risk." Studies have shown though that risk rises significantly once a plateau of 200mg/100ml is reached.

Diabetes

Diabetes appears most frequently during middle age, usually in individuals who are overweight and live sedentary life-styles. Diabetes can sharply increase the risk of heart attack, making control of the other risk factors even more important. (Diabetes is discussed at length later in this chapter.)

Other Contributing Factors

As mentioned, the other contributing factors to heart disease include obesity, lack of exercise, and stress. Obesity usually results from eating too much and/or exercising too little. Excess weight places a heavy burden on the heart, but it is associated with coronary heart disease primarily because of its influence on blood pressure, blood cholesterol, and diabetes. A lack of exercise has been shown to be a risk factor for heart attack and lack of exercise combined with overeating can lead to excessive weight—which is clearly a contributing factor. Some evidence also suggests that stressful living habits contribute to a higher incidence of heart attack.

To better understand how to prevent cardiovascular disease and cope with disease that does occur, it is useful to know something about each of the major cardiovascular diseases.

Arteriosclerosis

Arteriosclerosis is the general term for three patterns of vascular disease, all of which cause thickening and a loss of elasticity of arteries. The most prominent pattern is atherosclerosis, calcific sclerosis (calcium deposits on the arteries), and then arteriolosclerosis (diseases of the small arteries and arterioles). The focus of this section is on atherosclerosis.

Atherosclerosis, also called hardening of the arteries, is a degenerative disease that contributes to the development of high blood pressure, heart attack, and stroke. During the disease process, the arteriole linings become thickened and roughened by deposits of fat, cholesterol, fibrin (a clotting material), cellular debris, and calcium.

The buildup on the inner walls eventually becomes hard and thick, and the arteries lose their ability to expand and contract. When this occurs, the blood has difficulty moving through the narrowed channels. It is then easier for a clot to form, which may in turn block the channel and deprive the heart, brain, or another body organ of blood. The deposits may grow for many years before the vessel becomes clogged enough to cause trouble (fig. 13.2). When this does occur, however, that part of the body served by the clogged vessel is deprived of its blood supply. If blockage occurs in a coronary artery, the result may be a heart attack. If it occurs in a vessel leading to the brain, the result may be a stroke.

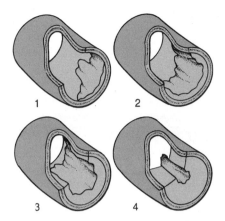

Figure 13.2

Progressive atherosclerotic buildup on artery walls.

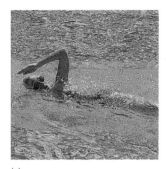

(a)

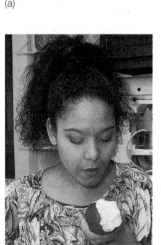

(b)

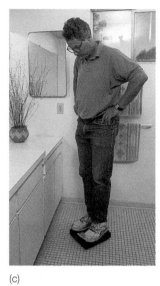

(c)

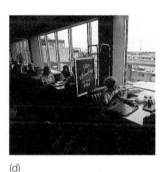

(d)

You can significantly and positively affect your future health and quality of life by developing prevention strategies in the following areas of your life: (a) exercise, (b) eat a diet low in cholesterol and saturated fat and high in fiber, (c) watch your weight, (d) make wise decisions about exposure to tobacco products.

The atherosclerosis disease process is far from being totally understood. Part of the mystery being studied is the ratio of good cholesterol, called **high-density lipoprotein (HDL),** to bad cholesterol, labeled **low-density lipoprotein (LDL),** or **very low-density lipoprotein (VLDL).** High levels of HDL have been associated with a lower risk of atherosclerosis. The exact function is not known, but it appears that HDL prevents plaque buildup and atherosclerosis. HDL is thought to carry the fats to the tissues of the liver, where it is excreted in the bile. High levels of LDL are associated with an increased risk of atherosclerosis because it seems to promote plaque buildup in the arteries. VLDL is associated with the triglycerides, also a fat, and also seems to contribute to atherosclerosis and coronary artery disease. Consequently, most physicians agree that the higher the HDL level and lower the LDL level, the less risk there is of coronary artery disease. A ratio of four to one is considered a good ratio for total cholesterol to HDL. For example, if a total cholesterol was 200 and an HDL was 50, then that would be a good ratio (four to one). The higher the ratio the better. For example, if total cholesterol was 150 and HDL was 50, that would be a three to one ratio, which would be even better.

Hypertension (High Blood Pressure)

In the United States, more than sixty-three million people have some elevation of blood pressure (American Heart Association 1992). Even more alarming, 25 percent of those with hypertension are unaware of it, 25 percent are aware but are doing nothing to control it, and 25 percent are not receiving adequate treatment. Thus, only 25 percent of those people with high blood pressure are actually getting adequate treatment (American Heart Association, *How You Can Help* 1986).

Understanding Blood Pressure

With each beat of your heart, blood pressure rises and falls within a limited range. Blood pressure is directly related to the amount of blood pumped through the heart, multiplied by the resistance of the vessels through which it is pumped. If either the amount of blood or the resistance increases, as with atherosclerotic buildup, your blood pressure rises. If your blood pressure remains elevated, you have high blood pressure.

High blood pressure adds to the work load of the heart and arteries, and the narrowed blood vessels may not be able to deliver enough oxygen to the body's organs. When the heart is forced to work harder for a long period of time, it tends to enlarge and can't keep up with the demands made on it. The arteries also show the wear and tear of high blood pressure by becoming hardened, less elastic, and scarred. When this happens, the blood is not delivered to the body's organs as it should be.

Causes of High Blood Pressure

In 90 percent of all high blood pressure cases, the cause is unknown, or idiopathic (Robbins and Kumar 1987). This type of high blood pressure is called **essential**

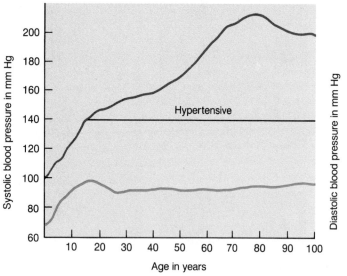
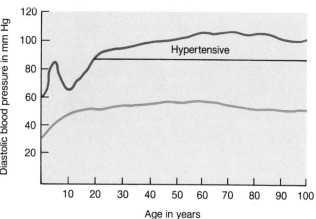

Figure 13.3

Range of normal and hypertensive pressures for different ages in the population.

hypertension. In the other 10 percent of cases, the high blood pressure is known as secondary hypertension; that is, with the correction of the primary health problem, generally renal disease, blood pressure usually returns to normal. The use of oral contraceptives is a common cause of hypertension. Oral contraceptives can raise blood pressure by increasing the blood volume, although the elevation is usually only slight. Overweight women who take birth-control pills are particularly susceptible to high blood pressure.

Determining Blood Pressure

The only sure way to know if you have high blood pressure is to have it measured with a **sphygmomanometer,** which consists of an inflatable rubber cuff that is placed around the arm and then inflated with air. The arm is squeezed with the cuff until the flow of blood momentarily stops. Then the air is released, and the blood again begins to flow. With a stethoscope, a trained person can record both the systolic pressure and diastolic pressure. To record a person's blood pressure, begin first by pumping up a pressure cuff so that it cuts off the circulation in the arm. The **systolic pressure** is the first number recorded and is the highest pressure that occurs when the heart beats. It is noted on a readout on the sphygmomanometer (pressure recorded in millimeters of mercury) when the first beat is heard through the stethoscope during the process of reducing pressure from the constricting cuff. It marks the beginning of blood flowing again during the heart contraction. The **diastolic pressure** is the pressure of the blood flow between heart pumps or when the heart is relaxed. It is recorded when the last beat can be heard. Both numbers are then recorded as the blood pressure measurement (e.g., 120/80).

What is a normal blood pressure? Researchers have collected data on blood pressure, evaluated it statistically, and determined that 120/80 is the typically "normal" blood pressure for an adult. Lower and higher values are within the normal range. Blood pressure can be considered high if the systolic is considered normal but the diastolic is high (e.g., 130/105), when the systolic is high and the diastolic is normal (e.g., 180/80), or if both values are high (e.g., 160/100). The upper limits of normal are about 140/90 (fig. 13.3).

Treatment of High Blood Pressure

Many medications are available for the treatment of high blood pressure, including **diuretics,** which eliminate excess fluid and salt, and **vasodilators,** which widen narrow blood vessels. In most cases, these drugs lower blood pressure, but often other actions must also be taken. If you are overweight and have high blood pressure, you can lower the pressure some by losing weight.

A controversial prevention strategy is the regular consumption of small amounts of alcohol. The effects of alcohol in reducing blood pressure are clear, but the studies do not consider the dangerous effects on the liver or on drinking behavior (Russell et al. 1991). Reducing the amount of salt in the diet may also help.

Heart Attack

Heart attack is a term that describes the result of coronary artery disease or atherosclerosis of the coronary arteries. If a blood clot forms in one or more of these narrowed arteries and blocks the flow of blood to that part of the heart, a heart attack, or **myocardial infarction,** may occur (fig. 13.4). That part of the heart begins to die. Luckily, the

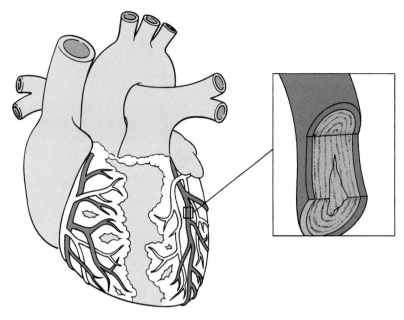

Coronary arteries (showing blocked artery)

Figure 13.4
Blocked coronary arteries cause heart attack.

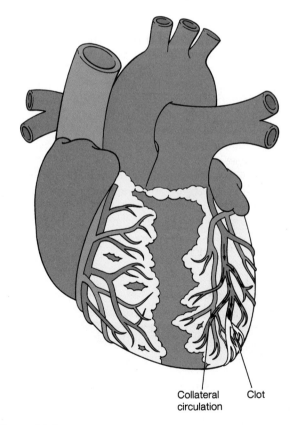

Collateral circulation   Clot

Figure 13.5
Collateral circulation.

heart has its own method of repair. If the damage is not too severe and the person does not die, other blood vessels begin to supply that area of the heart served by the blocked artery. One purpose of exercise is to enlarge the arteries and facilitate the development of **collateral circulation,** in which smaller blood vessels allow blood to flow to that part of the heart muscle served by a blocked main vessel, sometimes even before a heart attack occurs. Examination of the hearts of runners has shown that, in some cases, they suffered heart attacks during their lifetimes and never knew it because of the collateral circulation created by exercise (fig. 13.5).

Another result of coronary artery disease may be chest pain, or **angina,** which warns of narrowed or blocked arteries before a heart attack occurs. Angina usually occurs at times of emotional excitement or unusual physical exertion.

Symptoms of Heart Attack

Unfortunately, many who have heart attacks actually deny they are having a problem. It is important for us to know the warning signals of a heart attack.

Heart attack is the nation's number-one killer. When an attack occurs, there is no time for delay, since many individuals survive only if they get immediate medical care. Certain signs may indicate that a heart attack is occurring: an uncomfortable pressure, fullness, squeezing, or pain in the center of the chest, lasting two minutes or more; pain that spreads to the shoulders, neck, jaw, or arms; and severe pain, dizziness, fainting, sweating, nausea, or shortness of breath. Not all of these signals are always present, and they sometimes subside and then return. If some or all of these signals do occur, get help immediately.

What to Do

You should know exactly what to do when a heart attack occurs. Many communities have emergency rescue services to call. Many cities have a 911 number to call paramedics, who can administer **cardiopulmonary resuscitation (CPR).**

Sometimes the heart attack is so severe that the person's heartbeat and breathing stop. If you are trained to administer CPR, then you may save a life. If you are not, quickly find someone in the neighborhood or dorm who can help after you have called for emergency personnel. The four or five minutes it may take emergency personnel to arrive are critical. Many people are trained in CPR, so you may be lucky and find someone who can start the procedure. If you are not trained to administer CPR, you can check for breathing and a pulse at the carotid artery.

It is a good idea for parents and children to be trained in CPR given the number of lives that have been saved by brothers and sisters, roommates, and parents who have been trained.

After a Heart Attack

The actual diagnosis of heart attack is made by a physician and is based on the results of several tests taken at a hospital, either in the emergency room or in the coronary care unit (CCU). These units offer specialized treatment and around-the-clock care. A physician uses an **electrocardiogram (EKG),** a test that graphs the electrical impulses within the heart, along with blood tests to identify levels of cardiac enzymes, to determine whether a heart attack has occurred and whether there are any abnormalities caused by heart damage (American Heart Association, *After a Heart Attack* 1986).

In some cases, heart damage is extensive and special **bypass surgery** is needed. A special technique called **angiography** shows the cardiologist where and how great the obstruction is. A vein is removed from the leg and grafted to the coronary artery above and below the obstruction. Many times, more than one bypass is needed.

Another technique to facilitate the unrestricted flow of blood through the arteries is called **angioplasty.** This process is much like cleaning a sewage line with a "snake." A small balloonlike instrument on the end of a wire is forced through the artery and flattens the clogs or buildup against the arterial wall to allow for a better flow of blood.

New classes of heart drugs are leading the revolution in treating heart disease. The beta-blocking drugs, first made available in the late 1960s, are effective in preventing second heart attacks and sudden cardiac arrests in patients who have had previous attacks. The calcium-blocking drugs prevent the coronary arteries from contracting and having spasms that block the flow of oxygen to the heart muscle. Physicians can now treat heart attack victims by injecting a specific enzyme into the heart that prevents further damage to the heart muscle. Other drugs, including anti-arrhythmia agents, are now being tested.

Stroke

Stroke is a sudden loss of brain function, usually the result of some interference (either permanent or temporary) with the brain's blood supply. The extent of damage determines whether the stroke is minor and transient with no lasting effects, one that leaves the individual with some degree of disability, or one so major that the individual dies. The brain and its nerve cells depend on the oxygen and food brought to them by the bloodstream. When this supply is cut off for a period of time, the nerve cells die. Once these cells have died, they cease to fulfill their tasks of making a body part move, reporting on sensations, or operating one of the senses.

Stroke is perhaps the most devastating and disabling of all human disorders. It has afflicted some 3,020,000 persons in the United States and kills more than 145,000 annually (American Heart Association 1992).

Causes of Stroke

There are four causes of stroke (fig. 13.6). One of the more common causes is a **cerebral thrombosis,** which occurs when a clot **thrombus** forms inside one of the arteries supplying blood to the brain and blocks it. These clots occur in arteries damaged by atherosclerosis. Another form of stroke—**cerebral embolism**—may be caused by a wandering clot **embolus,** which is carried in the bloodstream until it becomes wedged in one of the arteries leading to the brain.

When a defective artery in the brain bursts, another form of stroke, **cerebral hemorrhage,** occurs. Blood supply to the cells is cut off, and the cells can't function. In addition, accumulated blood from the burst artery can pressure the surrounding brain tissue. This pressure can interfere with brain function, causing mild or severe symptoms of stroke.

Arterial hemorrhage in the brain may be caused by a burst aneurysm. **Aneurysms** are blood-filled pouches that balloon out from weak spots in the artery wall; they are often associated with high blood pressure. Aneurysms do not always cause trouble, but when one bursts in the brain, the result is a stroke (American Heart Association 1992).

A stroke can occur at any time or place, during activity or rest. Typically, those who have a cerebral hemorrhage suffer a sudden, severe headache and fall unconscious. When a cerebral embolism is the cause, the stroke comes

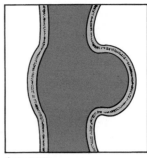

Aneurysm

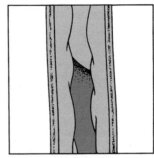

Thrombus

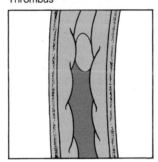

Embolism

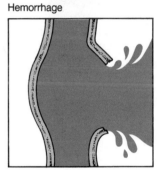

Hemorrhage

Aneurysm (ruptured)

Figure 13.6

Causes of stroke.

on even more suddenly and without warning. A cerebral thrombosis is similar to a cerebral hemorrhage but usually occurs after inactivity.

Risk Factors

The risk factors of stroke are slightly different from those discussed for heart disease. Two of them, sex and race, can't be changed. The risk of stroke is greater in men than in women; however, women who take oral contraceptives increase their risk of stroke, and women who smoke heavily further increase this risk.

There are certain modifiable risk factors for stroke, however. Controlling high blood pressure or diabetes reduces the risk, as does wise management of heart disease. An increase in the red blood cell count may be a risk factor of stroke, but this too can be modified through medical management.

Warning Signals

The warning signals of an impending stroke are a sudden, temporary weakness or numbness of the face, arm, and leg on one side of the body; a temporary loss of speech, or trouble in speaking or understanding speech; a tempo-

rary dimness or loss of vision, particularly in one eye; and unexpected dizziness, unsteadiness, or sudden falls (American Heart Association 1992).

Typically, the most visible sign of stroke is paralysis on one side of the body. Paralysis of the right side results from damage to the left hemisphere of the brain. These persons are likely to have problems with speech and language, which is called **aphasia,** and to be slow and cautious when approaching an unfamiliar problem. Paralysis on the left side indicates damage to the right hemisphere of the brain (fig. 13.7). These persons have difficulty with spatial perception and tend to be quick and impulsive, often attempting unsafe activities.

After a stroke, some of the damaged nerve cells may recover, or their function may be taken over by other nerve cells in the brain. In this way, the part of the body affected by the stroke may eventually improve or even return to normal. Some persons recover quickly; others, however, suffer such serious damage that even a partial recovery takes a long time.

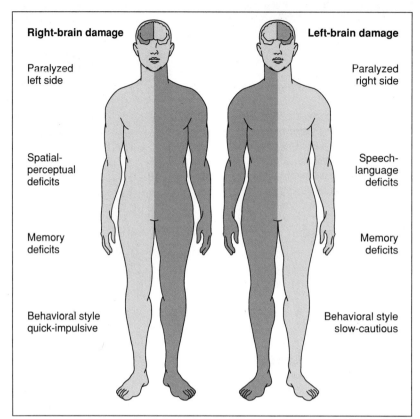

Figure 13.7

Brain damage affects the opposite side of the body.

Reproduced with permission. © "How Stroke Affects Behavior," 1992 Copyright American Heart Association.

Treatment and Rehabilitation

Treatment may include surgery and/or drugs. If a block-age has occurred in the carotid arteries of the neck, surgery called **carotid endarterectomy** is used to remove the atherosclerotic plaque buildup. If a blood ves-sel has been blocked by a clot, anticlotting drugs may be used either to prevent new clots from forming or to pre-vent an existing clot from becoming larger (American Heart Association 1992).

Most stroke patients can be rehabilitated with a pro-gram that teaches new skills to replace those lost and that maintains and improves the patient's physical condition—another example of tertiary prevention.

Other Types of Heart Disease

An untreated streptococcal infection can develop into rheumatic fever, which can in turn damage many of the body's tissues, especially in the heart, joints, brain, and skin. Rheumatic fever may cause permanent heart dam-age, known as **rheumatic heart disease.** People of all ages can develop rheumatic fever, but it is found most often in children aged five to fifteen.

Congenital heart defects are abnormalities in the structure of the heart that are present at birth. Most of these defects either obstruct the flow of blood or reroute the blood. Unusual heart defects also occur, upsetting the electrical impulses responsible for the heartbeat. In most cases, the cause of these defects is unknown, although German measles—if contracted by the mother during the first three months of pregnancy—is one identified cause.

Congestive heart failure occurs as a result of dam-age to the heart muscle caused by rheumatic fever, con-genital heart defects, heart attack, atherosclerosis, or high blood pressure. The heart muscle lacks the strength to cir-culate the blood properly, so the blood flow is inadequate to meet all of the body's needs.

Advances in Cardiovascular Medicine

The first heart transplant was performed in 1967. Within a few years, however, almost all of the early advocates of the procedure had abandoned the operation because of a mortality rate of up to 80 percent within a year following surgery. To prevent the body from rejecting the "new" heart, patients were often given huge doses of powerful

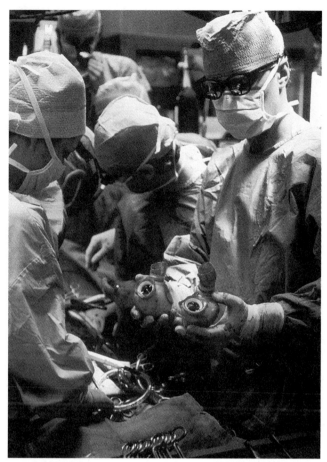

The Jarvik artificial heart.

immunosuppressive drugs. These drugs made patients more susceptible to other diseases, and the vast majority of transplant patients died from infection.

Transplant surgery has now been revived, however, because of a new drug called cyclosporine. This drug is a fungal compound that blocks the production of white blood cells that cause rejection but not of those that fight infection. So the heart transplant now seems to be a more successful operation. The transplants are now covered by Medicare.

So much progress has been made in cardiovascular medicine that many Americans now receive new hearts, with 70 percent surviving more than one year. Surgeons can even do combined heart and lung transplants, also with a 70 percent survival rate.

In December 1982, medical history was made in Salt Lake City with the implantation of an artificial heart into the chest of a sixty-one-year-old retired dentist, who was suffering from congestive heart failure. The plastic heart, called the **Jarvik 7,** was attached to the patient's atria, after the ventricles had been surgically removed. The artificial heart, slightly larger than the average heart, was connected by tubes to a compressor to keep it pumping.

Life was not easy for this first artificial heart recipient. He was permanently tethered to 375 pounds of equipment, including two compressors, a backup compressor,

a three-hour supply of pressurized air to operate the heart in case of power failure, a drier to dehumidify the air, and mechanisms that controlled the air pressure and heart rate. All this equipment rested on a cart that had to be kept six feet from the patient. The patient lived over three months with this artificial heart, and the information learned was extremely helpful for future advances.

Since that time, many patients have received transplants with Jarvik 7 or **Jarvik 7–70** (a smaller version of the Jarvik 7) artificial hearts. The Jarvik 7–70 was developed because the spherical shape of the ventricles in the Jarvik 7 did not fit easily into the chest. The Jarvik 7–70 fit better but had a 30 percent reduction in stroke volume (the amount of blood pumped with each beat). The latest version of the artificial heart is the Utah 100. Like the Jarvik 7–70, the Utah 100 is pneumatically powered and has a more oval shape to fit into the chest cavity better, but it has the same stroke volume as the original Jarvik 7 (Olson 1987).

The function of artificial hearts at this point is to allow the patient to live until a donor heart is found for transplantation. The average time that an individual has an artificial heart is ten to thirty days. The longest time a person has been on an artificial heart is two hundred days (Olson 1987).

The artificial heart has not been perfected. The hearts are prone to thrombosis, stroke, bleeding, clotting around artificial biomaterial, and destruction of red blood cells (Grieger 1986). In late 1989 and 1990, the FDA placed several medical devices under scrutiny (Jones 1990). In January 1990, the FDA withdrew approval for use of the Jarvik 7 artificial heart (Merz 1990), largely for sloppiness in manufacturing and complications with some patients. Researchers at the University of Utah Artificial Heart Laboratory and Humana Medical Center in Louisville, Kentucky, continue to refine the hearts with softer pumping action to prevent destruction of red blood cells, better anticoagulant drug balances, and better monitoring for early detection of stroke and other problems (Grieger 1986).

Cancer

The term **cancer** refers to a large group of diseases characterized by the uncontrolled growth and spread of abnormal or malignant cells. Cancer strikes at any age, but more frequently at advanced ages. Even so, cancer kills more children between the ages of three and fourteen than any other disease. In fact, after cardiovascular disease, cancer is the leading cause of death in the United States; about 24 percent of all deaths in this country are caused by cancer. About 30 percent of people now living will eventually get cancer (American Cancer Society 1990).

There are more than one hundred basic, recognized forms of cancer, but the one characteristic they share is their malignant nature. Normally, the body's cells reproduce themselves in an orderly manner. Worn-out tissues are replaced, injuries are repaired, and bodily growth proceeds

TABLE 13.1

Types of Cancer and Their Characteristics

Type of Cancer	Types of Cells That Give Rise to Each	How Spread	Most Common Sites
Carcinoma	Epithelial tissue	Lymphatic system	Skin, mucous membrane; glandular tissue of breast, liver, stomach, intestine, uterus, mouth, lung
Sarcoma	Connective tissue	Bloodstream	Bone, cartilage, fat, subcutaneous tissue, muscle
Lymphoma	Lymph nodes	Lymphatic system	Neck, armpits, groin, chest, abdomen
Leukemia	Blood-forming tissue	Bloodstream	Bone marrow, white cells
Melanoma	Wart, mole	Lymphatic system and bloodstream	Foot
Glioma	Brain tissue	Into brain tissue	Brain

From George E. Moore, *The Cancerous Disease*. Copyright © 1970 Wadsworth Publishing Company, Inc., Belmont, Calif. Reprinted by permission.

normally. Occasionally, however, certain cells undergo an abnormal change and begin the process of uncontrolled growth. These cells can grow into **tumors,** which are masses of tissues that are either benign or malignant. **Malignant tumors** are cancerous; **benign tumors** are not.

Benign tumors should also be watched carefully because they can change and become cancerous. Malignant tumors invade the surrounding normal tissue, kill it, and eventually spread to tissue in other parts of the body, where the invasive process is repeated. Malignant tumors are classified according to the types of cells that give rise to them. Table 13.1 lists the types of cancers, how they are spread, and the most common sites of each.

In the beginning stages of cancer, cancer cells usually remain at their original site, and the cancer is said to be localized **cancer in situ.** If untreated, some cells may invade neighboring organs or tissue by direct extension, which is called regional involvement. If still untreated, the cancerous cells become detached and are carried through the lymph or blood systems to other parts of the body. This is called **metastasis.** When cancer metastasizes, it usually results in death.

Causes of Cancer

The basic causes of most cancers are still unknown. Extensive research, however, has uncovered some predisposing factors that are connected to abnormal growth in certain cells and thus may cause cancer. Some of these factors are hereditary; others are environmental.

Our heredity plays a major role in the transformation of normal cells to malignant ones. In some unfortunate families, certain cancers occur with a frequency up to four times that of the general population.

Certain environmental factors, such as radiation, seem to cause genetic changes, or **mutations,** by directly damaging the **DNA** one of the substances that makes up our genes. A wide variety of chemicals, and perhaps even viruses, can also cause these changes.

Cancer-causing substances, **carcinogens,** regularly create problems in whole populations. Asbestos fibers can produce cancer, for example, so those who work in asbestos factories are at high risk. There is also a relationship between industrial solvents and bladder cancer. And, as we well know, there is a powerful connection between smoking and lung cancer.

Viruses have been isolated that cause cancer in animals. For instance, a virus obtained from mice with breast cancer can cause the same malignancy in a second animal. So far, a specific cancer-causing virus has not been isolated in human beings, but researchers continue to explore this possibility. It seems only a matter of time until we find a virus that can be definitely linked to some forms of cancer (Robbins and Kumar 1987).

Common Cancer Sites and Specific Risk Factors

Because prevention, detection, and treatment are site specific in many cancer cases, we will examine each of the major cancer sites separately. Figure 13.8 shows the American Cancer Society's 1992 estimates of cancer incidence and death by site and sex. As the figure shows, lung cancer has the highest overall death rates in the population. Notice how patterns vary between males and females. The risk factors and early symptoms of cancers by site are listed in table 13.2 on page 292.

Consumer Decisions for Prevention and Early Detection

We can actually prevent some cancers. For example, if we abandon smoking, we can prevent most lung cancers. We can also prevent certain cancers caused by occupational or environmental factors if we eliminate contact with the

Cancer Incidence by Site and Sex*

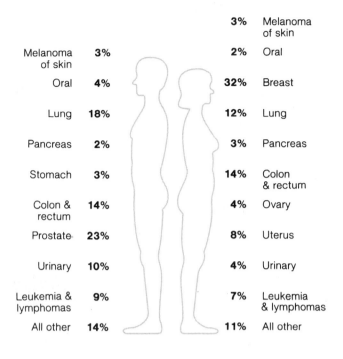

		3%	Melanoma of skin
Melanoma of skin	3%	2%	Oral
Oral	4%	32%	Breast
Lung	18%	12%	Lung
Pancreas	2%	3%	Pancreas
Stomach	3%	14%	Colon & rectum
Colon & rectum	14%	4%	Ovary
Prostate	23%	8%	Uterus
Urinary	10%	4%	Urinary
Leukemia & lymphomas	9%	7%	Leukemia & lymphomas
All other	14%	11%	All other

*Excluding nonmelanoma skin cancer and carcinoma in situ.

Cancer Deaths by Site and Sex*

		1%	Melanoma of skin
Melanoma of skin	1%	1%	Oral
Oral	2%	19%	Breast
Lung	34%	22%	Lung
Pancreas	4%	5%	Pancreas
Stomach	3%	12%	Colon & rectum
Colon & rectum	11%	5%	Ovary
Prostate	12%	4%	Uterus
Urinary	5%	3%	Urinary
Leukemia & lymphomas	9%	9%	Leukemia & lymphomas
All other	19%	19%	All other

Figure 13.8

Cancer incidence and deaths by site and sex—1992 estimates.

Courtesy of the American Cancer Society.

particular carcinogenic agents. Melanoma is on the rise (32,000 Americans diagnosed each year), largely due to sun exposure and the damaged ozone layer (Saltus 1992). Most cancers are not preventable, however, so early detection is a necessity. The American Cancer Society recommends safeguards for the prevention and early detection of cancer (fig. 13.9 on page 294; box, bottom of page 295). As with many chronic diseases, cancer has specific warning signals that can alert us to possible problems. These are also listed in the accompanying box.

Individuals twenty to forty years old should get a cancer-related physical examination at least once every three years; those over forty should get one annually. Special tests and procedures are listed in the accompanying box. Individuals can be examined for cancers of the thyroid, lymph nodes, oral region, and skin, as well as for nonmalignant diseases. Women can have pelvic examinations, and men can be examined for cancer of the testicles.

If cancer is suspected, a sample of a tumor is usually obtained through a **biopsy,** a simple surgical procedure in which a small section of the tumor is removed and examined under a microscope. Presence of cancer is determined on the basis of the quantity and type of cells and their relative proportions to normal cells. Malignant cells are irregular in shape, size, and growth patterns. They invade the surrounding tissue and spread to local and distant tissues. As the tumor grows and spreads, various symptoms may appear. If the tumor grows in soft tissue, a lump may become evident; if it blocks the opening of a vessel, such as the bowel or the bronchi of the lung, some pain may be evident. Abnormal weight loss can also indicate cancer, because malignant cells tend to compete more successfully for nutrients than do normal cells. Naturally, the earlier the detection, the more likely there is a cure.

Cancer Treatment

The goal of cancer treatment is complete cure; if that is not possible—and often it is not—treatment is aimed at controlling the disease and giving the patient as long and as full a life as possible. Surgery, radiation, and chemotherapy, alone or in combination, are the major means of treating cancer (American Cancer Society 1990).

Cancer is most often treated surgically. The surgeon removes not only the malignant tumor or organ but also a wide margin of normal tissue and often nearby lymph nodes. If all cancer cells can be eliminated at their site of origin, and if none has escaped into the bloodstream or lymph system, surgery can effect a cure. Surgery is currently used to treat cancers of the lung, breast, colon and rectum, uterus, prostate, bladder, head and neck, kidney, ovary, and thyroid.

Radiation is the second most common method of treating cancer. Today, about half of all cancer patients receive radiation therapy, either alone or in combination with some other therapy. X-ray machines of the past have

TABLE 13.2

Risks and Warning Symptoms of Major Cancers

Type of Cancer	Risks	Warning Symptoms
Lung	Cigarette smoking (the more you smoke, the higher the risks; over two packs a day is a significantly higher risk) History of smoking (the longer you have smoked, the higher the risk) Exposure to industrial substances Involuntary smoking Exposure to radiation Combination of smoking and working around industrial substances is a very high risk	Persistent cough Sputum streaked with blood Chest pain Recurring attacks of pneumonia or bronchitis
Colon and Rectum	Personal or family history of colon and rectum cancer Personal or family history of polyps in the colon or rectum Inflammatory bowel disease Diet high in fat Diet low in fiber	Bleeding from the rectum Blood in the stool Change in bowel habits
Breast	Over age fifty Personal or family history of breast cancer Never had children First child after age thirty	Breast changes that persist such as a lump, thickening, swelling, dimpling, skin irritation, distortion, retraction scaliness of the nipple, nipple discharge, pain or tenderness
Uterine/Cervical	Early age at first intercourse Multiple sex partners Endometrial cancer, history of infertility Failure of ovulation Prolonged estrogen therapy Obesity	Intermenstrual or postmenopausal bleeding or unusual discharge
Ovarian	Increases with age, peaking at sixty-five to eighty-five Women who do not have children Late age of first live birth Late age of first pregnancy Low number of pregnancies Low number of years of ovulation Already have had breast, colorectal, and endometrial cancer You are a nun, Jewish, or never married	No obvious signs or symptoms until late in its development Enlarged abdomen caused by the collection of fluids Vague digestive disturbances in women over forty (stomach discomfort, gas, distention) that persist and cannot be explained
Oral	Cigarette, cigar, and pipe smoking Use of smokeless tobacco Excess use of alcohol	Sore that bleeds easily and doesn't heal A lump or thickening in the mouth A reddish or whitish patch that persists Difficulty in chewing, swallowing, or moving tongue or jaws
Prostate	Increases with age (over sixty-five) Black Americans Some familiar association High dietary fat Working with cadmium	Signs and symptoms similar to infection or prostate enlargement Weak or interrupted flow of urine Inability to urinate frequently, especially at night, blood in the urine Urine flow that is not easily stopped Painful or burning urination Continuing pain in lower back, pelvis, or upper thighs

TABLE 13.2—*Continued*

Risks and Warning Symptoms of Major Cancers

Type of Cancer	Risks	Warning Symptoms
Bladder	Smoking (greatest) twice	Blood in the urine
	Men (four times more for men than women)	Increased urination
	Live in urban area	
	Work with dye, rubber, leather	
	Drink coffee	
	Artificial sweeteners	
Skin	Excessive exposure to sun	Any unusual skin condition
	Fair complexion	Change in the size, color, or shape of a mole or darkly pigmented growth or spot
	Occupational exposure to coal, tar, pitch creosote, arsenic compounds, or radium	Scaliness
	White (blacks rarely have skin cancer)	Oozing, bleeding, or the appearance of a bump or nodule
	Severe sunburn in childhood may have effect later in life	The spread of pigment beyond the border
		A change in sensation, itchiness, tenderness, or pain
Pancreatic	After age thirty (most are aged seventy to ninety)	No early symptoms
	Smoking	
	Male	
	Blacks (50 percent more common)	
	Incidence of chronic pancreatitis, diabetes, and cirrhosis	
	High-fat diet	
	Coffee (possibly)	
Leukemia	Down syndrome and other hereditary abnormalities	Fatigue
	Excessive exposure to radiation	Paleness
		Weight loss
		Repeated infections
		Easy bruising, nose bleeds or other hemorrhages

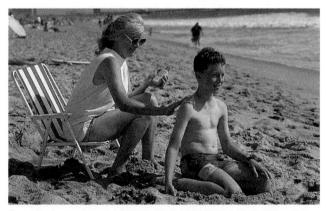

Sun blocks may provide some protection to help reduce the risk of skin cancer.

been replaced with supervoltage equipment, such as the linear accelerator, which allows deeper penetration. The beams don't kill malignant cells outright but instead destroy their reproductive mechanism, so that once they die, no new cancer cells develop. Radiation is often the primary treatment for a number of cancers, including cervical cancer, head and neck cancer, Hodgkin's disease, brain cancer, and cancers of the larynx, pharynx, esophagus, oral cavity, bone, prostate, testes, and skin. Radiation treatment can cause unpleasant side effects, however, including diarrhea, difficulty in swallowing, itching, and a diminished sense of taste.

Chemotherapy, the use of drugs and hormones, is the preferred treatment when cancers have spread beyond the reach of surgery or radiation. Thus far, it has proved most effective among rarer forms of cancer, including melanomas, acute leukemia, and testicular cancer. At present, some fifty different drugs are used, either alone or in combination. These drugs work because they interfere with the reproductive ability of the cancer cells. Unfortunately, chemotherapy can also cause serious side effects, including nausea, vomiting, diarrhea, anemia, lowered resistance to infection, and loss of hair.

In cancer treatment, the real hope for the future lies in earlier detection. Of course, the long-range hope in research is to be able to prevent the disease.

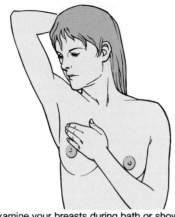

Examine your breasts during bath or shower; hands glide easier over wet skin. Fingers flat, move gently over every part of each breast. Use right hand to examine left breast, left hand for right breast. Check for any lump, hard knot or thickening.

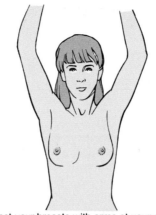

Inspect your breasts with arms at your sides. Next, raise your arms high overhead. Look for any changes in contour of each breast, a swelling, dimpling of skin or changes in the nipple.

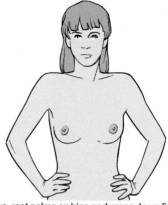

Then, rest palms on hips and press down firmly to flex your chest muscles. Left and right breast will not exactly match—few women's breasts do.

Regular inspection shows what is normal for you and will give you confidence in your examination.

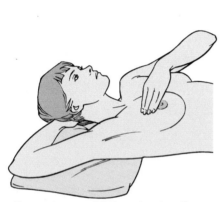

To examine your right breast, put a pillow or folded towel under your right shoulder. Place right hand behind your head—this distributes breast tissue more evenly on the chest. With left hand, fingers flat, press gently in small circular motions around an imaginary clock face.

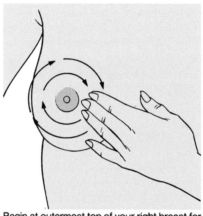

Begin at outermost top of your right breast for 12 o'clock, then move to 1 o'clock, and so on around the circle back to 12. A ridge of firm tissue in the lower curve of each breast is normal. Then move in an inch toward the nipple, keep circling to examine every part of your breast, including nipple. This requires at least three more circles.

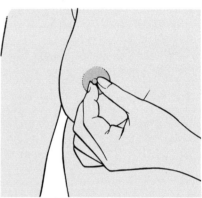

Now slowly repeat the procedure on your left breast with a pillow under your left shoulder and left hand behind head. Notice how your breast structure feels.

Finally, squeeze the nipple of each breast gently between thumb and index finger. Any discharge, clear or bloody, should be reported to your doctor immediately.

Figure 13.9

How to examine your breasts.

Used by permission, American Cancer Society, Inc.

Nutrition and Cancer

There is significant research being conducted to show the relationship between cancer and diet. Although several dietary carcinogens have been identified through laboratory studies with rats, no direct cause and effect relationships have been made. There is strong evidence through statistics that the following dietary guidelines might reduce your risk of cancer.

1. Maintain an ideal weight. Obese persons (40 percent or more overweight) increase their risk of colon, breast, prostate, gallbladder, ovary, and uterine cancer.

2. Reduce the total amount of fat you consume. A diet high in fat may be a factor in breast, colon, and prostate cancers.

3. Eat more high-fiber foods such as whole grain cereals, fruits, and vegetables. It may reduce the incidence of cancer of the colon.

4. Eat foods with high amounts of vitamin A and C daily. Sweet potatoes, oranges, spinach, peaches, apricots, carrots, grapefruit, strawberries, peppers, and other yellow and dark green vegetables supply these vitamins and may help reduce the risk of cancer in the larynx, esophagus, and lung. Do not use excessive vitamin A supplements because of the potential toxic buildup.

5. Eat cruciferous vegetables in your diet. Cruciferous vegetables include cauliflower, brussels sprouts, broccoli, and cabbage.

6. Eat low amounts of salt-cured, smoked, and nitrate-cured foods such as hams, pork, or bacon. There is more incidence of cancer of the esophagus and stomach in those who eat high amounts of these foods.

7. If you drink alcohol, drink only moderate amounts and especially do not drink in conjunction with the use of tobacco. Use of alcohol in conjunction with tobacco in any form increases cancer in the upper digestive areas and liver.

Used by permission, American Cancer Society, Inc.

Strategies for the Prevention of Cancer

1. Reduce exposure to sunlight and tanning salons especially if fair skinned.

2. Wear a strong sunblock (number 15) when in the sun.

3. When possible, avoid breathing polluted air. If necessary wear face mask or air filter due to chronic or occupational exposure.

4. Do not smoke any form of drug.

5. Avoid refined sugars, flours, and other forms of junk food.

6. Eat a low-fat diet.

7. Avoid carcinogenic (cancer-causing) chemicals found in some processed foods (i.e., sodium nitrite in bologna, hams, and bacon) and other sources (i.e., vinyl chloride, insecticides, and others). See the chapter on environmental health for a more comprehensive list of chemical carcinogens.

8. Avoid X rays, when possible.

9. Avoid obesity.

10. Keep alcohol consumption moderate if you drink.

11. Include vegetables from the cruciferous vegetables (broccoli, brussels sprouts, cauliflower, and cabbage) family in your diet.

12. Do not smoke cigarettes.

13. Eat plenty of fiber.

14. Practice monthly breast self-examination.

15. Have a pap test annually.

16. Have an annual test for colorectal cancer, especially after the age of fifty.

17. Practice regular testicular examination.

18. Have a regular physical examination from a physician.

19. And note the warning signs of cancer (below):

   C Change in bowel or bladder habits

   A A sore that does not heal

   U Unusual bleeding or discharge

   T Thickening or lump in breast or elsewhere

   I Indigestion or difficulty in swallowing

   O Obvious change in wart or mole

   N Nagging cough or hoarseness

Used by permission, American Cancer Society, Inc.

Performing a Three-Minute Testicular Self-Examination

The time to examine the testicles is when the scrotum is loose, relaxed, and warm (e.g., during a shower or bath). Roll each testicle gently between the thumb and fingers of both hands, and if you find any hard lumps or nodules or any changes from the previous examination in surface contours, then check with your physician soon. Do this exam monthly.

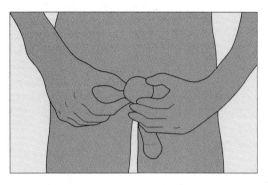 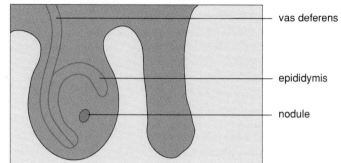

Used by permission, American Cancer Society, Inc.

The Difference Between a Melanoma and an Ordinary Mole

A normal mole is an evenly colored brown, tan, or black spot in the skin. It is either flat or raised. Its shape is round or oval and it has sharply defined borders (fig. 13.A).

Here's the simple ABCD rule to help you remember the important signs of melanoma:

A. **Asymmetry.** One half does not match the other half (fig. 13.B).

B. **Border irregularity.** The edges are ragged, notched, or blurred (fig. 13.C).

C. **Color.** The pigmentation is not uniform. Shades of tan, brown, and black are present. Red, white, and blue may add to the mottled appearance (fig. 13.D).

D. **Diameter greater than six millimeters.** Any sudden or continuing increase in size should be of special concern (fig. 13.E).

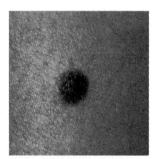 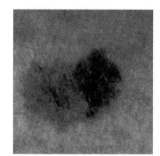 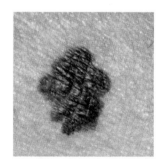

Figure 13.A   **Figure 13.B**   **Figure 13.C**

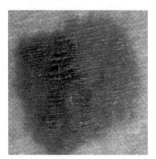 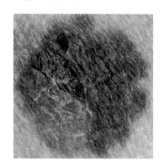

Figure 13.D   **Figure 13.E**

Source: Courtesy of the American Cancer Society.

The Devastation of Melanoma

Gregg was a high school athlete who became a coach, married, and had five children. He became an FBI agent. He was tall, strong, and a good father. Gregg had a mole on his back that he didn't watch carefully. When he and his wife finally noticed that it looked strange, melanoma had already progressed to the second stage of the disease, which is an infection of the lymph nodes. Gregg had some fifty operations on the lymph nodes to remove cancerous lumps. Unfortunately, it did not stop the disease. It progressed to the third stage and moved into the bloodstream and attacked the vital organs. Gregg went through chemotherapy. He lost his hair, vomited regularly, could not hold food down, and it almost killed him. He survived the chemotherapy and hoped that the disease was arrested. The disease did go into remission for a short time, but finally after three years of agony for Gregg and his family, he died. He had good insurance and was able to relocate his family near extended family members, but he left a widow and five children, ages five through seventeen, to recover from the three years of misery.

Gregg's wife, Joy, now looks at the positive aspects of the experience. During those three years, they became closer than they ever were, and her religious convictions have become stronger. Her children still feel like they have been cheated.

Could this devastation have been avoided? Maybe. Survivability increases the earlier cancer is detected. Joy now checks each child regularly for any of the danger signals of cancer.

Diabetes Mellitus

Diabetes mellitus, with an annual death toll of about thirty-five thousand, is the seventh leading cause of death in the United States (Robbins and Kumar 1987). It is difficult to know exactly how many people have diabetes in the United States. This is because there are varying degrees of the disease, and many people have diabetes but do not know it, but it is estimated at about fifteen million Americans (Randal 1992). The estimate means that 1 percent to 2 percent of the population has diabetes. There has been a dramatic increase in the number of people diagnosed with diabetes, which has been estimated at approximately 600,000 each year, representing a 6 percent annual increase. A major reason is the survivability of those with the disease. At the turn of the century, before insulin was prescribed, those with diabetes died at an early age, before they had the opportunity to have children. With the discovery of insulin, diabetics can live long and productive lives and bear children. These children of diabetics are carriers of the diabetic genes, although not all are diabetic. Genetic researchers may have found the diabetic gene, which provides hope for diabetics in the future (Bishop 1991).

Understanding Diabetes

Diabetes mellitus is a chronic disorder affecting the natural metabolism of carbohydrates, fats, and protein (Robbins and Kumar 1987). The cause of the ineffective use of carbohydrates in particular is defective or deficient insulin production. **Insulin** is a hormone produced by the pancreas that has several functions, including protein synthesis, glycogen (the form in which carbohydrates are stored in the body) formation in the liver and muscles, and glucose (simple sugar formed from carbohydrates) conversion to triglycerides (fats). The most critical function as it relates to diabetes is that insulin facilitates the crossing of glucose across cell membranes so that the cells can use the glucose for energy. Insulin is normally released into the bloodstream when blood glucose levels are high. This means the insulin functions to reduce the level of blood sugar by transporting it into the cells or storing it for later use. In diabetes, the lack of insulin results in the buildup of dangerously high levels of sugar in the blood.

The inability to use the sugar in the blood is accompanied by the breakdown of glycogen (stored form of carbohydrates) to additional blood sugar, which is normally inhibited by insulin. The high sugar level results in the overload of the kidneys, which are trying to reabsorb the glucose, and the result is excretion of sugar in the urine. Since sugar can't be used for energy, the major sources become fatty acids stored in fat deposits. In the liver, fatty acids are oxidized into ketone bodies, which are used by the muscle, heart, kidney, and brain. In type I diabetes, in particular, the formation of ketone bodies may exceed the rate of their utilization. **Ketosis** may result, which is excessive ketone bodies to the point of becoming toxic, which can lead to coma and death. Since tissues seem to be starving for glucose, protein supplies from the diet and tissues are diverted from their primary function of building to breaking down proteins to be used as an energy source for the cells.

Type I and Type II Diabetes

Type I diabetes, also called insulin-dependent diabetes mellitus (IDDM), was formerly called juvenile onset diabetes. It accounts for 10 percent to 15 percent of all diabetic cases. Type I diabetes is the more severe form of diabetes, characterized by an absolute lack of insulin. This is due to a reduction in the **beta cells** mass in the pancreas. These diabetics require supplemental insulin for survival. The loss of beta cells is thought to be caused by an interaction of environmental influences (viruses, stress), genetic vulnerability, and autoimmunity (Robbins and Kumar 1987).

Type II diabetes, also called noninsulin-dependent diabetes mellitus (NIDDM), accounts for 85 percent to 90 percent of all diabetic cases. This form of diabetes is not as severe and generally occurs later in life (generally after forty). Insulin is produced by the beta cells but is insufficient to deal with the glucose load. Often, strict diets, weight loss, and exercise can control type II diabetes. Warning signs of diabetes are shown in table 13.3.

Causes of Diabetes

Diabetes mellitus, in part, is a genetic disorder, but the direct method of inheriting the trait is not known. Until recently, it was assumed that there was a single pattern of genetic predisposition for both type I and type II diabetes, but studies with identical twins reveal that there is a difference. Among identical twins, there is a 50 percent chance that both twins will be affected, but for type II diabetes there is a 90 percent chance that both will be affected. This means that there are environmental influences, particularly for type I diabetes.

A number of factors may contribute to diabetes among those who are genetically predisposed. Viral infections such as mumps, measles, and mononucleosis have been implicated for many years as attackers, directly or indirectly, of beta cells to reduce their mass and ability to produce insulin.

Most important among type II diabetics is obesity. Approximately 80 percent of type II diabetics are obese. Sometimes, when type II diabetics attain an optimal weight, their symptoms of diabetes go away. Pregnancy, as a stress on the body, may result in temporary diabetes, and the body reverts to normal after the baby is delivered. Other major stressors, including trauma, infections, and hyperthermia, may unmask diabetes in those harboring the hereditary trait. It is well known that insulin requirements increase under stress.

TABLE 13.3

The Warning Signs of Diabetes

The following symptoms are typical. However, some people with noninsulin-dependent diabetes have symptoms so mild they go unnoticed.

Insulin-Dependent Diabetes	Noninsulin-Dependent Diabetes
(usually occur suddenly)	(usually occur less suddenly)
Frequent urination	Any of the insulin-dependent symptoms
Excessive thirst	Recurring or hard-to-heal skin, gum, or bladder infections
Extreme hunger	
Dramatic weight loss	Drowsiness
Irritability	Blurred vision
Weakness and fatigue	Tingling or numbness in hands or feet
Nausea and vomiting	
	Itching

Reprinted with permission from the American Diabetes Association. Copyright © 1984 by the American Diabetes Association.

The classic symptoms of the disease include the three "polys": polyuria (passage of excessive amounts of urine), polyphagia (excessive eating), and polydipsia (excessive thirst). The three polys are accompanied by weight loss, fuzzy vision, and fatigue.

Outcomes of Diabetes

The detrimental outcomes of diabetes depend on two factors: the severity of the disease and duration of the disease. Most problems result from the vascular system, as indicated by the fact that 80 percent of diabetics die from vascular disorders. Diabetics with the disease for fifteen or more years probably display one or more of the following conditions in mild or severe forms:

1. Myocardial infarction caused by atherosclerosis of the coronary arteries is the most common cause of death in diabetics.
2. Hypertension is more prevalent and severe in diabetics.
3. Kidneys are prime targets for diabetes. Renal failure is second only to myocardial infarction as a cause of death. Atherosclerosis of the kidneys and inflammation of the kidneys also occur.
4. Visual impairment and sometimes total blindness results from the thickening of capillaries of the retina of the eye.
5. Neuropathy is a disease of the peripheral nervous system, generally of the lower extremities and resulting in motor and sensory disfunction (e.g., sexual impotence, bladder and bowel dysfunctions).
6. Stroke, which again results from vascular problems.

7. Gangrene of the extremities from the lack of adequate blood supply to the hands and feet.

Decisions for Prevention

With autoimmune disorders such as diabetes, specific strategies for prevention are difficult to recommend. It is helpful to maintain ideal weight and eat nutritious food. Scientists at Berkeley and Stanford universities offer direct evidence that physical activity may help prevent noninsulin-dependent diabetes ("Running Away from Diabetes" 1992).

Studies with mice have provided other suggestions for prevention. Some Boston researchers identified two types of immune cells with opposing effects that determine whether diabetes-prone mice develop the disease. By injecting the mice with a toxin that destroys the cell type that destroys the body's insulin factories, they have tipped the balance in favor of the insulin-protecting cell type, halting diabetes onset. In the future, individuals with a predisposition to diabetes may receive an injection to prevent the onset of diabetes (Cowen 1990).

Hypoglycemia

Hypoglycemia is low blood sugar, which is just the opposite of the hyperglycemia, or high blood sugar, evident in diabetes. Hypoglycemia reflects a malfunction of the body's mechanisms that regulate glucose balance. It may result from a variety of causes and is accurately diagnosed by a glucose-tolerance test. Symptoms include anxiety, hunger, heart palpitations, sweating, headache, weakness, and fatigue. Those who suffer from hypoglycemia are subject to emotional mood swings, depression, and trouble thinking and recalling.

Individuals suffering from this disorder are usually helped with a strict diet regimen. Frequent small meals that are high in protein and include starches rather than simple sugars often bring about marked improvement of symptoms.

Kidney Disease

The normal human being has two kidneys located in the small of the back along both sides of the spine. They perform the vital processes of removing fluids and waste compounds from the blood and regulating the internal body chemistry by selective excretion or retention of various compounds. More than eighteen gallons of blood pass through the human kidneys each hour, carrying nutrients to the body's tissues and waste products from the tissues, as well as transporting compounds necessary for internal chemical balance.

Each kidney has more than a million microscopic filters called **glomeruli.** If these filters cease functioning, the body retains increasing amounts of water, salt, and other substances. The body tissues then begin to swell, and waste products accumulate, causing a condition called **uremia.** If uremia grows progressively worse, death can result (Robbins and Kumar 1987).

1. If the person is conscious, ask if he or she is diabetic and if you can help.

2. If the person is not conscious, check to see if there is some form of identification by looking on the wrist or seeing if he or she is wearing a diabetic bracelet. Call for medical help.

3. If the person is having an *insulin reaction* or insulin shock, he or she has not eaten enough food, has exercised too hard, or has received too high a dose of insulin. If the person is conscious, he or she may experience emotional changes, headache, numbness, poor coordination, slurred speech, a staggering gait, a cold sweat, and rapid heart beat. Many diabetics having a reaction have been falsely cited for driving while intoxicated. Provide the diabetic some candy or fruit juice, sugared (not diet) pop, or another sugar drink. Oftentimes the person has candy or honey packets. If unconscious, call for medical help and do not give the person anything he or she would have to swallow. A sugar cube under the tongue is okay if carefully observed and may help (Thygerson 1986).

4. *Diabetic coma* can result from overindulgence in food, too little insulin, injury, or decreased activity. The high blood sugar and ketosis cause the breath to have a peculiar sweetish odor. The diabetic may be thirsty, have abdominal pain or nausea, and vomiting may occur. You can provide fluids and get medical help.

5. If you can't distinguish between diabetic coma and a diabetic reaction, try giving the person a small amount of sugar, recognizing that the sugar helps the reaction, yet the small amount of sugar does not have a measurable effect on the diabetic coma (Thygerson 1986).

Warning Signs of Kidney Disease

Several of the kidney diseases can be diagnosed at an early stage if we clearly understand the warning signs and promptly seek medical help. The warning signs of kidney disease are as follows: (1) swelling of body parts, especially the ankles; (2) lower back pain, just below the rib cage; (3) puffiness, especially around the eyes and particularly in children; (4) increased frequency or changes in the pattern of urination; (5) pain or unusual sensation associated with urination and bloody or tea-colored urine; and (6) high blood pressure, affecting the efficiency of the body's waste-elimination process (Robbins and Kumar 1987).

Diagnosis and Treatment of Acute Kidney Disease

The symptoms listed previously may indicate an acute kidney disease, but only a physician can know for sure. Laboratory tests will confirm this. Treatment of acute kidney disease and some less serious chronic kidney disease includes diet, drugs, and sometimes surgery. The diet is modified to lower the intake of salt, water, and protein because the kidneys cannot do their job. Diuretics are used to help avoid fluid buildup in the body, and antibiotics are given to control any infection that might be present. In cases where problems are caused by birth defects, any obstructions are surgically removed.

Chronic Kidney Disease and Kidney Failure

In patients with chronic kidney disease, kidney function deteriorates gradually. When the kidneys fail, the individual has two courses of action: kidney transplantation or hemodialysis. A **kidney transplant** can be performed successfully in the patient who has lost most or all kidney function. A major reason that more kidney transplants are not done is that the kidney tissue of the donor and recipient must be matched. Many medical centers have waiting lists, and potential recipients must go on hemodialysis until a donated organ with a compatible tissue type becomes available. A donor and recipient who are closely related usually have the best chance for compatible tissue types and successful transplantation. The principal barrier to successful transplantation is the body's own immune system. If the defensive immune response of the body is not suppressed, it can destroy the foreign tissue within a short time. The development of more effective and less toxic drugs to suppress the destructive immune response has increased the chances of successful transplantation.

Hemodialysis is the only hope of survival for a large number of persons who suffer from kidney failure. Hemodialysis is performed by an artificial kidney machine, a machine that takes over the blood-purifying function of the damaged kidneys. The machine is connected through a tube to the patient's arm or leg. The blood flows through the machine to be cleansed and is then returned through another tube to the patient's blood vessel. Dialysis treatments are administered several times per week for a period of approximately nine hours (Burton and Martin 1978).

Chronic Diseases of the Respiratory System

Chronic respiratory disease is usually caused by inhaling a harmful substance, such as bacteria, industrial pollutants, or organic matter to which you may be allergic. Major diseases include chronic bronchitis, emphysema, and asthma.

Chronic Disease

The likelihood of your experiencing chronic disease in your life depends partly on your genetic predisposition and partly on your health actions of mind, body, and soul and their interdependence. It is extremely important to take action to maximize your potential to avoid cardiovascular disease, cancer, and the other chronic diseases cited in this chapter. Between two people of equal hereditary risk for a chronic disease, the person with positive states of mind, body, soul, and interdependence will resist chronic disease better than the person with negative states. Consider the following suggestions for mind, body, and soul and their interdependence in avoiding chronic disease.

Mind

When problems and negative situations arise in your life, you will either effectively handle the problem or struggle with it over time. The ability to do self-counseling and creative personal problem solving, to mange time, and to perform the other skills of the mind described in chapter 2 determines whether you resolve, learn, and grow from the problem or negative situation or whether you end up frustrated, upset, and depressed. Enhance your creative personal problem-solving abilities, your ability to manage time effectively, and your ability to ask yourself good questions and then come up with solutions. The positive mind state that results will help you control your problems and you will be able to fortify your immune system to prevent chronic disease.

Body

You may notice that the physical prevention strategies for all chronic diseases, including heart disease, cancer, arthritis, and diabetes, are common for all diseases. If you (1) attain and maintain optimal weight, (2) do aerobic exercise four to five times a week for a duration of thirty minutes, (3) eat regular, low-fat, high-fiber, high-complex-carbohydrate, balanced meals, (4) do flexibility and strength maintenance exercises, and (5) get adequate rest and sleep, then the likelihood of experiencing chronic disease is greatly lessened. In addition, the quality of your life will be greatly improved.

Soul

Positive states of the soul also help you avoid chronic disease and ensure a higher quality of life. To love others, to feel loved, and to have a means of releasing pent up emotions such as anger in positive ways (walking it off) can fortify your defenses against chronic disease. A spiritual orientation and faith in positive forces greater than yourself also help. From psychoneuroimmunology (PNI) we know that a fighting spirit, optimism, hope, and a good laugh periodically fortify the body against chronic disease. Reflect on those skills of the soul described in chapter 2 and adopt them into your life-style.

Interdependence

It may be hard to believe, but a guard against disease is to provide service to others. Case studies in PNI have shown that even watching humanitarian acts (Mother Teresa doing service to people in India) fortifies the immune system. In your own life, doing acts of service and expressing unconditional love to others (giving without any expectation of receiving) not only makes you feel good emotionally, but it also helps to fortify your body.

Chronic bronchitis results from chronic inflammation in the bronchi of the lungs, which causes mucus to form, with resultant coughing. In many instances, this disease is due to cigarette smoking. It often precedes or occurs concurrently with emphysema (Purtilo 1978).

Emphysema is a form of lung disease that takes a number of years to develop. Emphysema is characterized by overinflation of the lungs and the destruction of the alveoli (air sacs), which is the site where gases are exchanged between the lungs and the bloodstream. Few people under the age of fifty have emphysema, but the average age is getting lower, probably because many people are starting to smoke at an early age. Overstretched air sacs and an inability to breathe normally are characteristic of the disease. At first, the shortness of breath is hardly noticeable, but the condition gradually worsens until the victim has to limit physical activity. A person with advanced emphysema is often unable to walk up a flight of stairs without stopping (Robbins and Kumar 1987).

Asthma occurs because of a hypersensitivity (allergy) to a particular substance or substances. When the allergic person inhales this substance, the lungs' airways narrow, and mucous tends to form and obstruct the airways; exhaling is impaired, and wheezing occurs.

Warning Signs of Respiratory Disease

Numerous signs and symptoms can indicate respiratory problems. Shortness of breath is a warning signal if it occurs during everyday activities that have not caused breathing difficulty in the past. Coughing may also be a significant symptom, especially if it lasts for any period of time. Sputum production (particularly in the early morning) and coughed-up blood are signs of a serious problem that should receive medical attention. Chest pain can have a number of causes, including chronic lung disorders or infection, and should be reported to a physician.

Decisions for Prevention

You can protect your lungs and other organs of the respiratory system in various ways. First and foremost, you can decide not to smoke. Second, you can work to keep the atmosphere clean, since environmental pollutants can damage the respiratory system. If you work in an atmosphere with pollutants, wear a mask to protect the respiratory system. You can avoid becoming overweight, because the heavier you are, the harder your lungs must work.

Genetic Disease

Genetic diseases are disorders of the hereditary material—the genes and chromosomes. Those with genetic diseases are either born with the disorder or born with a susceptibility to develop the disorder later in life. Some genetic diseases are inherited in a complex manner involving multiple genes. Others involve multiple genes plus certain environmental factors. About 20 percent of all birth defects are genetically induced, 20 percent are environmentally influenced, and the rest result from the interaction of heredity and environment.

Genetic diseases create the nation's most serious child health problem. The defects that occur are characterized by abnormalities of body structures and/or functions.

Detection and Diagnosis

Physicians can now detect many birth defects and genetic abnormalities before birth. Detection techniques include **amniocentesis,** which is the analysis of the amniotic fluid taken from the intrauterine environment; **ultrasound,** which involves the use of sound waves; and **fetoscopy,** the insertion of a viewing instrument into the womb to observe the fetus. Physicians can plan treatment before the baby is born, if necessary; they can determine fetal maturity to eliminate birth hazards; or they can suggest abortion in cases of severe problems.

Relatively few genetic defects can be completely corrected, but many can be treated to slow, stop, or partly reverse harmful effects. Available types of treatment include corrective surgery; chemical regulation by drugs, hormones, vitamins, and dietary supplements; transplantation, including bone marrow for immune-deficiency disorders; and rehabilitative training to help compensate for mental, physical, and sensory handicaps.

Decisions for Prevention

For couples who suspect that their future children may be at risk of inheriting a disorder, genetic counseling is a necessity. One or both parents may know of a particular defect in the family history or may belong to an ethnic group at relatively high risk for a specific disease. If there is some risk of a defect, a genetic counselor can define the odds and explain the potential for treatment or care if the couple chooses to have children. This decision is one that only the parents can make, but they should have access to all the latest information before making their choice.

Arthritis

Arthritis is humanity's oldest known chronic disease. There are several types, all of which attack the body's joints, and the effects vary from slight pain to severe crippling and total disability. The word *arthritis* means inflammation of a joint. The three most common types are rheumatoid arthritis, osteoarthritis, and gout.

Rheumatoid arthritis is the most difficult rheumatic disease to control and can do the most damage to the joints. The condition usually begins between the ages of twenty and fifty, with twice as many women as men afflicted. It generally affects many joints but most commonly the small joints of the hands. Joint inflammation causes pain and swelling and, if uncontrolled, may cause destruction of the bones, deformity, and eventual disability. Its course is unpredictable. It flares up suddenly (perhaps the result of emotional distress) and just as suddenly returns to remission. Usually, the first signs are fatigue, muscle stiffness (especially in the morning), and joint pain. Painful swelling begins, with nodules from the size of a pea to a walnut appearing under the skin. Joint motion is gradually lost and deformities occur.

Osteoarthritis seems to result from a combination of wear and tear on the joints and other unknown factors. It is much more common and less damaging than rheumatoid arthritis. Older people most frequently develop osteoarthritis. The disease is characterized by degeneration of the joint cartilage. The cartilage develops small cracks and wears unevenly. Disability most often results from disease in the weight-bearing joints of the knees, hips, and spine. Common symptoms are pain and stiffness, especially in the fingers and in the joints that bear the body's weight.

Gout is the easiest form of arthritis to detect and treat and is the best understood. It usually occurs in men and commonly affects the joints of the feet, particularly the big toe. Gout results from the deposit of too much uric acid (a body chemical) in the tissues. Uric acid crystals form in the joints, causing inflammation and severe pain. Attacks of gout may follow minor injury, excessive eating or drinking, overexercise, or surgery. Sudden attacks often occur for no apparent reason and may last for days or weeks.

Diagnosis and Treatment of Arthritis

Accurate diagnosis of rheumatoid arthritis can be made only by a physician after a careful physical examination. The treatment regime may include rest, physical therapy (including heat and corrective exercises), one of many drugs that control pain and inflammation, and, in some cases, surgery. The same general methods of diagnosis, treatment, and care are used for osteoarthritis. Surgical correction of deformed weight-bearing joints, especially the hips, has been effective in helping many osteoarthritic patients walk again without pain.

Gout responds more satisfactorily to treatment and is more effectively controlled than the other types of arthritis. The goal of treatment is to reduce the level of uric acid in the blood through drug therapy (Arthritis Foundation 1986). Exercise is recommended for arthritis sufferers, preferably in water (Levin 1991).

Decisions for Prevention

Although it is not yet possible to cure rheumatoid arthritis, it is possible for patients to cope successfully. The prime objective of treatment is to prevent joint destruction. The possibility of remission makes it crucial that all efforts are made to prevent joint destruction during the active stage. Rheumatoid arthritis usually lasts a lifetime; therefore, physicians try to avoid the use of toxic drugs as much as possible. This demands that patients undergo treatment with lesser drugs at the earliest sign of occurrence. If rheumatoid arthritis is diagnosed early, and if prompt and individualized treatment is begun, severe crippling can usually be prevented or minimized.

Since osteoarthritis results from wear and tear on the joints, any protective care we can give our joints may deter the onset of this disease. This includes attention to weight, poor posture, or injury or strain from your occupation or recreation.

Drugs can reduce excessive uric acid in the blood and prevent further attacks of gout. Though medical treatment is the most important area in the management of this disease, life-style also affects gout to some extent. Persons susceptible to gout should avoid or limit alcoholic beverages, maintain normal weight, get sufficient exercise, and avoid using drugs that are not absolutely necessary, because many drugs elevate the uric acid level (Arthritis Foundation 1986).

Summary

1. Prevention can be divided into three stages: primary prevention (taking steps to avoid the disease before symptoms occur), secondary prevention (treatment at an early stage of the disease), and tertiary prevention (rehabilitation).

2. Risk factors associated with heart disease include smoking cigarettes, obesity, hypertension, a diet high in fats and cholesterol, high cholesterol, and lack of exercise.

3. Heart attack is the nation's number-one killer.

4. Stroke is a devastating disease characterized by a sudden loss of brain function that can lead to paralysis, loss of speech, and even death.

5. Other types of heart disease include rheumatic heart disease, congenital heart disease, and congestive heart failure.

6. The latest advances in cardiovascular medicine include heart transplantation, Jarvik 7 and 7–70 artificial hearts, cardiovascular risk identification and reduction, and angioplasty.

7. Cancer is characterized by uncontrolled growth and spread of abnormal, or malignant, cells.

8. The cause of cancer is unknown, but risk factors are poor diet, exposure to industrial chemicals, smoking, ultraviolet light, and others.

9. The major sites of cancer include the skin, colon, lungs, rectum, breast, uterus, and mouth.

10. Treatment and research in cancer include chemotherapy, radiation treatment, and experimental studies using interferon and genetic engineering.

11. Diabetes mellitus is a disorder in which the body does not produce enough insulin, which enables the sugar in the blood to reach the cells for energy.

12. There are two types of diabetes: type I, which is insulin-dependent diabetes, and type II, which is noninsulin-dependent diabetes.

13. Diabetes has warning signs and treatments. In addition, first aid for diabetics is important to know.

14. A number of different diseases can attack the kidneys, potentially leading to chronic kidney disease and kidney failure.

15. Chronic respiratory disease may be environmentally induced by cigarette smoking and industrial pollutants.

16. Genetic diseases cause more health problems for young children than any other type of disease. Many genetic diseases can be detected before birth.

17. Various diseases affect the neuromuscular-skeletal systems, the most common of which affect the joints of the body, including osteoarthritis, rheumatoid arthritis, and gout.

Commitment Activities

1. Learn to take blood pressure. It is likely that someone else in the class knows how. Ask your instructor to provide some sphygmomanometers and stethoscopes so you can learn. After you know how to take it, you can purchase a blood pressure kit so you can monitor your blood pressure throughout your life.

2. As you prepare to do your life-style contract in this section, become aware of the available resources in your community to help you. You and your class may want to go to the American Heart Association to help you understand how to modify the cholesterol or salt in your diet, lose weight (see the chapter on weight control), quit smoking (see the chapter on tobacco), or control blood pressure. This organization has several pamphlets to help you reduce the risks of heart disease.

3. There are often clubs or meetings of people who have experienced bypass operations or who are rehabilitating from heart attacks. Either attend one of the meetings or invite someone who has had one of these operations to talk to your class.

4. Many who suffer heart attacks are saved by those who are trained to do CPR. The local chapters of the American Heart Association and American Red Cross

offer CPR classes. It is well advised that you take the opportunity to become trained in CPR. It is likely that your college or university has classes in first aid and CPR. You never know when you will need this skill.

5. Gather information about organizations in your community that help women who have had mastectomies and parents of children with leukemia. Offer some hours to help spread information about the work of these organizations.

6. Genetic counseling should be available to all persons in the community. Determine where genetic counseling is available in your community. If such counseling is not available at your university health center, perhaps you could help develop a program. If it is available, what kinds of promotional activities can help students become aware of this service?

7. Find out if any industries in your area produce carcinogens. Which carcinogens are produced? What has the industry done to lower risk or inform employees of the risk involved? Is there a risk to the community?

8. If you have not had a physical examination in the last year, decide to have one before the end of this semester. Develop a list of questions to ask your doctor about your own personal risk with respect to the diseases covered in this chapter.

References

American Cancer Society. *1990 Cancer Facts and Figures.* New York: American Cancer Society, 1990.

American Heart Association. *After a Heart Attack.* Dallas, Tex.: American Heart Association, 1986.

American Heart Association. *How You Can Help Your Doctor Treat Your High Blood Pressure.* Dallas, Tex.: American Heart Association, 1986.

American Heart Association. *1992 Heart and Stroke Fact Statistics.* Dallas, Tex.: American Heart Association, 1992.

Arthritis Foundation. *Basic Facts: Answers to Your Questions.* Atlanta, Ga.: Arthritis Medical Information Series, 1986.

Bishop, J. E. "Gene that Causes a Diabetes Type May Be Found." *Wall Street Journal,* February 15, 1991, p. 84(w), B2.

Burton, B., and Martin, A. A. "What You Should Know About Kidney Dialysis." *Pharmacy Times* (January 1978).

Cowen, R. "Mouse Study Suggests Diabetes Prevention." *Science News* 137 (March 31, 1990): 198.

Grieger, L. "MDs Hit FDA Restrictions on Artificial Heart Cases." *American Medical News* (February 21, 1986).

Humble, C. G. "Oats and Cholesterol: The Prospects for Prevention of Heart Disease." *American Journal of Public Health* 81, no. 2 (February 1991):159–60.

Jones, L. "House Panel Puts FDA Regulation of Medical Devices under Scrutiny." *American Medical News* 33 (March 9, 1990):2–3.

Levin, S. "Aquatic Therapy." *The Physician and Sportsmedicine* 19, no. 10 (October 1991):119–24.

Levy, R. I., and Moskowitz, J. "Cardiovascular Research: Decades of Progress, a Decade of Promise." *Science* 217 (1982):121–29.

Merz, B. "FDA Cities Deficiencies, Withdraws Approval for Jarvik 7 Artificial Heart." *American Medical News* 33 (January 26, 1990):1–2.

Olson, D. "ISAO International Registry: Bridge-to-Transplant Experience with the Jarvik 7 and the Jarvik 7–70 Total Artificial Heart." *Artificial Organs* 11, no. 1 (1987):63–68.

Purtilo, D. T. *A Survey of Human Diseases.* Reading, Mass.: Addison-Wesley, 1978.

Randal, J. "Insulin Key to Diabetes But Not Full Cure." *FDA Consumer,* 26, no. 4 (May 1992):15–20.

Robbins, S. L., and Kumar, V. *Basic Pathology.* Philadelphia: W. B. Saunders, 1987.

"Running Away from Diabetes." *Berkeley Wellness Newsletter* 8, no. 4 (January 1992):6.

Russell, M.; Cooper, M. L.; Frone, M. R.; and Welte, J. W. "Alcohol Drinking Patterns and Blood Pressure." *American Journal of Public Health* 81, no. 4 (April 1991):452.

Saltus, R. "Genetic Damage and Skin Cancer." *Technology Review* 95, no. 2 (February-March 1992):11–12.

Thygerson, A. L. *The First Aid Book.* Englewood Cliffs, N.J.: Prentice-Hall, 1986.

Additional Readings

American Cancer Society readings are many and very good, including the following. Each of these booklets contains information about the incidence, types, prevention, treatment, and prognosis of each of the types of cancer.

Facts on Bladder Cancer

Facts on Bone Cancer

Facts on Breast Cancer

Facts on Cancer of the Brain

Facts on Cancer of the Larynx

Facts on Childhood Cancer

Facts on Colorectal Cancer

Facts on Hodgkin's Disease

Facts on Leukemia

Facts on Lung Cancer

Facts on Lymphomas and Multiple Myeloma

Facts on Oral Cancer

PNI: Choices and Disease

Psychoneuroimmunology (PNI) is the study of the interaction of the mind, the central nervous system, and the body's immunological system. It has been shown that people with a fighting spirit, optimism, hope, and faith can actually build their immune systems. The brain has the capability to self-medicate and to release a variety of mental and physical painkillers and motivating substances (neuropeptides) when the demand is there.

You have learned in these chapters on disease that there are some things you can do to help prevent disease, such as avoiding contact with microorganisms, practicing "safer" sex, maintaining immunizations, having regular medical examinations, eating nutritiously (high fiber, low fat, low salt, low sugar), exercising, controlling stress, monitoring cholesterol and hypertension levels, avoiding tobacco and drugs, maintaining ideal weight, and reducing your exposure to sun and other carcinogens. Even if you are living an optimal life-style, the fact is, because of genetics and other uncontrolled variables, you may still get sick. So, what does PNI tell us?

Most of the research in PNI has been with diseases. AIDS patients have lived longer with positive mental states, patients have helped to throw cancer into remission believing that treatment will work, and immune systems have been fortified because people just didn't have time to get sick.

It is important to note here a major caution. How you think can in fact either weaken or fortify your immune system. This is *not* to suggest that you can think diseases away, but you can help the process. If you are sick, *it is important to follow a physician's treatment plan,* but you can supplement the plan by believing that treatment will work, that with proper treatment you will overcome the problem, and that mentally you will feel medicines and treatments working. If you are not sick, *it does not mean that you do not need periodic physician examinations* just because you are thinking yourself well. It means that positive thinking helps to keep you well.

Consider the following suggestions to help fortify you against disease and to help you when you become sick.

1. Believe in the treatment prescribed by your physician or, for minor illnesses, believe in your personal therapy (bed rest, positive thinking, etc.). For an illness, you may receive a prescription from your physician, such as penicillin for strep throat; then you should start with positive thoughts. When you take the prescription, feel it working, imagine the pain going away, believe that it will work, and feel yourself becoming stronger, overcoming the illness.

2. Formulate a cause in your life. Work vigorously toward some goal, whether it be your studies, athletics, service, or another cause that demands that you function optimally. This is not to be frustrating or overloading, but something that is exciting for you. Make yourself comfortably too busy to get sick. Many case studies have

been reported that, while working vigorously on a project, performance, or other cause, people may have been tired but not sick. At the moment when the performance was through, they would take a deep breath and relax. Shortly, they would feel a cold, sore throat, or other minor illness.

3. When you do behaviors to make you feel healthier (exercise, eat high-fiber foods, meditate, etc.), do some imagery and picture the power of the positive behavior. Imagine the fiber cleaning the digestive system, the exercise clearing arteries and expelling all the stress, and meditation calming and allowing your body to rebuild.

4. Challenge yourself. Do something you haven't tried and work at it until you do it well. Try a new activity such as skiing, roller blading, playing an instrument, speed reading, etc.

5. If you get sick, you may want to try repeated imagery. As you lay in bed with the illness, picture your immune system attacking the foreign antigens, imagine the battle, and see yourself winning. Repeat the scenarios until you feel better.

Life-Style Contract

After reading and pondering the last two chapters, you should have a good understanding of:

1. the nature and devastating consequences of communicable, cardiovascular, and other chronic diseases and cancer;
2. how to prevent some of the diseases through life-style change;
3. the importance of taking action by becoming immunized, avoiding stress, and avoiding the consumption of food or beverages that facilitate disease.

You have been provided an opportunity to assess your health status as it relates to disease prevention. Based on the results of these assessments and information you have been provided, it becomes important for you to act on the information you have received. In a specific way, the following are some suggested behaviors that you could employ to enhance your health as it pertains to the prevention of disease.

1. Avoid mucous contact via glasses, toothbrushes, sexual intimacy, sharing needles, etc. of anyone infected with a communicable disease.
2. Before becoming sexually intimate with someone, get to know them very well—to the point that you can discuss past sexual histories.
3. Have regular physicals to determine the health of organs, the existence of any communicable diseases, or the identification of any chronic diseases for early detection and treatment.
4. Don't infect others—stay at home, cover your mouth, and keep your distance with an infectious disease.
5. Make sure you are immunized against all appropriate diseases.
6. Practice STD preventive measures.
7. Don't smoke or drink coffee.

8. Attain and maintain an ideal weight (body fat composition).
9. Reduce your cholesterol level if it is high (exercise, diet, or prescription medication).
10. Manage stress levels.
11. Monitor, and reduce if necessary, your blood pressure.
12. Eat low-fat foods and a balanced diet with lots of vegetables and fiber.
13. Avoid hazardous chemical and carcinogens (sun, asbestos, etc.).

Life-Style Contracting Using Strength Intervention

I. Choosing the desired health behavior or skill

A. Keeping in mind the purposes in life and goals you identified in the mental-health chapter, consider one or two health behaviors related to disease prevention (from the list here or your own creation) that will help you reach your goals. To assess the likelihood of success, ask yourself questions similar to those used in previous sections, such as:

1. Is my purpose, cause, or goal better realized by adoption of this behavior?
_____ yes _____ no
2. Am I hardy enough to accomplish this goal? (This means I feel I can do it if I work hard, am committed to do it, am challenged by it, and see myself in control enough to make it happen.) _____ yes _____ no
3. Is this a behavior I really want to change and that I feel I can change?
_____ yes _____ no
4. Do I first need to nurture a personal strength area? _____ yes _____ no (If yes, be sure to include this as a part of the plan.)

5. Do I need to free myself from the negative effects of a behavior (break a bad habit)? ____ yes ____ no (If yes, be sure to include this as a part of the plan.)

6. Have I considered the results of the assessments in the two previous chapters? ____ yes ____ no

(Yes answers to the first three questions are a must to be successful. It might be wise to consider a different behavior if you cannot honestly answer yes to these questions. Your answers to questions 4–6 ought to provide insights for your consideration in making your plan.)

B. Behaviors I will change (no more than two)

_____

_____

II. Life-style plan

A. A description of the general plan of what I am going to do and how I will accomplish it. Consider apperceptive experiences—successes you have had in the past—since they may help you consider the best ways to carry out this plan.

_____

_____

_____

_____

_____

_____

B. Barriers to the accomplishment of the plan (lack of time, materials, support, etc.).

1. Identify the barriers _____

_____

_____

2. Means to remove the barriers (use problem-solving skills or creative approaches such as those described in the mental-health chapter)_____

_____

_____

_____

C. Implementation of the plan.

1. Substitution (putting positive behaviors in place of negative ones)_____

_____

_____

2. Confluence (combining a mental and a physical activity for time efficiency if possible)

_____

_____

3. Systematic enhancement (using a strength to help a weakness)_____

_____

_____

4. When _____

5. Where _____

6. Preparation _____

_____

7. With whom _____

_____

_____

III. Support groups

A. Who _____

_____

_____

B. Role _____

_____

_____

C. Organized support _____

_____

IV. Trigger responses _____

_____

_____

V. Starting date _____

VI. Date/sequence the contract will be reevaluated _____

_____

VII. Evidence(s) of reaching goal _____

_____

_____

VIII. Reward(s) when contract is completed_____

_____

_____

IX. Signature of student _____

X. Signature of facilitator _____

XI. Additional conditions/comments _____

_____

_____

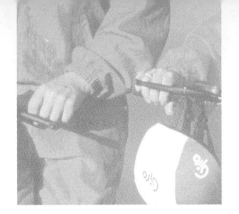

PART VI

Choices and the Aging Process

T HE QUALITY OF THE AGING PROCESS AND THE DEATH EXPERIENCE ARE TREATED IN CHAPTER 14. YOU CAN CHOOSE TO ENJOY THE PROCESS AND EXPERIENCE OF AGING. YOU CAN ALSO CHOOSE TO MAXIMIZE THE QUALITY OF YOUR AGING PROCESS BY ADOPTING HEALTHY BEHAVIORS, WHICH CAN ALSO LEAD TO A QUALITY DEATH. UNDERSTANDING THESE PRINCIPLES WILL ALSO HELP YOU BE A BETTER HELPER TO THOSE IN NEED.

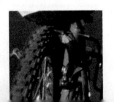

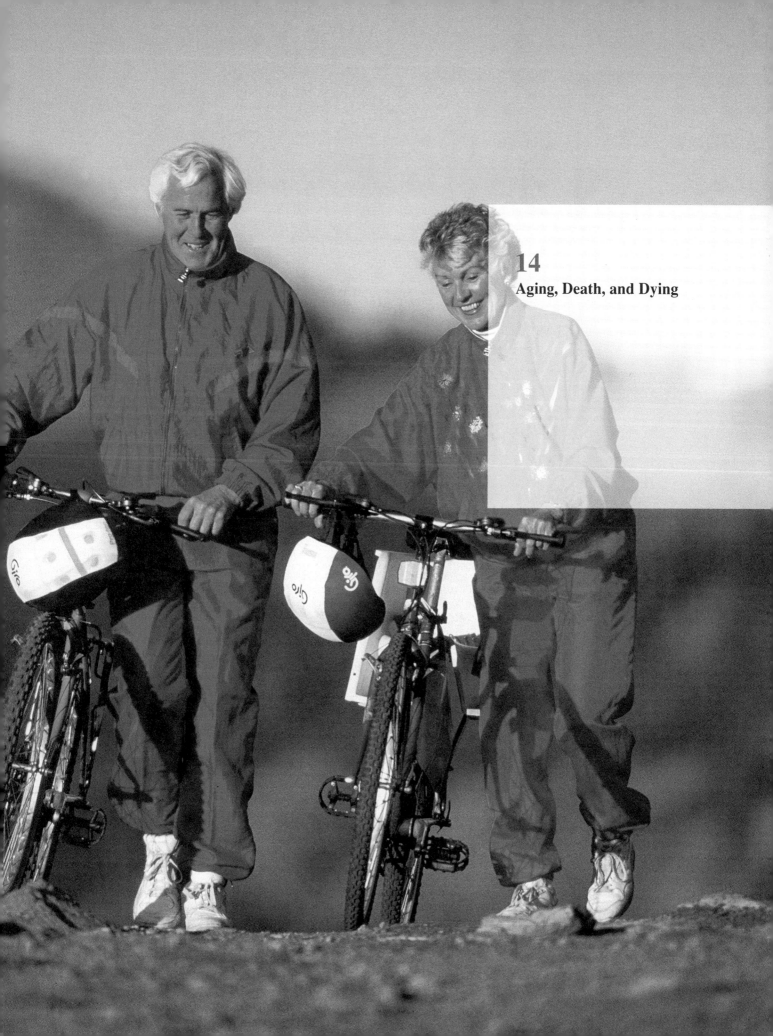

CHAPTER 14

Aging, Death, and Dying

Although every chapter in this text is concerned with the process of aging through the life cycle, this chapter helps you gain a healthy perspective on aging and death—something missing in many areas of our society. Aging and death are a part of life, and creative and healthful aging is the process of leading a healthy life-style and practicing wise consumer habits. Death is as natural a process in the life cycle as birth and can be viewed as a fulfilling completion to the life experience.

Aging

Without the process of aging, we would never enjoy the variety that comes with changing physical and psychological experiences in the world. Unfortunately, many people in our culture have forgotten or never learned how to age healthfully and creatively.

The Multidimensional Perspective of Aging

Some individuals define aging negatively, focusing only on the biological process of physical decline. An example of the biological definition of aging is, a "post maturational process that correlates over time with increasing functional losses" (Phillips and Gaylord 1985). Other definitions are simple, such as "the process of becoming physiologically and mentally older." In this text, **aging** is viewed as a multidimensional process, with many of the dimensions of health growing stronger or purer. Even the dimensions of health in older years that do not grow stronger, such as the physical dimension, can be optimized within some limitations.

For an example of a dimension that grows stronger, consider the spiritual dimension of health. In religious literature, both Western and Eastern, spiritual enhancement is viewed as a refining process. Over time, spiritual experiences enhance the spirituality of the individual. Those who live the longest have the greatest opportunity to refine their spiritual selves.

Intellectually, a look at most cultures shows that wisdom is viewed as a product of age and experience. The more decisions and outcomes a person experiences, the better prepared he or she is to make wise decisions in the future. The elder is often sought after for that wisdom. It is unfortunate that our society on the whole does not tap the valuable resources of the elderly.

Likewise, social skills and mental skills can be refined and maintained if they are continually used. Some of the most graceful, gracious, and mentally competent individuals in our society are well past retirement years. Even physical decline can be slowed and maintained at a functional level if people work at it (see the accompanying box, "Optimal Physical Health").

A thorough understanding of the multidimensional view of health will lead you to conclude that aging is desirable. It is through experience and time that your full potential can be reached. Young people today should be aware of the rich resources this society has that are sometimes found in a nursing home. This section focuses on this precious human resource and how students can effectively live life-styles so that they may also reach their potentials in their later years.

The Growing Aging Population

The number of people who are reaching retirement age and living well beyond this age is growing rapidly. This group also enjoys a higher quality of life than in the past, with more retirement communities and centers available.

Older Americans, those sixty-five years and older, number over 30 million, representing 12.4 percent of the U.S. population, or one in every eight Americans. The ratio of women to men is 18 million to 12.4 million, with women outliving men. The older population is getting older itself, with the sixty-five to seventy-four-year age group eight times as numerous as in 1900, the seventy-five to eighty-four-year group twelve times as large, and the eighty-five and older group twenty-three times more numerous (Cavanaugh 1993).

The Baby Boom generation is rapidly progressing toward retirement, and estimates are that 21.8 percent of the population, or 65.5 million Americans, will be over the age of sixty-five by the year 2030 (U.S. Bureau of the Census 1989). In light of the increasing numbers, it has been noted by many that the elderly are becoming a major social, political, and economic factor in our society. It is noteworthy that our older people are more educated, are predominantly female, are usually still in households, and are mostly not in the work force.

There are numerous reasons why people are living longer, including better medical care, better nutrition and fitness practices, and the vitality of retirement communities. This is a compliment to educational programs and medical science. This information is valuable to young people who also want to have healthy elderly years. You can begin to deal with the aging process when you are very young. There are still many questions about the aging process, and when they are answered, others will be helped to grow old in a healthy manner. **Gerontology** is the study of the elderly and aging. Those who study the needs and impact of this expanding group are called gerontologists. These specialists are attempting to deal more effectively with the emotional, social, physical, mental, and spiritual needs of the elderly.

The Nature of Aging

Gerontologists have described several aspects of the aging process as they have studied older populations. Here we describe the physical aspects of aging, the mental aging process, some theories on why people age, and some interesting ongoing research to better understand the aging process. It is important to note that the characteristics that follow do not necessarily apply to all older people. Many older people remain energetic and mentally alert until death.

Physical Aging

With increasing numbers of older people, millions of dollars each year are granted to study the aging process. The following are some of the areas that are affected by aging and are being studied to see why people might lose some functions (Andres and Hallfrisch 1989):

1. Vision—in our forties can decrease in range of color, intensity, distance, and width of field; our ability to adapt to darkness also lessens.

2. Hearing—loss begins at approximately age twenty and is progressive. As we grow older, we begin to lose our capacity to hear particular sound frequencies, especially the very high and very low frequencies.

3. Other sensory areas are affected as well. The balance center (cochlea) becomes less sensitive, and people may lose their balance more often. Taste buds become less sensitive, and the number of buds declines. Touch sensations may also diminish.

Osteoporosis Risk Assessment

Indicate which of the following categories apply to you:

_____ 1. Postmenopausal woman and not taking estrogen.

_____ 2. Premenopausal woman.

_____ 3. Over seventy years of age.

_____ 4. Between sixty and sixty-nine years of age.

_____ 5. Between fifty and fifty-nine years of age.

_____ 6. Caucasian.

_____ 7. Slight bone frame.

_____ 8. Medium bone frame.

_____ 9. Intake of milk and dairy products is less than equivalent of two glasses of milk per day (one ounce cheese = one glass of milk).

_____10. Intake of milk and dairy products is equivalent of two to four glasses of milk per day.

_____11. Life-style allows you to be exposed to one hour of sun per day or you routinely drink a quart of vitamin D fortified milk per day.

_____12. Regular vigorous exercise four times per week or have a physically demanding job (loading, walking stairs, and so on).

_____13. Your water supply is fluoridated or take a supplement of one milligram per day.

_____14. Take glococortides for long-term treatment of asthma or rheumatoid arthritis, or you take anticonvulsive drugs for long-term treatment of seizure disorder.

Scoring/Interpretation

Total the points as follows:

Add one point for each if you checked numbers 2, 5, 6, 8, 10, 14.
Add two points for each if you checked numbers 1, 4, 7, 9.
Add three points for each if you checked number 3.
Subtract one point for each if you checked numbers, 11, 12, 13.

If your total is more than eight, you are at high risk of bone loss disability. If your total is four to seven, you are at moderate risk, and a score of three or less puts you in the low-risk category.

Healthy Aging Assessment

_____ 1. I take time to relax.

_____ 2. I am active.

_____ 3. I eat nutritionally balanced meals.

_____ 4. I love life (enjoy nature, other people).

_____ 5. I control my stress levels.

_____ 6. I learn new skills all the time.

_____ 7. I get adequate, but not too much, sleep.

_____ 8. I have good communication skills.

_____ 9. I am service-oriented and like to do things for others.

_____10. I have a safe living environment.

_____11. I am creative.

_____12. I accept and like myself.

_____13. I have a purpose to my life.

Scoring/Interpretation

Total the items you have checked. If you have checked ten or more, then you are in a healthy aging mode. If you have checked six to nine items, then you are in a moderately healthy aging mode. If you have checked less than six, then you are in an unhealthy aging mode.

Comfort Scale

Respond to the following questions in a way that reflects how you feel. Respond with one of the following:

a = comfortable

b = somewhat comfortable

c = somewhat uncomfortable

d = uncomfortable

1. How comfortable do you feel talking about death and dying? a b c d

2. How comfortable would you feel if called upon to visit and support someone you cared about who had been declared terminally ill? (Mark the degree of comfort for each of the states listed.

   Denial (thinks he or she will beat the disease) a b c d

   Anger (mad at you, physicians, and/or others) a b c d

   Bargaining (pleading with God to change the situation and a pledge to do better) a b c d

   Depression (sadness, may not even talk) a b c d

   Acceptance (wants to get affairs in order and bid farewell to loved ones) a b c d

3. How comfortable would you be in providing support for a friend or relative who had someone close to them die? Mark the degree of comfort for support in the cases listed:

   Child losing parent a b c d

   Parent losing child a b c d

   Loss of someone who was in his or her later years (e.g., grandparent) a b c d

4. If you were to die and someone else could use one of your organs, what degree of comfort would you feel in making your organs available for donation upon your death? a b c d

5. If it was your misfortune to have something happen to you that would leave you in a coma and only kept alive through artificial life support, with little hope for survival, how comfortable

would you be in signing (before the coma) a statement indicating that you would not like to be kept alive in that state?   a b c d

6. If someone you felt responsible for was kept alive only by life support, and you knew that the person would not want to remain in this state, how comfortable would you be in ordering the withdrawal of the life-support equipment?   a b c d

Death Preparation Scale

Please check all the things you have done; leave blank if you have not done these things.

_____ Completed an organ donor card

_____ Made out a living will

_____ Talked to clergy or spiritual mentor about life, death, and life after death.

_____ Made out a personal will.

_____ Talked with parents about how they would like their funerals to be: memorial versus funeral, cremation versus burial, type of casket, where they would like to be buried, viewing versus nonviewing, music selections, and so on.

_____ Talked with parents or grandparents, other family members, and friends about their beliefs about death and life after death.

_____ Completed a funeral arrangement form that you can get at a funeral home in your community so that in the advent of your death others will know your wishes.

_____ Have mentally rehearsed (imagery) counseling or visiting with someone who has been declared terminally ill.

_____ Mentally rehearsed how you would comfort someone who had a family member or friend die (e.g., child losing parent, parent losing child, loss of grandparents, sudden and tragic versus expected losses).

_____ Talked with parents or grandparents about their will. I have learned who the executor is, how the estate would be divided, how the surviving spouse would be cared for, if underaged children were involved, who would take custody, and so on.

Scoring/Interpretation

Comfort Scale: Score as follows and total your score:

a = 4
b = 3
c = 2
d = 1

This scale measures your comfort in dealing with death and death-related experiences. The interpretation of your score is as follows:

18–24 = high degree of comfort
12–17 = moderate degree of comfort
0–12 = not comfortable in handling death-related experiences (The behaviors and concepts suggested in this chapter may help you become more comfortable.)

Death Preparation Scale: Total the number of items you have marked.

This second scale helps you determine how prepared you are to deal with the death of a loved one. All of the activities will make very difficult situations more manageable. Any of you who has experienced the death of a loved one will recognize how important these items are. Interpret as follows:

9–10 items checked   = very well prepared
5–8 items checked   = moderately prepared
5 or fewer items checked = poorly prepared

Complete the life-style contract at the end of this chapter to help you become better prepared to deal with death.

Optimal Physical Health

The following was a typical day for Larry Lewis of San Francisco. Larry woke up in the morning and jogged five to seven miles through Golden Gate Park. He then walked to work where he was on his feet most of the day working as a waiter, logging an additional five to six miles. Larry entered a senior olympics track meet and ran the one-hundred-yard dash in seventeen seconds. This is not all that exceptional until you consider that Larry is 103 years of age.

Source: BYU Films, *Run Dick, Run Jane*, 1974.

The capability of a person to retain good mental functioning is exemplified by Stephen Powelson, a seventy-year-old man who has memorized twenty-two of the twenty-four books of Horner's *Illiad,* in Greek.

4. Psychomotor skills—the ability to move and coordinate muscle groups—can decline.

5. Reaction time—the time it takes to receive a sensory stimulus and have muscle groups respond—increases.

6. Speed and accuracy of movement decrease.

7. Learning skills and short-term memory decrease slightly.

8. Problem-solving abilities can decline with age.

9. Creativity levels can diminish.

10. Habit patterns can become more rigid; that is, we tend to persist in our habitual ways.

11. Hunger drives are diminished—older people have smaller appetites than younger people.

12. Sexual drives may decrease.

13. Activity levels may decline.

14. Nutritional needs include the R.D.A. requirements and also more calcium, vitamin B-6 and vitamin B-12 (because the aging body absorbs and utilizes these nutrients less efficiently) in addition to assuring adequate intakes of folic acid, zinc, magnesium, and vitamin D.

Many researchers feel that the loss of many of these functions is a product of disuse. Some of the physical symptoms do not appear until retirement, when someone quits exercising, reading, or actively listening. Older people who have used their physical skills in their professional work rarely lose their abilities.

There are some physical diseases that are feared by the elderly, most notably **osteoporosis.** The Health Assessment at the beginning of this chapter cited the risk factors associated with osteoporosis. The habits you acquire in youth may affect whether or not you get osteoporosis in old age. Osteoporosis is a disease that mainly affects the elderly, or, more specifically, postmenopausal women. Osteoporosis is a reduction in bone mass that increases the susceptibility to fracture. About 700,000 fractures a year are attributed to osteoporosis. The primary risk factors associated with osteoporosis include consuming too little calcium, lack of exercise, and lack of estrogen therapy for postmenopausal women (Lindsay 1987). Other contributing factors include excessive protein consumption, lack of fluoride, and smoking.

A syndrome called asthenia/cachexia manifests itself by the "wasting away" of a person. Obvious signs of this condition are frequent falling, weight loss, decreased activity, decreased food intake, and some less obvious signs such as poor wound healing, recurrent infections, and ulcers (Verdery 1990). Sometimes the process can't be reversed, but in most cases, depending on the cause, reversal can occur. Some care givers do not attempt to turn asthenia/cachexia around and merely let the person waste away.

Mental Aging

Individuals who are well prepared for old age will be happier than those who are not. Those who focus on the loss that occurs in older years generally have more mental-health problems. When physiological losses occur for older people, some perceive a loss of control and autonomy. The inability to get somewhere, perform a task, or even remember something may result in frustration. At older ages, family and friends of similar ages die more frequently, and the loss of lifelong loved ones may cause difficulty in coping. Another loss may occur when, because of medical problems, the elderly person needs constant monitoring. The person may need to go to a nursing or retirement home, which results in a loss of privacy. Most elderly individuals are retired, so there is a loss of productivity, wage-earning ability, and even their homes.

On the positive side, individuals who are prepared for old age will be able to cope because many of the losses will be avoided. Good financial planning will result in being able to keep a house and wage-earning ability. The aging process can be seen as a gain for the mentally healthy person—a gain of time and opportunity to see the world or develop new hobbies and interests. Many people start new businesses after retirement from their lifelong careers. Although there may be deaths of close friends and relatives, the socially active elderly person will have a strong support system to help him or her cope.

Sexuality and the Elderly

Some people suggest that a loss of sexuality is characteristic of old age. On the contrary, mental aging does not include the loss of the desire to be loved and nurtured and give love. One study of people sixty to ninety-one years of age reported that 83 percent were still sexually active (Botwinick 1984).

Males might show a gradual decline in sexual interest with age, but sex drive does not cease unless they decide to let it cease. It may take males a longer period of time to have an erection and to ejaculate, but barring organic problems, they are still quite capable of sexual intercourse at any age. Many times, men experience the self-fulfilling prophecy phenomenon; that is, they have erectile failure just because of society's distorted values that sexual

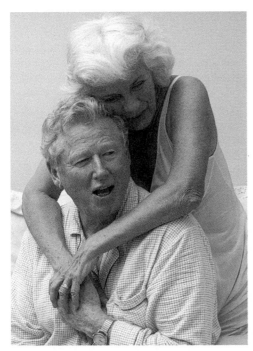

Older individuals have needs to give and receive love and to be nurtured; sexual activity among the elderly is much more prevalent than society acknowledges.

activity is for young people and that "dirty old men" should not participate. Men who ignore social views can have long and enjoyable sexual lives.

Women's sexual activity does not decline until after age sixty, and then it may decline at a gradual rate. Women become less sexually active in many cases merely because they do not have a sexual partner or their partners are no longer sexually active. Many women still masturbate. One survey showed that 88 percent of older women can still achieve orgasms (Botwinick 1984).

Menopause

Women's feelings about **menopause** have a bearing on their degree of sexual activity. Menopause is characterized by the cessation of the release of eggs by the ovary, clearly a signal to a woman that her reproductive years are over. This life change signals different messages. Some women feel a great sense of relief and freedom that they no longer have to use birth control to avoid pregnancy. As a result, sexual interest increases. Unfortunately, other women perceive menopause as losing their feminine identity and purpose, and this is followed by depression and major life disruption. In the negative case, there may be a decreased interest in sexual activity, at least until psychological adaptation has occurred.

Alzheimer's Disease and Other Dementias

The mental diseases most dreaded by the elderly are Alzheimer's disease and dementia. They are, perhaps, the most emotionally draining and demanding diseases of the

elderly. **Dementia** is the loss of mental functions in an alert and awake individual characterized by a group of symptoms, including short-term memory loss, loss of language functions, inability to think abstractly, inability to care for oneself, personality change, emotional instability, and loss of a sense of time or place that results from numerous causes. Three quarters of the cases of dementia are caused by Alzheimer's disease (55 percent to 65 percent of cases) and strokes.

Alzheimer's disease is a chronic, degenerative, dementing illness that has no known cause. There is no known cure or intervention to stop the progression of the disease. Specific symptoms of Alzheimer's patients include memory and intellectual impairment, wandering and agitation, depression, delusions, and family stress (Light and Lebowitz 1989).

More than seventy conditions can cause dementia, including the following:

1. degenerative diseases: Alzheimer's disease, Parkinson's disease, Huntington disease, and others;
2. vascular dementia: cerebral embolisms, blood clotting, infarctions;
3. anoxic dementia: cardiac arrest, cardiac failure, carbon monoxide;
4. traumatic dementia: head injuries;
5. infectious dementia: AIDS, herpes, encephalitis, meningitis, brain abscess, neurosyphilis;
6. space-occupying lesions: brain tumors, hematomas, cancers;
7. toxic dementias: alcohol, poisons;
8. others: epilepsy, posttraumatic stress disorders, heat stroke, multiple sclerosis, and other autoimmune disorders.

An estimated two million Americans suffer from severe dementia, which means that someone must care for them continually. An additional one to five million have mild or moderate dementia. There has been a dramatic increase in the number of cases of dementia as evidenced by the fact that there are ten times as many people affected today as there were at the turn of the century. By the year 2000, there is a 60 percent increase expected and five times as many cases by the year 2040, when many college students reading this text will be at susceptible ages.

The progression of the disease varies with each case, but generally dementia is noticed by family, friends, or co-workers and not physicians. Although sometimes the disease appears suddenly, most cases become evident in a slow, hidden fashion. A minor loss of memory, mental ability, or judgment that gets progressively worse is a common scenario.

The emotional and financial drain on the families of those with dementia are enormous. The average length of time that people have Alzheimer's disease is eight and a half years before they die, and cases have occurred where twenty-five years of constant care was required before death. To help those who must care for someone with dementia, national organizations such as the Alzheimer's Disease and Related Disorders Association (ADRDA) have been formed to provide support. National attention has focused on the disease, which has been described in *Newsweek* and *Life* magazines and on prime-time television (*Do You Remember Love?*, a made-for-television movie aired by CBS in 1985). The book *36 Hour Day* on caring for patients with dementia has sold over a half million copies. Dementia is becoming one of the most dreaded diseases of our elderly and is projected to become an even more prevalent problem in the future.

Mental aging is largely in the control of the individual. Actively using the senses and emotions, having a positive outlook on life, and planning for old age will, for many individuals, keep them mentally vital. Only in the cases of disease will some of these functions be lost. When there is a greater understanding of why people age, some of these diseases may be eliminated.

Aging Theories

It is easy to observe the external bodily changes that occur with increasing years, but it is not so easy to pinpoint why these changes occur. Many theories have been proposed to explain the natural phenomenon of aging, but none has been proved to be the only correct one.

1. *Brain size theory:* The idea that brain size determines longevity is based on studies comparing body and brain sizes of eighty-five different species of animals.
2. *Biological clock(s):* The theory is that a biological or genetic clock(s) predetermines how long we live.
3. *Disposable soma theory:* This theory suggests that aging results from the allocation of resources (intake of energy) among the various tasks to be performed by the body (growth, foraging, defense, repair). The optimal condition is to allocate as little energy as possible to somatic (body) repair and divert to other functions. Over time, the need for repair becomes evident and, in the end, insurmountable, which is reflected as aging and death.
4. *Pleiotropy theory:* Pleiotropic genes are those that may have good effects in a young body but become harmful later in life due to a mutation or change. For example, a gene may play a positive role in the calcification of bone during development but contribute to the calcification of arteries in later life.
5. *Wear-and-tear theory:* The body is much like a machine in that by design it breaks down. The theory supposes that through constant use, cells, tissues, or whole organs just break down through several means, such as accumulated damage or error.
6. *Genetic theories:* Several genetic theories of aging have been proposed. According to one, over time the body's cells lose the genetic information required to make the proteins necessary to rebuild the body.

7. *Immunological theories:* Scientists have also proposed theories linking aging to the immune system. Two of these theories suggest that the immune system is, in a sense, destroying the body from within. According to the third, the immune system may simply lose its vigor and no longer be able to fight off disease.
8. *Error accumulation theory:* Cellular reproduction is not perfect, and cells with defective components are occasionally generated. Assuming that the defective parts are stable and are passed on when the cell reproduces again, they could eventually build up and impair cell function. Also, the accumulation of harmful metabolic wastes implies that certain compounds are formed for which the cells have inadequate removal mechanisms.
9. *Cell loss theory:* The cell loss theory supposes that the rate at which cells die daily varies for each individual and determines our longevity.
10. *Nutritive theories:* Animal experiments demonstrate that cutting down on food consumption by taking in only essential vitamins, minerals, and proteins prolongs life radically. As a result, some suggest that our nutritive habits contribute to how rapidly we age.
11. *Environmental theories:* Water pollution, radiation, the declining ozone layer, and smog may cause cells to be destroyed or cell walls to break down, thereby speeding the aging process.
12. *Brain chemistry theory:* According to the brain chemistry theory, aging is directly related to chemicals that transmit messages in the brain. With age, the number of transmitters decreases, which prevents the important centers in the brain from signaling other areas to produce the hormones necessary for bodily functions.
13. *Cross-linking:* Outward aging occurs as increasing numbers of proteins join connective-tissue fiber molecules in the skin, which forms wrinkles.

Ageism

With a basic understanding of the nature of aging, the social aspects of aging are presented next. The following sections include a discussion of ageism and stereotyping, ageism and retirement, and combating ageism.

Ageism and Stereotyping

Ageism—discrimination based on age—is a powerful, socially reinforced prejudice in this society. Ageism is often a product of **stereotyping**, which is a shared, conventional expectation of how people in a certain group behave, think, and relate. When an athlete on a sports scholarship walks into class, we are likely to form a set of images of what that person is like—"not too bright," "interested only in sports," and so forth. We may find that we also have a set of expectations about this person. Stereotyping affects the way we vote, raise children, select doctors, teach in schools, and make other decisions.

The concepts of "young" and "old" as well as "healthy" and "unhealthy" are defined in the Western culture as polar opposites. If we value youth, we are not likely to value old age as well. If we value activity and productivity, we probably do not also value physical restriction or a slower pace. One day an executive is seen as a competent, productive, healthy professional at age sixty-nine; the next day, the executive's seventieth birthday, the same person is seen as fickle, senile, and unhealthy and is consequently forced to retire.

Stereotyping is socially unhealthy for optimum human growth because it ignores individual variation. As a society, we must examine our views of growing older so we can overcome cultural barriers and promote a healthier perspective on what it means to age in the United States.

Ageism and Retirement

Competition for jobs, money, and other resources is fundamental to understanding ageism in our society, where productivity and independence are prime measures of the value of human worth and dignity (Jose and Richardson 1980). The elderly no longer compete for jobs and money, and by retirement they are considered dependent and nonproductive. Where does this place the retiree on the Western continuum of human worth? Unfortunately, not highly esteemed. Contrast this with Eastern societies, in which the elderly are valued for their experience and wisdom.

Upon retirement—reflect on the associative weight of this word—individuals may experience several traumatic changes. With our first childhood step, independence has been ingrained in us as an inherent and valued part of individual strength (Jose and Richardson 1980). Retirement may reflect financial dependence on the Social Security system and pension funds even though every wage earner contributes throughout their lifetimes. Retirement can be a visible declaration to supportive children that it is now their turn to take care of their parents. This may be a welcomed concept in some cultures but not in the Western culture, which so highly values independence and self-sufficiency.

For many individuals, their jobs are a major source of identification. During the working years, we accumulate a valuable store of knowledge that is found only in life, not in textbooks. Yet when retirement occurs, the teaching role may be denied when individuals are best qualified to give advice. Research on creative approaches to retirement indicates that a good retirement plan should be directed toward building a future and should begin well before the transition into retirement begins. Part of retirement planning ideally should include: (1) examining and evaluating the present situation, (2) determining what satisfaction in retirement means, (3) developing short-range plans and a set of goals or objectives, (4) clarifying long-term objectives, and (5) evaluating progress.

It is not surprising that secondary impotence—erectile failure due to psychological causes—is experienced by some older men at retirement age. The sense of uselessness and powerlessness they experience in the work arena extends into the area of sexual activity. Women, too, suffer particular difficulties. Middle-aged women are often viewed as less desirable than men the same age. For women in the United States, a youthful appearance appears to be the single standard of beauty; so as a woman's face and body mature, she tends to lose esteem in both her own eyes and in those of others.

Combating Ageism

What can be done to help eliminate ageism and make the lives of older individuals more satisfying? First, we can improve the conditions and levels of wellness of retired or nearly retired individuals who are making age- and work-related adjustments. Young people can more actively draw on the experience and wisdom of the elderly, and the elderly can strongly seek creative outlets for their wisdom.

Second, we can clarify our values regarding independence, competition, and productivity and reexamine the premiums we put on youth and beauty. These values are deeply embedded in the structures of Western society. The United States school system is based on competition; there is competition in men's and women's athletics, physical education classes, and recreation, as well as in the grading system. Such extracurricular activities as choirs, bands, student body offices, and clubs also promote competition.

Self-actualization is a noncompetitive ideal that we can fully realize only if we have the time to work through Erikson's last life crisis: ego integrity versus despair. It is almost impossible to stand back from one's life and examine it with complete objectivity while working. Creative retirement offers the gift of unprogrammed time in which to realize fully this ultimate challenge of assessing, owning, and giving true meaning to life's activities. This is as important as any competitive undertaking or external productivity.

Third, we can view giving and receiving nurturing as both a masculine and a feminine characteristic. Also, we can equally value giving and receiving. Men who learn to nurture others may find it easier to receive nurturing whenever they need it, especially in their later years.

Spirituality and a sense of meaning and purpose in life are important values to be considered in the prevention of ageism. This seems to be particularly truc for those who are approaching death and reaching out to deeper dimensions for comfort and strength. Spiritual experiences can be evoked through music, meditation, reading, religious activity, and the natural world, but often they arise through our contact with others who have experienced their own spirituality. Older people usually have come to terms with the last developmental crisis—ego integrity versus despair—and association with them helps prepare us for our own resolution of this crisis.

Guidelines for Healthy Aging

The assumption is that if we live longer, we will enjoy a longer quality of life. Russell (1989) projects that although we will live longer, 80 percent of that additional time will be spent sick or disabled. To better the odds of a longer and higher quality of life, some guidelines should be followed. One perspective of healthy aging is proposed by Dychtwald (1989), who suggests that retirement can result in either boredom or a "cycle life." Cycle life means redoing in retirement what occurred in the early part of the life cycle. In other words, retirees should return to school, change careers, and take part in sports and other skill-enhancement activities.

The following basic conditions for healthy aging (adapted from Robinson 1981) apply at any age. If you want to lead a more enjoyable life both now and in the future, you might consider these conditions now, as you make decisions about your life-style.

1. Accepting leisure—taking time in your life to enjoy relaxation.
2. Being active—exercising, reading, going to cultural events.
3. Eating properly—following a good nutritional program.
4. Taking interest in life—enjoying nature, meeting others, maintaining relationships.

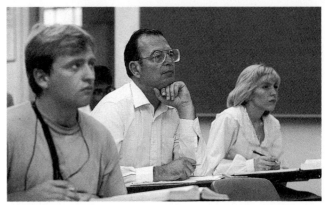

Being active, taking an interest in life, and learning new skills are important components of healthy aging.

5. Controlling stress levels—paying heed to the stress management strategies described in chapter 2.
6. Learning new skills—learning to write better, play noncompetitive games, do crafts, garden, and so on.
7. Getting adequate sleep but not too much—determining the amount of sleep (seven to eight hours in most cases) that makes you feel good.
8. Communicating feelings openly—men especially need to learn freedom of emotional expression; pent-up emotions are stressful.
9. Doing things for others—servicing others is gratifying, healthy, and life-prolonging.
10. Selecting a safe living environment—avoiding pollution, crime areas, and other unsafe and unhealthy environments, if possible.
11. Adding freshness to your life—acting and thinking creatively.
12. Knowing yourself—accepting, exploring, and liking yourself.
13. Establishing a unifying philosophy of life, whether it be based on principle or religion—establishing a sense of purpose that causes you to value life and motivates you to be productive.

Options for Care

What happens when people you love—parents or grandparents—become debilitated, perhaps as an indirect result of old age, and need care? Providing constant care is a difficult responsibility that requires an outlay of time, energy, and money. In this society, there are four basic options for care of the debilitated elderly.

Medicare: Government Aid to the Elderly

Even with healthful living practices, medical problems may arise. Because many elderly are not able to afford medical care, the government developed the Medicare program. **Medicare** is the largest health insurance program in the country for people sixty-five and older, disabled people covered by Social Security, and individuals with end-stage renal disease. Medicare, with its sister program Medicaid (health insurance for the poor), was instituted in 1965 by the U.S. Congress. It is clear that the program has done much to reduce the financial burdens of the elderly and to allow them access to state-of-the-art health-care services. With an annual federal budget of over $75 billion, nearly thirty million elderly and disabled citizens benefit from the program. The program is not free to the elderly. They must purchase the insurance much like other policies, except at more reasonable rates.

The current system of Medicare, with all of its benefits, is still inadequate, particularly in the prevention of disease. The costs of a physical exam that might detect a disease in its early stages would necessitate a patient paying an annual deductible amount plus a portion of the remaining costs. On a Social Security income of a few hundred dollars a month, where money must be spent on food and shelter, the "luxury" of a physical exam, eyeglasses, hearing aids, and other preventive measures is beyond many elderly individuals' budgets.

Home Care by Relatives

Home care may require that a family member be home at all times; if both spouses work, perhaps one must quit. The result of this sacrifice might well be that the elderly person's love and care needs are provided for, but the family's financial resources for taking care of themselves and the relative are seriously reduced.

Geriatric or Adult Day Care

Many communities have day care centers for older people similar in function to those for children. The elderly receive care during the day but are home alone or with families in the evening. This frees the family to work, while satisfying the love, responsibility, and companionship needs of the elderly.

Nursing Homes

Many individuals have determined that they can't provide adequate home care for older people and so have placed them in nursing homes. Nursing homes generally provide adequate physical care, but do they satisfy their clients' psychological and emotional needs?

Many older individuals in this society are in unfortunate situations, while many others live productive and happy lives until the day they die. There is something special about older individuals who live full lives. They have abilities developed in their resolutions of life crises and in their decisions to follow certain life-styles and life habits.

Principles of Aging Applied to the Young

A main purpose of this chapter is to help you improve your relationships with older people by talking with them and learning from them. The elderly have basic needs just like younger people—to be needed, to feel secure, to be loved, and to be productive. You can help the elderly accomplish these basic needs.

Another purpose is to help you prepare for your elderly years. It is difficult for most students to imagine ever being old, but unless some unforeseen circumstance takes your life early, you will become old. Granted, this is obvious, but the reality of the statement does not enter many young minds. Preparation for the late years begins as a young adult. Physically, the guidelines to successful aging apply to students in youth. Eating right, exercising for a lifetime, controlling stress, avoiding drugs and tobacco, and other healthy behaviors are important.

Planning for retirement is important. When job hunting, carefully examine retirement programs and benefits. Developing activities outside of your work life is extremely important. It is obvious to an onlooker which people enjoy retirement and which don't. Some individuals are anxious from having nothing to do, and others create a whole new life of hobbies and other pursuits. With good health, strong relationships, hobbies, and financial security, retirement can be a welcome, productive, and joyful time.

Death and Dying

The American culture is caught in a paradox. We are fascinated with death, as evidenced by the popularity of television shows and movies that include significant amounts of violence and death. At the same time, we deny that we are mortal or that others close to us could die until faced with a life-threatening situation. Americans are a death-denying society, and therefore we do not prepare for our own death or the death of a loved one.

Many college students, for example, have not talked with their parents or grandparents about where they want to be buried, what kind of funeral or memorial service arrangements they would prefer, whether they want to be buried or cremated, whether or not they want their organs donated, what death means to them, and their beliefs in life after death. College students may not have a will because they deny that death could happen to them at a young age. With the combined fascination with death and denial of death in society, we are often ill prepared to psychologically cope with the death of a loved one. Death is a natural part of life. This section provides guidelines for those who may be grieving and helps prepare for the financial and psychological losses that accompany the death of a loved one.

The Concept of Death

Death is the natural outcome of life, whether we live healthily or unhealthily, yet the thought of a loved one dying or of dying ourselves is so unpleasant that we often repress it. When we do discuss death with others, we tend to avoid direct description in favor of such euphemisms as "passed away," "taken away," "gone to the great beyond," or even "kicked the bucket" or "knocked off."

When does death actually occur? At first the question seems simple. The historical common law definition was that "death occurs when the lungs and heart cease to function." By this definition, however, those who have had heart attacks and have been revived by cardiopulmonary resuscitation would have "died." Today's life-support machines can keep us "alive" if we cannot breathe on our own or if our hearts cannot beat on their own. Machines can clean the blood if the body's organs cannot do it and feed us if we cannot eat. Even when individuals do not emit any brain waves, they can still "function" artificially. When, then, is a person actually dead?

The Harvard Medical School has developed a definition of death, based partly on our ability to measure the brain's electrical activity (Ad Hoc Committee 1968). According to this definition, an individual is declared dead when the following four criteria are met:

1. Unreceptiveness and unresponsiveness: The patient is totally unresponsive to applied painful stimuli, such as poking with pins.
2. Unresponsiveness in breathing: For over an hour, the patient shows no spontaneous muscular contractions or breathing.
3. Lack of reflexes: The knee-jerk reflex is absent, or the pupils do not contract when light is pointed in the eye.
4. Flat electroencephalogram (EEG): For twenty minutes, the patient's brain does not generate an electrical impulse or brain wave.

According to this definition of death, a person kept functioning by life-support systems is considered "alive" until the machines are shut off.

Death and dying are part of health decisions and feelings. If we repress thoughts and discussions of death, we will be unprepared when death does occur and have difficulty recovering or helping someone else recover from such a traumatic experience. By understanding the issues and feelings that arise in dying and mourning, we can help ourselves cope with the eventuality of death.

Stages of Dying

Many individuals never know consciously that they are dying. People who die from traumatic injuries or massive coronaries do not have time to prepare to disengage with life, as far as we know. Many others, however, do have some advance notice of death due to terminal illness. In these cases, they can come to terms with the inevitability of their situations in a very immediate sense. Elizabeth Kübler-Ross (1969) has worked for years with terminally ill and dying patients and has observed that many pass through five psychological **stages of dying:** (1) denial, (2) anger, (3) bargaining, (4) depression, and (5) acceptance. Given enough time, most terminally ill patients can and do pass through these stages, although not all go through them in the same order. Some may skip a stage, revert to an earlier stage, or get stuck in one stage. A person copes with death either through these stages or in his

or her own unique way. Each person experiences the dying process with the same individuality that distinguished him or her as a healthy person.

1. Denial: When the news comes that death is at hand, denial is the easiest way to cope—"It can't be true, not me." Individuals may believe that a cure will be found for their disease or that they will be the exception to the rule.
2. Anger: When people realize they are really going to die, they are likely to become angry—"Why me?" Such anger is often directed at the medical staff, the family, or God. They may feel that they are unjustly being taken from the living and should not have to go through the ordeal of dying.
3. Bargaining: Bargaining is a final attempt to avoid the inevitable. Individuals may plead with God, promising to reform their lives in exchange for a miraculous recovery. Promises are made if, and only if, the death can be stayed.
4. Depression: When bargaining fails and people realize that the last hope is dimming, they are likely to feel depression and self-pity. They feel the loss of friends and loved ones, good health, and the freedom of home. It is natural in this stage to grieve.
5. Acceptance: Acceptance of the inevitable fate of dying is difficult, but eventually this arrives for most if time is allowed. The dying are likely now to want to make sure that all personal and professional matters are taken care of, including wills and funeral arrangements, and to bid farewell to special people in their lives.

Understanding these stages can help us talk to and aid loved ones who might be dying. For example, if your loved ones are in the denial stage, you can respond by listening. Ordinarily, you shouldn't encourage denial, but neither should you force someone into premature acceptance. The dying person is attempting to cope, and you can support the attempt if not the present outcome. Understanding that an angry stage is common can help you be tolerant and feel less hurt if the anger is directed toward you. When the dying individual is in the bargaining stage, you might encourage the development of the person's spiritual dimension and self-forgiveness. During the depression stage, you should continue to express love and not allow the person to be left alone.

When the dying individual has reached the acceptance stage and wants to be open about dying, it is frustrating to have loved ones showing denial, depression, or anger. If the person has accepted the actuality of death, then you must accept it as well and help put everything in order.

Hospices

Many people die in hospitals, often alone or with medical staff and away from their families. Most people, however, want to die at home with loved ones or in homelike

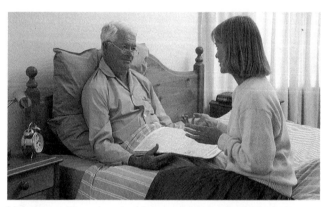

Hospices, although not widely available to all, aim to help individuals to die with dignity away from institutional settings.

surroundings. This desire has given rise to the **hospice** concept. To make dying a fulfillment of life rather than a tragic end, the hospice provides either home care or a homelike atmosphere for the terminally ill. A hospice is a comfortable place with a cheerful atmosphere. Volunteers visit and talk with dying patients, helping them to cope and offering a sympathetic ear. Families visit freely without the restrictive hours or age limits common in hospitals. Within this temporary caring community, family and friends have the opportunity to encounter each other at the deepest levels and find mutual sustenance. Volunteers within the hospice program also make home visits for those who wish to die at home.

Remember that hospice is really a concept more than a place. There are hospice places, but, in most cases, patients are at home with volunteers or family. They spend time together with the goal of being supportive and also to provide pain management. Most hospice patients are those who have painful degenerating diseases such as cancer and AIDS. In the almost two decades of hospice care in America, the movement has moved from an alternative health-care approach to an accepted part of the

American heath-care field (Rhymes 1990). Medicare and other insurances now cover the cost of hospice care. To be reimbursed for hospice benefits the patient must, among other qualifications, have a terminal illness with a life expectancy of six months or less; have elected the hospice benefit, relinquishing other benefits except for the attending physician (i.e., no more curative treatments); and have more than 80 percent of the payments be for home care (Rhymes 1990).

Access to hospice care has been limited to some degree by unavailability, ignorance, and some restrictions of providers. The public and health-care systems need to be continually educated about hospices so that death with dignity may occur.

Euthanasia

A doctor's Hippocratic oath dictates that the ultimate purpose in medicine is to preserve life. Doctors encounter situations, though, that mercifully would dictate otherwise. An entire issue of the **Hastings Center Report** (1992) is on euthanasia and covers the ethics of regulating death, a common practice in Germany and the Netherlands, and other ethical issues surrounding the merciful taking of a life. The pros and cons of letting people live in pain or relieving them of their suffering is expressed in the words of one physician ("Euthanasia" 1990):

> How often have we encountered a patient in the last stages of a terminal disease? There are no mornings or evenings, no day or night, just the time between the narcotics that are necessary to relieve their unbearable pain. There are no thoughts of the future; just memories of the past and those are often clouded by the narcotics.

This issue involves the survivors as well. When dying is prolonged and painful, as in some forms of cancer, or when the recovery of a patient on life support seems impossible, the issue of euthanasia may arise. **Euthanasia** (from the Greek words for "good death") means the promotion of an easier, swifter death for reasons of mercy. Because of the various circumstances involved, four types of euthanasia can be distinguished.

In **indirect voluntary euthanasia,** a patient on life-support machines or drugs asks the physician (or sometimes another trusted person) to withdraw the support if a change in his or her condition merits it. For example, a patient may ask that support be removed if recovery becomes impossible, or a terminal cancer patient may refuse treatment except for pain to die more quickly. This is indirect euthanasia because the physician does not actively promote death (as by a fatal drug), yet no special treatment is used to keep the patient alive. If death comes, it is natural. It is voluntary because the patient requests it.

Indirect involuntary euthanasia usually involves a comatose patient on life support. In this instance, relatives arrange to have the patient's life support removed. The term *involuntary* is applied because the patient did not personally choose to have life support removed.

In **direct voluntary euthanasia** (or voluntary mercy killing), the patient asks to have a fatal drug administered if his or her condition worsens. **Direct involuntary euthanasia** (involuntary mercy killing) occurs when the patient lapses into a coma and the relatives arrange for administration of the fatal drug. Both forms of direct euthanasia are illegal.

Cases involving the possibility of euthanasia show the complexity of the personal and ethical decisions we may face. On the one hand, we want to cling to the life of a patient, particularly that of a loved one. The medical profession and religious perspective point to preserving life at all costs. On the other hand, keeping a person on life-support systems is expensive, and medical bills can mount quickly, leaving survivors in severe financial difficulty.

One approach to resolving the problem of euthanasia has been enacted by an organization called Concern for Dying. They have developed the **living will,** a simple statement you can make to indicate that if a condition requires life support, you wish to have no life-support systems and to let nature alone decide.

Life-after-Death Experiences

Our modern ability to snatch individuals from the jaws of death by technological means is partly responsible for the resurgence of claims of life after death. Traditionally, life after death was considered a religious topic, beyond the realm of psychologists, medical doctors, and health educators. Raymond Moody's books *Life After Life* (1975) and *Reflections on* (1977) and K. Osis and E. Haraldsson's book *At the Hour of Death* (1977) have given credence to the issue for other professionals. And controversial discussions of life after death by Kübler-Ross (1974) have heightened this debate. Whether the life-after-death experience is a preview of after-death experiences or a psychological or physiological reaction to the void created at death continues to be debated. What is important is not whether these reported experiences are true but what they mean

---

ISSUE

Euthanasia: To Pull or Not to Pull

One of the dilemmas we face in this time of advanced technology is the capability of keeping people "alive" through life-support machines. If the brain does not have the capability to send messages to the heart and lungs to keep them working, a machine can do it. There are several questions you may want to ask.

Is it a disservice to let a person with almost no hope for recovery survive as a vegetable?

Would you want to be kept alive by a machine if you had little hope of recovering with your mental facilities intact?

Do you think others you care about would want to live or die in this situation?

Does "pulling the plug" constitute taking a life, or is the life already taken? Have you talked with your loved ones and learned their feelings? Is it a good idea to raise the topic with them just in case?

- **Pro:** Taking people off life support is the natural thing to do if there is no chance for survival. Medical intervention should not take away the person's right to die. If left on life-support machines, they would accumulate thousands of dollars of medical bills.

- **Con:** Medicine should do everything to keep someone alive. There have been numerous cases of people suddenly coming out of comas and surviving. Pulling the plug is taking a life.

What are some things you can do to avoid making a difficult decision like this? What would you do?

---

to people (Richardson 1979). Do these experiences increase hopes, fears, the sense of caring, and purpose or cynicism?

Life-after-death experiences include seeing others who have already died, being out of their bodies and able to look down upon themselves with great interest, seeing beings of light, experiencing a peaceful existence in a beautiful setting, having instantaneous panoramic playbacks of their lives, and traveling through dark tunnels. These experiences reportedly have occurred just as the person was dying or between the time he or she "died" (heart stopped) and were revived.

The following three factors are common to these reports:

1. The patient enjoys the death experience; it is peaceful, serene, and, in most cases, positive.

2. The patient "returns" with a new zest for living and a sense of the meaning of life, including a strong desire for knowledge and an increased emphasis on loving.

3. People who come back would not take their own lives to recapture the death experience because they have a renewed sense of purpose among the living; they no longer fear death.

Many people in the world could see if they were to receive a transplant with donated eyes. Many people on dialysis machines would be less restricted if they received a new kidney. You can arrange to donate your vital organs after death. Many people are now arranging to do this, although some religious groups oppose the practice.

Donation needs to be arranged before death. If you decide to donate, fill out a uniform donor card (as shown here) so that medical personnel and the mortician are alerted. Carry the card with your identification so that it can be easily found.

Any state that has passed the Uniform Anatomical Gift Act makes the uniform donor card legal if signed in the presence of two witnesses who also sign. You must be at least eighteen years of age. If you have questions, contact the Humanities Gifts Registry in your state or call (215) 922–4440. If you desire, a spouse or parent may also donate your organs before or immediately after your death, either for transplant or to a research or teaching institution for anatomical study.

MINNESOTA DEPARTMENT OF PUBLIC SAFETY
Driver and Vehicle Services Division/108 Transportation Building/St. Paul, Minnesota 55155

In the hope that I may help others, I hereby make this anatomical gift, if medically acceptable, to take effect upon my death. I give any needed organs or parts for the purpose of transplantation.

(PLEASE PRINT) Donor's Name _____
First   Middle   Last

Date of Birth _____
Month   Day   Year

SIGNED BY THE DONOR IN THE PRESENCE OF THE WITNESSES SET FORTH BELOW
If donor is under 18 years of age BOTH parents, a legal guardian or parent or parents having legal custody must also sign in the presence of these witnesses.

Signature of Donor _____ Date _____

Address _____
Street   City   Zip   State

Signatures of both parents,
legal guardian or parent(s) _____ _____
having legal custody.

_____   _____
Witness   Witness

THIS IS A LEGAL DOCUMENT UNDER THE UNIFORM ANATOMICAL GIFT ACT OR SIMILAR LAWS. You are hereby notified that all personal data furnished on this document is part of a public record and transcripts may be issued to anyone.
PS-33204-03 Donor Card

GIFT OF LIFE ORGAN DONOR PROGRAM

Transplantation of some human organs is now a reality because of advances made in medical technology. One of the major problems is the shortage of transplantable organs. The Minnesota Department of Public Safety, Driver and Vehicle Services Division, through an act passed by the State Legislature, now give anyone the opportunity to indicate on the Driver License or Minnesota Identification Card that, upon death, needed body organs may be used for transplantation, if medically acceptable.

If you desire to register in the Organ Donor Program, complete the form on the reverse side and present it **with** your Driver License or Minnesota Identification Card application.

PLEASE NOTE:
1. **PRINT** your first, middle and last name.
2. **PRINT** your date of birth. (Month, day and year)
3. **In the presence of two witnesses, WRITE your name in the space provided for "signature of donor" and if under 18, BOTH parents, a legal guardian or parent(s) having legal custody WRITE their names in the spaces provided and have the two witnesses sign the document.**
4. **PRINT** your complete residence address.

The "DONOR" designation will then be indicated on your Driver License or Minnesota Identification Card. The designation may be removed by applying for a duplicate license or **new** Minnesota Identification Card.

If the donor cannot sign, the Donor Document may be signed for the donor at the donor's direction, in the donor's presence, and in the presence of two witnesses who must sign the document in the donor's presence. **If the donor is under 18 and cannot sign no "Donor" designation may be added to the Driver License or Minnesota Identification Card.**

If you do not wish to register in the Organ Donor Program, proceed with the Driver License or Minnesota Identification Card application as indicated thereon, disregarding this document.

Source: State of Minnesota.

If you feel that you would not like to be kept alive through life-support mechanisms when your chances of recovery are negligible, then you might want to make out a living will. To get free information about writing a living will, you can contact the following organization:

Choice In Dying, Inc.
200 Varick St., 10th Floor
New York, NY 10014–4810

It is important to specify your resident state so the documents will be relevant to your state laws. The following is a sample living will.

ADVANCE DIRECTIVE
Living Will and Health Care Proxy

Death is a part of life. It is a reality like birth, growth and aging. I am using this advance directive to convey my wishes about medical care to my doctors and other people looking after me at the end of my life. It is called an advance directive because it gives instructions in advance about what I want to happen to me in the future. It expresses my wishes about medical treatment that might keep me alive. I want this to be legally binding.

If I cannot make or communicate decisions about my medical care, those around me should rely on this document for instructions about measures that could keep me alive.

I do not want medical treatment (including feeding and water by tube) that will keep me alive if:
- I am unconscious and there is no reasonable prospect that I will ever be conscious again (even if I am not going to die soon in my medical condition), or
- I am near death from an illness or injury with no reasonable prospect of recovery.

I do want medicine and other care to make me more comfortable and to take care of pain and suffering. I want this even if the pain medicine makes me die sooner.

I want to give some extra instructions: *[Here list any special instructions, e.g., some people fear being kept alive after a debilitating stroke. If you have wishes about this, or any other conditions, please write them here.]*

The legal language in the box that follows is a health care proxy.
It gives another person the power to make medical decisions for me.

I name _____ , who lives at _____
_____ , phone number _____ ,
to make medical decisions for me if I cannot make them myself. This person is called a health care "surrogate," "agent," "proxy," or "attorney in fact." This power of attorney shall become effective when I become incapable of making or communicating decisions about my medical care. This means that this document stays legal when and if I lose the power to speak for myself, for instance, if I am in a coma or have Alzheimer's disease.

My health care proxy has power to tell others what my advance directive means. This person also has power to make decisions for me, based either on what I would have wanted, or, if this is not known, on what he or she thinks is best for me.

If my first choice health care proxy cannot or decides not to act for me, I name _____
_____ , address _____ ,
phone number _____ , as my second choice.

(over, please)   LWGEN

I have discussed my wishes with my health care proxy, and with my second choice if I have chosen to appoint a second person. My proxy(ies) has(have) agreed to act for me.

I have thought about this advance directive carefully. I know what it means and want to sign it. I have chosen two witnesses, neither of whom is a member of my family, nor will inherit from me when I die. My witnesses are not the same people as those I named as my health care proxies. I understand that this form should be notarized if I use the box to name (a) health care proxy(ies).

Signature _____

Date _____

Address _____

Witness' signature _____

Witness' printed name _____

Address _____

Witness' signature _____

Witness' printed name _____

Address _____

Notary [to be used if proxy is appointed]_____

Drafted and Distributed by Choice In Dying, Inc.—the National Council for the right to Die. Choice In Dying is a National not-for-profit organization which works for the rights of patients at the end of life. In addition to this generic advance directive, Choice In Dying distributes advance directives that conform to each state's specific legal requirements and maintains a national Living Will Registry for completed documents.

CHOICE IN DYING INC.—
the national council for the right to die
(formerly Concern for Dying/Society for the Right to Die)
200 Varick Street, New York, NY 10014 (212) 366-5540

5/92

Reprinted by permission of Choice In Dying (formerly Concern for Dying/Society for the Right to Die), 200 Varick Street, New York, NY 10014-4810, 212/366–5540.

If the life-after-death phenomenon is accepted, an additional stage might be added to Kübler-Ross's stages of dying. The additional stage might be called "mood elevation" (Richardson 1979), because the dying person would not only accept death but move into a positive state of happiness, love, and peacefulness. **Thanatologists,** those who study death and dying, report that fear of the unknown is a major problem when we try to cope with death. If we accept the fact of death and the idea that death might be a pleasant passing into another existence, the coping may become easier and fear reduced. For example, members of religious groups with strong beliefs in postmortal existence seem to have low anxiety levels about death and have an ability to adjust sooner following a death than those without such beliefs.

The Purpose and Price of Funerals

For the survivors of a death, recuperation can be a slow, painful ordeal. One of the most difficult tasks to accomplish when a loved one has died is making funeral arrangements. Many people find it hard to make sensible consumer decisions in the midst of their grief. Some have found later that they spent more than they could afford to bury their dead.

Religious Perspective of Death

Because religions vary in their beliefs about the nature of death, burial rituals also vary. Many Christian religions believe in the resurrection that was described in the New Testament. The belief is that Christ was the first to be resurrected and other people would also be resurrected after they die. The resurrection belief is that at death, the spirit leaves the body and after resurrection, the spirit and body are reunited to live a life in a glorified state in heaven.

Many Eastern and American religions believe in reincarnation. In reincarnation, the spirit or soul is eternal and the refining process is through multiple rebirths in different bodies. Some groups believe that the spirit or soul begins in lower forms of animal life and progresses to human form, while others think that rebirth only occurs in human forms. Still other people believe that there is no afterlife and that life ends at death.

Funeral rituals may vary according to beliefs. Many people believe that cremation is immoral because people should not intentionally destroy a body that is to be resurrected. On the other hand, believers in reincarnation feel that the body will be disposed of anyway, so cremation is appropriate.

Other beliefs peculiar to particular religions or cultures include burial at sea, placing the body in a high place so that natural environmental elements will dispose of the body, burial underground, cremation and burying or spreading ashes, placing the body in a tomb, or freezing.

ISSUE

Funerals: A Consumer and Personal Dilemma

Many people pay for their funerals before they die rather than forcing their families to take care of it later on. Many others leave requests in their wills that no funeral be held, either for personal reasons or to save the family the expense and time of a funeral.

- **Pro:** It is a good idea for people either to pay for their funeral before they die or to arrange for no funeral at all. A death is hard enough for a family without going through the financial and/or physical burden of a funeral. It is a loving thing to do.

- **Con:** It is a waste of money to pay for a funeral before you die. People should spend their money on things that make their lives happier, not on things that make their death easier for others. Let their families arrange the funeral. Funerals allow people a healthy expression of grief.

What are some things you can do now to resolve a potential dilemma that may arise when someone close to you dies and you must arrange for the funeral?

Americans are beginning to purchase less expensive funerals, however. Many people feel that normal funeral costs are far beyond their income levels and that the emphasis on "last respects" is mainly a sales pitch by funeral directors and morticians. In many states, **embalming**—the process of replacing the blood with preserving fluid—is required if burial does not occur within twenty-four hours of death. This is one expense many can avoid. Rather than purchasing an expensive casket, people today often use inexpensive wooden caskets or build their own. Rather than renting a funeral chapel, some have their loved ones buried and then hold the memorial service in their church or home. The reason for these changes to save on funeral costs is that many find they grieve over the financial burden as much as for the loved one.

Some may choose **cremation** as an alternative to burial in the ground. The body is usually placed in an inexpensive casket (although this is not necessary) and then burned in a special furnace called a retort. The body and casket are reduced to ashes, which are usually placed in an urn (a stone or metal container) and stored in a columbarium (a special place in a cemetery) or a mausoleum (a building designated specifically for cremated remains).

You may choose to be cremated or have your loved ones cremated because many feel it is sanitary, economical, and preserves land. Some religions have sanctions against cremation, however, and some individuals feel that cremation isn't natural. Survivors may see cremation as destruction of the loved one, or they may want a grave to visit. It is important to talk with loved ones who are likely to die before you so you can make arrangements in accordance with their desires.

Grieving

When we know a loved one is dying, we often go through stages of grief similar to those Kübler-Ross describes for the dying person. Survivors, too, may deny that death is occurring and become angry, sometimes at the patient, especially if they depend on the dying person. They may spend much time in prayer, bargaining for the person to recover; they get depressed; ultimately, they usually accept their lonely state.

When someone close to us dies, we experience **bereavement,** the objective fact of loss. Bereavement may bestow the label of orphan, widow, widower, or survivor on us. **Grief** is a normal reaction to bereavement; it is also a coping process for adjusting to life without the deceased. Symptoms that often accompany grief are tightening of the throat, shortness of breath, sighing, an empty feeling in the stomach, weakness, tension, or pain. Anger or indifference are other possible responses to

Sudden Infant Death Syndrome (SIDS) is "the sudden death of any infant or young child, which is unexpected by history and in which a thorough postmortem examination fails to demonstrate an adequate cause for death" (proceedings of the International Conference on Causes of Sudden Death in Infants 1970).

Infants who die of SIDS are generally discovered by a parent or babysitter early in the morning or at a periodic check. Instinctively, the infant is taken into the arms of the parent or care giver, who frantically attempts to resuscitate the baby.

SIDS is rarely reported in infants prior to one month of age with peak incidents at two to three months and 90 percent of SIDS victims at under twenty-five weeks of age. It is the largest single cause of postnatal death, accounting for two to three deaths per one thousand live births each year (Smith 1985).

Although there are no apparent causes of SIDS, the most likely SIDS victims, based on several studies, are those born prematurely, during winter months, to young mothers, to smoking or drug-dependent mothers (particularly to those using methadone), and to mothers who have had little or no prenatal obstetrical care. One final factor that links the majority of SIDS victims is that they die while they are sleeping.

Numerous theories have arisen to explain the mystery of SIDS. The theory that has the greatest support is the apnea theory, which refers to the interruption of breathing or respiratory function generally during rapid eye movement (active sleep), creating a situation of greater vulnerability to asphyxiation.

SIDS is one of the most traumatic crises parents may face. The infant's death is so unexpected and the explanations about cause are so vague that parents are ill prepared, guilt ridden, and stunned by the loss. A SIDS death magnifies the normal grieving process, which may prolong the recovery process.

---

bereavement. **Mourning** is a social response to the state of bereavement. People wear black, have funerals, and follow other cultural patterns of expression.

Normal Grieving

C. M. Parkes defined the grief process as a progression of psychological and social experiences (Smith 1985). The first phase is a period of numbness. This is the first reaction of feeling stunned, paralyzed, and dulled by the news of a death. This stage serves an anesthetizing, or protective, function. The numbness stage is measured in hours or days before entering the second stage, called searching.

Searching occurs after we recognize the reality of the loss and set in motion the psychological process of adjusting. Anxiety, yearning, preoccupied thinking about the deceased, sobbing, crying, and delusions typify this stage. Many times these delusions are hypnagogic, that is, they happen when the person is falling asleep. For example, widowed persons report hearing the spouse's voice in the other room and even getting up, almost expecting them to be there. Others hear their spouse drive up in a car and wait for them to come up the stairs. The searching phase takes five to fourteen days but may linger up to a year. The emotion from this stage is anger, which may be directed to the deceased, family members, or physicians but is more often repressed. The anger, which may seem unjustified to the grieving person, results in the other dominant emotion, guilt. During the searching process, the person often discovers missed opportunities in relationships, which also results in guilt. Anger and guilt require venting, which is where another person can help someone who is grieving.

The third stage is reactive depression, which is characterized by "sleep and eating disruptions, apathy and

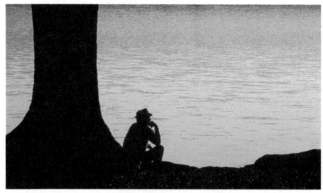

When you know a loved one is dying, you may feel very much alone and begin to experience stages of grief similar to those of the dying person.

malaise, dysfunctions in higher mental activities, and disorganization in certain other behaviors" (Smith 1985). The death of a loved one throws an individual's life out of focus, changes goals, adds new responsibilities, and results in other major shifts in life-style.

In the final stage, readjustment, the bereaved person gradually assumes certain roles and functions that were previously performed by the deceased. He or she creates a new life, and the depression is reduced or ceases. Researchers suggest that many people adjust after one year, but others may take as long as two years to reach a fully functional life-style.

Talking with Children About Death

The death of a significant person in the life of a child has immeasurable impact, largely because of the lack of preparation for a death (Marks 1991). To help you talk

Aging, Death, and Dying

The guidelines for healthy aging and for having death be a positive fulfillment to an enriching life are functions of mind, body, and soul and their interdependence. The essence of each of the following actions is that if you use your mind, body, and soul and also maximize your interdependent relationships, then you will have abilities for a longer period of time.

Mind

To effectively plan your multidimensional goals, consider for a moment a eulogy performed at your funeral or memorial service. How do you want to be remembered? What will you be known for? Whom have you helped? What will others say about you? Plan your goals to be in harmony with that eulogy.

Body

Like disease prevention, the common thread to healthy aging and delaying death is to (1) attain and maintain optimal weight, (2) do aerobic exercise four to five times a week for a duration of thirty minutes, (3) eat regular, low-fat, high-fiber, high-complex-carbohydrate, and balanced meals, (4) do flexibility and strength maintenance exercises, and (5) assure you get adequate rest and sleep.

Soul

Talk with religious leaders, read philosophical or spiritual literature, and get in touch with your spiritual source of strength. Ponder important questions in life, such as What is the purpose of my life? What is the purpose of the lives of those I love? Why am I here? Where am I going after this life, if anywhere? What is the meaning of death? How can death be a positive event?

Interdependence

Talk with those you care about and get their feelings about the same questions you pondered for your own soul.

1. Here are my feelings about the purpose of life. What are your feelings about the purpose of life?
2. Why are we here?
3. What happens at death?
4. How would we want our memorial or funeral experiences to be—that is, who would talk, what should they talk about, how do we want to be remembered, what music should there be, etc.?

---

with a child about death, the following are some considerations and guidelines:

1. The ideal person to talk with a child about death is someone the child can trust, has confidence in, and feels is both open and sincere (Savicki 1985).
2. Prior to a significant death, prepare the child by talking about the ill person (Hansen and Frantz 1985): for example, "Since Gramma became sick, what have you been feeling or thinking?"
3. Consider the age and development of the child. At ages three to four, there is a lack of clear understanding of death; death is a temporary departure. At ages five to nine, children have a more realistic concept of death and accept its definitiveness, but the deceased may also be viewed as changed to a spirit ghost or as living in heaven. After age nine, the irreversibility of death is finalized (Savicki 1985).
4. While each person has his or her own way of talking with a child, a helpful starting point is to review the meaning the deceased had for you and for the child. Phrases such as, "Do you remember when? . . . " or "What do you remember most about? . . . " or "If you could tell . . . one more thing, what would you say?" (Savicki 1985).
5. Talking about the future stresses the permanence of death and how the child will be affected: "Things will be different now, but we'll always remember the good times together . . . " or "We're really going to miss . . . " or "What will you miss the most?" (Savicki 1985).
6. Be honest in answering the simple questions that come from the child, such as "Why do people die?" or "Do you still eat and breathe when you die?" (Savicki 1985).
7. Protecting children from a funeral when they understand what is happening is generally not advised, unless the child chooses not to attend. Leaving children out of a family event increases insecurity and results in missed opportunities to grieve (Savicki 1985).
8. Preparation for the funeral is important. Tell the child, "Gramma will look different now" and grown-ups will be "silent, sad, and weepy" (Hansen and Frantz 1985).
9. Remember that a child's grief, not properly faced, can resurface unexpectedly (Hansen and Frantz 1985).

Helping a Grieving Adult

To help an older person grieve, you can listen, hold, touch, and understand anytime during the grieving process, which may be one to two years. Some people may never recover completely. Let the person share the grief with you. They may be angry with you one day and need to hold you the next, so be prepared. Reassure a grieving

My dad had diabetes since he was a teenager but in spite of it had lived a full life. He had raised his four children so that each was independent with their own children. Dad was sixty-seven and had been feeling the long-term effects of diabetes—his vision was poor and he had to receive laser treatments regularly to try and save his sight, but he really couldn't drive anymore and go off to the mountains like he wanted. The circulation in his extremities was poor; in fact, he had dry gangrene in his toes. The doctors had told him that he would have to have his feet amputated someday. He also had a series of minor strokes, none seriously debilitating, but they were worrisome. He still tried desperately to be productive and although it might take him an hour to put in one screw with his poor vision, he was able to continue to make things, dreaming of the next time there would be a family reunion in the mountains.

Two weeks before he died, he and Mom came to visit me in my new house that I had been landscaping. He helped me load rocks and debris left from construction. He was happy when he could help. His life was a life of service to his wife, his children, his religion, and boy scouts. His major goal in life was to make sure Mom was left financially secure when he died and that his children were independent.

The night before he left on the plane, Dad and I sat under a big Texas sky and talked for hours. It was reminiscent of the many times we had talked under the stars in the Sierras, Rockies, and deserts on boy scout and family camping trips. This time we talked about the impending amputation, his determination not to lose his legs, his life as he had lived it, and not wanting to lose his dignity. "If it kills me, then let it be," he stated. It was at that time that Dad and I talked like we had never talked before. We had always hugged, kissed, and expressed love, but this time it was deeper, a sense of finality was in the air. We told each other how much we loved each other. I told him how he was my hero. I told him that much of what I had accomplished in sports, as a family man, and as a professional was just to try and make him proud of me. He always said he was proud of me and I lived for that. We talked about Mom's security, how he'd thought he'd lived an okay life. We shared our beliefs of life after death. We shared everything I would ever want to share. I am so grateful for that night. I still cherish that night.

There was a good possibility that I would see him in a few months when we would make our annual vacation out West to visit family. He was still working around the house and no one had said he might not live long, but somehow each of us knew that this would be the last time I would see my dad alive.

The next day, when I took Mom and Dad to the airport, we tried to talk lightly, planning our next outing, but each knew that we had had our last outing together. As he and Mom walked toward the gate, I snapped one last photograph, and he disappeared into the plane. Two weeks later, Mom called and said that Dad had experienced a heart attack and may not make it through the night. We hurried to make a trip out to see him, but before we were able to leave, we received the news that Dad had died.

Dad had insisted that there not be a funeral, that he be buried immediately. We flew out immediately and buried him as he requested with only family members present. We then had a memorial service. A lot of people came to the memorial service—people we hadn't seen in years. It was a sad, yet joyous occasion. I felt so peaceful and grateful that I spoke at the memorial, giving me an opportunity to publicly acclaim the greatness of this humble man. I was so proud of the relationship we had and proud of the simple, but wonderful life this man had led. It seemed to me, and I expressed it, that his life was much like Camelot, a brief shining moment in history that will be remembered forever.

It was a time to rally around Mom. Each of the four children from all over the country and their spouses came, and we shared then, the love for each other that we hadn't shared in some time. It was a renewing—a new zest for living.

Although there was much sadness—and, oh, how I missed my dad—there was a peace that I had not felt before, knowing that if death has to occur, what better way to part. I have thought of that moment many, many times since his death, and each time I was strengthened, comforted, and grateful.

Source: Condensed from G. E. Richardson, Personal Journal, March through June 1985.

---

adult that their feelings of guilt, sadness, despair, and any other feelings are normal. Try to put them in touch with others who are grieving. Parents who have lost a child through a particular disease or suicide should share their experiences with others in similar circumstances.

Stillbirth and Perinatal Death

Pregnancy and birth are normally joyful experiences for parents and families. When a couple is pregnant, they begin to dream, fix up rooms, make purchases, select names, and tell many people about the upcoming birth. Unfortunately, in 1 percent to 2 percent of cases, a baby is **stillborn** (dead at birth) or experiences **perinatal death** (dies within hours or days after delivery) (Smith 1985). Obviously, many parents are not ready for the death and are devastated. Psychologically, parents grieve differently than with someone they have known well, since they have few memories of the child to cherish. Therapists recommend that the child be named, be seen by the parents (if not, take photographs for later viewing), and have formal funeral services, which provide a mechanism for grieving and identification (Smith 1985).

Death as a Positive Force in Life

With all the negative emotions and readjustments that accompany death, there are some positive outcomes. When families are close and communicate feelings openly, death can be rewarding. It can draw the survivors closer together, help individuals to reform, change behaviors, and grow from the experience. The accompanying box entitled "Peace and Rewards in Death" typifies the feelings of a survivor after the death of his father.

Summary

1. Aging is not just a physical experience but a social, emotional, intellectual, and spiritual experience as well.

2. The percentage of older people in our society is growing rapidly.

3. There are some physical functions that seem to decline with age.

4. Mental aging can result in either depression or a healthy outlook on life, depending on the makeup of the individual.

5. Both men and women experience healthy sexual relations well into their senior years.

6. Ageism is discrimination against the elderly and should be combated by our society.

7. There are guidelines for the elderly and young people to follow to promote healthy aging.

8. At some time, we must deal with the death of a loved one and our own eventual death. There are ways to be better prepared for death.

9. People who die gradually often pass through five identifiable stages: denial, anger, bargaining, depression, and acceptance.

10. Hospices provide a more humanistic approach to death than is possible in hospitals.

11. Euthanasia is an issue that many of us must face.

12. The life-after-death phenomenon is reported by many people who have approached death, and their experiences have positive implications for everyone.

13. Funerals can be very commercialized. Consumers must be aware of unnecessary expenses and, before death, learn the wishes of loved ones in regard to funerals.

14. Grieving is a difficult coping task that generally consists of numbness, searching, reactive depression, and readjustment.

15. Death can be a positive experience for the survivors under the right circumstances.

Commitment Activities

1. If you have relatives who are old, make a better effort to be with them, learn from them, and give to them. If you do not have someone nearby, volunteer to spend an hour a week at a retirement village or rest home to help out and learn from the residents.

2. Examine the list of creative aging guidelines. Contract with yourself to modify your life-style to fit the healthy aging life-style.

3. Locate two people in your community who have recently retired or are about to retire, perhaps a professor at school and a member of your family. Arrange a time to interview them, if they are willing, on their views of retirement. How do their attitudes toward retirement reflect their attitudes toward their lives thus far?

4. Imagine yourself graduating from college, selecting an occupation or life's work, and then training to become the best at whatever work you decide to do, whether a trade, profession, or unpaid job. Imagine selecting a dream partner—the romance, the emotions—and making a commitment to marriage or another arrangement. Visualize your professional and homemaking skills. Imagine that you become what you want to become in your mid-years and have the life-style you want. Imagine now you are approaching old age. Perhaps you decided to have children; visualize those children. Imagine the life-style that you would ideally have in retirement. Visualize where you would want to live and what activities you would like to do. Have you had a good older life in your imagination? Are you in a rest home or your own home? What are some of the things you do? Are you doing anything now to help an older person enjoy the kind of life you have just envisioned for yourself in old age?

5. In your state there are laws that regulate funerals, donation of organs, euthanasia, and living wills, as well as a statute that defines when a person is legally dead. Find out what the laws are in your state regarding death-related procedures.

6. Is there a hospice near you? If so, arrange a time to visit and volunteer to help out for an afternoon to get the feel of the place. If they have time, talk with staff members about their attitudes toward death and dying. How do they compare with your own? If there is no local hospice, read about other communities that do have such services and write a brief, but comprehensive, proposal suitable for submission to your county.

7. Draw a decision tree that outlines all the possible choices related to life-support systems and outcomes of those choices. For example, one choice you have is to refuse any kind of support, the consequences of

which are quick or prolonged, but nevertheless certain, death. What are your other choices? Now examine the tree. Which of these options would you choose for yourself? for an older family member? for your own child?

References

Ad Hoc Committee of the Harvard Medical School to Examine the Definition of Brain Death. "A Definition of Invisible Coma." *Journal of the American Medical Association* 205 (1968):337–40.

Andres, R., and Hallfrisch, J. "Nutritional Intake Recommendations Needed for the Older American." *American Journal of the American Dietetic Association* 89 (1989) 1739–42.

Botwinick, J. *Aging and Behavior.* New York: Springer Publishing, 1984.

Cavanaugh, J. C. *Adult Development and Aging.* Pacific Grove, Calif.: Brooks/Cole Publishing, 1993.

Dychtwald, K. "Age Wave: The Challenges and Opportunities of Aging America." In S. Walton, "A Ride on the Age Wave." Health 40 (July 1989):88.

"Euthanasia." *American Medical News* (July 27, 1990):24.

Hansen, J. C., and Frantz, T. T., eds. *Death and Grief in the Family.* Rockville, Md.: Aspen Publications, 1985.

Hastings Center Report, March-April 1992.

Jose, N. L., and Richardson, G. E. "Ageism: Need We Discriminate?" *Journal of School Health* (September 1980):419–21.

Kübler-Ross, E. *On Death and Dying.* New York: Macmillan, 1969.

Kübler-Ross, E. *Questions and Answers on Death and Dying.* New York: Macmillan, 1974.

Light, E., and Lebowitz, B. D. *Alzheimer's Disease Treatment and Family Stress: Directions and Research.* Rockville, Md.: U.S. Department of Health and Human Services, Public Health Service, 1989.

Lindsay, R. "Managing Osteoporosis: Current Trends, Future Possibilities. *Geriatrics* 42, no. 3 (1987):35–40.

Marks, J. "We Have a Problem." *Parents Magazine* 66 (January 1991):47.

Phillips, H. T., and Gaylord, S. A. *Aging and Public Health.* New York: Springer Publishing, 1985.

Rhymes, J. "Hospice Care in America." *Journal of the American Medical Association* 264 no. 3 (1990):369–72.

Richardson, G. E. "The Life After Death Phenomenon." *Journal of School Health* 49 (1979):451–53.

Robinson, F. M., Jr. "Leisure Well-Being for Longer Living People." *Health Values: Achieving High Level Wellness* 5, no. 2 (1981):55–60.

Russell, C. "I Hate To Be a Party Pooper But . . ." *American Demographics* 11 (March 1989):2.

Savicki, S. D. "Talking with Children about Death—Six Pragmatic Guides." In *Loss, Grief, and Bereavement.* ed. O. S. Margolis et al. New York: Praeger, 1985.

Smith, W. J. *Death in the Human Life Cycle.* New York: Holt, Rinehart, and Winston, 1985.

U.S. Bureau of the Census. Current Population Reports, series p. 23, no. 159. *Population Profile of the United States; 1989.* Washington, D.C.: U.S. Government Printing Office, 1989.

Verdery, R. B. "Wasting Away of the Old Old: Can It—and Should It—Be Treated." *Geriatrics* 45, no. 6 (1990):26–31.

Additional Readings

Botwinick, J. *Aging and Behavior.* New York: Springer Publishing, 1984. The psychological aspects of aging are described in detail with supporting theories in this book.

Congress of the United States. *Losing a Million Minds: Confronting the Tragedy of Alzheimer's Disease and Other Dementias.* Congressional Summary, Office of Technology Assessment (April 1987). For those interested in Alzheimer's disease, this document provides an overview of this dreaded disease of older people.

Hansen, J. C., and Frantz, T. T., eds. *Death and Grief in the Family.* Rockville, Md.: Aspen Publications, 1985. This provides a good understanding of the bereavement process and describes how to cope with the loss of a loved one.

Hastings Center Report, March-April 1992. Several articles cover the different dimensions of euthanasia, including European practices, the physician's role, and the ability to regulate life.

Jose, N. L., and Richardson, G. E. "Ageism: Need We Discriminate?" *Journal of School Health* (September 1980):419–21. This article focuses on social ageism and its effect on society and the elderly.

Kalish, R. *Death, Grief, and Caring Relationships.* Monterey, Calif.: Brooks/Cole, 1981. A sensitive book that treats the issues of mourning, bereavement, and the psychological coping process accompanying the death of a loved one.

Kübler-Ross, E. *On Death and Dying.* New York: Macmillan, 1969. This is a classic in the field of thanatology, describing in detail the psychological stages of dying.

Moody, R. A. *Life After Life.* New York: Bantam Books, 1975. A fascinating book of several descriptions of "life after life" experiences by people who had been declared dead but then were revived.

Psychoneuroimmunology (PNI), the study of the interaction of the mind, the central nervous system, and the body's immunological system, has shown that people with a fighting spirit, optimism, hope, and faith can actually build their immune systems. You have learned about the grieving process, the experience of death, and coping with death. You should also understand that the nature of healthful aging is favored by the positive mental states of a fighting spirit, optimism, hope, and a cause and purpose in life.

As this section pertains to PNI, it should be noted that research has been done that shows the relationship between ill health and bereavement, grieving, and depression as a result of a death of a loved one (Stein, Miller, and Trestman 1991). To suggest that we can cope optimistically with the death of a loved one and not grieve, feel lonely, and depressed is to suggest the unhealthy denial of feelings. Research has also demonstrated that positive outlooks for the elderly improve their quality of living. The following are some suggestions to fortify the immune system or at least minimize the negative effects and some ways to ensure quality aging for you and those you care for.

1. In the event of the death of someone you care about, plan for your grieving, mourning, and depression. It is something that is inevitable. You understand the process—it is something you must go through. When you feel sad, feel sad—don't fight it. When you need to cry, cry. Go through the adjustment process with as much natural feeling and denial as you need. This facilitates the rapid and successful mourning experience. It reduces the amount of time that your immune system is down.

    Here, for example, is the story of an incredible young widow. Her husband died of melanoma. The year-long struggle from diagnosis to chemotherapy to death was extremely difficult for this mother of five children. It took her a year to begin to function optimally. She reentered the university, where she hoped to become a dietitian. As a single parent, she could only go part-time but began to set new goals and dreams. Three years after her husband died, her father died. This time she coped much better; granted, the father did not live with her, and, though she missed him dearly, she continued to function.

    Then two years after her father died, she met one of the most difficult tests in coping with death. She was about four weeks away from graduating from college and taking her Registered Dietitian examination. Her seventeen-year-old son, who had assumed many of her husband's duties around the home in the absence of his father, was suddenly killed in an automobile accident. The powerful protective instincts of the mother, particularly in the absence of a spouse, made this particularly difficult. She went through the funeral experience with much support, then analyzed what she had to go through. She had done it twice and knew what had to happen. By choice, she put the grieving out of her mind and went into a state of denying her feelings. She concentrated quite well on her studies and taking the examination. After she received her diploma and took her examination, she put on her backpack and went solo into the mountains for two weeks, where she cried, prayed, and agonized. When she returned, even though her heart ached for a while and she still had some occasional times to grieve, she was in control and functioning.

2. It may be time to create a cause or purpose in the spirit of the person that passed on. What you may want to do in the name of that purpose is to do some good and benefit others.

3. It is best to counteract the negative mental states of depression with the death of a loved one by maximizing those things that fortify the immune system while you are grieving. It is extremely important to sustain a physical exercise program, get enough sleep and rest, eat properly, and keep as active as possible during the grieving process.

4. As it pertains to healthy aging and the immune system, see if you can do something that gives a brighter outlook on life to those older people who you would like to help as your cause. Take over a funny or heartwarming video, and watch it together. Tell funny stories and listen. Try to take them for a walk as often a possible, and then fix up their living space so that it is health enhancing (from their perspective).

5. As it pertains to your own healthy aging, be sure that your avocational and recreational pursuits have life-lasting implications. If you enjoy writing, reading, gardening, playing an instrument, or other pursuits, be sure to continue those throughout your life. Choose a cause or purpose in life that can last beyond the years of retirement. For example, there is an interesting story of a woman who had

been widowed in her sixties. She served in the Peace Corps and then started doing volunteer work since her financial situation was very secure. She made a statement that several people overheard as she headed off to conduct a group for seventy- and eighty-year-old women who had just lost their spouses: "You must excuse me because I have to run down and help these little old ladies." Being eighty-eight at the time of the comment, she was their senior by a decade.

Reference

Stein, M.; Miller, A. H.; and Trestman, R. L. "Depression and the Immune System." In *Psychoneuroimmunology*, 2d ed., ed. R. Alder, D. L. Felton, and N. Cohen. San Diego: Academic Press, 1991, pp. 897–923.

Life-Style Contract

After reading and pondering the last chapter on choices and the aging process and death and dying, you should have a good understanding of:

1. the nature of healthy aging;
2. what some of the things are that you can do to prepare mentally and fiscally for your own death or the eventual death of someone close to you;
3. the nature of the death and dying process;
4. what some things are you can do now for your own healthy aging experience.

You have been provided an opportunity to assess your health status as it relates to aging and death and dying. Keeping in mind some of the things that you have read in this chapter, the following list includes behaviors that you can do to enhance your health in these areas.

1. Become an organ donor.
2. Make out a living will.
3. Talk to clergy/spiritual mentor about life, death, and life after death.
4. Talk with parents or significant others about how they would like their funerals to be planned: memorial versus funeral, cremation versus burial, viewing versus nonviewing, music selections, and so on.
5. Adopt recreational pursuits that you really enjoy and will be able to do for a lifetime.
6. Make someone's retirement pleasant and rewarding by working on projects together, visiting, traveling together, making things with them, writing often, etc.
7. Adopt a grandmother or grandfather at a local rest home and visit periodically, take the person to a ball game, musical, etc.
8. Mentally rehearse how to comfort someone who may be dying or when someone has had someone close to them die.
9. Purchase a family burial plot or mausoleum space.

10. Complete your own funeral arrangements and keep them in a place near your will so others do not have to guess what you would like or feel obligated to buy an expensive service.

Life-Style Contracting Using Strength Intervention

I. Choosing the desired health behavior or skill

A. Keeping in mind the purposes in life and goals you identified in the mental health chapter, consider one or two health behaviors related to aging and death and dying (from the list here or your own creation) that will help you reach your goals. To assess the likelihood of success, ask yourself questions similar to those used in previous sections, such as:

1. Is my purpose, cause, or goal better realized by adoption of this behavior?
____ yes ____ no
2. Am I hardy enough to accomplish this goal? (This means I feel I can do it if I work hard, am committed to do it, am challenged by it, and see myself in control enough to make it happen.) ____ yes ____ no
3. Is this a behavior I really want to change and that I feel I can change? ____ yes ____ no
4. Do I first need to nurture a personal strength area? ____ yes ____ no (If yes, be sure to include this as a part of the plan.)
5. Do I need to free myself from the negative effects of a behavior (break a bad habit)? ____ yes ____ no (If yes, be sure to include this as a part of the plan.)
6. Have I considered the results of the assessment in the previous chapter?
____ yes ____ no

(Yes answers to the first three questions are a must to be successful. It might be wise to consider a different behavior if you can't honestly answer yes to these questions. Your answers to questions 4–6 ought to provide insights for your consideration in making your plan.)

B. Behaviors I will change (no more than two).

_____

_____

II. Life-style plan

   A. A description of the general plan of what I am going to do and how I will accomplish it. Consider apperceptive experiences—successes you have had in the past—since they may help you consider the best ways to carry out this plan.

_____

_____

_____

_____

_____

_____

   B. Barriers to the accomplishment of the plan (lack of time, materials, support, etc.).

     1. Identify the barriers _____

_____

_____

     2. Means to remove the barriers (use problem-solving skills or creative approaches such as those described in the mental health chapter)

_____

_____

_____

   C. Implementation of the plan.

     1. Substitution (putting positive behaviors in place of negative ones) _____

_____

_____

     2. Confluence (combining a mental and a physical activity for time efficiency if possible)

_____

_____

   3. Systematic enhancement (using a strength to help a weakness) _____

_____

   4. When _____

   5. Where _____

   6. Preparation _____

_____

   7. With whom _____

_____

_____

III. Support groups

   A. Who _____

_____

_____

   B. Role _____

_____

_____

   C. Organized support _____

_____

IV. Trigger responses _____

_____

_____

V. Starting date _____

VI. Date/sequence the contract will be reevaluated _____

_____

VII. Evidence(s) of reaching the goal _____

_____

_____

VIII. Reward(s) when contract is completed _____

_____

_____

IX. Signature of student _____

X. Signature of facilitator _____

XI. Additional conditions/comments _____

_____

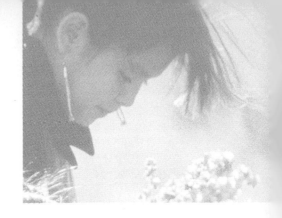

PART VII

Choices and the World Around You

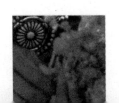

C HAPTER 15 DEALS WITH MANY TOPICS RELATED TO YOUR ENVIRONMENT. EN-VIRONMENTAL POLLUTION, THREATS TO YOUR HEALTH RELATED TO THE ENVI-RONMENT, AND PERSONAL SKILLS AND ACTIONS NEEDED ARE PRESENTED. CHAPTER 16 PULLS TOGETHER SKILLS AND KNOWLEDGE NEEDED TO MAKE HEALTHY DECISIONS.

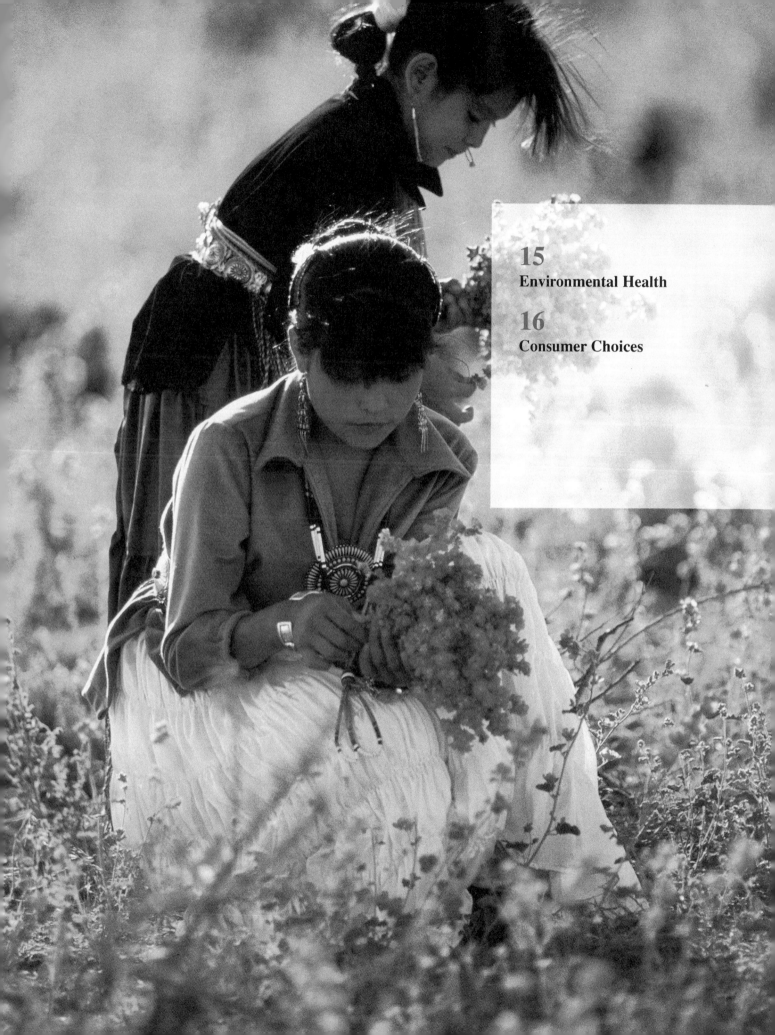

CHAPTER 15

Environmental Health

Key Questions

- What progress was made at the Earth Summit to protect the natural environment?

- What government regulations control the quality of public drinking water?

- What are the threats to our drinking water?

- What health hazards are associated with air pollution?

- What effects did the most devastating nuclear accident have on the world?

- What can you do about the environment?

- Can exposure to loud noise cause hearing impairment?

- What is acid rain?

- What effect does global warming have on the world?

- What can you do to promote environmental health?

Chapter Outline

Population Growth
Toxicity
Water Pollution
    Bacterial Contamination
    Chemical Contamination
    Regulation of Water Pollution
    Acid Rain
Air Pollution
    Kinds of Air Pollution
    The Nature of Air Pollution
    The Greenhouse Effect and Global
       Warming
    The Thinning of the Stratospheric
       Ozone Layer
    Health Effects of Global Warming
       and Ozone Layer Depletion
    Reducing Air Pollution
Land Pollution
    The Love Canal and Other Incidents
    What and How to Recycle
Noise Pollution
Environmental Threats from Nuclear
      Power Plants
    The Chernobyl Disaster
    The Threat of Nuclear Explosion
Personal Action

I n June of 1992, in Rio de Janeiro, the world came together to what could have been a major worldwide agreement to preserve the environment. Over one hundred world leaders and thirty thousand participants gathered to consider these questions: What kind of planet will our children inherit? Will they have room to roam, air to breathe, and food to eat? Will they ever see an eagle flying free or enjoy the solitude of a pristine mountain lake ("Earth Summit" 1992).

These questions arise in this era because we hear information such as the following: the world has lost 500 million acres of trees since 1972 (one-third the size of the United States); over ten thousand animal species are extinct; in Brazil the rain forest is burned for farmland, which will promote global warming; oceans are littered with plastics and tar balls and are rapidly losing fish; the garbage dumps, oil spills, sewage discharges, drift nets, and factory ships are only the visible problems with the sea, because 70 percent to 80 percent of maritime pollution comes from the sediment and contamination that flows into the seas from land-based sources, topsoil, fertilizers, pesticides, and industrial waste ("Earth Summit" 1992).

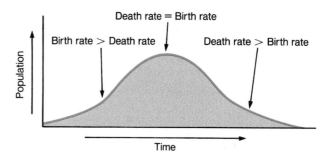

Figure 15.2

The normal growth curve.

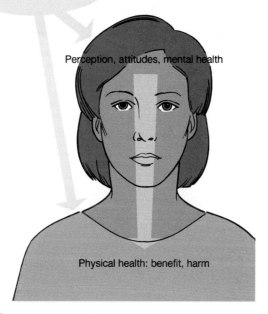

Figure 15.1

The effect of environmental factors on perception, mental health, and physical health.

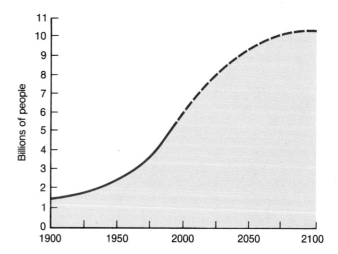

Source: United Nations Population Division

Figure 15.3

World population growth, 1900–2100.

From *World Population Prospects as Assessed in 1980* (United Nations publication, Sales. No. #E.81.XIII.8). Reprinted by permission.

One purpose of the Earth Summit was to sign the Biodiversity Treaty, which would call upon industrial nations to give the developing world financial incentives to protect their natural ecosystems, endangered plant and animal species, and rain forests. There appeared to be a difference of perspectives between the Northern Hemisphere and the Southern Hemisphere: in the north the forests are seen as a treasure to deal with the greenhouse effect by absorbing carbon dioxide and keeping global warming in check; in the south the developing nations see the same forests as a source of farmland, exotic woods, fuel, and lumber. The United States was the only country not willing to sign the agreement.

The decision we must make as a world community is between (1) economic growth, which necessitates producing steel, cutting trees for lumber, and other forms of industrialization and (2) protecting the world from environmental pollution, acid rain, the destruction of the protective ozone layer, the elimination of thousands of endangered species of plants and animals, and the warming of the planet. As Margaret Thatcher, then Prime Minister of England, put it in her famous "Green Speech" to the Royal Society, "With all these enormous changes in population, agriculture, use of fossil fuels concentrated into such a short period of time, we have unwittingly begun a massive experiment with the system of the planet itself" (Woodell 1989).

We each exist in an environment that is either conducive to health or detrimental to health. The conditions where we live can be either environmental stressors or positive factors, both of which affect mental health, stress level, and physical well-being (fig. 15.1).

Air pollution, noise, water pollution, chemicals, trash, land abuse, and other environmental conditions can negatively affect our outlook on life and our mental health and ultimately destroy us. Figure 15.2 demonstrates the normal growth curve and how after a certain population is reached, a species ultimately destroys itself.

Population Growth

Many people are concerned about the projected world population growth (fig. 15.3). It appears that the world has reached its peak in growth. On a positive note, humans are not mice in a confined cage; the world is very large, with huge areas of land that have not been developed. We have the ability to adapt, destroy waste products, and

Directions: Circle the number in front of the items that you have done or are doing.

1. When camping or when I do not have access to culinary water, I purify water (or would purify water) using tablets according to instructions or boil it before drinking.
2. On high pollution days, I wear a mask with extended exposure to the smog.
3. During temperature inversion, I try to reduce the build-up of air pollution by not burning in fireplaces and reducing automobile travel as much as possible.
4. I have visited my water or sewage treatment facilities and water sources.
5. I try to avoid known carcinogens such as vinyl chloride, asbestos, benzene, mercury, X rays, and so on.
6. I make sure my car is tuned and has functional emission control equipment.
7. I avoid noise pollutants (sit away from speakers at concerts, select an apartment away from busy streets or airports, and so on).
8. I have written my representative in state or federal government about environmental issues.
9. I avoid using aerosol sprays.
10. I recycle plastics.
11. I recycle metals.
12. I recycle aluminum.
13. I reuse materials such as grocery shopping bags, cardboard boxes, etc.
14. I recycle tin cans.
15. I recycle glass containers.
16. I recycle newspapers.
17. I recycle cardboard.
18. I purchase recycled products.
19. I use products that have minimal packages and avoid plastics.
20. I use as few paper products as possible.
21. I dispose of hazardous materials (old car batteries, used oil, or used antifreeze) at gas stations or other appropriate sites.
22. If I have children or when I have children, I will use a diaper service as opposed to disposable diapers.

Scoring/Interpretation

Total the items that you have circled. Ideally, you can be doing all these things, but if you are trying to do at least some, you can score yourself as follows:

17–22	=	Good contributions to maintaining the environment
12–16	=	Moderate contributions to maintaining the environment
Below 12	=	Need to consider the recommendations made in this chapter to help the environment

---

develop chemicals that can sterilize and disinfect. How far our resourcefulness will take us, though, is a concern of many environmental health specialists. Limiting family size, increasing efficient food production, and removing waste are worldwide concerns. This is of particular concern in densely populated areas. In some places of the world, overpopulation results in multiple families in single dwellings. Life expectancy is shortened because of improper waste removal, poor sanitary conditions, and the rapid spread of disease. The population explosion is not only a medical, economic, and political issue but a moral issue.

The more people there are, the more air pollution there is from autos; the more waste there is to be removed; the more homes to be built, which uses up wood from the forests; the more development and expansion into the ever-decreasing natural landscape; the more factories to be built; and so on. With more people, the higher our chances are of breathing bad air, drinking contaminated water, and being exposed to toxic substances. This picture sounds dismal, but it is difficult to find a positive outcome of natural resource waste. The positive side of the picture is that there are measures that we can take to avoid toxic substances and demand good control from federal, state, and local governments. In more developed countries, for example, the population growth is much less than that of less developed countries (fig. 15.4).

Before understanding how the air, water, and land are being threatened by contamination, a basic understanding of the concept of toxicity is necessary.

Toxicity

Almost any chemical can become toxic (poisonous) if you are exposed to excessive amounts. **Toxicity** depends on the exposure level and the dose at which various negative effects occur. Because we are constantly exposed to chemicals, it is important to know as much about them as possible to avoid overexposure.

You will not suffer from toxicity from a chemical without exposure to that chemical. **Exposure** is the pathway or means a person comes in contact with the chemical. Understanding how exposure occurs is an important step in preventing toxicity. **Risk assessment,** as it applies to the study of environmental health, is the scientific estimation of the likelihood of health problems as a result of exposure to chemicals. The estimation of risk is based on

Population Control

Some countries are now imposing mandatory birth-control measures to help control the population (India and China). Couples are only allowed to have one or two children. Many health professionals feel that the United States should also put a limit on family size. Although the likelihood of that happening from a constitutional perspective is slim, do you favor it for other countries, where this can happen? Do you favor it for people on welfare in this country?

- **Pro:** In countries where they can hardly feed their people, it certainly makes sense to limit the family size. If they don't limit the size, then they will probably starve to death. This should be particularly true for low-income people. Even in this country, if people on welfare are going to be subsidized by the government, then perhaps they should be limited while they are on welfare, in light of the economic deficit facing the United States.

- **Con:** This is a moral and spiritual issue first and economic and political issue second. Restricting family size is a major infringement of human rights and is inhumane. This policy is not in reference to dogs or cats but loving couples who want offspring to carry on traditions and family names and to create family units. Just because someone is on welfare does not mean they should also lose their dignity, their need for family, or their need to be loved.

How would you react to governmentally imposed restrictions on family size?

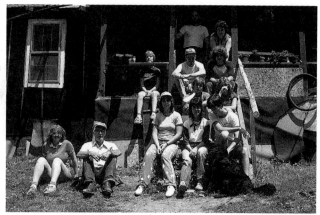

The worldwide population explosion is a medical, economic, political, and moral issue.

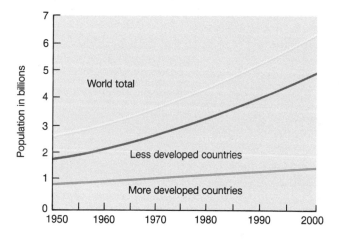

Figure 15.4

World population growth, 1950–2000.

From *World Population Prospects as Assessed in 1980* (United Nations publication, Sales. No. #E.81.XIII.8). Reprinted by permission.

studies that show amounts of exposure and consequential health problems that have resulted over time. Risk assessment is the key to determining safe working conditions, products that will be sold on the open market, building materials, and other government-controlled materials.

Whether a chemical is toxic is also dependent on potency. Potency is the ability of the chemical to cause cancer or other problems. Potency is expressed when the chemical is in the body in terms of milligrams of chemical per unit of body weight (kilograms) per day. For example, benzene has a potency or an ability to cause cancer at an exposure of 0.052 milligrams/kilogram/day. Potency may also be determined by a cumulative analysis. For example, exposure to 93 milligrams of benzene over a lifetime increases the risk of cancer to 1 in 1,000, or 241,000 people in America. Sometimes the potency of exposure is based on the surrounding water or air that we drink or breathe. The units then become parts of the chemical to total parts in the air or water. For example, cancer risks increase when the amount of benzene that will be inhaled with the air is 5,500 parts per million or when the amount ingested with water is 550 parts benzene per million.

Chemicals are moved from one place to another in a variety of ways, and we can be exposed to the same chemical from a variety of sources. The chief mediums for chemicals include air (gases or vapor), water (liquid substances in the ground, on the surface, or in rainwater), soil or sediments (chemicals mixed with dirt), and food (fish, animals, or plants).

Movement between mediums is dependent on the chemical properties of the substance; but, chemicals can be changed or moved through metabolism (bacterial change or eating), chemical transformation (such as in the exposure to ultraviolet light), exposure to heat (liquid to gas forms), and in conjunction with other chemicals (nontoxic sodium nitrite to carcinogenic nitrocimines). Chemicals can then be moved into the human body by inhalation, absorption, or ingestion.

Water Pollution

By now, we should be fully aware that we cannot take safe drinking water for granted.

Bacterial Contamination

Most municipal water-treatment facilities are equipped only for bacterial decontamination, which is accomplished by chlorination of the water. Thus, water leaving these facilities is tested only for absence of **coliform bacteria** and presence of a **chlorine residual.** The chlorine residual is the amount of chlorine added minus the amount used up in the decontamination process. A chlorine residual in a water sample indicates that the bacteria have been killed and that some chlorine remains in the water to kill bacteria that enter after the water leaves the plant. Too many dangerous bacteria in drinking water may spread waterborne diseases.

Chemical Contamination

Routine daily tests for possible chemical or radiological contaminants in a water supply are impractical, so these tests are conducted only in special instances. Consequently, facilities that discharge chemical and radioactive waste have a heavy responsibility to institute at least minimal pollution controls. If you know of any industries that discharge wastes into local lakes, rivers, or streams, you should find out about their pollution-control policies.

Threats to human health posed by chemical contamination of water supplies are much more serious than those posed by bacterial contamination, because chemicals may persist in the environment for a much longer time.

Though much of the bacterial contamination of water supplies can be treated at municipal water-treatment facilities, the effects of chemical contamination can be virtually irreversible. For instance, widespread use of high-nitrate fertilizers in cattle-feeding areas has contaminated many underground water sources with nitrates to levels that exceed drinking water standards. Once an underground water supply is contaminated, purification is practically impossible. If young children ingest water high in nitrates, methemoglobinemia (a fatal blood disease) can result (U.S. Environmental Protection Agency 1973). In addition to acute disease episodes, the effects of chemical contaminants can be chronic. Low levels of chemical contaminants in water may not be noticed until they are ingested and concentrated in the body over a long period of time.

Thermal and radioactive pollution of water are other ways we pay for industrialization. In **thermal pollution,** excessive heat is added to the natural water supply, causing detrimental changes in the aquatic balance. This excess heat is usually derived from power plants situated near rivers, lakes, or streams that use the inexpensive nearby water source to cool their equipment. Raising the water temperature even a few degrees, however, may change how fish and plants obtain their food. For example, if the water temperature is too high, the fish may have to migrate; if the fish are enclosed in a lake, they are "stuck." Heated water also contains less dissolved oxygen, which plants need for respiration, because heat drives it out of the water and plants. Without enough oxygen, water plants die and the fish that depend on them for food must also migrate.

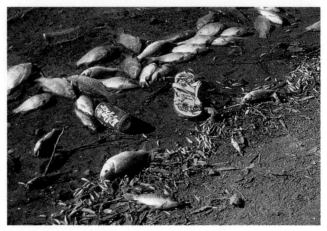

Often water pollution occurs because of laziness or carelessness.

Radioactive pollution of water can be even more insidious than thermal pollution. Radioactive wastes discharged into natural waters by nuclear plants are the most common source. This influx of radiation may make the water unusable for humans or for water life.

Regulation of Water Pollution

The 1972 amendment to the **Federal Water Pollution Control Act** of 1948 is considered landmark legislation. For the first time, national goals for water quality were announced. These national goals were to improve water quality so that all navigable waters (interstate and intrastate) would be clean enough for swimming, recreation, and fish and wildlife by July 1983 (Willgoose et al. 1979).

The **Clean Water Act** of 1977 and subsequent legislation provided federal support to implement the provisions of the 1972 amendment to the Federal Water Pollution Control Act. The most effective program to improve water quality funded efforts to upgrade municipal sewage-treatment facilities. As a result, fish have returned to waters they had abandoned, and the recreational appeal of Lake Erie, for example, which was a dying lake, has been revived.

Besides governmental efforts, we can see progress by the chemical industry in water pollution control. One particular example of industrial initiative has been the use by Dow Chemical of certain bacteria that turn specific chemical wastes into harmless end products.

Governmental efforts and industrial initiatives, however, are not enough by themselves to improve our water quality. We must all participate. To start, we can learn more about the water pollution problems in our communities and express our concerns to elected officials. One letter at the federal level is believed to have as much effect as twenty-five votes on influencing policy. Further, we can make our life-style compatible with improved water quality by using water frugally and not littering our natural waters. Whether and how we extend a heritage of cleaner water is up to us.

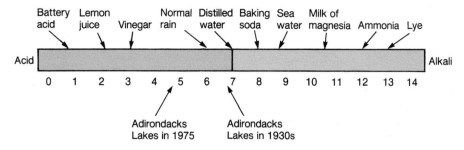

Figure 15.5

A pH scale showing acid rain in relation to other substances.

From Anne Nadakavukaren, *Man and Environment: A Health Perspective, Second Edition* (Prospect Heights, Illinois: Waveland Press, Inc., 1986) p. 281. Reprinted by permission.

Acid Rain

Acid precipitation in the form of snow, rain, hail, and fog is a concern that wasn't even recognized when the Clean Air Act was passed in 1977. **Acid rain** has a pH that is less than 5.6 on the pH scale, which ranges from 0 to 14, with 0 representing the strongest acids and 14 representing the strongest alkali. The pH of distilled water is 7.0. Rain is usually slightly acidic at 5.6 because of its tendency to react with atmospheric carbon dioxide (fig. 15.5).

The extent of the problem of acid rain was originally thought to be only near industrial centers. Now the phenomenon occurs hundreds of miles from the original source, causing the pH of unpolluted lakes to change from normal to acidic and killing fish and other forms of wildlife. For example, the sparkling Adirondacks lakes in New York, once known for their excellent trout fishing, are now devoid of fish. Minnesota's Boundary Waters Canoe Area is on the brink of suffering the same fate. Reports of mysterious disappearance of fish come from Ontario and Quebec (140 Ontario lakes are now devoid of fish) to the waterways of Scandinavia (10,000 lakes no longer have fish). The Black Forest of Germany and Roan Mountain of North Carolina have also been affected by acid rain. The Rockies and Sierra Nevada mountains are under threat, too. Such lakes have been poisoned by sulfuric and nitric acids falling from the sky (Nadakavukaren 1986).

Air Pollution

The **Clean Air Act** is the most important federal law protecting the air we breathe. It establishes ambient (outside) air standards for six pollutants and emission standards for those six and other chemicals. The act does not have jurisdiction over indoor pollutants. The six noncarcinogenic pollutants have been labeled **criteria air pollutants** because they are threshold chemicals and safe levels can be established (i.e., scientists know at what level they become dangerous). The pollutants include carbon monoxide, lead, nitrogen dioxide, hydrocarbons, ozone, particulates, and sulfur dioxide. Sources of pollutants covered under the Clean Air Act include emissions from auto-mobiles, which carry significant amounts of all the criteria pollutants except ozone and sulphur dioxide.

The **Environmental Protection Agency (EPA)** has identified **hazardous air pollutants** that are generally considered to be carcinogenic. Those hazardous air pollutants include asbestos, benzene, beryllium, mercury, radionuclides, and vinyl chloride. The Clean Air Act requires the EPA to set emission standards with an ample margin of safety to protect the public health. The EPA does not have authority to regulate the release of chemicals other than criteria and hazardous air pollutants. Indoor air quality (random accumulation, carbon monoxide, and formaldehyde, for example) is generally not controlled.

Kinds of Air Pollution

Air pollution can have both natural and artificial origins. Because of the natural sources of pollution, the air in our atmosphere has probably never been pure. Naturally generated air pollution—such as volcanic eruptions, wind-blown dust, and pollen—is unavoidable. Artificially generated air pollution, such as factory smoke and auto exhaust, began on a large scale about the time of the Industrial Revolution and quickly affected human health and the environment.

Visible air pollution, such as smoke and soot from factories, was recognized and even accepted as the price of industrialization in Europe in the 1700s. It took only about twenty-five years before artificially generated pollution exceeded nature's capability to purify the air in heavily industrialized areas. When weather conditions accentuate the effects of artificially generated air pollution, the number of human illnesses and deaths rises. In the 1800s, air pollution ordinances were passed that seemed to be effective in reducing smoke.

Perhaps the real reason for the improvement in the visible air quality during the 1950s was the shift from coal to petroleum as our primary energy source. But this change in energy sources did not solve the air quality problem. By the middle of the twentieth century, "invisible" air pollution emerged as the leading culprit of unhealthy air, and air quality actually deteriorated even

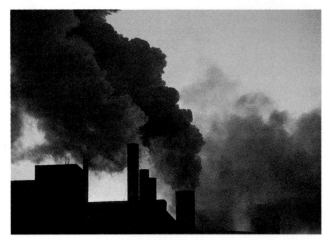
Avoid as much air pollution as you can, particularly on smog alert days.

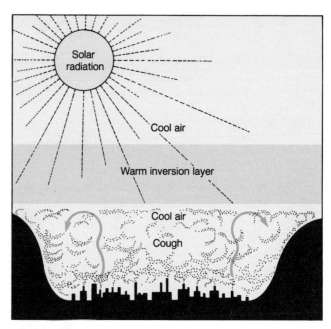

Figure 15.6

Thermal inversion, triggered by a high pressure area, traps pollutants in a layer of cool air that cannot rise to carry the pollutants away.

further. This deterioration resulted from the proliferation of the motor vehicle and the availability of relatively inexpensive fuel. Americans became addicted to the personal convenience that motor vehicles offered. Work and leisure revolved around the car. At one point, the rate of vehicle registrations even surpassed the birth rate!

The Nature of Air Pollution

When a concoction called **photochemical smog**—the product of sunlight acting on auto and industrial exhausts—became our major air pollutant, nature's job of cleaning the air became even more demanding. Not surprisingly, transportation is still the single greatest contributor to air pollution in this nation. Chemically, the major gaseous air pollutants are carbon monoxide, nitrogen oxides, and the sulfur oxides, while the major solid components of air pollutants are hydrocarbons and particulates. (Figure 15.6 shows how smog gathers in a populated area.)

Here, again, lies the root of the debate over industrialization versus preserving the forests. To clean the air, we need forests, but we also need forests for industrialization.

The danger posed by these air pollutants lies in their invisibility. Without formal testing, we never know where the chemicals are being emitted or how much is present. Air pollutants can affect the human body in many ways, some of which are shown in figure 15.7.

The Greenhouse Effect and Global Warming

The **greenhouse effect** (fig. 15.8) refers to the "effect that the accumulation of carbon dioxide and other gases in the earth's atmosphere has on the balance between the energy the earth receives from solar radiation and the energy it loses by radiation from its surface back to space" (Leaf 1989). The Industrial Revolution focused on the use of fossil fuels (coal and oil), whose byproduct is, among other gases, carbon dioxide. Carbon dioxide, along with other "greenhouse gases" like methane, nitrous oxide, and chlo-

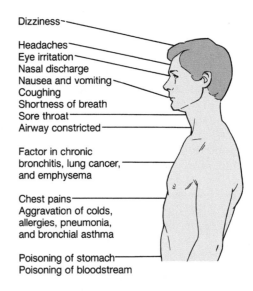

Figure 15.7

Some possible effects of air pollution on the human body.

rofluorocarbons, are largely transparent to the sun's rays, including ultraviolet light, which warm the earth's surface. Unfortunately, when the warmth is bounced off the earth's surface the greenhouse gases act like water vapor, absorb the longer infrared waves emitted from the earth, and trap the warmth.

This balance of gases is critical. If there were no gases, there would be another ice age since no warmth would be retained, but as we produce more gases than necessary to maintain the earth's warmth, a slow warming

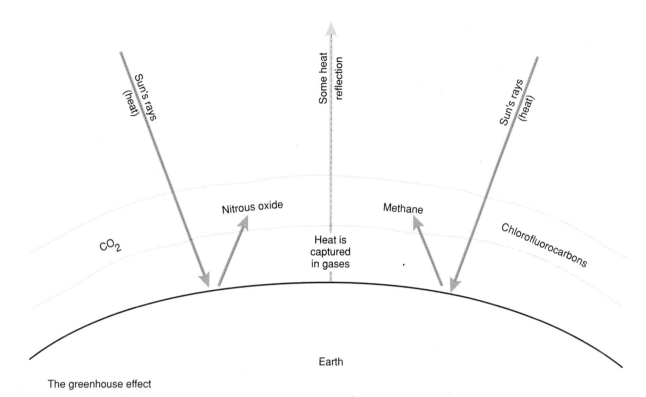

Sun's rays (heat)

Some heat reflection

Sun's rays (heat)

Nitrous oxide

Methane

CO_2

Heat is captured in gases

Chlorofluorocarbons

Earth

The greenhouse effect

Figure 15.8
The greenhouse effect.

occurs. Experts suggest that we are witnessing a slow warming rate of about three-tenths of one degree Celsius every decade. This amount may seem trivial, but a warming of between two and five degrees Celsius is about the difference between current conditions and the last ice age. The effects of this **global warming** may

1. turn fertile and arable areas into deserts and move prime agricultural areas north (e.g., Canada) and to higher elevations;
2. melt the polar ice caps and, depending on the amount of melt, raise the sea level by three to twenty feet;
3. increase the sea level and displace millions of people living near the coasts;
4. increase precipitation, since heat increases evaporation but would likely be unevenly dispersed; where winter normally holds water in snow, it would result in quick run-offs and increased flooding;
5. with population displacement, turn agricultural lands into deserts, causing wider famine.

The Thinning of the Stratospheric Ozone Layer

Another environmental disturbance that humans are causing is the depletion of the ozone layer in the stratosphere. The **ozone layer** is a kind of shield protecting us from the sun's ultraviolet radiation. Ultraviolet light is divided into three types based on its place on an electromagnetic spectrum. Ultraviolet C includes wavelengths of 200 to 290 and is the most damaging to life, but fortunately the ozone shields us from exposure. Ultraviolet B (wavelength

of 290 to 320) is not as damaging to life as ultraviolet C but many times more damaging than A (over 320). The pathological consequences of ultraviolet B and C are chiefly attributable to its disruption of DNA and proteins in the body (Leaf 1989). The ozone layer blocks it from reaching the earth's surface.

It has been only in the last few years that scientists have understood what we are doing to the ozone. **Chlorofluorocarbons** (used in aerosols), refrigerants, nitrous oxide (from internal combustion engines), and other industrial products rise to the stratosphere, become reactive with the ozone, and destroy it. Ozone is formed naturally by the action of sunlight on the rare molecules of oxygen in the stratosphere. It does regenerate but very slowly. The half-life of recovery of ozone is three to five years.

In the spring of 1985, a hole in the ozone layer was discovered and thereafter has grown to the size of a continent. In March of 1988, the thinning of the ozone layer was noted over the North Pole. The ozone layer continues to decrease at the rate of 4 percent to 5 percent per decade ("Earth Summit" 1992).

Health Effects of Global Warming and Ozone Layer Depletion

The health effects of global warming via the "greenhouse effect" and the holes in the ozone have been forecasted by Leaf (1989) as the following:

1. There will be an increased production of respiratory irritants that will add to the already polluted air and lead to increases in lung diseases such as

While the world community fights to limit waste, recycle, conserve, and protect, it is amazing how one man can cause so much destruction in such a short time. At the end of the Persian Gulf War, when troops from Iraq were withdrawing from Kuwait, the orders from Hussein were to destroy the oil wells of Kuwait before they left. The consequences were devastating.

1. One thousand oil wells were destroyed.

2. Approximately six hundred were set ablaze like orange fireballs all over the desert. It took until the fall of 1991 for these fires to be extinguished, after having consumed enormous amounts of crude oil.

3. Oil was dumped into the Gulf waters, leaving a major oil slick that threatened extinction of several species of sea life.

4. The smoke from the oil fires caused black clouds to cover areas of Kuwait. It appeared as night at noon. Soot from the fires fell like snowflakes, and oil droplets fell like greasy black rain. Temperatures were twenty degrees Fahrenheit hotter under the black clouds (Elmer-DeWitt 1991).

These selfish, thoughtless acts will take years to recover from. What should the world leaders do with such a criminal?

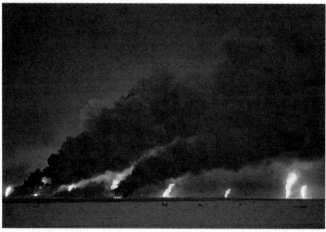

Selfish, thoughtless acts by individuals can undo much of the world community's efforts to protect and conserve the environment.

---

bronchitis, asthma, and chronic obstructive pulmonary disease.

2. The breakdown of the ozone layer will also result in greater ultraviolet D radiation and raise the incidence of skin cancers and cataracts.

3. Excessive ultraviolet light will also compromise the immune system and in combination with the increasing unsanitary conditions caused by other sources of pollution, this will lead to an increase in infectious diseases.

4. As the ocean levels rise from glacial melting, waterborne infections will also multiply.

5. Decreased food supplies will be the most serious repercussion of global and climatic environmental changes.

Reducing Air Pollution

Reducing air pollution from any one source is not a simple task. Vehicle emissions alone involve several pollutants, and different pollutants require different reduction methods, each with technological problems. The greatest hindrance to real progress in reducing air pollution, however, is that we currently value economics and energy above the environment. Until we rearrange our priorities, no fundamental progress will result. As members of this society who care and are concerned about the environment, we must each contribute to making everyone more environmentally conscious.

Attempts to clean up the air were spurred by the environmental movement, which had its most profound impact in the early 1970s. The U.S. Environmental Protection Agency was established during these years, and many environmentally related laws were passed. Among these laws were the Clean Air amendments, which specified auto emission standards for cars produced after 1975 and 1976.

Though major strides in auto air pollution control were made, none of these goals was entirely attained. In part, this is because of our life-style values. For example, the Arab oil embargo of 1973–74 forced a greater change in life-style than perhaps any other event in the 1970s. Gone were the days when gasoline cost only 25 to 35 cents per gallon. The days of dollar-plus per gallon gasoline and uncertain availability began. When a decision had to be made whether to add the costs of environmental quality to the rising cost of gasoline, politics and economics won out. Auto manufacturers were permitted to delay implementation of costly pollution-control efforts in favor of energy efficiency. Economics and energy dictated decisions rather than environmental quality. Hence, our life-style values seemed to shift.

If we are to reverse this trend, we must act to preserve environmental quality, making it as important as economic and energy considerations. There is no reason why goals related to economics, energy, and environment cannot be pursued simultaneously.

Land Pollution

Ironically, efforts to abate water and air pollution have made land pollution even worse. This is because there are only three repositories for the wastes of society: the earth, its water, and its atmosphere (U.S. Environmental Protection Agency 1973). The environment is an interconnected system, and restrictions imposed on any one of these three repositories inevitably lead to an overflow on the other two. For example, restrictions on water disposal of sludge (organic wastes from the treatment of water) have meant that land disposal was the next alternative. The ban on open burning of garbage and debris to reduce air pollution has meant that the burden of disposal has been transferred to the land. Furthermore, the trend is to look more and more to earth as the ultimate repository for hazardous chemical and radioactive wastes. The earth has literally become a pit for all undesirable substances. According to a recent U.S. Environmental Protection Agency estimate, more than thirty thousand dump sites in the United States pose a significant risk to human health (American Public Health Association 1980).

The sheer increase in the bulk and weight of solid waste has further aggravated the disposal problem. In 1960, each person in this country generated approximately 2.7 pounds of solid waste per day; by 1980, that amount had risen to approximately 3.9 pounds per day. This trend represents about a 1 percent increase in solid wastes per person per year (Grisham 1986). Consider all the packaging and wrappings for food, the boxes and bags for clothes, and the plastic we dispose of daily without thinking. It adds up. While the amount of solid waste has grown steadily, the means for its disposal have been limited.

Traditionally, solid waste has been incinerated, buried in **sanitary landfills,** or converted by resource recovery (**recycled**). Each method has inherent benefits and risks. No one method of solid waste disposal is best for all kinds of waste. For example, resource recovery is usually the most environmentally responsible method; however, potential health hazards require incineration rather than recycling of hospital wastes. In selecting the best disposal method, we must consider energy and economics; how-ever, as with air quality enhancement, life-style values should guide our attitudes and actions. The time for solid waste to be "out of sight, out of mind" has passed. We must exercise our insight to minimize the hazardous effects of land pollution on health and environment.

The Resource Conservation and Recovery Act (RCRA) and the Comprehensive Environmental Response, Compensation, and Liability Act (CERCLA, or Superfund) are the two federal laws governing regulation of present and future land disposal practices and cleanup. The Toxic Substances Control Act (TSCA) is the federal law that regulates production and use of new chemicals and previously unregulated chemicals. Before a new chemical can be produced for industrial or commercial use, the EPA must review the available toxicological data base. The EPA has the power to regulate any chemical judged to pose an unreasonable risk of injury to human health or to the environment. Types of control include labeling, banning, disposal methods, exposure precautions, and required consumer information.

The Love Canal and Other Incidents

The indiscriminate use and careless disposal of hazardous material became shockingly evident in 1978 in a small residential suburb of Niagara Falls, New York. The Love Canal was a dream of William Love, who dug the seven-mile navigable canal from above Niagara Falls to below the falls. His dream was to build a model industrial city using hydroelectric power. Mr. Love's dream faded when he went bankrupt in 1927, but the canal was used for fishing and recreation and was annexed by the city.

In 1947, Hooker Chemical Company bought the land and received permission to dump chemical wastes into the canal. Over the years, twenty-one thousand tons of chemical wastes, acids, alkalis, solvents, and chlorinated hydrocarbons were disposed of at this sight. By 1953, waste filled the canal and it began to grow over with grass and weeds. Not many homes were near the area at the time, but Hooker then sold the site to the city for a token $1. In 1955, a school was built, followed by several hundred modest homes. Residents smelled odors, but that was not unusual in an industrial city.

In the mid-1970s, during some heavy rains, chemicals began oozing through basement walls in these homes, puddles of chemical wastes stood and never evaporated, vegetation became scorched, and lawns died. Holes opened up in fields revealing large, corroded, leaking chemical drums. Complaints and fears by the citizens were not initially responded to and instead they received assurances that everything was okay. In 1978, the EPA began to test the area and found twelve known carcinogens in basements of houses and in the soil. Benzene, dioxin, and numerous other chemicals were found. Finally, the area was condemned, and President Carter proclaimed the area a national emergency. The state purchased the homes and over five hundred families moved. Studies of these families remain highly controversial, but indications of elevated rates of miscarriage, birth defects, and chromosomal damage are evident.

In 1990, the houses on Love Canal went up for sale with a statement that "the homes are safe, but not guaranteed." Lawsuits are still pending against Hooker Chemical, which ultimately became a subsidiary of Occidental Petroleum.

In 1989, another widely publicized event was the oil spill along the Alaskan coast of Prince William Sound. The *Exxon Valdez* oil tanker struck ground and spilled eleven million gallons of oil. The captain was found to be intoxicated, and the result was a $2.5 billion cleanup operation and a devastating impact on the environment and wildlife. Some three hundred lawsuits were filed against Exxon and individuals, and settlements have exceeded a billion dollars (Lemonick 1992). Again in January of 1993 a tanker wrecked on the Shetland Islands of Scotland and spilled its entire oil cargo into the sea. Birds and animals were killed, and gale winds whipped the oil and sea into a foam mist that covered sheep and humans alike on the island.

Other hazardous sites include the "valley of the drums" near Louisville, Kentucky, where seventeen thousand drums (of which six thousand were full of chemicals) were discovered. Apparently the owner of the land had been paid by industrial firms to haul their wastes to an approved site. Instead, he pocketed the money and dumped the chemicals on his own land, in some cases dumping the chemicals on the soil to reuse the drums. In Iberville Parish, Louisiana, a nineteen-year-old man was killed when a load of the chemical he dumped into a waste pit reacted with other chemicals there. A cloud of hydrogen sulfide gas formed, which enveloped him and paralyzed his lungs. The pit was operating without a permit. In Montague, Michigan, the Hooker Chemical Company built a factory that produced the highly toxic pesticide C-56. The factory had allowed the C-56 to be vented into the air near the tourist town of White Lake and also to ooze through the floor and onto the work areas below. Two billion gallons of ground water were contaminated and one million gallons of carcinogenic water flowed into White Lake daily (Nadakavukaren 1986).

What and How to Recycle

New industries all over America are helping to recycle materials for continued use, thereby reducing the demand on landfills. As consumers, we can all try to purchase products that have been recycled, which encourages reuse and the formation and profitability of recycling companies. We can also recycle a variety of products that we use on a regular basis. Check your local community for locations to deposit recyclable materials. The following list identifies recyclable materials and how to prepare them for return.

1. Metals—scrap metal dealers may accept some large appliances. Call first. Higher prices may be given if metals are separate and clean.
2. Aluminum—siding, cans, gutters, and other materials can be recycled at centers in most communities. Squash the cans and place in a reusable trash barrel.
3. Tin cans—rinse cans out. Remove ends and labels. Carefully smash cans to flatten.
4. Plastics—plastic beverage containers such as two-liter pop bottles (#1 PET) or plastic milk and

water containers (#2 HDPE) are currently accepted at some local supermarkets if washed and crushed.

5. Glass containers—separate according to color (clear, brown, green) and rinse. Labels are okay to leave on.

6. Newspapers—bundle newspapers with string for convenience and drop off at recycling bins, some stores, or recycle centers.

7. Cardboard—must be unwaxed and corrugated (like a pizza box).

8. Paperboard—unwaxed boxes such as those for crackers, cereal, and powdered laundry detergent. Just remove the inner linings before recycling.

9. Magazines—take magazines to doctor's offices, hospitals, nursing homes, day-care centers, hair salons, laundromats, tire stores, and other places with waiting rooms where others may enjoy them (check with the organization first). Some communities also recycle glossy paper magazines and catalogs.

Noise Pollution

With technology, increasing populations, more air travel, and industrialization comes more noise. With construction equipment, amplifiers, jet engines, street traffic, trains, school bells, vacuum cleaners, televisions, compact disc players, and other noise makers, we are abusing our ears. This abuse often results in hearing dysfunctions. Hearing loss results from the destructive effect of noise on the delicate hair cells in the inner ear. These hair cells convert fluid vibrations in the inner ear into nerve impulses that are carried to the brain, resulting in the sensations of sound. With the damage to the hair cells, hearing loss may be partial, as noticed by either a softening of sound or loss of certain frequencies (generally the higher frequencies), or loss may be complete. Hearing loss is generally associated with prolonged exposure to noise over 70 to 85 decibels (Nadakavukaren 1986).

Noise-induced hearing loss is progressive and is usually not accompanied by such overt symptoms as pain or bleeding. Noise has been implicated in both temporary (acute) and cumulative (chronic) effects on human health. Sudden noises can produce immediate blood vessel dilation, increases in blood pressure, heart rate changes, and hormonal secretions. Continuous noise can exact a toll on mental health and increase our susceptibility to infection and gastric disorders. Steady levels of loud noise have led to a higher incidence of cardiovascular and balance problems among exposed workers than among nonexposed workers (Evans 1982). In addition to these problems, nerve damage from loud noises may produce hearing impairment that cannot be restored by hearing aids or surgical procedures.

How irritating and damaging sound is depends on frequency (pitch) and amplitude. Pitch measures the speed of the vibrations in **hertz (Hz).** We can hear from 10 to 20,000 Hz. Amplitude measures the force behind the vibration or loudness. Amplitude is measured in **decibels (db),** which range from 0 (where normal ears can begin to hear) to 194 (the theoretical maximum loudness of pure tones). Decibels are logarithmic, which means that 20 decibels is one hundred times as loud as 0, 30 decibels is one thousand times as loud as 0 decibels, and so on. Comparative sounds and measured decibels are shown in table 15.1.

Excessive noise not only results in hearing loss but is a safety hazard as well. It is responsible for many accidents. For example, a worker in an auto glass factory caught his hand in a piece of equipment and screamed for help, but no one could hear him because of excessive factory noise, and he lost his hand. Two people were struck by a locomotive while watching Senator Robert Kennedy's funeral train pass through the city because they hadn't heard the warning whistle, which had been drowned out by the noise of the news media helicopters and secret service. While jogging or walking on streets, many people listen to music with headphones and never hear oncoming cars. They are frequently hit.

The federal government has tried to reduce excessive noise with the passage of the Noise Control Act, which regulates new commercial products that are considered to be major noise sources. Regulations mandating mufflers on cars have greatly reduced city noise.

More importantly, we can control how much noise we are exposed to and how much hearing damage occurs. If we are forced to work around or be around loud noises, then ear protectors can be worn. We can choose to be in front of the speakers at a concert or dance or farther away.

Environmental Threats from Nuclear Power Plants

The benefits of nuclear energy are unquestioned. In a day of diminishing oil reserves, when there is a need to have oil shipped from countries experiencing political unrest, nuclear power is a good supplement. The dangerous part of nuclear power plants is the potential for massive destruction if accidents occur. The first major nuclear power disaster occurred in Russia.

The Chernobyl Disaster

In April of 1986, in Chernobyl, a one thousand megawatt nuclear power plant suddenly broke down and resulted in the world's worst nuclear accident. The resulting fire billowed smoke, gas, and radioactive particles in the air, causing radioactive fallout all over Europe and even in parts of the United States. It will be years before the total loss of life is known because all resulting cancers have not yet occurred. The process leading to the disaster occurred in six steps:(1) the cooling system for the reactor failed; (2) the uranium fuel melted; (3) the graphite overheated and flammable gases resulted; (4) the mix exploded; (5) radiation billowed; and (6) emergency measures faltered.

The Threat of Nuclear Explosion

Radiation fallout can kill someone immediately or linger in the body for decades. The *rem* is the unit of measure for radiation. The following represents the dosage and health consequences:

Exposure	Effect
5,000 rem	Kills almost immediately
1,000 rem	Causes death within days
400 rem over several days	Kills half of its victims within a month
150 rem over a week	Survivable

Radiation from fallout affects people differently but is often characterized by loss of appetite, nausea, and diar-

TABLE 15.1

Sound Levels and the Human Response

Common Sounds	Noise Level (db)	Effect
Air raid siren	140	Painfully loud
Jet takeoff	130	
Discotheque	120	Maximum vocal effort
Pile driver	110	
Garbage truck	100	
City traffic	90	Very annoying, hearing damage
Alarm clock	80	Annoying
Freeway traffic	70	Phone use difficult
Air conditioning	60	Intrusive
Light auto traffic	50	Quiet
Living room	40	
Library	30	Very quiet
Broadcasting studio	20	
	10	Just audible
	0	Hearing begins

Source: U.S. Environmental Protection Agency.

rhea. Often these initial symptoms disappear after a week, inducing a false sense of recovery. Then high fever sets in and affected individuals lose weight and become lethargic as their gastrointestinal tracts lose the ability to absorb nutrients. Damage to blood-forming tissue produces a drastic lowering of the white blood cell count, leaving the individual prey to infection.

It is important to be aware of these threats and be active politically, demanding that these energy-producing plants are careful monitored and maintained.

Personal Action

In the spirit of Earth Day 1990, it becomes extremely important to make a decision and encourage local, state, and national governments to deal effectively with the environmental dilemmas we face. Should we try and do something to help prevent continual pollution, the destruction of the ozone, and the greenhouse effect? Granted, on an international level, we need to continue to provide active political support for the international attempts at dealing with these problems, but it is here in the United States that we can make a significant impact. The United States, by its unwillingness to sign the Biodiversity Treaty, has set itself up as a negative influence on the world's cooperative efforts to preserve the earth's natural resources. The United States has only 5 percent of the

Nuclear Power Accidents

More than a dozen serious accidents have plagued the U.S. effort to tame nuclear power. Among the worst:

July 24, 1959: A blocked cooling system caused melting of twelve of the forty-three fuel elements in an experimental power reactor at Santa Susana, California, near Los Angeles. Radioactivity was contained.

January 3, 1961: Control rods were removed in error from the core of a military experimental reactor near Idaho Falls, Idaho. This caused a steam explosion that killed three technicians, one of them impaled by a control rod. These were the only deaths so far in U.S. reactor operations. Radiation levels were very high in the plant, but the damage was contained.

October 5, 1966: Failure of a sodium cooling system caused a partial core meltdown at the Enrico Fermi demonstration breeder reactor thirty miles from Detroit. Radiation was contained.

June 5, 1970: A false signal from a meter at Commonwealth Edison's Dresden II plant in Morris, Illinois, was blamed for a two-hour loss of control. A buildup of radioactive iodine at one hundred times the permissible level was contained.

November 19, 1971: The waste storage space at the Northern States Power Company's reactor in Monticello, Minnesota, filled to capacity and spilled over. Above fifty thousand gallons of radioactive waste water flowed into the Mississippi River, and some was taken into the St. Paul water system.

March 22, 1975: A technician using a candle to check for air leaks set fire to electrical insulation at the Brown's Ferry reactor in Decatur, Alabama; cables controlling safety equipment burned out, and the cooling water fell to dangerous levels before a makeshift system was devised. No radioactive material was released.

March 28, 1979: In the worst U.S. commercial nuclear accident so far, a series of equipment failures and human mistakes led to a loss of coolant and partial core meltdown at the Three Mile Island reactor in Middletown, Pennsylvania. The Nuclear Regulatory Commission later concluded that the plant came within an hour of catastrophic meltdown. Some radiation escaped into the air, but health risks were found to be minimal.

August 7, 1979: Highly enriched uranium was released from a secret nuclear-fuel plant near Erwin, Tennessee, and about one thousand people were contaminated with up to five times as much radiation as they would normally receive in a year.

February 11, 1981: Eight workers were contaminated when 110,000 gallons of radioactive coolant leaked into the containment building of the Tennessee Valley Authority's Sequoyah plant in Tennessee.

January 25, 1982: A stem-generator pipe broke at the Rochester Gas & Electric Company's Ginna plant near Rochester, New York. Radioactive water spilled into the containment vessel, and some radioactive steam escaped into the air.

June 9, 1985: At least sixteen equipment failures and human error started a sequence similar to the Three Mile Island failure at Toledo Edison's Davis-Besse plant in Oak Harbor, Ohio. But auxiliary cooling pumps averted damage to the core.

January 4, 1986: A cylinder of uranium hexafluoride, a chemical used in nuclear-fuel production, was improperly heated at a Kerr-McGee plant at Gore, Oklahoma. One worker died and one hundred were hospitalized; small levels of radiation were detected in the area.

---

world population but uses 25 percent of the world's energy and emits 22 percent of the carbon dioxide produced. The U.S. Interior Secretary, for example, gave permission to loggers to cut down 1,700 acres of ancient forest in the Pacific Northwest, which is home to the threatened northern spotted owl, an endangered species. This will add to the thousands of animal species that are already extinct.

We are making some progress. As a result of the Earth Summit in Rio, all agreed that polluters should pay for the cost of pollution, that poverty should be eradicated, and that appropriate demographic policies should be adopted (birth control). Additionally, in 1982, after ten years of hard negotiation, the Convention on the Law of the Sea was signed by 119 countries (with only 35 ratified at this point), to give each country a two-hundred-mile zone from its coast for exclusive economic purposes but also the responsibility to improve and maintain. The Montreal Protocol on substances that deplete the ozone layer was established in 1987 and has been signed by 35 countries. It froze the production of chlorofluorocarbons at 1986 levels and mandates a 20 percent reduction by 1993 and a further decrease by 1998. Other conferences and meetings such as the International Council of Scientific Unions and the World Meteorological Organization are all trying to deal with the issue of ozone layer destruction.

On a personal basis, we all must help behaviorally by recycling paper, aluminum, and other products; car pooling; using public transportation; walking more; and engaging in other activities to help preserve our world.

HEALTH ACTIONS

Environmental Health

Intuitively, many of us sense some benefit from being in natural environments. Although there is limited scientific evidence demonstrating such an energy transfer, something happens when we embrace natural surroundings. Those of us who try this and become advocates through first-hand experience realize that it takes us to a higher level of consciousness and energy. These insights as they pertain to interdependence in the environment will become truths for you as you participate in and experience them. If when you are done, you feel the benefit, then it is a truth and benefit for you, and you will want to continue. Jean Shinoda Bolen stated, "If we personally realize that harmony between ourselves and the elements of the environment is at work in our lives, we feel connected rather than isolated and estranged from others. We feel ourselves as part of a divine, dynamic interrelated universe." Some of this may sound strange, but try it and see how you feel.

Mind

When managing time and planning your daily activities, include activities that will help to reduce your exposure to pollution or write a letter to a local, state, or national leader expressing your concerns. Allow yourself to experience the benefits of a natural environment as described following.

Body

Avoid exposure to pollutants as much as possible. Wear earplugs when you anticipate being exposed to loud noises (rock concerts, construction equipment, etc.), wear a filter mask on high air pollution days, and assure your drinking water is clean. In a positive sense for your body, enjoy the refreshing nature of clean water either when drinking it or when emersed in a shower, a pool, or natural body of water. Go to an area with lots of trees and clear air and breathe deeply and reflect upon the refreshing nature of the air.

Soul and Interdependence

Combining actions of the soul and interdependence is appropriate here. Using environmental surroundings as a trigger is the first step. Reflecting on the enrichment of soul is the second step, making these two dimensions inseparable. Try any of the following.

1. Meditate in stillness. In a natural setting, immerse yourself in the landscape, relax your body, do some relaxation techniques, and observe the natural flow of your breath—do not try to control it. During the pauses between inhalation and exhalation, focus on what you are feeling in the present.

2. Gaze at stars. Select music that makes you feel in harmony with nature, take a portable audio cassette player, lie down on a blanket away from street lights on a clear night, and gaze at the stars. Then turn on the music softly and marvel at the magnificent universe.

3. Gaze at a campfire or fireplace. If you have a chance to sit around a campfire or a fire in your home, gaze into the naturalness of the fire. Feel the warmth, watch the mesmerizing flames dancing, and listen to the crackling. It is warm, assuring, and cleansing and provides a natural type of meditation.

4. Become part of nature. Go to a place in a natural setting and sit motionless for twenty minutes. When you arrive, you generally disrupt or scare animals, so just sit motionless for a time and wait for nature to return to its natural state. Try to blend in. Try to be in the present moment. Then listen for the silence between the sounds.

Summary

1. In this day of rapid world population growth and high technology, the concern over food supplies, waste disposal, and nuclear accidents is evident.

2. Water from both ground and surface sources is being contaminated from the air (acid rain) and through dumping waste into our water supplies.

3. Legislative efforts have been enacted to prevent some dumping, but more must be done.

4. Much has been done in the fight for pure water, but more must be accomplished.

5. The air we breathe is contaminated by numerous chemicals, and it is wise for us on particularly smoggy days to stay indoors or breathe through a mask.

6. Concern over indoor air is also more evident today.

7. Noise pollution is a subtle form of pollution with no real painful symptoms, but it gradually results in hearing loss. Noise is also responsible for numerous accidents.

8. Land pollution came to the forefront of American awareness during the Love Canal incident in the 1970s.

9. Perhaps the most devastating threat to our environment is uncontrolled nuclear energy, such as the world saw during the Chernobyl incident.

10. With all these potential dangers, it is important for citizens to be aware and active in politics to control the threats to our environment.

11. A pollution-free environment is critical to physical health as well as to positive attitudes and outlooks.

Commitment Activities

1. The Environmental Protection Agency carefully monitors the water supplies of cities. Some sources are completely safe, others marginal, and other water supplies contain chemicals or elements that are above recommended standards. Cities are given imperatives to clean up the water supply by certain dates. As a class, find out about the water source in your community and compare its safety to that of other communities.

2. A good class project is to assess the environmental condition of your campus or community. Team up and examine the water treatment plant and the method of waste disposal (track your waste from your apartment or dorm to where it is deposited), determine acid rain threat, and assess the degree of air pollution. Report back to class.

3. When you go to your home or apartment, do a safety check. Look for anything that could cause an accident and check to see if you are prepared in case of an accident. For example, is there loose carpet that could cause someone to trip, particularly around stairs? Do you have a fire extinguisher and smoke alarm? Do you know how to call for emergency vehicles (911) or have other numbers posted? Do you have any exposed electrical wires, overloaded circuits, or dangerous appliances? Have you recently had your gas line checked for leaks? Are there any potential fire hazards, such as turpentine or gas in cans that are not in sealed metal containers?

4. Locate the nuclear plant nearest to where you live. If close, visit it and ask questions regarding its safety and maintenance.

5. Learn to purity water several ways: boiling, water purification tablets, or chlorine. Outdoor stores or sporting goods outlets often carry literature and tablets.

6. Learn about sewage treatment. How is sewage treated in your community? Learn how people not on sewer lines deal with waste. Learn about septic tanks and drainage (leech) lines and how much someone needs for particular kinds of soils (percolation tests). You can learn about this from your local health department.

References

American Public Health Association. "Love Canal Situation Raises Policy Issues." *The Nation's Health* (July 1980).

"Earth Summit" *Time*139, no. 22 (June 1, 1992):42–65.

Elmer-DeWitt, P. "A Man-Made Hell on Earth: The Ecological Devastation of Kuwait Is Worse than Imaged, but It Is Not the Planet-Wide Catastrophe that Some Predicted." *Time* 137 (March 18, 1991):36.

Evans, G. W. *Environmental Stress.* Cambridge, Mass.: Cambridge University Press, 1982.

Grisham, J. W., ed. *Health Aspects of the Disposal of Waste Chemicals.* New York: Pergamon Press, 1986.

Leaf, A. "Potential Health Effects of Global Climatic and Environmental Changes." *New England Journal of Medicine* 321, no. 23 (1989):1577–83.

Lemonick, M. D. "Alaska's Billion Dollar Quandry." *Time* 140, no. 13 (September 28, 1992):60–61.

Nadakavukaren, A. *Man and Environment: A Health Perspective.* Prospect Heights, Ill.: Waveland Press, 1986.

U.S. Environmental Protection Agency. *Health Effects of Environmental Pollution.* Washington, D.C.: U.S. Environmental Protection Agency, 1973.

Willgoose, C. E., et al. *Environmental Health.* Philadelphia: W. B. Saunders, 1979.

Woodell, S. R. J. "Forecasting Our Environmental Future (And That Was the Future)." *Futures* 21 (1989):547–59.

Additional Readings

Fields, R.; Taylor, P.; Weyler, R.; and Ingrasci, R. *Chop Wood Carry Water.* Los Angeles: Jeremy Tarcher, 1984. A book that helps you to become more sensitive to the environment through poetry and readings.

Freudenberg, N. *Not in Our Backyards: Community Action for Health and the Environment.* New York: Monthly Review Press, 1984. A good book on how to be active in controlling environmental pollutants from a political and community standpoint. The focus is on waste removal.

Kaplan, M. *Earth Song.* Berkeley, Calif.: Crystal Heart Press, 1988. A book on how to become more sensitive to the natural environment.

Nadakavukaren, A. *Man and Environment: A Health Perspective.* Prospect Heights, Ill.: Waveland Press, 1986. A good overview of environmental health, providing details that have been overviewed in this chapter.

CHAPTER 16

Consumer Choices

Key Questions

- How do health consumer skills relate to health decisions?

- How should the truth of advertisements be evaluated?

- What guidelines should you follow when taking over-the-counter and prescription drugs?

- What rights do consumers of health products have and what should be done about consumer complaints?

- When and how should medical specialists be selected?

- What alternative medical systems might be considered?

- In what ways can we pay for medical care?

- What rights do patients have?

- What is quackery, and why is it so common?

- How can quackery be recognized?

Chapter Outline

 e are all consumers. Understanding total health and the factors motivating our health behavior and learning to base our health decisions on sound questions and procedures are basic to every facet of health. For example, all topics in this text involve consumer decision making. These decisions might relate to health information, health products, or health services.

Because total health relates to continual growth and improvement, there are several steps to creating a personal plan for better health: (1) assessing health-producing and health-destroying behaviors, (2) adopting health-producing behaviors in a systematic way so the behaviors are reinforced, (3) recognizing and accepting good feelings associated with high-level wellness, and (4) cognitively understanding why certain behaviors are related to health and positive feelings (Corry 1983).

All these steps can be accomplished by intelligent health consumers. The idea is the same whether considering decisions about drugs, exercise programs, stress management, or other health matters. In the

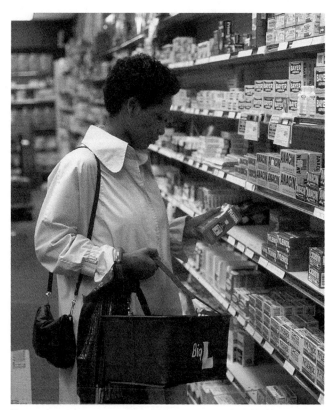

Every day there are opportunities to assess health-producing and health-destroying behaviors.

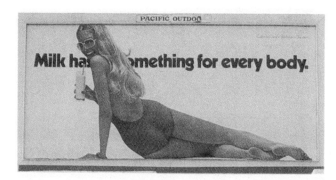

We receive a steady diet of advertisements related to our health.

past, we may have felt like health consumers only when buying a product or service related to medical care, but today consumer decisions are made when starting an exercise program, learning breast self-examination, stopping smoking, selecting health insurance, and so on.

An example of the four-step process described can be seen by considering physical fitness. A personal assessment of health-producing and health-destroying behaviors (step 1) might reveal breathlessness when participating in moderate physical activity, a tendency to be completely exhausted at the end of the day, and an undesirable shape. Adopting health-producing behaviors in a systematic way (step 2) might mean walking up steps instead of using the elevator, initiating a daily exercise program, and controlling food intake a little better. Recognizing and accepting the good feelings that result from the increase in health-producing behaviors (step 3) might be seen in greater personal confidence, increased energy throughout the day, and an improved self-image resulting from a change in body contours. Understanding why certain behaviors are related to health and positive feelings (step 4) is fundamental to the first three steps. This also makes it likely that there will be attempts to increase the incidence of other health-producing behaviors as well.

The entire contents of this text indicates the many topics that require intelligent consumer health decisions. Think for a moment how consumers make decisions about such a variety of health topics. As decisions are made, certain information about health products, advertising, con-

sumerism, health care, and quackery is basic. In this chapter, this information is provided in the hope that it will be applied to health decisions about the many other topics in the text. For consumers of life, it can be no other way.

The Vulnerable Consumer

Caveat emptor means "let the buyer beware." Even in this age of warranties and money-back guarantees, most of us have bought a product that didn't work or didn't perform as promised and have found that there was little that could be done about it. Like it or not, *caveat emptor* still applies today. Government regulations do not protect us from being cheated in the marketplace or ensure that health advertisements in magazines, on television, and on radio are accurate.

Advertising

Because of advertising, we often buy health products we don't need or that don't perform according to our expectations. Advertisers exploit our psychological needs and emotions. An example of where advertising has helped convince us of the need for a product is facial cleansers. Women spend more than half a billion dollars a year on facial cleansers because advertising claims indicate that brand X leaves the skin "retexturized and younger looking," brand Y "nourishes dry skin to give it more youthful elasticity," and brand Z provides a "refreshing first step to younger-looking skin." As with many cosmetic products, numerous claims are made, but the truth is, like soap and water, they just take off makeup ("Facial Cleansers" 1989).

Another example is tanning pills. These pills use a food-coloring agent that, if taken in extremely high doses, actually colors the skin. Not only are the major ingredients illegal for this use, but tanning pills can cause numerous health problems, such as allergic reactions, nausea, diarrhea, and itching and welts on the skin. In addition, they offer no protection from the sun ("Beware of Tanning Pills" 1991).

In a given day, around 23 percent of television time is advertisements. About 31 percent of these commercials contain health messages (Wallack and Dorfman 1992).

Directions: Circle the number in front of the following things you do.

1. I make buying choices largely because of the advertisements I've seen or heard.
2. I read and understand labels on packaged foods before I purchase them for the first time.
3. I use laxatives regularly.
4. I use mouthwashes regularly.
5. I would purchase a name brand aspirin before I would buy a generic or cheap brand.
6. I follow directions carefully when taking medications like aspirin or cold remedies.
7. If a physician gives me a prescription, I always ask about possible side effects of the drug.
8. If a prescription works for me and someone else has the same problem I had, I would share my medications to help him or her get better.
9. I ask friends and family to see if anyone has a prescription medication to treat a problem that I have.
10. I take prescription medications only until I feel better.
11. If I purchased a health product that did not do what it was supposed to do, I would contact the Food and Drug Administration (FDA), the Federal Trade Commission (FTC), or the National Advertising Division (NAD).
12. I take antacids regularly.
13. I almost always take cold remedies when I get a cold.
14. I take sleeping aids.
15. I really don't keep track of how much medicine I use.

Scoring/Interpretation

Use the following key to total your scores. Give yourself the indicated value if you marked an item. Give yourself a zero if you didn't mark an item.

1. = −3	6. = 3	11. = 3
2. = 3	7. = 3	12. = −3
3. = −3	8. = −3	13. = −3
4. = −3	9. = −3	14. = −3
5. = −3	10. = −3	15. = −3

0 to 12	=	You are practicing good consumer skills.
−1 to −16	=	You will need to read this chapter carefully to improve your consumer skills.
−17 to −33	=	You are practicing several poor consumer skills.

Directions: Circle the letter in front of all responses that apply.

1. In selecting a physician, I would
   a. ask my friends.
   b. pick someone who was geographically close.
   c. check to see with which hospital the physician is affiliated and call the administration for a recommendation.
   d. check to see how available he or she would be in an emergency and if out of town, how patients would get treatment.
   e. ask how much he or she charges for a visit.
   f. call the local or state medical society, and ask for recommendations in my area.
2. Under which of the following situations would you seek medical help? (Mark all that apply.)
   a. a stomachache
   b. a persistent cough or sore throat
   c. a headache
   d. severe bleeding or deep cut
   e. persistent chest pain
   f. swallowing some mild poison
3. From which of the following health professionals would you feel comfortable and confident receiving treatment for a serious disease? (Mark all that apply.)
   a. allopathic physician (prescribes drugs or chemotherapy to treat diseases)
   b. osteopathic physician (heats, manipulates, or massages the musculoskeletal, nervous, and circulatory systems in addition to methods such as chemotherapy)
   c. chiropractor (aligns back to relieve impinged nerves)
   d. acupuncturist (inserts and manipulates needles to treat disease)
   e. naturopath (treats disease with natural herbs)
   f. faith healer (cures the disease through divine help)

Scoring/Interpretation

1. If you circled letters a, b, d, and e, which are good things to consider, then it appears you are assuming that the physician is well-respected among his or her peers. It is important to consider if friends are satisfied, and if the physician is reasonably priced, closely located, and readily available for convenience and comfort.

   To determine competency, you should have selected c and f to check how hospitals and the professional society view the physician in terms of respect and competence. Find out information like the number of malpractice lawsuits against him or her and so on.
2. All of the reasons could be indicators of serious illness, but a and c would need to persist over some time before most doctors would recommend that you visit them. In most cases, these pass in a short amount of time. When in doubt, call and ask whether or not you should see the doctor.

   Letters d and f would necessitate immediate help by either traveling to an emergency room (if someone can drive you) or calling paramedics.

Letters b and e are conditions that should be checked by a physician by appointment.

3. Only a and b are licensed to practice medicine. C, d, and f can supplement medicine but cannot treat a serious disease. E is extremely questionable from a medical perspective and in treating a serious disease would be considered quackery.

HEALTH ACTIONS

Consumer Decisions

When making consumer decisions, it is helpful to consider influences related to the mind, body, and soul. Certainly one dimension influences another, but questions such as those listed here need to be considered. Perhaps you can think of additional questions that also need consideration.

Mind

1. When selecting this product or service, how influenced was I by advertising?
2. What is my motive for buying this product? For example, am I trying to get rid of a headache? Am I trying to avoid headaches in the future?
3. What can I do to avoid the need for this product or service in the future?

Body

1. Have I tried natural means of solving my problem before using medications? For example, do I have a proper diet, follow a healthy exercise program, or use sound techniques to control stress?

2. Do I "listen to my body" so I learn when things seem to be functioning well and when they don't?

Soul

1. Are my consumer habits in harmony with my basic values and what I think is important in life? For example, do I do what I say, and do I act consistently with what I think is important?
2. Are my consumer choices consistent with my cause and purpose in living? For example, do I buy products that impact the environment, or do I use substances instead of positive health behavior to prevent problems?

Finally, summarize what you need to do to improve your health skills and make them consistent with your values. Combine areas to improve similar skills at the same time. Prioritize what you need to do, and explain how you will do it. Pick your top priorities and begin improving your consumer skills.

Most of these messages are not designed to provide accurate and useful health information but are supposed to make us feel good about a certain product. Think of all the ads you have seen during the past week on television, in magazines, and in newspapers that concerned health-related products.

To understand our vulnerability to ineffective health products, we can't look at advertising pitches alone. After all, no one forces us to buy that new type of deodorant or that supposedly medicinal soap. To understand why we buy products that don't do any significant good, we must also look at why we are so susceptible to advertising in the first place.

Consumer Insecurities

We can be cheated when we are not well informed, are anxious about health, or are desperate for an affordable solution to a health problem. Many individuals are convinced that using sleeping pills or "pep" pills is safe without medical supervision. Others believe that copper bracelets cure arthritis, that extra vitamins supply energy, or that garlic cures anything. Some women have been convinced, by advertising and through myths handed down from one generation to the next, that douching is necessary. Interestingly, douching is more common among women who live in poverty. Also, women with less than a high school education are more likely to report douching than those with sixteen or more years of schooling (56 percent versus 16 percent). Not only is douching unnecessary, but it has been associated with pelvic inflammatory disease (PID) and ectopic pregnancy (Aral, Mosher, and Cates 1992).

We are also vulnerable because we all have some anxiety that something serious could happen to our health or even that we will be disliked if we don't use that special mouthwash. Who hasn't felt some pain or other symptom and wondered if some dreadful disease had finally taken hold? We might hesitate to seek competent medical attention for fear of knowing the truth and head for the drugstore shelf instead.

The high cost of medical services further complicates the issue of consumer vulnerability. Regardless of whether we pay directly for health services or pay higher insurance premiums to get quality service, the cost is going up. As costs rise, it becomes increasingly tempting to try health products that appear to be less expensive and provide a quick fix.

Evaluating Advertisements

As consumers, we must learn how to evaluate the advertising claims made for a product systematically. Here are a few helpful guidelines (adapted from Shipley and Plonsky 1980):

1. Determine the purpose of the advertisement.
2. Determine the audience for which the advertisement is intended.
3. Determine the type of psychological approach being used—related to emotions, needs, or wants.
4. Evaluate the source of the advertisement, both the person who placed the ad and the medium carrying it.
5. Determine the basic content of the ad. For example:
   a. Which statements are true?
   b. Is any information left out?
   c. What are the positive and negative effects of the product?
   d. What are the ingredients of the product?
   e. Is there a guarantee? If so, what kind?
   f. What is the credibility of the people and the organization associated with the product?
6. Determine whether the medium used to carry the ad has influenced the presentation of the information (photographic techniques, makeup, and so on).

Fortunately, there is help for consumers when it comes to evaluating advertisements and controlling them to some extent. The **Federal Trade Commission (FTC),** an agency of the federal government, has the power to halt what it deems deceptive or unfair advertising. A classic example of this occurred when mouthwash manufacturers claimed that their products not only helped combat bad breath but also prevented sore throats and colds, or at least eased their symptoms. The FTC decided that these claims were misleading and that the manufacturers could no longer make them.

Nearly forty other government agencies have some say in how certain types of advertising are presented. For example, the Civil Aeronautics Board looks at airline ads, and the Food and Drug Administration reviews pharmaceuticals.

There is also some self-regulation. In 1971, several advertising associations and the Council of Better Business Bureaus created a **National Advertising Division (NAD)** to promote standards and handle complaints. The program is voluntary, but the NAD can turn over its findings to a regulatory agency for action ("Advertising Watchdogs" 1984).

The media also help, but how carefully ads are screened before they appear on radio and television and in newspapers and magazines varies a great deal. The process often involves specialists in areas such as pharmaceuticals or children's food who look at thousands of ads each year. Children's ads receive special attention.

Some of the best scrutiny comes when the NAD responds to complaints about competitors misrepresenting the facts, especially when two products are compared. The NAD also initiates its own investigations. Some people feel that advertising in general is now probably fairer, more accurate, and more honest than it has ever been. Many corporations, thanks to the consumer movement, have been forced to be more public-minded than they were years ago ("Advertising Watchdogs" 1984).

Because there is no guarantee that advertisements and other sources of health information are totally accurate, it is important for consumers to be able to identify differences between accurate and inaccurate information. The checklist in the accompanying box can be very helpful for this purpose. The first part of the checklist is used to evaluate the qualifications of individual authors, the second part is to be used when an organization, agency, or other institution is the information source, and the third part focuses on the information itself (McKenzie 1987).

Decisions About Common Drugs

Common drugs provide an excellent example of how we must make daily health decisions. Americans live in a drug-oriented society. Early in life we learn that if we don't feel well, we can take a pill to help and if we are hurt, we can use medicine to relieve the pain. Later, we learn we can even take pills if we feel too tired or not tired enough. Eventually, we may believe that pills or other medicines can take care of almost every problem. In an earlier chapter, drugs that individuals use simply because they like their effects were discussed; here the focus is on drugs used mainly as health products.

Drugs used primarily as health products are either **over-the-counter (OTC) drugs** or prescription drugs. Over-the-counter drugs, or proprietary drugs, can be purchased without a doctor's signature. Prescription drugs, by contrast, require a written order from a medical doctor to be purchased and can only be sold by a licensed pharmacist.

We need drugs of either type only when we have real health problems. Most of the time, making good health-related decisions and choosing a suitable life-style can greatly reduce the likelihood of needing any drugs at all—even in old age. Contrary to what the ads might say, a healthy life-style and a little time do cure many ills.

OTC Drugs

Self-medication with over-the-counter drugs is widespread. Most of these drugs are relatively ineffective, they are frequently used unnecessarily, and they may have adverse side effects. Some of the OTC drugs most frequently used and abused are laxatives, mouthwashes, and cold remedies.

Checklist for Evaluating Health Information

Question	Response		
	Yes	*No*	*Not sure/Don't know*
Part I. The author A. Background information on the author is provided.			
B. The author's educational background is in the discipline in which the author is writing. (Note: Be cautious of impressive titles easily confused with qualified professionals.)			
C. The author is a recognized expert in the discipline in which the author is writing.			
D. The author is a recognized member of a professional health organization in the area in which he/she is writing.			
Part II. The source A. The source is a recognized organization in the health field.			
B. The source is interested in sharing information, not in making a profit.			
Part III. The information A. The author uses misleading comparisons to encourage consumers to draw conclusions, such as "contains twice as much" and "up to eight hours relief."			
B. The information is based on "personal observations" and not sound scientific data.			
C. The author uses testimonials of "cured" or "satisfied" consumers.			
D. The author uses statements including the words "new," "quick," "secret," or "amazing" as they relate to health.			
E. The information contains all-inclusive statements such as "this approach always works."			
F. The information is an advertisement used to make a profit.			
G. The information is inconsistent with other information on the same topic.			
H. The author uses few or no references to substantiate the point.			
I. The author uses sensationalism to emphasize points, such as "a product like this has never before been available to the public."			
J. The information defies common sense and seems unbelievable.			
"Yes" answers are desired in Parts I and II. "No" answers are desired in Part III.			

Source: J. F. McKenzie, "A Checklist for Evaluating Health Information" in *Journal of School Health,* Vol. 57, No. 1, January 1987, p. 31. Reprinted with permission. American School Health Association, Kent, Ohio.

Laxatives help eliminate feces and relieve constipation. Often, however, constipation can be relieved by changing dietary patterns, and regular physical exercise can promote regularity as well. Regularity does not necessarily mean a daily bowel movement must occur; thus, laxatives are usually not needed. Moreover, their continued use can be habit forming.

Cold remedies of the past included applying kerosene plasters to the chest or wrapping a dirty sock stuffed with salted pork and onion around the neck. Today's remedies smell better, but they come no closer to curing colds or shortening their duration than the old remedies did. The potency of over-the-counter cold products rivals anything requiring a prescription. All of these remedies, no matter how effective, only relieve symptoms. The infection must run it course ("Cold Remedies" 1989). When colds are treated, they are cured in about seven days: if left untreated, they last about a week.

Television commercials give the impression that a wide variety of OTC drugs to relieve pain exist, but there are really only three choices: aspirin, acetaminophen, and ibuprofen. Aspirin, discovered in 1899, is quite common. It is available in several forms—tablets, capsules, buffered, coated, and time-release. Acetaminophen (marketed as Tylenol, Anacin III, and Datril) was not widely used until it became a nonprescription drug in 1955. Acetaminophen and aspirin are equally effective for relief of minor pains, but unlike aspirin and ibuprofen, acetaminophen does not suppress inflammation. It does not irritate the stomach, as aspirin can, but it can upset the stomach. Ibuprofen, available as Advil, Nuprin, and Medipren, is the newest nonprescription pain medicine on the market. In practice, aspirin and acetaminophen relieve pain as effectively and usually cost less than ibuprofen ("OTC Pain Medications of Only Three Types Available" 1987).

Dangers of Self-Medication

There is a big difference between self-care and self-medication. Using OTC drugs is a form of self-medication. According to an old proverb, people who are their own doctors have fools for patients. Even with the current emphasis on optimal health, which includes self-care, this statement retains some truth, particularly when it comes to taking drugs.

What are the potential dangers of self-medication? One is that if we use drugs based on our own advice, we may use them longer than necessary. Also, chemical substances may repress symptoms and delay us from seeking medical treatment until a problem is serious or even uncontrollable. Further, because similar symptoms result from different problems, the wrong condition may be treated. No one likes to have disease symptoms, but they serve a purpose by showing that a health problem exists.

Self-medication can also result in taking drugs in doses that cause bodily damage. If we use more than one medicine at a time, we may alter the effects of each and end up with unintended side effects. In short, when putting chemicals into our bodies, we are betting we will benefit. Self-medication may diminish our chances of winning the bet.

Precautions

No medication is completely harmless, and any chemical substance has potential problems. Consistent with other health-related decisions, we must decide if any potential risk, no matter how small, is worth the probable benefits from taking a substance.

The first precaution is to use only relatively harmless substances for self-medication (even though no substance is totally harmless). Aspirin, sodium bicarbonate (for simple indigestion), calamine lotion (for mild skin irritations and bites), milk of magnesia (as a laxative), and alcohol (as an antiseptic and for rubbing) can be used for minor problems. Intelligent use is not likely to cause harm.

A second precaution is to pay close attention to OTC drug labels. The labels must list the name of the product, the symptoms the product relieves, the contents, the quantity, the name and address of the manufacturer or packer, directions for use, warnings (such as limits on the length of use, possible side effects, total dosage in a day), and possible drug interactions. In addition, note the expiration date on the label; after that date, the product is not safe to use.

A third precaution is to check with the pharmacist about the OTC medication chosen. The letters *NF* or *USP* appear on some OTC drug labels: official standards for strength, purity, and identity are found in two reference books, the *National Formulary (NF)* and the *United States Pharmacopeia (USP)*, written by pharmaceutical experts. When a drug label contains either set of letters, the drug has been manufactured according to official standards. If your OTC drug labels do not contain all of the information cited here, take the medications back to the place of purchase and find out why.

A fourth precaution is to follow label directions exactly; instructions for the use of a drug are given for good reasons. If you exceed the quantity or rate of dosage, you may harm yourself. Any negative reactions to medicine should be reported immediately to a physician or nurse practitioner.

Prescription Drugs

Prescription drugs are usually more powerful than OTC drugs. Prescriptions are required by law because only a trained and appropriate physician can correctly diagnose a specific problem and know the proper medicine and dosage. If you go to a doctor and get a prescription, mention all medications you are using (both OTC and other prescription drugs) and any negative reactions you have had to any drug. Drug interaction can be harmful.

The general points made about OTC drugs also apply to prescription drugs. The labels on prescription drugs, however, do not give some of the basic information found on OTC drug labels. What the drug does, the possible side effects, and appropriate precautions are not usually on the label because it is assumed this information is provided by the physician. The label is likely to have information on how much to take and how often. Check with your physician and/or druggist about the method of taking a drug and its possible side effects.

Drugs have three different names. One name is based on chemical structure, there is a shorter generic name used by pharmacists and physicians, and there is a brand name used by the manufacturer. For example, a variant of penicillin, which fights bacterial infection, is 6-amino-penicillanic acid, or ampicillin. Some brands are Amcill, Omnipen, and Polycillin. Several companies also make "generic" versions of the drug, which contain the same active ingredients as drugs sold under a brand name. In recent years, consumer interest in **generic drugs** has increased because they are often significantly cheaper than brand-name drugs.

There is a real payoff for shopping for the best price on prescription drugs. Prices for the same drug can vary by 100 percent or more in the same community. A brand-name drug in one pharmacy can cost twenty-two times more than the generic version in another ("Prescription for Savings" 1990).

Generic drugs are supposed to be of the same quality as drugs sold under specific brand names. If generics were always prescribed for the roughly 75 percent of major drugs available in that form, patients and insurers would cut their costs about $1 billion a year. Yet, the FTC estimates that no more than $236 million per year is saved. The consumer can help by reminding the physician that generics can save money.

Emphasis on the money-saving power of generic drugs raises questions about their quality. The FDA ana-

lyzed samples of the thirty most widely prescribed generics, however, and concluded that generics as a class are not inferior to brand-name drugs ("Update on Generics" 1990).

Guidelines for Best Results

Once you have detected a potential medical problem, consulted with a physician, and obtained a prescription drug to help deal with the problem, follow these guidelines to get the best possible results from the medication:

1. Follow the physician's instructions for taking the medicine. The dosage and length of time you take the drug are dictated by your individual situation. Don't stop taking the drug just because you feel better; there is probably a good reason why you are supposed to take it for a certain time period.
2. Ask the physician about possible side effects from the medication. If you have unexpected symptoms or side effects, report the problem to your physician at once.
3. Don't start taking new drugs without your physician's knowledge. Harmful drug interactions may occur.
4. Carefully follow label instructions about storing the medicine. Some drugs need to be refrigerated; others need to be kept dry.
5. Don't take a prescription meant for someone else, and don't allow someone else to use one meant for you. The same drug can affect different individuals quite differently. Furthermore, you or the other person may have seriously misdiagnosed the problem.
6. Never mix different tablets or differently dated tablets in one bottle. You or someone—even a child—may take the wrong tablet and treatment would be difficult to diagnose.
7. When prescription drugs are no longer needed, dispose of them. This removes the temptation to let someone else try them or to use them yourself when they are no longer safe.
8. Find out what to do if you inadvertently miss a dose.

Drugs can serve a useful purpose in society. We must respect their value and power, however, and avoid the temptation to take them casually or without good medical cause.

Decisions About Home Health Testing

One relatively new health decision relates to the use of do-it-yourself medical testing. Individuals test their eyesight, stool, urine, blood, and blood pressure in search of health clues related to vision problems, gastrointestinal diseases, infection, ovulation, pregnancy, diabetes, hypertension, and other conditions.

Home Health Testing

Home health testing is a tremendous help to consumers. Tests done at home save time and money and help us to be healthier than ever.

- **Pro:** The availability of an increasing number of home health tests helps consumers pay closer attention to their health. Tests provide information crucial to improving levels of health and decision making.
- **Con:** Home health tests may be of some use, but consumers need to use caution. Tests are not 100 percent accurate. They are also just one indicator and not a measure of overall health. Health decision making involves much more than just information obtained from home health tests.

Should home health tests be used? If so, under what circumstances?

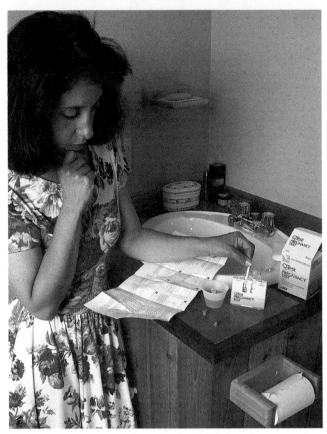

Although home pregnancy tests have become easier to administer, their accuracy rates vary. They are not foolproof tests.

In general, there are three categories of self-testing products: (1) tests that help diagnose a specific condition or disease in those with symptoms, such as pregnancy test kits (used after a missed period); (2) screening tests that identify indications of disease in those without symptoms (e.g., testing stools for hidden blood); and (3) monitoring devices that provide ongoing checks for an existing condition used on the advice of a physician (e.g., blood glucose test kits for diabetics).

Benefits of Home Tests

To consumers, this trend of self-reliance in health care can mean lower medical costs, a closer watch on chronic conditions, and earlier detection of health problems. A positive pregnancy test may prompt a woman to seek medical care early in her pregnancy; a woman being treated for infertility problems can pinpoint her time of ovulation; and regular blood pressure readings can provide helpful information to both patient and doctor. Thanks to convenient portable tests, individuals with some chronic health problems can maintain testing regimens away from home. An example is glucose monitoring, which has long helped diabetics keep their disease under control so they can live healthier and more normal lives.

Problems with Home Tests

The biggest problem with home tests is the risk of misinterpreting or overrelying on test results. A single abnormal reading is often taken as a "diagnosis" of a problem, or a return to a normal reading is taken as a "cure." Another problem is that once results of a home test are known, a person might not seek medical care. For example, a pregnant woman might not see her doctor for appropriate prenatal care, whereas in the past she would have at least seen the doctor to have a pregnancy test performed.

Making medical decisions without professional medical advice can be dangerous. Using the results of one test as a diagnosis is risky. A usual diagnosis by a physician involves an evaluation of the patient's medical history, a physical examination, other tests, and sometimes consultation with other medical experts.

No home test is 100 percent accurate, even under the best conditions, and results can differ from brand to brand. With a pregnancy test, for example, if enough of a certain hormone is present in a urine specimen, a signal should occur to indicate a possible pregnancy. But kits from different companies may indicate this signal at different hormonal levels, and all women don't produce the hormone at the same rate. The accuracy of three brands of home pregnancy tests ranged from 45.7 percent to 89.1 percent, depending on how early after a missed period the tests were performed (Blaylock 1986).

Hints for Using Home Testing Kits

Despite problems with some home tests, including questions about their accuracy, the future looks bright for manufacturers of home testing kits. On the horizon are plans for tests for cholesterol, syphilis, herpes, strep throat, and perhaps even AIDS. Since these tests are likely to be around for quite some time, it is wise to be aware of the guidelines for their use (Farley 1986).

Consumer Protection

Considering the many health products used and the many companies that produce them, it might seem a matter of luck that there aren't more problems. But there is much more than luck involved. Protection for the consumer does exist, even though it is not likely it will ever be perfect.

One informal type of consumer protection has been the close scrutiny of research findings. Typically, researchers publish their findings in medical journals. Supporters of this practice contend that this helps ensure credibility by allowing peers to identify inaccurate testing. Critics say the process, which takes many months or even more than a year, can cause serious delays in the application of new treatments. They feel the delay puts patients in greater danger than allowing information and treatments to be released quickly. You will probably hear more about this issue. In the meantime, when do you think research information should be released?

Our Rights as Consumers

The consumer's *right to safety* has been partly protected by such agencies as the Consumer Product Safety Commission and the Environmental Protection Agency. In addition, specific laws and regulations require the safety and effectiveness of prescription drugs, medical devices, and OTC medicines; the safety of buildings and mobile homes; the remedy by auto makers of safety defects found in cars; and other protections.

The *right to be informed* is basic, because we cannot make intelligent consumer decisions without enough information to protect ourselves from deception. There is a mandated and voluntary trend toward plain language in

credit agreements, insurance policies, and other contractual forms. In grocery stores, nutrition values and content statements now appear on food packages, as do unit prices on shelves. Consumer organizations have become more prominent in gathering and distributing practical information of value to shoppers.

The *right to choose* has been supported by efforts to break up monopolies and encourage marketplace competition. Manufacturers can no longer set retail prices, as some once did under fair-trade laws. Bans that once kept prescription drug prices from being advertised are now illegal. The outlawing of mandatory fee schedules in general has given the consumer greater choice of health services.

The *right to be heard* has been more evident than ever in recent years, both in government and business circles. **Class action suits,** in which one consumer can pursue a remedy on behalf of all who have had the same problem, are commonly heard in the courts. Consumer affairs offices are often found in departments of the federal, state, and local governments, and within businesses.

How can you exercise your rights as a consumer? First, you must know where to go for assistance and how to seek redress for problems.

Consumer Protection Agencies

No one has the time or expertise to check the contents, safety, and advertising of all health products. Fortunately, many government agencies at the federal, state, and local levels, as well as numerous private agencies, possess some of the resources needed to protect consumers from fraudulent claims and dangerous products. The most prominent agencies involved in consumer protection follow.

Food and Drug Administration (FDA)

The FDA's major responsibility is to enforce laws designed to ensure that foods are wholesome, drugs and medical devices are safe and effective, cosmetics are harmless, and the labeling of such products is truthful. The FDA also has authority to require that manufacturers of medical devices prove the safety and effectiveness of their products before they put them on the market.

The development and approval of a new drug product comprise a long and involved process. Here is a simplified view of the steps the FDA takes.

1. A new drug is developed through research and is then subjected to screening tests and testing on animals. If it has the desired effects, more animal tests are done to see what dosage levels are poisonous, what the safe dosage level for humans might be, and whether there is a reason for human testing.

2. If tests indicate the drug can safely be tested on humans, the sponsor applies to the FDA for permission to conduct tests on humans. The sponsor must submit results of the animal studies and show that no human test subject will be exposed to an unreasonable risk.

3. Human testing is divided into three phases. Phase I determines what chemical action a drug has, how it is absorbed by the body, how it should be given, and what the safe dosage range is. Phase II involves testing on a limited number of patients for treatment or prevention of a specific disease. Phase III is the most extensive testing stage. Studies are done to assess the drug's safety, effectiveness, and most desirable dosage in treating a specific disease in a large number of people.

4. If all stages are successful, the sponsor applies to the FDA for approval to market the new drug. The FDA reviews all available information to determine if the benefits of using the drug properly outweigh the risks.

5. Once the FDA gives approval, the company is required to keep records relating to production methods for the drug and its safety and effectiveness. Any negative information must be reported to the FDA.

To ensure product safety, the FDA can take a number of possible actions. It can prevent the sale of a product, require that it be redesigned, demand that it be relabeled or packaged in a safer way, and take action against false or misleading labeling. The FDA can order the recall or removal of products from the marketplace or go to court to seize illegal products. It can also obtain injunctions against violators or prosecute manufacturers, packers, or shippers.

Federal Trade Commission (FTC)

The FTC was established in 1914 to protect consumers by keeping competition in the marketplace free and fair. The FTC is a consumer protection agency. In the area of health products, it is concerned with preventing misbranding, mislabeling, and fraudulent advertising.

The FTC's enforcement power is limited to issuing *cease and desist* orders, requiring that those responsible for deception stop their deceptive practices. Such orders can be appealed to the courts, however, and it may take months for a deceptive practice to be stopped.

In recent years, the FTC has dealt with such problems as advertisements for vitamin preparations that promise users increased sexual responsiveness, health books containing claims of unproven or questionable methods for curing cancer or heart disease, and advertisements for drugs promising cures for arthritis or other noncurable conditions. From a practical standpoint, the FTC is most likely to focus on deceptive practices in life-threatening situations.

U.S. Postal Service

The Postal Inspection Service of the U.S. Postal Service is responsible for preventing the mails from being used to defraud the public. It investigates mail-order fraud and protects consumers from harassment and from certain types of junk mail.

The Postal Service can refuse to deliver mail from a promoter, thus forcing the shutdown of a mail-order operation. The Postal Service can also take legal action, though it is more likely that such action results from a consumer complaint.

State and Local Government Agencies

Many states and municipalities have agencies with responsibilities similar to those of national agencies. Almost every city and state has a Department of Consumer Affairs that provides general consumer information and referrals. State and local health departments often have divisions regulating food and drugs, health facilities, medical care licensing and services, veterinary health, product safety, occupational safety, and radiation control. These agencies may be more responsive than federal ones in dealing with a specific problem because they tend to be less bureaucratic.

Better Business Bureau

The Better Business Bureau is supported entirely by private business. Local bureaus assist with misunderstandings between customers and business firms, and they investigate questionable business activity and instances of apparently false advertising. While these bureaus can provide information on a specific company or charity, consumers must draw their own conclusions. Bureaus will not endorse a company, product, or person or offer legal advice.

Chamber of Commerce

The Chamber of Commerce is a voluntary organization interested in publicizing, developing, and promoting commercial opportunities in communities. It acts as a communication vehicle between businesses and consumers and often has a business-consumer relations code. The Chamber strives to protect the health and safety of consumers by monitoring the design and manufacture of products as well as eliminating fraud and deception.

Consumers' Union

Consumers' Union is the most important of a number of independent testing organizations designed to inform Americans about the quality of products we buy. Information from the Union is printed in its magazine, *Consumer Reports.* Consumers' Union does not accept paid advertisements or endorse products.

Consumer Complaints

When dissatisfied with a product or service, we should first honestly ask ourselves whether we used the product as labeled, carefully followed instructions, and had realistic expectations. If, after answering these questions, further action is needed, there are several relatively informal and appropriate steps to take.

Informal Actions

First, gather all relevant facts about the product or service, including names, dates, and circumstances. Any written evidence, such as a receipt, is helpful. In general, keep receipts, unused products, and records of transactions until the complaint is handled in a satisfactory manner. Then, if possible, go to the place where the product or service was received. If put off by a salesperson or clerk, ask to see the manager. If the manager does not provide satisfaction, talk to someone of higher and higher authority until a solution is found.

If it is not possible to return to the place of purchase, make a phone call or write a letter. Be clear about the complaint and related facts. When connected with the proper person, ask the person's name and position and write it down for future reference. Ask to speak with that person's superior if necessary, but listen to what the person on the other end of the line says. If wrong about the complaint, admit it. Ideally, you will be satisfied with the corrective action suggested; if not, more formal action can be pursued.

Formal Actions

If direct contact with the company or appropriate individuals does not lead to satisfactory results, the National Consumers' League (*Consumer Almanac* 1975) recommends the following:

1. Photocopy your original letter and send copies to city, county, or state voluntary consumer groups or governmental consumer agencies; your state's attorney general; the local Better Business Bureau; the appropriate business or professional association;

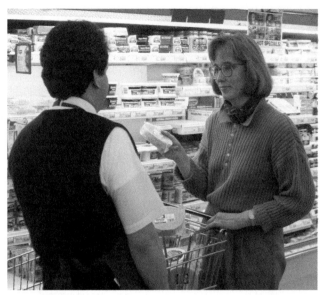

There are many ways to register a consumer complaint.

national consumer groups; and the state and national office of Consumer Affairs.

2. If the company in question does business in interstate commerce, contact the appropriate federal government agency.

3. If the problem has to do with unfair or deceptive advertising or business practice, contact the FTC, and if the deceptive advertisement appears in the local media, contact the broadcaster or newspaper and request that they stop running the ad.

4. Advise the company in question that you are taking these steps and send them copies of all letters sent. Many companies fear the adverse publicity of letters and will provide satisfaction concerning the complaint.

5. If all these efforts prove ineffective, your local voluntary or governmental consumer agency may assist you by writing letters and visiting the company. Government agencies often send out investigators and will take remedial action if it is justified.

6. As a last resort, you can sue the business in small claims court (the ceiling on recovery, depending on the state, is usually $500–$1,500). No lawyer is needed, and the filing costs are small. Contact the Small Claims Study Group, c/o John H. Weiss, Room 1, Quincy House, Cambridge, Massachusetts 02138, for advice on using these courts.

Consumer Responsibility

The ultimate responsibility for consumer protection is in your hands. Today, help is available from legal sources, as well as from public and private agencies designed to help protect you. But it is a mistake to sit back and assume that everything is being taken care of for us. The size of the population, combined with the thousands of products and services available to consumers, makes it impossible for regulatory agencies and consumer interest groups to protect us fully.

How can you help promote consumer protection? First, keep informed on consumer issues by gathering and using information on health in general, using consumer protection organizations and legislation and the decision-making process. If consumer problems develop, take action on them. The solution to your problem might assist other consumers as well. Everyone has a responsibility to help rectify difficulties with health products or services. In the final analysis, we are our own consumer protection agency.

Making Decisions About Medical Care

Practically everyone at some time needs to see a medical specialist or use a medical facility or is called upon to help someone with a medical problem. In certain situations, such as a serious car accident or the sudden development of a severe pain, immediate medical care is needed. In other situations, such as when a person has had a sore throat or been coughing for a few days, it is harder to determine whether or not to seek medical care.

When to Seek Medical Care

Some individuals rely too much on self-care, believing that a symptom will go away if left alone or if treated with over-the-counter medicine. The dangers of self-medication have been discussed. At the other extreme, some individuals rush to a physician the moment they feel a muscle twitch or get a headache. How can we know when to seek professional advice or care? Medical care should be sought in the following situations:

1. When a life-threatening situation exists. For example, any of the following conditions can lead to immediate death: severe bleeding, stopped breathing, ingestion of a poison, shock, or chest pains (which may precede a heart attack). In these situations, go to a hospital emergency room or call an ambulance.
2. When any bodily symptom (e.g., pain, swelling, fever) lasts for an unusually long time. For example, a sore throat usually lasts only two to seven days.
3. When there is uncertainty. Call a physician's office and explain the problem.

You are the expert on your own body. You are the most sensitive to your bodily changes and are consequently the best early warning system to any changes in well-being. If you experience unexplained symptoms, consult a physician as soon as possible.

Deciding on Kinds of Medical Help

When a medical emergency occurs, there isn't time to choose a hospital or personal physician; sometimes there is no choice about who to see or where to go. But for reg-

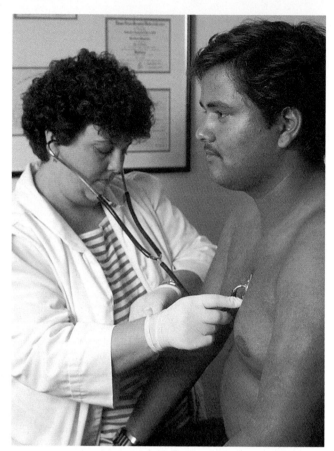

For regular care, it is important that we make informed decisions about our use of health professionals' services.

ular care, it is important to make informed decisions about a personal physician and dentist.

Both **allopathic physicians** (those with doctor of medicine—M.D.—degrees) and **osteopathic physicians** (those with doctor of osteopathy—D.O.—degrees) are licensed to practice medicine and have had the required medical education. How, then, do you choose between them? They both had to pass the same examinations for state licensure, and in most cases, they would treat a patient similarly. The major difference between an M.D. and D.O. lies in their philosophical approach to medicine. Allopathic physicians generally emphasize drugs and other forms of chemotherapy as the preferred means to treat disease. Osteopathic physicians emphasize the roles of the musculoskeletal, nervous, and circulatory systems in the management of bodily ailments. Consequently, some D.O.s would apply manipulative therapy, such as massage or heat treatment, in addition to chemotherapy. Another factor to consider is accessibility. This might be the distance of the doctor's office from your home or workplace, the practitioner's office hours, the practitioner's weekend or vacation substitute, and financial costs. When you narrow the field to one practitioner, a visit allows you to consider such personal qualities as personality, patience, and a willingness to answer questions clearly. If you feel uncomfortable with a physician's opinion or personal qualities, seek out another physician.

Tips for Choosing a Physician

1. Call the local county or state medical society and ask for names of physicians in the area.
2. Find out what hospital the physicians on your list are affiliated with.
3. Find out whether the physician can be reached easily in an emergency.
4. Inquire about the physician's fees.
5. Make a get-acquainted visit— an appointment before you get sick.

Get to Know the Physician

1. Does the physician listen to the things you have to say?
2. Is he/she willing to share his/her overall view of medical care?
3. Will he/she help you stay healthy as well as treat you when you're sick?
4. Does his/her philosophy concerning use of drugs, reliance on tests, and so forth, agree with yours?
5. What is his/her background and education?
6. What specialists is he/she likely to send you to for surgery or other unusual problems?

Source: The Associated Press, as printed in the *Birmingham News,* May 5, 1987, pp. 6G–7G.

A **nurse practitioner** can extend a physicians' services. Usually this individual is a registered nurse (R.N.) who has had additional education and experience and who can assess patients' health histories, conduct physical examinations, and order and interpret diagnostic tests. The nurse practitioner works under the guidance of a licensed physician, but some states allow nurse practitioners to engage in private practice. Depending on their area of study, nurse practitioners may be called family nurse practitioners, pediatric nurse practitioners, geriatric nurse practitioners, or surgical nurse practitioners.

A **physician assistant (P.A.)** can also extend physicians' services. Under the supervision of a physician, the P.A. can do many things usually done by a physician. For example, they can perform physical exams, treat some ailments, prescribe some medications, and talk with patients about health problems. Most P.A.s work in physicians' offices, but some work in hospitals or other medical care settings.

How to Help the Medical Specialist Help the Patient

Medical care involves a partnership between patient and practitioner, not a one-way contract. Patients must articulate their problems, clearly state their needs and expectations, and fully cooperate in getting well. Remember, the physician-patient relationship is confidential, and only health professionals with a "need to know" are authorized access to medical records.

After the problem is described, the practitioner examines and tests the patient and may order certain lab tests or X rays to help diagnose the problem before prescribing treatment. Throughout the visit, the patient needs to understand exactly what is going on. Ask for clarification of any prescribed treatment or medications, such as whether a medication can cause drowsiness or other side effects, what the dosage is, and when to take the medication. The cost of recommended tests, treatments, or prescriptions should also be learned, along with possible alternative and less costly options.

The practitioner may need to refer the patient to a specialist. In addition to family medicine or general practice, there are five major clinical specialties: (1) **internal medicine** includes such subspecialties as the study of heart problems, endocrine diseases and metabolism, and the digestive system; (2) **obstetrics and gynecology** is concerned with childbearing and diseases of women; (3) **pediatrics** is concerned with infants, children, and adolescents; (4) **psychiatry** deals with mental problems; and (5) **surgery.** A physician's training can be verified by calling the county medical society or checking the *Directory of Medical Specialists,* available in many public libraries. Other suggestions for shopping for a physician are found in the accompanying box.

A patient may be referred by a physician or go directly to one of these specialists or to another health professional, such as a **clinical psychologist** or a **licensed clinical social worker.** Licensed clinical psychologists hold a Ph.D. degree from an accredited school and specialize in emotional and psychological adjustment, as well as in temporary or chronic emotional difficulties and disturbances. The psychiatrist, who is also a physician, is likely to see patients who require medication as well as psychotherapy. The psychologist is more likely to see patients who do not require constant prescription medication for their specific emotional problems. Licensed clinical social workers specialize in the same areas as clinical psychologists.

Other health professionals include **optometrists** and **ophthalmologists.** An optometrist specializes in measuring visual acuity and prescribing corrective lenses. An ophthalmologist is an M.D. who specializes in the treatment of eye disorders and diseases. Clinical psychologists, optometrists, and other health professionals function independently and outside a physician's realm of supervision, though they may choose to work with a physician to help a patient. Other health professionals include medical (lab) and X-ray technologists, as well as respiratory, physical, and occupational therapists.

Emergency care centers are located nationwide. Their mission is to treat minor injuries or short-term illnesses of patients who have no physician or whose doctor is unavailable. They have a licensed medical doctor present at all times, promise to deliver prompt treatment to walk-in patients, and claim to cost less than a hospital emergency room. They are typically open evenings, weekends, and holidays in addition to normal daytime hours. Here's how to decide in advance whether to use a certain center:

1. Ask your family physician what he or she knows about the center, its doctors, and staff.

2. Check on the center's reputation—how long has it been in operation and how is it regarded in your community?

3. Visit the center, meet the physician, and tour the facilities. Talk to patients, note professional credentials, request literature, and learn how the center functions.

4. Find out how the center maintains its records. Will the center communicate directly with your physician?

5. Ask how the center works with local hospitals and emergency ambulance services, and ask if there is life-support equipment available.

6. Find out whether an emergency center physician can bypass a hospital emergency department and admit a patient directly into the hospital if needed.

7. Ask how the center handles follow-up care.

Your decision about whether to use an emergency center or a hospital ultimately depends on your judgment of the seriousness of the problem, the cost, convenience, and your trust in the facility. We will probably see more of this new consumer orientation to health care in the future.

New Options for Medical Care

In the past, treatment in either a physician's office or a hospital were our only real choices. As medical care has become more of a business, however, other delivery systems are available as consumer products.

Ambulatory care centers are growing very rapidly. The National Association for Ambulatory Care indicates that in 1982, there were 600 urgent care centers (for minor injuries and family care) in the United States, by 1985 there were 2,500, and by 1990 over 5,000. The number of "surgicenters" (for outpatient surgery) has also increased rapidly.

Urgent care centers provide treatment without an appointment. Minor problems, such as sprained ankles, sore throats, and cuts needing stitches, are handled. Urgent care centers do not have the same sophisticated medical equipment or medical specialists found in a full-service hospital. The centers are usually open twelve to sixteen hours per day. Critics have called them "Docs-in-a-box" or even "Medical McDonalds."

Surgicenters are capable of providing minor, low-risk, outpatient surgery. For operations such as a biopsy or removal of tonsils, the patient usually goes home within a few hours after surgery. Costs are less at a surgicenter because they can operate at fixed hours, with scheduled appointments, and don't require the expensive equipment of a hospital. Surgicenter patients must be referred by a physician or a hospital.

In the summer of 1991, there was another new development—medical information by telephone. In one case, members of a Massachusetts community health plan are able to use a home computer to get nonemergency medical information. In another case, which is much more controversial, individuals in New York and New Jersey can call

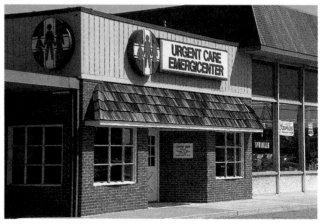

Should we accept convenience and possibly lower prices offered by this urgent care center?

a 900 number and ask questions of a licensed physician (Zoler 1991). Some feel medical information by telephone is a sign of a deteriorating relationship between physicians and patients. Others think it is a good way to get medical information. What do you think?

Alternative Medical Systems

Some individuals argue that the Western system of medicine is not the only acceptable way to deal with medical problems. They point out that other systems have been used with interesting results. In fact, some alternative therapies, such as acupuncture and chiropractic, are gaining respect from the medical establishment and from insurance companies ("Alternative Medicine Is Catching On" 1993).

ISSUE

Should You Use the Services of a Chiropractor?

You will hear many pros and cons about chiropractic. Here are some examples.

- **Pro:** Many individuals report good results from using chiropractic services. Since chiropractors specialize in problems of the back and spine, it makes sense to use a chiropractor if that type of problem exists. If chiropractors weren't legitimate, they wouldn't be allowed to practice.

- **Con:** The chiropractor's training is inadequate. Legitimate medical (M.D.) specialists are available to take care of problems related to the back and spine. There is no good reason to use a chiropractor.

Would you use chiropractic services?

The dangers of improper medical care are real and common; however, the danger of labeling something as improper simply because we do not understand it is equally great. While we must always be careful not to place our mental or physical health in the hands of a fraud, we must be equally careful to remain open and curious about new procedures. For example, D.O.s (osteopaths) were once thought of as quacks because their work was misunderstood. In the same way, chiropractors are often labeled as quacks when, in fact, they might perform important services in certain circumstances.

Chinese medicine, including the use of herbs and acupuncture, was long thought to be superstitious hocus-pocus until some open-minded American physicians traveled to China and began investigating Eastern treatment methods from a Western perspective. We are now discovering that Chinese medicine has much to offer the West and vice versa. Similarly, medicine from India is receiving increasing interest and respect from the West, and Western-trained doctors are studying age-old Indian techniques.

What is most important is to choose practitioners and methods consistent with our needs, and these individuals should have good training, demonstrate their competence, and be respected in their fields of expertise.

Chiropractic

Chiropractic is based on the theory that deviations from health are caused by dislocations of the spinal column (subluxations). Chiropractors locate subluxations by spinal analysis and X ray and then manipulate and adjust the spinal column. The goal is to realign the vertebral column properly to remedy disease or other problems.

Chiropractors in the United States are basically of two types—straights and mixers. Straights use spinal manipulation and massage only, and mixers use these techniques as well as heat, light, and diet therapy. Chiropractors are not legally authorized to perform surgery, prescribe drugs, or practice obstetrics, and they are not permitted to practice in any hospital accredited by the Joint Commission on the Accreditation of Hospitals. Chiropractors often claim they can treat acne, goiter, heart disease, obesity, prostate trouble, angina, and ulcers, among other conditions (Price, Galli, and Slenker 1985).

No scientific proof supports the theory of chiropractic practice. Orthodox medicine has always violently opposed chiropractors. The attitude of some physicians is changing, and in some instances physicians and chiropractors now work together; however, chiropractors are not generally accepted by most medical and health groups (Price, Galli, and Slenker 1985).

After reading the information here about chiropractic, the assistant to the executive vice-president for professional affairs of the American Chiropractic Association took the liberty to write what he called a "more factual, balanced article regarding chiropractic" (American Chiropractic Association, personal correspondence, 1990). Consistent with our decision-making theme and emphasis on considering varying points of view, here is his information:

> Chiropractic is based on the premise that the relationship between structure and function in the human body is a significant health factor and that the relationships between the spinal column and the nervous system contribute to the disease process. The doctor of chiropractic conducts systematic physical, neurological, and orthopedic examinations using the methods, techniques, and instruments standard with all health professions. Chiropractors also include postural and spinal analysis unique to their profession. Diagnostic X-ray and standard and special laboratory procedures and tests are used to arrive at a differential diagnosis. The chiropractor corrects, reduces, mobilizes or immobilizes articular abnormalities, particularly of the spine and pelvis, to normalize structural and functional relationships and relieve attendant neurologic, muscular, and vascular disturbances. These methods do not include prescription drugs or major surgery, thus avoiding the dangers therein. Patient care is conducted with due regard for environmental, nutritional and psychotherapeutic factors as well as first aid, hygiene, sanitation, rehabilitation, and physiological therapeutic procedures designed to assist in the restoration and maintenance of neurological integrity and homeostatic balance.

> There are approximately fifty thousand licensed chiropractors in the United States. Each state has a licensing board which governs the scope of practice. Every state and the District of Columbia license chiropractors upon completion of a minimum of two years prechiropractic education in the basic sciences and four years of chiropractic college, some states require more education. Additional time is spent in internships, residency or other specialty programs.

Chiropractors have hospital privileges in many hospitals throughout the United States although not yet in every state.

When deciding whether chiropractic medicine can help you, Dr. Dean Edell's (1990) observations might be helpful: "Chiropractors, it's safe to say, are a mixed bunch. Some are good ones who are content to deal with muscular and skeletal problems that frustrate ordinary physicians. Then there are ones I call embarrassments, the ones who want to be primary care physicians. This brand of chiropractor honestly believes that all diseases are caused by a pinched nerve or a misaligned spinal column."

Edell feels the consumer is caught in the middle, since some physicians would gladly refer a patient with neck or back pain to a good chiropractor—after first ruling out more serious problems. On the other hand, most doctors simply don't trust practitioners who haven't earned a medical degree.

If you feel it might be appropriate to consult a chiropractor, Edell (1990) offers the following advice:

1. Try a chiropractor for neck or back pain after first visiting an internist to rule out cancer and other more serious ailments.

2. Be aware that chiropractors work best for people suffering moderate, chronic pain. Spinal manipulation can actually worsen many serious disorders, including herniated discs or arthritis.

3. Make sure to find a good one. Many doctors still publicly refuse to refer patients to chiropractors, but you'll probably find that quite a few doctors "secretly" know of a few you can trust. These are the chiropractors you'll want to patronize.

Acupuncture

Acupuncture existed as long as 4,500 years ago in ancient Chinese civilizations. In the early 1970s, when acupuncture became known in the United States, Western doctors seriously questioned the theory behind it.

Acupuncture is a medical technique that involves inserting and manipulating needles in the body to relieve pain and treat disease. The needles are much finer than syringe needles and seldom cause pain or bleeding. By inserting needles at points often far from the area to be treated, the Chinese claim to stop pain and restore health by rebalancing the life force. Needles are inserted at any of over 367 points where there may be blockages. The objective is to balance forces necessary for health.

Traditionally, the Chinese used acupuncture for back pain, arthritis, cancer, headache, nerve deafness, ulcers, blindness, and mental disorders. Today, the Chinese have generally modified their claims and indicate it is not appropriate for all diseases and cannot be used for structural damage or infection. How it stops pain is a mystery; however, it does seem to be helpful in some cases of deafness, narcotics withdrawal, and chronic pain. In addition, it can provide effective anesthesia in some situations.

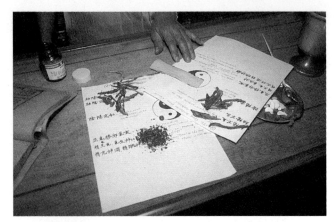

An example of a Chinese herbalist cure for AIDS.

Herbal Medicine

Herbal medicine has been practiced for centuries. Ancient Egyptians established pharmacies based on myrrh, peppermint, olive oil, licorice, and other herbs, in addition to plants, roots, and seeds.

Very little is actually known about the effectiveness of herbal medicines or for what conditions they might be effective. Herbal medicine has increased in popularity in recent years, perhaps because of the soothing effects of treatments and claims of being "natural." One danger is that some herbs are known poisons, and it is almost impossible to control dosages. In addition, there is a danger of self-diagnosis and failure to use more appropriate medical techniques.

Faith Healing

Faith healing is based on the belief that the mind, which controls the body, can cure disease through divine help. A basic premise is that the patient must have faith in healers because they are God's instruments. Techniques used include prayer, laying on of hands, witchcraft, and trance. Some who believe in the healing power of faith say that sickness does not exist except as a mental condition. Others turn to faith healing only when medical science has failed to cure them (Price, Galli, and Slenker 1985).

Many people now follow a wide range of beliefs and practices not sanctioned by mainstream medicine. More than 130 different groups of healers of five broad healing types have been identified (table 16.1). Most individuals who use faith healing also use conventional health care. In general, those who use any of the five broad healing types view health, illness, and healing from a perspective much broader than medicine's main focus on biological functioning (McGuire 1989–1990).

The mainstream medical profession recognizes the power of faith to influence both psychological and physiological functioning. There are also times when diseases reverse or cure themselves without medical intervention. This is referred to as **spontaneous remission.** If a sick person has been seeing a healer, it might appear that the healer is responsible for the cure.

TABLE 16.1

Five Types of Faith Healing Groups

Group Name	Who Belongs	What They Practice
Christian	Most are middle-aged, middle-class and men outnumber women.	Most base healing on Jesus' healing ministry and the place of healing in early churches.
Metaphysical	Tend to be diverse groups—some made up of mostly older people with others having a range of ages. Women are more common than men.	These groups came from Christian Science, Unity, and Religious Science. They maintain church buildings and control religious teachings. Many of their beliefs are similar to psychic and occult groups.
Technique Practitioners	Mostly middle-class including all ages— even children.	Techniques are usually applied one-on-one. Many are used including acupuncture, reflexology, naturopathy, rolfing, and other nonorthodox medicine.
Eastern Meditation and Human Potential Groups	Upper middle-class and very well educated. Most are between twenty-five and forty and women predominate.	They draw from Eastern forms of meditation and popular psychotherapy methods. Examples are sensitivity training, Transcendental Meditation, Jain yoga, and meditation.
Psychic and Occult Groups	Some have a broad age spectrum, but middle-aged are most common. Some groups have many men, but women are more common.	They emphasize gaining power and control over life. Groups are quite diverse and include Eckankar, Great White Brotherhood, Spiritual Frontiers Fellowship, and many unaffiliated psychic healing circles.

Source: Meridith B. McGuire, "Healing Rituals in the Suburbs" in *Psychology Today* 23 (1/2):57–64, January/February 1989.

Faith healing has existed throughout history. In recent years, though, as individuals have realized that science cannot cure everything and that there is a strong connection between emotional and bodily disorders, there is an increased interest in faith healing. There is no proof of the efficacy of faith healing, however, because confirmed medical conditions are difficult to obtain (Price, Galli, and Slenker 1985).

Paying for Health Care

The average cost of a hospital room continues to increase, but room charges are only part of the cost of a hospital stay. Medical costs in the United States increase by over 15 percent per year. The average hospital stay costs close to $4,000. Next to house payments and transportation costs, the largest outlay of money may well be for medical expenses.

Methods of Payment

By planning ahead, we can make wise decisions about how to pay for medical expenses—decisions that meet our needs and are within our budgets. Remember, good health today does not protect you from a sudden catastrophe tomorrow.

College students are often underinsured or not insured at all. Find out whether or not your university or workplace provides a student insurance plan. Family health insurance policies or an employer's medical plan may not necessarily cover all your medical needs. Extra insurance or extra savings may be needed. Medical expenses are too high to be taken for granted!

Paying for medical care directly is no longer feasible, given the high cost of health services, but anticipated medical expenses can be financed in various ways. One way is through a traditional health insurance plan; another is through a **health maintenance organization (HMO).** Health insurance plans are much more common than HMOs, which are only recently available in many communities.

What are the differences in charges between health insurance plans and HMOs? Very little. Both charge very similar monthly fees; thus, some employers offer either option to their employees. There is also little difference in objectives—both provide subscribers with ways to pay for many medical expenses—but they achieve these objectives differently. For example, under a health insurance plan, you are reimbursed for medical expenses after you use the service. Under an HMO, you pay a fixed membership fee (instead of health insurance premiums) in advance. You pay a very small charge for seeing a physician, and all other health-care services are paid for. HMOs make higher profits if they can avoid incurring major medical expenses (for which they must bear the cost), so they actively work toward keeping people well through timely curative services and appropriate preventive care.

Another difference between medical insurance plans and HMOs is the choice of physicians. Under a health insurance plan, you choose your physician, but under HMOs you must choose or are assigned to physicians who are part of that HMO. Furthermore, whenever you are within the geographic service area of the HMO, you must

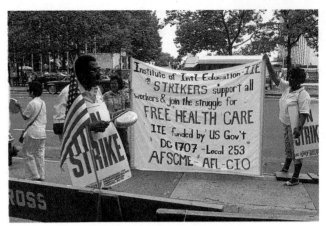

With the rising cost of health care, many people support the development of a national health-care system. The debate over this continues.

use the HMO for services to be covered. If you are outside the HMO's service area, however, the HMO arranges for payment to another physician.

In practice, the line between health insurance plans and HMOs is becoming less and less distinct, and there are as many varieties of HMOs as there are insurance plans. To make the distinction even more ambiguous, major health insurance companies such as Blue Cross and Blue Shield have already established or are in the process of establishing HMOs.

HMO enrollments have been rising each year, but patient dissatisfaction seems to have increased with HMO efforts to hold down costs. Some individuals favor conventional pay-as-you-go doctoring because of shorter waiting periods for appointments, easier access to specialists and hospitals, and more stable relationships between patients and their physicians ("Second Thoughts on HMOs" 1987).

What Is Received for the Payment?

What can you expect from the money you put into the medical care system now and in the future? Unfortunately, because the cost of health care certainly continues to rise, less and less can be expected. The upward spiral of health-care delivery costs has not been matched with equivalent improvements in general health or health-care delivery. In a few instances, slight declines in ill health have been detected. This problem became even more obvious in 1993, when Hillary Rodham Clinton was given an actual and visible role in the health-care cost problem.

The rising costs of health care and the relative stagnation or even decline of delivery suggest that fundamental changes are needed in the health-care delivery system. Various forms of national health insurance have been proposed and debated in Congress, but to date no form of national health insurance has been approved. The ideal plan would include "womb-to-tomb" universal coverage of all Americans, but how such a project might be financed remains unresolved. Supporters of national health insurance feel it is needed because of the rapidly rising costs of medical care, the maldistribution of medical services, and

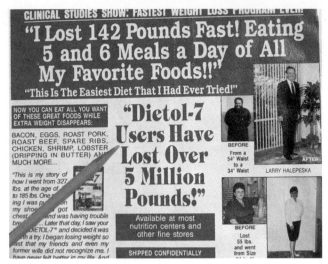

We can be susceptible to quackery because of our strong desire to look and feel better.

many other factors. Opponents feel nationalization and further institutionalization of an already depersonalized system would harm the consumer. Chances are, as you read this, debates about national health insurance continue.

Patients can influence the quality of care by exercising patient rights. The American Hospital Association has suggested the Patient's Bill of Rights that appears in the accompanying box.

Quackery

In television movies, the traveling "pitchman" of old is still seen proclaiming from the back of a covered wagon the wonders of his potions and pills. Covered wagons have long since been replaced by slick ad campaigns, but the same basic attempt is still seen to get money by providing useless or unneeded health products and services. **Quackery** uses discredited or unproven methods or devices to diagnose and/or treat a variety of diseases and other disorders. Today's pitchman is known as a *quack*— a practitioner or other individual who uses these methods or devices to deceive the public.

The most obvious danger of quackery is the loss of money, but there are also other serious consequences. First, using quack treatments can delay receiving legitimate medical services, which may mean the difference between needing a simple, relatively inexpensive treatment and needing a complex, expensive treatment or even being beyond the point of successful treatment altogether. Second, patronizing a quack may lead directly to additional harm or even death, because some quack treatments and devices cause very serious problems. Third, quackery can promote dangerous self-medication.

The Lure of Quackery

Quacks find a receptive audience because we want to be vibrant, attractive, and interesting. We are often anxious about our health and want to find quick, inexpensive

A Patient's Bill of Rights

Introduction

Effective health care requires collaboration between patients and physicians and other health care professionals. Open and honest communication, respect for personal and professional values, and sensitivity to differences are integral to optimal patient care. As the setting for the provision of health services, hospitals must provide a foundation for understanding and respecting the rights and responsibilities of patients, their families, physicians, and other caregivers. Hospitals must ensure a health care ethic that respects the role of patients in decision making about treatment choices and other aspects of their care. Hospitals must be sensitive to cultural, racial, linguistic, religious, age, gender, and other differences as well as the needs of persons with disabilities.

The American Hospital Association presents *A Patient's Bill of Rights* with the expectation that it will contribute to more effective patient care and be supported by the hospital on behalf of the institution, its medical staff, employees, and patients. The American Hospital Association encourages health care institutions to tailor this bill of rights to their patient community by translating and/or simplifying the language of this bill of rights as may be necessary to ensure that patients and their families understand their rights and responsibilities.

Bill of Rights*

1. The patient has the right to considerate and respectful care.

2. The patient has the right to and is encouraged to obtain from physicians and other direct caregivers relevant, current, and understandable information concerning diagnosis, treatment, and prognosis.

   Except in emergencies when the patient lacks decision-making capacity and the need for treatment is urgent, the patient is entitled to the opportunity to discuss and request information related to the specific procedures and/or treatments, the risks involved, the possible length of recuperation, and the medically reasonable alternatives and their accompanying risks and benefits.

   Patients have the right to know the identity of physicians, nurses, and others involved in their care, as well as when those involved are students, residents, or other trainees. The patient also has the right to know the immediate and long-term financial implications of treatment choices, insofar as they are known.

3. The patient has the right to make decisions about the plan of care prior to and during the course of treatment and to refuse a recommended treatment or plan of care to the extent permitted by law and hospital policy and to be informed of the medical consequences of this action. In case of such refusal, the patient is entitled to other appropriate care and services that the hospital provides or transfer to another hospital. The hospital should notify patients of any policy that might affect patient choice within the institution.

4. The patient has the right to have an advance directive (such as a living will, health care proxy, or durable power of attorney for health care) concerning treatment or designating a surrogate decision maker with the expectation that the hospital will honor the intent of that directive to the extent permitted by law and hospital policy.

   Health care institutions must advise patients of their rights under state law and hospital policy to make informed medical choices, ask if the patient has an advance directive, and include that information in patient records. The patient has the right to timely information about hospital policy that may limit its ability to implement fully a legally valid advance directive.

5. The patient has the right to every consideration of privacy. Case discussion, consultation, examination, and treatment should be conducted so as to protect each patient's privacy.

6. The patient has the right to expect that all communications and records pertaining to his/her care will be treated as confidential by the hospital, except in cases such as suspected abuse and public health hazards when reporting is permitted or required by law. The patient has the right to expect that the hospital will emphasize the confidentiality of this information when it releases it to any other parties entitled to review information in these records.

7. The patient has the right to review the records pertaining to his/her medical care and to have the information explained or interpreted as necessary, except when restricted by law.

8. The patient has the right to expect that, within its capacity and policies, a hospital will make reasonable response to the request of a patient for appropriate and medically indicated care and services. The hospital must provide evaluation, service, and/or referral as indicated by the urgency of the case. When medically appropriate and legally permissible, or when a patient has so requested, a patient may be transferred to another facility. The institution

*These rights can be exercised on the patient's behalf by a designated surrogate or proxy decision maker if the patient lacks decision-making capacity, is legally incompetent, or is a minor. Reprinted with permission of the American Hospital Association, copyright 1992.

to which the patient is to be transferred must first have accepted the patient for transfer. The patient must also have the benefit of complete information and explanation concerning the need for, risks, benefits, and alternatives to such a transfer.

9. The patient has the right to ask and be informed of the existence of business relationships among the hospital, educational institutions, other health care providers, or payers that may influence the patient's treatment and care.

10. The patient has the right to consent to or decline to participate in proposed research studies or human experimentation affecting care and treatment or requiring direct patient involvement, and to have those studies fully explained prior to consent. A patient who declines to participate in research or experimentation is entitled to the most effective care that the hospital can otherwise provide.

11. The patient has the right to expect reasonable continuity of care when appropriate and to be informed by physicians and other caregivers of available and realistic patient care

options when hospital care is no longer appropriate.

12. The patient has the right to be informed of hospital policies and practices that relate to patient care, treatment, and responsibilities. The patient has the right to be informed of available resources for resolving disputes, grievances, and conflicts, such as ethics committees, patient representatives, or other mechanisms available in the institution. The patient has the right to be informed of the hospital's charges for services and available payment methods.

The collaborative nature of health care requires that patients, or their families/surrogates, participate in their care. The effectiveness of care and patient satisfaction with the course of treatment depend, in part, on the patient fulfilling certain responsibilities. Patients are responsible for providing information about past illnesses, hospitalizations, medications, and other matters related to health status. To participate effectively in decision making, patients must be encouraged to take responsibility for requesting additional information or clarification about their health status or treatment when they do not fully understand information and instructions. Patients are also responsible for ensuring that the health care institution has a copy of

their written advance directive if they have one. Patients are responsible for informing their physicians and other caregivers if they anticipate problems in following prescribed treatment.

Patients should also be aware of the hospital's obligation to be reasonably efficient and equitable in providing care to other patients and the community. The hospital's rules and regulations are designed to help the hospital meet this obligation. Patients and their families are responsible for making reasonable accommodations to the needs of the hospital, other patients, medical staff, and hospital employees. Patients are responsible for providing necessary information for insurance claims and for working with the hospital to make payment arrangements, when necessary.

A person's health depends on much more than health care services. Patients are responsible for recognizing the impact of their life-style on their personal health.

Conclusion

Hospitals have many functions to perform, including the enhancement of health status, health promotion, and the prevention and treatment of injury and disease; the immediate and ongoing care and rehabilitation of patients; the education of health professionals, patients, and the community; and research. All these activities must be conducted with an overriding concern for the values and dignity of patients.

---

solutions to health problems. We might visit a reputable physician and be unhappy with the results. Physicians can't guarantee results or speedy recoveries, but quacks do, and we can easily take the bait. Or, in the case of terminal illness, we might turn to a quack as the last resort. We want to have hope, and quacks offer a promise.

The claims of quacks often appear plausible partly because of our relative ignorance of health matters, the inability to filter through the flood of information about new developments in health care, and the frequent tendency to take what is seen in print as truth. Quack claims also appear believable because they play on modern fascina-

tion with technology. Humans have walked on the moon, life has been nurtured in test tubes, and polio has been virtually wiped out—if science and technology have brought these developments, why not a quick cure for cancer or instant relief from arthritis?

Another interesting aspect of quackery is the **placebo effect.** Scientists running controlled studies in laboratory settings discovered that subjects given, for example, a simple sugar pill were almost as likely to show subjective signs of improvement—and in some cases even objective improvement—as the subjects given an actual test drug for their problems. Apparently, expectations of receiving

The Top Ten Health Frauds

Americans spend an estimated $27 billion a year on quack products and treatments. Over thirty-eight million Americans have used a fraudulent health product within the past year. Here is the FDA's list of the top ten health frauds (but keep in mind that health fraud is not limited to these ten):

1. Fraudulent arthritis products
2. Deceptive cancer clinics
3. Bogus AIDS cures
4. Instant weight-loss schemes
5. Fraudulent sexual aids
6. Quack baldness remedies and other appearance modifiers (such as cream to remove wrinkles or a device to "develop" the bust)
7. False nutritional schemes
8. Chelation therapy (This is an injection or tablet that is supposed to clean out the arteries. Both the FDA and the American Heart Association agree that there is no scientific evidence that chelation therapy works.)
9. Unproven use of muscle stimulators (Claims are made that stimulators can remove wrinkles, perform face-lifts, reduce breast size, and remove cellulite. Claims are even made that they can reduce one's beer belly with no effort. They can't do any of these things.)
10. Candidiasis hypersensitivity (Candida is a fungus found naturally on the body. It can multiply and infect the skin or mucous membranes. Promoters recommend antifungal drugs and vitamin and mineral supplements. They don't work, and the idea that some people are hypersensitive to candida has not even been proven.)

Source: "The Top Ten Health Frauds" in *Consumers' Research* 73 (2): 34–36, February 1990.

help have a great deal to do with the actual effect of a drug, activity, or service. It is easy to see how quackery can take advantage of this placebo effect by raising expectations of the miraculous curative powers of some drug or procedure. In fact, it is the expectation of improvement that does the curing, not the drug or procedure itself.

The self-limiting nature of many diseases also contributes to the success of quackery. Many diseases (e.g., the common cold) go away even with no treatment. Other diseases are cyclic. For example, the cancer victim might think he or she is cured during a time that the disease is not as evident. It is easy to see how a person who has visited a quack or used a quack remedy might think it was successful if symptoms seem to disappear.

Major Areas of Quackery

Major target areas for quack promotions include arthritis, fitness, weight loss, and cancer. Nutrition and cosmetic quackery are also common (and phony supplements are a waste of money and can cause or mask real health problems ["Phony Health Supplements" 1993]). Even bogus AIDS treatments are increasing.

Arthritis quackery is common because over forty million Americans suffer from arthritis, and the nature of the disease (pain comes and goes and there is no cure) makes it fertile ground for fraud. Arthritis sufferers may actually believe they have been cured by a quack remedy during a time the disease is in remission.

More than $2 billion is spent annually on quack arthritis cures such as snake venom, lemon juice, milk from vaccinated cows, and steroids. Some treatments can be extremely dangerous. It is important to remember that pain relief and inflammation treatments are not the same. Serious arthritic conditions should be treated by a doctor.

Fitness is a prime area for quacks because many of us want the benefits of exercise without actually exercising. Recent years have brought all sorts of body toning devices, such as electrical muscle stimulators and machines that vibrate body parts. Such devices are worthless for body toning and can even be dangerous, but they are advertised and sold as substitutes for exercising.

Weight loss schemes might be the most popular form of quackery. Millions of individuals seek a painless and effortless way to win the battle of the bulge. Since proper diet and exercise take constant discipline and work, quack claims are especially appealing. The fact is you can't lose weight unless the amount of food you eat is reduced and the amount of exercise you do is increased. There are no medicines or devices that make this process effortless.

Cancer quack cures are probably the cruelest and most expensive. Seriously ill individuals may spend thousands of dollars on ineffective quack treatments. Among the most popular quack cancer remedies are immune-enhancing therapies (to improve the immune system), metabolic treatments, and special diets. None of these is effective (Cassileth 1991). There is no one device or remedy capable of diagnosing or treating all types of cancer. Cancer cannot be detected or treated solely through the use of machines. Before being treated at a cancer clinic or using a product that is supposed to cure cancer, it is wise to consult with a respectable physician and the American Cancer Society.

Recognizing Quackery

Considering the many health decisions made in the world of advancing technology, how can we tell which health products and services are legitimate? Few rules apply in every situation, but here are some warning signs that quackery may be present:

1. A cure for the disease is guaranteed.
2. A special or "secret" formula or machine is discussed.
3. A quick and easy treatment and speedy cure are promised.
4. Health services are advertised, using case histories and testimonials from patients.
5. We are warned of the dangers of orthodox drugs and treatments.
6. Claims are made of persecution by the medical community.
7. There is a refusal to accept proven methods of medical research.
8. Claims are made of treatment methods that are better than surgery, X rays, and medically prescribed drugs.
9. Ingredients are not identified.
10. Support from experts is claimed, but they are not named or fully identified.
11. Claims are made for effectiveness for a variety of conditions (the broader a claim, the less believable it is).
12. The product is declared as all "natural." This probably means the product is some combination of vitamins and minerals and no different from a typical multivitamin pill.
13. Vague illusions are made to "published research," sometimes with an offer to supply references by letter.
14. The product is only offered through the mail or door-to-door.

Some mail services, such as those that sell eyeglasses or dental plates, may not actually be fraudulent but are of dubious value because interpretation, adjustment, or quality control by a health professional is crucial. For example, a mail-order urinalysis has been promoted by some firms for many years. A urinalysis is an important part of a health examination but is of questionable value when conducted through the mail. Its results can also be misleading without a more thorough exam and interpretation by a licensed physician.

If you suspect quackery in any health-related product or service, consult a physician, pharmacist, or other health professional. In addition, one of the consumer protection agencies mentioned earlier might be contacted.

If you want to take legal action against a quack, you can get help from the National Council Against Health Fraud. This organization can refer you to an experienced lawyer, provide a registry of expert witnesses, give information on defense witnesses, and furnish a list of unproven, fraudulent, and potentially dangerous treatments. Contact Michael Botts, P.O. Box 33008, Kansas City, MO 64114; phone (816) 444–8615 ("How to Spot A Quack" 1990).

Even though the ultimate responsibility for wise health decisions falls on the shoulders of consumers, we are not alone in the process. Help is available if we seek it and know how to use it.

Summary

1. A personal plan for better health involves assessing health-producing and health-destroying behaviors, adopting health-producing behaviors in a systematic way, recognizing and accepting the good feelings associated with high-level wellness, and understanding why certain behaviors are related to health and positive feelings.

2. In part because of advertising, we often buy health products we don't need or want. To make wise consumer decisions, we must learn to evaluate advertising claims systematically.

3. Many OTC drugs are ineffective and are used unnecessarily. There are potential dangers from self-medication. There are also certain guidelines to follow for best results when using prescription drugs.

4. Consumers have the right to safety, the right to be informed, the right to choose, and the right to be heard. Many government and private agencies exist to protect consumers.

5. Consumer complaints can be handled formally or informally. In either instance, certain steps should be followed. The ultimate responsibility for consumer protection is in the hands of the consumer.

6. Decisions about medical care include when to use self-care, when to seek medical care, how to help the medical specialist help us, and how to find a suitable medical specialist or hospital.

7. Medical care should be used in a life-threatening situation, when bodily symptoms have lasted for an unusually long time, and when there is uncertainty. To choose medical care, the consumer must know what kind of medical help is available, how to check credentials, and how to evaluate personal responses.

8. New options for medical care include urgent care centers and surgicenters.

9. Alternative medical systems include chiropractic, acupuncture, herbal medicine, and faith healing.

10. Options for paying for medical care include individual insurance programs and various types of HMOs. There are many rights to remember as a patient.

11. Quacks find a receptive audience in the American population for a variety of reasons. Major areas of quackery include arthritis, fitness, weight loss, and cancer.

12. There are a number of ways to recognize quackery.

Commitment Activities

1. Collect at least six advertisements for health products. Evaluate the ads with the guidelines presented in this chapter. Does this activity affect your feelings about any of the advertisements?

2. Using the checklist for evaluating health information presented in the chapter, analyze health information you hear and see in the next several days. What can you conclude about the health information based on this analysis?

3. Find out which consumer protection agencies exist in your home or college community. Visit representatives from three of the agencies and briefly interview them. Use questions such as the following and add your own: How does your agency help protect consumers? What are the most common consumer problems you see? How can individuals best work with your agency? How can consumers help prevent the problems you encounter?

4. Collect information on several health insurance plans and an HMO, if one is in your area. What are the benefits and drawbacks of each? How would you choose among them?

5. Share your most recent experience as a patient in either a hospital or an office/clinic with other class members. Bring out your perceptions of the positive and negative aspects of your encounter with the medical care system.

6. Pay attention to advertisements in some popular magazines. Using this chapter's guidelines for recognizing quackery, identify instances where quackery seems to be present. Write to the editors of magazines in which suspected quack practices or products are advertised. Point out the apparent quackery to them and inquire about their policies for accepting advertising. Request a written explanation.

References

"Advertising Watchdogs." *Changing Times* (July 1984):53–54.

"Alternative Medicine Is Catching On." *Kiplinger's Personal Finance Magazine* 47, no. 1 (January 1993):98–99.

American Chiropractic Association, personal correspondence, March 2, 1990.

Aral, S. O.; Mosher, W. D.; and Cates, W. "Vaginal Douching Among Women of Reproductive Age in the United States." *American Journal of Public Health* 82, no. 2 (February 1992):210–14.

"Beware of Tanning Pills." *Consumers' Research* 74, no. 1 (January 1991):29–30.

Blaylock, B. "Home Health Testing Kits." *Birmingham News* (November 11, 1986):6D–7D.

Cassileth, B. R. "Questionable and Unproven Cancer Therapies." *Consumers' Research* 74, no. 9 (September 1991):20–23.

"Cold Remedies: Which Ones Work Best?" *Consumer Reports* 54, no. 1 (January 1989):8–11.

Consumer Almanac. Washington, D.C.: Consumers' League, 1975, pp. 15–22.

Corry, J. M. *Consumer Health.* Belmont, Calif.: Wadsworth, 1983.

Edell, D. "How to Find a Good Chiropractor." *Edell Health Letter* 9, no. 4 (April 1990):2.

"Facial Cleansers." *Consumer Reports* 54, no. 6 (June 1989):408–10.

Farley, D. "Do It Yourself Medical Testing." *FDA Consumer* (February 1986).

"How to Spot A Quack." *Consumers' Research* 73, no. 2 (February 1990):36.

McGuire, M. B. "Healing Rituals in the Suburbs." *Psychology Today* 23, no. 1/2 (January/February 1989–1990):57–64.

McKenzie, J. F. "A Checklist for Evaluating Health Information." *Journal of School Health* 57, no. 1 (January 1987):31–32.

"OTC Pain Medications of Only Three Types Available." *UAB Report* (January 30, 1987):5.

"Phoney Food Supplements." *Edell Health Letter* 12, no. 1 (January 1993):1.

"Prescription for Savings: Shop Around." *Changing Times* 44, no. 2 (February 1990):102.

Price, J. H.; Galli, N.; and Slenker, S. *Consumer Health.* Dubuque, Iowa: Wm. C. Brown Publishers, 1985.

"Second Thoughts on HMOs." *Changing Times* 41, no. 5 (May 1987):33–38.

Shipley, R. R., and Plonsky, C. G. *Consumer Health.* New York: Harper and Row, 1980.

"Update on Generics." *Changing Times* 44, no. 2 (February 1990):102.

Wallack, L., and Dorfman, L. "Health Messages on Television Commercials." *American Journal of Health Promotion* 6, no. 3 (January/February 1992):190–96.

Zoler, M. L. "Do Call-In Consults Enhance or Counterfeit Medicine?" *Medical World News* 32, no. 8 (August 1991):25.

Additional Readings

Kazman, S. "The FDA's Deadly Approval Process." *Consumers' Research* 74, no. 4 (April 1991):31–34. Outlines the FDA approval process for new drugs and gives examples of deaths that might have been caused by "too much safety."

Lohr, K. N., and Schroeder, S. A. "A Strategy for Quality Assurance in Medicare." *New England Journal of Medicine* 322, no. 10 (March 8, 1990):707–12. Summarizes the findings of a National Academy of Sciences report on medical care for elderly people. Emphasizes major issues needing consideration.

Quackery. U.S. Department of Health and Human Services Brochure. Publication no. 85–4200, n.d. Discusses the high price of health fraud, common targets for quack attacks, evaluating advertisements, and how to protect yourself.

Psychoneuroimmunology (PNI) is the study of the interaction of the mind, the central nervous system, and the body's immunological system. It has been shown that people with a fighting spirit, optimism, a sense of control, hope, and faith can actually build their immune systems. The brain has the capability to self-medicate and to release a variety of mental and physical painkillers and motivating substances (neuropeptides) when the demand is there.

The discussion of health-care providers and consumer health is extremely important as it relates to PNI. You have learned that modern medicine has become extremely sophisticated and specialized. Medicines and technology continue to become more and more sophisticated. Often, the power of touch, hope, and optimism are neglected, and the members of the medical profession rely almost totally on technology for healing. Those physicians who provide hope, optimism, touch, a sense of control, and other human caring traits facilitate the healing experience.

Generally speaking, quackery thrives largely because of the belief that a certain fraudulent cure works. Consumers believe something works, and it does, through their own self-efficacy or faith. The methods by themselves do not work, but in combination with a patient who believes, the patient's hopes, fighting spirit, control, and optimism are raised. This may fortify the immune system so the patient feels better. Faith healings among religions also promote the positive states that may result in feeling better. This process has been demonstrated repeatedly when modern medicine has been administered to someone of another culture.

Someone who is offering some form of quackery generally offers something more than a traditional doctor's office visit. They give substantial time and touching and take time to understand feelings. We can learn from that element of care giving and take advantage of alternative forms of healing that can supplement doctors' orders. It is with some hesitation that this recommendation is made in light of how we have treated quackery in the past. It has been viewed as totally negative and worthless. The fact is, it may provide hope in some cases. The caution is twofold.

Never use a quackery method instead of a physician's recommendation, but perhaps the method can be used in harmony with the prescription. This is particularly true if you have strong faith in the method.

Secondly, do not spend much money on a questionable product in spite of claims, unless you have money to throw away. You can create your own techniques to bolster your immune system.

With those cautions in mind, you may want to try some methods that are truly beneficial to reduce stress and provide a basis for hope, optimism, control, and a fighting spirit.

1. Take the opportunity to learn water therapy (Angelé 1980). Many of us know how good it feels to sit in a Jacuzzi and feel the benefits of water massage. The most famous form of therapy is the German Kneipp water application method and its therapeutic benefit. It is the four hundred-year-old science of warm and cold water applications to various parts of the body that results in a reduction of the stress response, a relaxing and calming effect, enriched circulation, and stimulation of the skin. In essence, the process is to apply cold water (46°–50° F) on the skin, beginning with the arms (from fingers to shoulders), the legs (from the toes to upper leg), the face, and finally the body. Lie down, relax, and feel the wonderful sensation of the tingling skin following the experience. There are 160 different Kneipp applications. Many involve special equipment and are beyond the scope of this text but would be a viable complement to traditional medical care.

2. Mentally feel the healing effects of acupressure massage. Massages in combination with acupressure can improve circulation, reduce muscle tension and pain, relieve pain, and help deeply relax the mind and body. Massage takes your mind off problems, lets you focus on the positive touching experience, and produces a subtle calm over the whole body. The Chinese thoroughly studied the body, isolating and recording the points where knots and bands of excessive muscle tension frequently occur.

3. Enhance your spiritual dimension of living (if comfortable with this concept) as it pertains to faith, belief in a higher power, and practice accessing that power through the means dictated by your own belief system. Rituals or symbols (prayer or charms) to aid in the healing or preventive sense can help complement medicine.

4. There are numerous other techniques that can make you feel good if you try them and believe that they will work, especially if used in harmony with medical guidance. Examples include deep-muscle therapy, meditation, and self-hypnosis (Feltman 1989).

References

Angelé, K.H. *Your Daily Health Care with Kneipp.* Bad Worishofen, Germany: Kneipp-Verlag GMBH, 1980.

Feltman, J., ed. *Hands-On Healing.* Emmaus, Penn.: Rodale Press, 1989.

By reading and working through the activities in the chapter on consumer health, you should have a good understanding of:

1. the influence of advertising on consumer health decisions as well as ways to evaluate advertising;
2. guidelines for the use of OTC and prescription drugs;
3. available consumer protection and ways for consumers to take action;
4. decisions that need to be made related to medical care;
5. alternative medical systems;
6. options for paying for medical care;
7. the threat of quackery and how to deal with it.

There has also been an opportunity to assess your feelings about many consumer health issues. Health-producing behaviors are enhanced by wise consumer health decisions. Examples of such decisions relate to every chapter of this text.

Since consumer health decisions are so basic to total health, it is appropriate to consider ways to strengthen your well-being related to consumer health. The model for preventing health problems presented in chapter 1 provides the framework within which to consider the relevance of the issues presented in this section.

The following list includes some sample behaviors related to consumer health. These are only possibilities, and there may be others more appropriate for you.

1. Assess your motivation and reasons for purchasing health products and utilizing certain medical services.
2. Examine the outcomes and scientific basis of any self-medications and/or self-treatment that you use.
3. Become a wiser consumer of health products and services. For example, keep informed about consumer issues, read labels carefully, check out products and services before purchasing them, and buy generic drugs when possible.
4. Use your rights as a consumer to take action if you experience a problem with a medical product or service.
5. Analyze your personal health insurance options and implement an insurance plan to cover you and your family in the best way possible.
6. Be alert for quackery and take action to prevent it. Analyze ads, articles, and medical claims from other sources in a manner appropriate for a wise health consumer.
7. Develop a plan for others to help them become wiser health consumers.
8. Think of a situation related to consumer decisions that has caused disorganization or disruption in your life. Develop a plan to promote resilient adjustment (see chapter 1 for a review of these terms) in your life to prevent potential health problems related to consumer decisions in the future.

Life-Style Contracting Using Strength Intervention

I. Choosing the desired health behavior or skill

  A. Keeping in mind the purposes in life and goals you identified in the mental-health chapter, consider one or two health behaviors related to consumer health (from the list here or of your own creation) that will help you reach your goals. To assess the likelihood of success, ask yourself questions similar to those used in previous sections, such as:

   1. Is my purpose, cause, or goal better realized by the adoption of this behavior?
      ____ yes ____ no
   2. Am I hardy enough to accomplish this goal? (This means I feel I can do it if I work hard, I am in control of what needs to be done, I am committed to do it, and the goal is a challenge for me.) ____ yes ____ no
   3. Is this a behavior I really want to change and that I feel I can change? ____ yes ____ no
   4. Do I first need to nurture a personal strength area? ____ yes ____ no (If yes, be sure to include this as part of the plan.)
   5. Do I need to free myself from a bad habit in order to accomplish this goal?
      ____ yes ____ no (If yes, be sure to include this as part of the plan.)
   6. Have I considered the results of the assessments in the consumer health chapter? ____ yes ____ no These results may be helpful in developing a plan.

   (Yes answers to the first three questions are a must to be successful. It might be wise to consider a different behavior if you cannot honestly answer yes to these questions. Your answers to questions 4–6 ought to provide information for consideration in your plan.)

  B. Behaviors I will change (no more than two)

   _____

   _____

II. Life-style plan

  A. A description of the general plan of what I am going to do and how I will accomplish it. (Consider apperceptive experiences—successes you have had in the past—since they may help you develop the best ways to carry out this plan.)

   _____

   _____

   _____

   _____

   _____

   _____

B. Barriers to accomplishment of the plan (lack of time, feelings of others, hesitation to take action, motivation, etc.).

    1. Identify barriers _____

    _____

    _____

    _____

    2. Means to remove barriers (use problem-solving skills or creative approaches such as those described in the mental-health chapter) _____

    _____

    _____

    _____

    _____

C. Implementation of the plan.

    1. Substitution (putting positive behaviors in place of negative ones) _____

    _____

    2. Confluence (combining activities for time efficiency if possible) _____

    _____

    3. Systematic enhancement (using a strength to help a weakness) _____

    _____

    4. When _____

    5. Where _____

    _____

    6. Preparation _____

    _____

    7. With whom _____

III. Support groups

    A. Who _____

    _____

    B. Role _____

    _____

    C. Organized support _____

    _____

IV. Trigger responses _____

    _____

    _____

V. Starting date _____

VI. Date/sequence the contract will be reevaluated _____

    _____

VII. Evidence of reaching goal _____

    _____

VIII. Rewards when contract is completed _____

    _____

IX. Signature of client _____

X. Signature of facilitator _____

XI. Additional conditions/comments _____

    _____

    _____

    _____

Appendix A
Health Objectives for the Nation

In 1979, the Department of Health and Human Services made public the "1990 Objectives for the Nation." Using the 1990 objectives as a foundation, in 1990, the year 2000 health objectives for the nation were presented in a publication entitled *Healthy People 2000: National Health Promotion and Disease Prevention Objectives.* These objectives outline the health goals for the country and also identify the health risk factors to eliminate to accomplish these objectives. Three broad goals were proposed to serve as overall measures of the nation's health. They were, by the year 2000, to

1. increase the span of healthy life for Americans;
2. reduce health disparities among Americans;
3. achieve access to preventive services for all Americans.

The specific priority areas to accomplish these goals were grouped in four categories: health promotion priorities, health protection priorities, preventive services priorities, and surveillance and data systems priorities:

Health Promotion Priorities
1. physical activity and fitness
2. nutrition
3. tobacco
4. alcohol and other drugs
5. family planning
6. mental health and mental disorders
7. violent and abusive behavior
8. educational and community-based programs

Health Protection Priorities
9. unintentional injuries
10. occupational safety and health
11. environmental health
12. food and drug safety
13. oral health

Preventive Services Priorities
14. maternal and infant health
15. heart disease and stroke
16. cancer
17. diabetes and chronic disabling conditions
18. HIV infection
19. sexually transmitted diseases
20. immunization and infectious diseases
21. clinical preventive services

Surveillance and Data Systems
22. surveillance and data systems

Approximately four hundred objectives are listed for the nation. Sample objectives related to some of the chapters in this text include the following:

1. Reduce overweight among people ages twenty through seventy-four to a prevalence of no more than 20 percent (baseline: 25.7 percent in 1976–1980).
2. Increase to at least 50 percent the proportion of people age six and older who regularly perform physical activities that maintain muscular strength, muscular endurance, and flexibility (baseline data unavailable).
3. Reduce cigarette smoking to a prevalence of no more than 15 percent among people age twenty and older (baseline: 29.1 percent in 1987).
4. Reduce alcohol-related motor vehicle crash deaths to no more than 0.9 per 100 million vehicle miles

traveled (VMT) and to 8.5 per 100,000 people (baseline: 1.2 per 100 million VMT and 9.7 per 100,000 people in 1987).

5. Reduce pregnancies among girls age fifteen to seventeen to no more than 55 per 1,000 (baseline: 73.2 pregnancies per 1,000 in 1982).

6. Reduce rape and attempted rape of women age twelve and older to no more than 107 per 100,000 women (baseline: 119.7 per 100,000 in 1986).

7. Increase to at least 40 percent the proportion of people age sixty-five and older who participate in moderate physical activities three or more days per week for twenty minutes or more per occasion (baseline: 31 percent in 1985).

8. Increase to at least 90 percent the proportion of people who live in air quality reporting areas that have not exceeded the Environmental Protection Agency standard for ozone in the previous twelve months (baseline: 68 air quality reporting areas, with 113 million people exceeding the standard in 1985-1987).

9. Reduce influenza-associated deaths among people age sixty-five and older to no more than 40 per 100,000 people (baseline: 70 per 100,000 in 1987).

10. Reverse the rising trend in the incidence of AIDS cases and reduce annual incidence to no more than the projected number of 80,000 new cases in 1992 (baseline: 32,971 cases in 1988).

11. Reduce gonorrhea to an incidence of no more than 225 cases per 100,000 people (baseline: 297 per 100,000 in 1988).

12. Reduce the mean serum cholesterol level for people age twenty and older to no more than 200 mg/dL (baseline: 213 mg/dL in 1976–1980).

13. Reduce breast cancer deaths to no more than 25.2 per 100,000 women (baseline: 27.2 per 100,000 in 1986).

14. Reduce to no more than 60 percent the proportion of adolescents age fifteen who have experienced dental caries (cavities) in permanent teeth (baseline: 78 percent in 1986–1987).

15. Reduce to at least 35 percent the proportion of people age eighteen and older who experience adverse health effects from stress (baseline: 44 percent in 1985).

Some of the groups that have helped and are helping to accomplish these goals are federal, state, and local organizations as well as private and voluntary groups. Some organizations where students can receive complimentary information about particular health problems include the following:

Voluntary Organizations

- Al-Anon Family Group Headquarters
  314 W. 53rd St., 2nd floor
  New York, NY 10012
  (800) 356–9996
  (212) 245–3151 (in New York and Canada)

- Alcoholics Anonymous
  P.O. Box 459, Grand Central Annex
  New York, NY 10017
  (212) 686–1100

- American Cancer Society
  19 W. 56th St.
  New York, NY 10019
  (212) 586–8700

- American Dental Association
  211 E. Chicago Ave.
  Chicago, IL 60611

- American Diabetes Association
  One W. 48th St.
  New York, NY 10020
  (800) 232–3472

- American Dietetic Association
  430 N. Michigan Ave.
  Chicago, IL 60611

- American Heart Association
  7320 Greenville Ave.
  Dallas, TX 75231
  (214) 750–5300

- American Lung Association
  1740 Broadway
  New York, NY 10019
  (212) 315–8700

- American National Red Cross
  17th and D Streets, NW
  Washington, D.C. 20006
  (202) 737–8300

- The Arthritis Foundation
  1314 Spring St. NW
  Atlanta, GA 30309
  (404) 837–3240

- Council on Family Health
  633 Third Ave.
  New York, NY 10017

- National Association for Sickle Cell Disease, Inc.
  245 S. Western Ave. Suite 206
  Los Angeles, CA 90006

- National Consumers League
  1028 Connecticut Ave., NW,
  Suite 522
  Washington, D.C. 20036

- National Council on Alcoholism
  733 Third Ave.
  New York, NY 10017
  (800) 622–2255

- National Foundation-March of Dimes
  1275 Mamaronek Ave.
  White Plains, NY 10605
  (914) 428–7100

- National Mental Health Association
  1021 Prince St.
  Arlington, VA 22314
  (703) 684–7722

- World Health Organization
  1501 New Hampshire Ave., NW
  Washington, D.C. 20036

Government Agencies

- Centers for Disease Control
  and Prevention
  Public Inquiries Office
  1600 Clifton Rd. NE
  Building 1, Room B63
  Atlanta, GA 30333
  (404) 639–3534

- Consumer Information Center
  18th and E Streets, NW
  Washington, D.C. 20405
  (202) 566–2794
- Environmental Protection Agency
  Public Information Center
  PM 211–B
  401 M St., NW
  Washington, D.C. 20460
  (800) 368–5888

- Food and Drug Administration
  Office of Consumer Affairs
  5600 Fishers Lane
  Rockville, MD 20857
  (301) 443–3170
- National Cancer Institute
  9000 Rockville Pike
  Bethesda, MD 20014
  (301) 496–6641
- National Center for Alcohol Education
  1601 N. Kent St.
  Arlington, VA 22201

Appendix B
Personal Safety

If you are between the ages of one and forty-five the following statement is critical: *Statistics Show That, If You Die Between The Ages Of One And Forty-five, It Will Most Likely Be From An Accident.* Frequently it is in an automobile accident, but it may be from a fall, drowning, electrocution, or one of many other "accidents" that occur thousands of times a day. Let's say you are one of the lucky ones and do not die in an accident this year. There will be more than ten million disabling injuries this year, accounting for a total financial loss of over $100 billion. This does not even take into account the accidents we recover from within a few weeks or the ones in which no one is hurt but property is damaged. How can you keep from joining these statistics? There are many things you can do to reduce your risk of having an accident and many more things you can do to lessen the damage and speed your recovery. That is what personal safety is all about.

Medical Emergencies

Medical emergencies are common in every community. You have probably been a bystander or personally involved in at least one medical emergency in the last year. It is a well-documented fact that, in 90 percent of all cases where CPR is performed by a nonprofessional care provider, the CPR is performed on a friend or family member of the provider. This means that you will probably be called upon to give first aid to someone you know. There is nothing more frustrating and guilt inducing than having to watch a friend or family member suffer or even die because you did not know what to do.

This appendix is written by Les Chatelain, Director of Emergency Programs and Deputy Director of the Health Behavior Laboratory, University of Utah.

First, know how to get help. Have emergency telephone numbers posted on or near all telephones. The 911 system is in operation in most communities but not all. Know the emergency number for your area. You may not need the 911 services. It may be the Poison Control Center or your family physician that you need, and 911 can't connect you with them. *All* emergency numbers should be posted. Other important information to post by your telephone includes work telephone numbers, your address, including number coordinates for both your house and street, and telephone numbers of friends and family members. These people may be of assistance with such things as tending younger family members, transportation, or food preparation. You will be surprised at how difficult it is to remember simple things like telephone numbers or where the kids are during an emergency.

Second, be prepared to give the needed information to dispatchers. They will ask for your name, the telephone number you are calling from, the exact location of the emergency, what happened, how many victims, what the victims' conditions are, and what help is being given. This means you need to assess the emergency briefly prior to making the call. Lack of information may delay the response of needed personnel.

Third, provide basic emergency care. This is very limited unless you are trained. You can obtain first aid and CPR training from many sources, including the American Red Cross, American Heart Association, hospitals, community adult education programs, colleges and universities, church groups, and civic groups. It is recommended that you receive CPR training yearly and first aid training at least every three years. There are some things that can be done with little or no training. Immediately assess the emergency. Is it safe for you, the victims, and others to be in the area? Ask the victim what happened. If he or she can talk to you, then the person probably has adequate airway, breathing, and pulse. These should be assessed throughout your treatment. If the person does not respond to you, determine if he or she is breathing and has a pulse. If there is no breathing or pulse, treat these according to your training. Look for any bleeding. Most bleeding can be slowed down or stopped by applying pressure to the wound with your hand. Some type of clean barrier (such as a towel or clothing) should be placed between your hand and the wound to prevent infection of the victim or yourself. *Important:* do not move the person unless you absolutely have to, either to treat the victim or because the scene is definitely unsafe (it is usually best to keep the victim of an automobile accident in the car and in the position you find him or her). Talk to the person and keep him or her calm. Be very reassuring. If the victim is too hot, try to cool him or her down. If the victim is too cold, try to warm him or her up. Always work within your training. Do all you can for the victim(s), but do not attempt things you are not trained to do or can't remember how to perform.

Lastly, while we hope that we will never be involved in a medical emergency, we still need to be prepared. Have a first aid kit available. You may want one at home, in your car, and at work. Obtain health insurance if at all possible. With the cost of medical treatment these days, an accident can become a financial burden from which you will never recover. Some relatively inexpensive sources for health insurance are your school and/or work. Even if your work does not provide health insurance for free, it is often available at reduced costs through your employer.

Auto Safety

Our automobile tends to be one of the most frequently overlooked areas in safety. Sure, we wash and wax it, and if we are going on a long trip we may have it checked out, but when was the last time you checked the air pressure in your spare tire? Most automobile accidents and breakdowns occur within five miles of our residence. Amost all companies with large fleets of vehicles require drivers to do a daily or weekly safety check, and yet most of us are comfortable with twice a year for big trips. We typically do not go as many miles per day as a fleet vehicle, but we should still check our vehicles every two to four weeks. This inspection should include checking fluid levels such as oil, coolant, transmission, and window washer; lights including front, rear, brake, hazard flashers, turn signals, and interior lights; fan belts; brakes; tires; battery; and the exhaust system.

Even with all of the maintenance and checking that we must do, you may still experience a breakdown or accident (also see "Travel Safety," "Automobile" later in this appendix). In these cases you should have an emergency kit in your vehicle. This kit should contain first aid supplies, flares (or other warning devices), a flashlight, blanket, tools, jumper cables, tow cable, fire extinguisher, warm clothing, and change/coins to make a phone call. Some extra fluids such as oil and coolant can be helpful, but carrying extra fuel is discouraged.

None of the equipment mentioned is of any use if you do not know how to use it. One of the best examples of this was the person who arrived at an accident, and decided to put flares out to warn oncoming traffic. After checking to see that there had not been any gasoline spilled, he preceded to go through two books of matches trying to light the flares. It is important that you know how to use your jack as well as how to change the tire; one without the other is useless. There are a variety of places that offer training in basic maintenance and repair of your vehicle and use of emergency equipment. Some of these include automobile clubs, automobile dealerships, community adult education programs, and church and civic groups. If all else fails, ask a friend, but do it *before* you get stranded.

Home and Apartment Safety

There are many safety concerns to consider when choosing where to live. Look at the area you have chosen. If it is a high crime area, it may not be your first choice; however, finances often dictate where we live. If this is the case, recognize the fact and do all you can to make your selection as safe as possible. Walk around the outside of the building. Are there a lot of bushes or trees that would provide dark hiding places or access points for burglars or attackers? Are there adequate lights, and do they work? Pay particular attention to walkways, parking, and entrances. If snow is a problem in your area, ask how snow removal is taken care of and how soon after the snowfall removal occurs. Is access controlled at the entrance to the building, or can anyone enter? How is that access maintained? If you are looking at a multiple story building, do not choose to live on the first floor or above the fifth floor. Burglaries and assaults occur most frequently on the first floor because access is much easier. Living above the fifth floor is a problem because it takes longer to evacuate from that height in case of a fire or disaster. Another problem with living above the fifth floor is that conventional rescue and fire fighting methods are of limited use above that height, and many towns do not have the specialized equipment needed. Look to see that exits are not used for storage. Those items may obstruct your path during a fire or disaster.

Washrooms and storage areas are frequent locations for assaults and rapes. Look at the location of these areas in your facility. Is help readily available; are they adequately lighted; are they frequently used? Many times this information is not completely accurate from the landlord or person trying to sell you this property. Don't be afraid to ask other tenants. These same things apply to your current home or apartment. Survey the outside of your home to see that all of these concerns are cared for.

After assessing the outside of your house or apartment, turn to the inside. Is there at least one smoke detector on each level of the house? Are stairways well lit and in good repair? Are exterior doors solid (as opposed to hollow) and do they have deadbolt locks and peepholes to

How Safe Are You?

The following assessment helps you to determine your "safety awareness" and to make choices that affect your daily life.

1. Have you taken a CPR (cardiopulmonary resuscitation) class within the last year?
2. Have you taken a first aid class within the last three years?
3. Do you keep emergency telephone numbers and instructions on or near your telephone at home and at work?
4. Have you checked the safety features in your car within the last two weeks to be sure that they are working properly?
5. Do you always wear a seat belt when traveling in a car?
6. Do you keep an emergency kit in your car including tools, jumper cables, flashlight, warm clothes, first aid kit, etc.?
7. Do you completely clear snow and ice from all windows and lights prior to driving in winter conditions?
8. Does your home/apartment/dorm have smoke detectors, fire extinguishers, deadbolt locks, and a peephole to see who is at your door?
9. Are all primary and secondary exit routes from your home/apartment/dorm well lit and clear of any obstructions?
10. Do you store, use, and dispose of chemicals in a safe and legal manner?
11. Do you live on the ground level of a building?
12. Do you live above the fifth floor of a building?
13. Do you know where the utility shut-offs are for your home/apartment/dorm and know how to use them if needed?
14. Do you have a "seventy-two-hour kit" in case of a disaster?
15. Do you choose day care for your children based on convenient location?
16. Have you taken appropriate steps to make your home/apartment safe for elderly visitors or occupants?
17. Did you look at safety factors such as location, lighting, windows, and exits when choosing your home/apartment/dorm?
18. Do you hike, bike, walk, or jog alone?
19. When choosing a route to bike, walk, or jog, do you drive along the route first to look for hazards?
20. When you go fishing, hunting, hiking, biking, walking, or jogging, do you tell someone where you are going and when you will return?
21. When traveling by air, do you keep medications, personal needs, money, and identification in your carry-on luggage?
22. When vacationing by car, do you plan your routes and stops ahead of time, and does someone know where you are and how to contact you every day?

The "safe" answers to questions 11, 12, 15, and 18 are no; all others should be answered yes.

If your answer was not the "safe" answer on

- Three or fewer questions, your personal safety awareness is good to excellent.
- Four to six questions, your personal safety awareness is moderate, and the sections covering those questions should be reviewed to see if new decisions should be made.
- Seven or more questions, it indicates a need to increase your personal safety awareness. This appendix is for you. Remember, these are choices and decisions that affect your life every day.

see who is at your door? Are all windows equipped with functioning locks? Do all throw rugs have nonslide backs? Do showers and baths have nonslip surfaces or mats? Is access available to shut off utilities if needed, and do you know how to shut them off? Are emergency exits (fire escapes, chain ladders, push-out windows) in good repair? Is the hot water heater set at a low enough temperature to prevent accidental scalding? Are outlets in the kitchen, bathroom, garage, and other areas where water is likely ground-fault protected? Is there air conditioning so that doors and windows will not have to be left open during hot weather?

These are all physical characteristics about your house or apartment, but the most hazardous thing you will face at home is you. All of the things we look at inside and outside of your home must be used and maintained in order to protect you. If you do not check them periodically and repair or report them as needed, you may as well not

have them. Your actions affect your safety around the home in many other ways. You should store guns separately from ammunition, and they should be where access is limited (preferably locked). Have first aid supplies available and emergency telephone numbers posted on or near the telephone (see "Medical Emergencies" section of this appendix). Household chemicals should be stored where small children can't gain access to them. All chemicals should be used in accordance with the label instructions and should be disposed of properly. If you or others smoke in your home, have plenty of ashtrays spread in convenient locations. *Never* allow people to smoke in bed. Never use extension cords in place of permanent wiring. Do not overload electrical circuits; if you are always blowing a fuse, there is a problem that should be evaluated by an electrician. Keep doors to bedrooms closed at night to slow the spread of smoke and fire (most deaths occur from smoke inhalation).

Dorm Safety

Most of the information in the home and apartment safety section is applicable to living in dorms. There are some additional problems frequently seen in dorms, though. Keep your door shut and locked when not in there and late at night. Do not use extension cords or "splitters" to provide additional electrical outlets. Do not cook in your dorm room unless the room is designed to allow cooking and specific authorization has been given. Do not have excessive combustibles such as posters and pictures on the walls. Always evacuate the building when a fire alarm sounds no matter how many false alarms there have been. Provide a medical history including any special medical problems and any prescription medications you are taking to the hall director in case you are involved in an accident. Know the quickest exit routes from your room, the bathrooms, the lounge, and other areas where you are likely to be spending a lot of time. Have someone that you can tell where you are going and when you will be back, so it will be noticed if you are missing, and keep track of each other.

Disaster Preparedness

Disasters come in many forms. They may be floods, fires, tornadoes, hurricanes, hazardous chemical spills, winter storms, or earthquakes. The one sure thing about disasters is that every location has the potential for at least one type of disaster. While there is little we can do to prevent them, we can do many things to lessen their effect and to allow us to return to normal as soon as possible.

One important thing to do is to recognize what hazards exist in your area. Most natural disasters have locations that are more seriously affected. For instance, floods affect river beds and low-lying areas. Earthquakes have fault lines and liquefaction areas. Avalanches and snow storms affect foothills and mountains. Even hurricanes and tornadoes show areas more prone to be involved when we look at past events. Take this information into consideration when choosing where to live. Building styles are affected differently, also. For example, a single-story wooden structure experiences less damage than a multi-story unreinforced brick building during an earthquake. This type of information can be gained about all natural disasters that you are likely to be exposed to. This information can be obtained from your local or state government, an emergency preparedness agency, local engineering firms, board of realtors, or university engineering, architecture, or environmental studies department.

Some important things to know during and immediately after a disaster are how and where to turn off damaged utilities such as gas, water, and electricity. Being trained in first aid is very important. Knowing where to go and how to protect yourself during a disaster is essential.

Probably the most important thing is to prepare for disasters. Not all disasters can be predicted nor will we get any warning before they occur. It is important, though, to use any warning we get. Know how and from where the warning will come. Will it be on television or radio or will it be sirens and/or individual contacts? Use what time you have to secure belongings, but never risk your life to save an object. If told to evacuate the area, do not question that decision; just leave the area. Have a seventy-two-hour kit available. A seventy-two-hour kit contains supplies necessary to live on your own for at least three days. Experience tells us that utilities and services are disrupted immediately after a disaster but will be resumed in most areas affected within seventy-two hours. You should have adequate supplies of food, medications, fuel for heat and cooking, water, and personal needs. A more in-depth description of a seventy-two-hour kit is available from the American Red Cross or your local emergency preparedness agency.

Safety and the Elderly

The elderly are a group frequently overlooked in safety considerations. Because they are older, there are many physiological changes that not only increase their risk of accidents but also cause the elderly to be more seriously affected by incidents and recover more slowly. Visibility is a concern with the elderly. Small steps and irregular surfaces are frequently not noticed. These should be very visibly marked or removed when possible. Night vision is often impaired, increasing the need for well-lighted walks, halls, and stairs. Elderly people often do not move or react as quickly. A task as simple as crossing the street can become a problem when traffic lights do not allow adequate time.

As we age we become shorter and tend to stoop, making it difficult to reach many items. Frequently used items should be stored on lower shelves, and secure step stools should be provided for access to higher items. Installation of handrails, nonslip backing on rugs, and nonslip surfaces in bathtubs and showers can prevent many falls. As we age we are unable to adapt to changes in temperature as quickly so particular attention needs to be given to the elderly during spring, fall, and particularly hot or cold spells. One of the most difficult decisions most of us will face is when to stop driving. It is very difficult to give up the freedom that our car affords us, but at some point the risks outweigh the freedom. The elderly are frequent targets for crime. Simply accompanying them on errands can prevent many of these attacks.

Assault

Assault, robbery, and rape have been a problem for as long as humans have existed. There are no solutions, but there are many things we can do to reduce the risk of these problems. At least a portion of each section in this appendix has related to preventing assaults, and many of the chapters in this text mention it. The information in this section can be applied to many situations also.

Whenever possible, travel in groups, particularly at night or in unfamiliar areas. Whenever handling money, such as at stores or in a bank, always put the money securely away before leaving the check stand or teller window. Carry purses with straps that go around your arm or carry wallets in inside pockets or pockets that button. Park in well-lighted areas. Always have your keys ready before you reach your door. Pause briefly before you reach your car, and look under the car and in the front and back seat. Always lock your car and house/apartment when not in it, even if you will be away just a minute. Carry valuable items in sacks or other coverings so others do not know what you have. Lock valuable items in the trunk of your car where they can't be seen. Choose routes to travel based on safety, not time or shortest distance. If you think you are being followed, go directly to a busy location such as a store and call the police. For more information on preventing assaults, contact your local police department.

Recreational Safety

While it never seems that we spend enough time recreating, it is often some of the most hazardous time we spend. Outside of the work environment, more accidents occur in the pursuit of recreation than any other activity. Many of the recreational activities that we choose gain their thrill from the risks associated with them. In this section, we can't discuss all recreational activities and their risks, but we can address some of the most common activities.

Hiking and Backpacking

Never hike alone. Tell others where you are going and when you will return. Always take any needed medications in case something happens and you are unable to return as scheduled. Whenever hiking in unfamiliar areas, carry a map and compass and know how to use them. Be prepared for the worst possible weather, not the best. Always carry a survival/first aid kit with you.

Hunting and Fishing

When not in use, equipment should be stored properly. Always unload guns when not actively hunting or when crossing fences, streams, or ditches. Be aware of others around you when casting or shooting. Take hunter safety classes every three to five years. Store guns and ammunition separately and locked away to limit access. Take a class and receive proper training prior to attempting to reload your own ammunition. Follow recommendations for hiking and backpacking.

Bicycling

Always wear an ANSI recognized bicycle helmet. Follow all traffic laws; bicycles are considered vehicles. Dress appropriately for temperatures; if you are riding at a speed of fifteen miles an hour and going into a five-mile-an-hour

breeze, the wind chill would be equivalent to a twenty-mile-per-hour wind. Have periodic tune-ups performed to ensure all parts are working properly. When riding in dim light or at night, be sure to have properly operating lights and reflectors. Wear clothing that increases your visibility to others. Never wear earphones or other devices that impair your hearing.

Jogging and Walking

Wear adequate clothing. Remember that it is easier to remove clothing than to put on clothing that you do not have. Wear clothing that increases your visibility to others. When walking or jogging in dim light or at night, wear or carry lights and/or reflectors. Always tell someone your route and when you expect to return. When choosing a new route, always drive the route first to look for hazards, including dogs, rough terrain, and possible areas for mugging, and note locations where help is available. Never jog or walk alone. Do not wear clothing or earphones that obstruct vision or hearing. When on vacation or traveling, always ask local running/walking clubs for suggested routes near your hotel. Ask hotel personnel for information on suggested routes. Watch for other joggers/walkers, and ask to join them.

Travel Safety

Travel safety is something that we either take for granted or choose not to consider. The consequences of both actions can range from discomfort to death. Most of our travels are by automobile or aircraft, so those are the two modes we will discuss. These same concerns can apply to travel by train, bus, or boat, also.

Aircraft

Always carry a bag with you. Whenever you check your bags, there is a chance of being separated from them or that someone will go through them. In the carry-on bag, take all medications you need, any personal needs such as contact solution and storage case, identification, money, and travelers' checks. Other things to consider putting in your carry-on bag are things to increase your comfort, such as toothbrush and paste, deodorant, a small bar of soap, and a change of clothes.

As soon as you get settled into your seat, identify the two exits nearest you, and determine which is the best in an emergency. Things to consider when choosing which is best would include proximity, ease of opening, who would be opening it (a trained flight attendant or an untrained passenger who didn't read the passenger safety card any better than you did), the age and health of passengers between you and the exit, and any obstructions such as the beverage cart. When choosing your seat assignment, choose a seat near an exit and know how to operate the exit.

If a hijacking should occur, there are a few basic rules to observe. First, don't be a hero. Never confront the hijackers or other passengers. Try to blend in. Always look down. Know where the exits are. Have a plan if things go wrong; don't think you will know what to do when things start happening all around you.

Automobile

Have your car checked out before traveling and take the repair person's advice. Having something repaired before the trip is less time consuming and less expensive than being towed to the nearest town and waiting for parts. Also, remember that the local Ford dealer in a small town is not going to have those special German wheels or Porsche carburetor. Plan your route and stops ahead of time. Give a copy of your route and schedule to a friend in case someone must get in contact with you. Stop frequently, even if it is just to walk around the car a couple of times. Check in with others at least every other day to get important messages and to let them know you are alright. Do not travel alone. Plan where to stay; do not leave it to luck. Plan how to get help if needed.

If your car does break down, try to get well off the road. Be aware of where you stopped. Are you just over the top of the hill or around a corner? Is it foggy, raining, or snowing? All of these things reduce the warning other cars have that you are stopped. Warn oncoming traffic with your emergency flashers as well as flares or reflectors in the direction of oncoming traffic. If your car is stranded all or part of the way in a traffic lane, then get out of the car and stand well off the road. If your car is well off the road, then stay in your car with the doors locked. If someone stops to help you, it is usually best to have them send qualified help (police, tow truck, etc.) to you rather than going with them for help. You are usually better to stay with your car and wait for help than trying to walk for help.

Motel/Hotel Safety

There are several things to be concerned about while at a hotel. The first thing is when making reservations or checking in, always request a room below the fifth floor. Most deaths in hotel fires involve guests above where standard rescue and fire fighting equipment are effective. Also, if available, stay above the first floor to reduce the access for thieves from outside. If they offer a nonsmoking wing, request a room there. Many fires start from guests smoking in bed. On the way to your room, familiarize yourself with the layout of the hotel. It will be very disorienting if you have to evacuate your room into a dark or smoky corridor. Notice where the emergency exits are and any alcoves or hallways you could get lost in between your room and the exit. Notice if there are fire extinguishers in the hallway and where they are located from your room.

Look for the fire alarms or sirens to see that one is close enough to your room to be heard. Locate the nearest alarm pull station in case of a fire.

Once in your room, familiarize yourself with the room. Remember that there are frequently no lights in an emergency. Note where the extra towels and blankets are; they may be critical in an emergency. Always carry a small flashlight in your luggage that can be used if the power goes out in your room. As soon as you have settled in, take valuables such as cameras and extra money to the front desk to be kept in their safe. Never leave your door open, even just to go to the ice machine. Whenever you are in the room, keep the security lock fastened also. Never open your door to anyone until you have seen them through the peephole, and always be cautious, even of hotel employees, unless you have requested their assistance.

When leaving a hotel in an unfamiliar city, always ask directions, even if you think you know where you are going. Inquire of the hotel staff as to the safety of walking near the hotel and of using transit systems. If you are a jogger, watch for other guests who jog and join them so you will not have to jog alone. Inquire with hotel staff and/or the local running club for good routes near the hotel. If you do jog or walk alone, leave your route and expected return time with hotel staff, and let them know when you return.

If the fire alarm is sounded while you are in your room, always evacuate no matter how inconvenient it is. When leaving, take your room key with you, and lock your door. Prior to opening the door, feel it for heat. If the door is hot or the corridor is full of smoke and fire, stay in your room. If you are trapped in your room, hang a towel out of your window to indicate that you are in there. Try to call the front desk to inform them that you are trapped. Immediately fill the bathtub with water that can be used to wet towels and blankets if needed. If smoke begins to come into the room under the door or through air vents, try to seal them with wet towels or bedding. If your room begins to fill with smoke, open a window a small amount. Smoke and flames can enter the room from the outside, also; therefore, only open the window a small amount and only if necessary. Try to attract the attention of people outside the hotel to arrange your rescue. Once outside the hotel, do not re-enter until you are told it is safe by hotel personnel and others have entered.

Conclusion

As you can see, simply living through each day without accidents or injuries is harder than we ever imagined. By increasing your safety awareness, you can reduce the risk of inconvenience, injury, disability, and even death. As with all of the information in this book, it is your decision whether to use it. Knowledge without action is of little use.

Glossary

A

abortion   The premature expulsion of a fertilized egg, embryo, or fetus from the uterus.

abstinence   The decision to refrain from drinking any alcoholic beverage.

acid rain   Rain that has a pH of less than 5.6.

active immunity   Immunity to a disease derived from having had the disease or from the injection of the infectious organism.

active listening   Paraphrasing a speaker's words to be sure that the message was communicated.

acupuncture   A medical technique that involves inserting and manipulating needles in the body to relieve pain and treat disease but also used in smoking cessation.

additive   A substance added to foods to enhance certain qualities, such as freshness, appearance, and taste.

adjustment disorders   Mental distress arising from an inability to cope with changes in the environment.

aerobics   Exercises that demand extra oxygen consumption but are performed at a rate below that needed to produce oxygen debt.

ageism   Discrimination based on old age.

aging   The process of growing older.

AIDS (acquired immunodeficiency syndrome)   A breakdown in the body's natural defenses that is spread primarily through sexual contact and is often fatal; there is no known cure.

alarm stage   First stage of the general adaptation syndrome characterized by an immediate increase in muscle tension, heart rate, blood pressure, brain activity, and other physical peaking responses.

alcoholism   Loss of control in drinking; the inability to refrain from drinking; the inability to stop drinking before becoming intoxicated.

allopathic physician   A physician who has received a medical doctor degree (M.D.).

alpha-fetoprotein (AFP)   Test done during early stage of pregnancy to determine neural tube defects.

Alzheimer's disease   A dementia marked by a distinctive loss or change of nerve cells that can be detected.

ambisexuality   *See* bisexuality.

ambulatory care center   Provides treatment for minor problems without an appointment.

amenorrhea   The absence of menstruation.

amino acids   The building blocks of proteins.

amniocentesis   Analyzing the amniotic fluid taken from the intrauterine environment; a test used to determine fetal defects.

amniotic fluid   Fluid surrounding the fetus.

amphetamine   Stimulant drug used to combat fatigue and suppress appetite; as drug of abuse, commonly called "upper."

anabolic steroid   A substance derived from the male hormone testosterone used to increase muscle bulk largely because of muscle tension, but with serious side effects.

analgesic   Medicine that relieves pain; painkiller.

aneurysm   A ballooning-out of the wall of a vein, an artery, or the heart due to weakening of the wall by disease, traumatic injury, or an abnormality present at birth.

angel dust   The street name for Phencyclidine, which is a hallucinogen in the form of a crystalline powder that produces bizarre and volatile effects.

angina   Chest pain associated with heart disease; can be brought on by smoking.

angiography   A diagnostic procedure through which the chambers and blood vessels of the heart are examined.

angioplasty The process of arteries being cleared by a small balloon-type instrument on the end of wire, much like cleaning a pipe with a "snake."

animal parasite Any animal (worms, lice, protozoa) that feeds on another organism.

anorexia nervosa The suppression of appetite rather than loss of appetite. It has been described as self-induced starvation or dieting gone out of control.

antabuse A drug that in combination with alcohol causes nausea, dizziness, and heart palpitations; used to deter persons from drinking.

antibody Substance manufactured by the body to destroy invading organisms.

anxiety disorders Excessive fears called phobias or panic disorders.

anxiety prone personality A person who sees problems as being worse than they actually are.

aphasia Loss of speech, usually caused by a stroke.

apperception Building on the success of earlier experiences.

appestat The feeding center of the brain that produces hunger pains.

arteriosclerosis A group of diseases characterized by thickening and loss of elasticity of artery walls.

arthritis A chronic disease characterized by inflammation in the joints.

artificial insemination The introduction of a male's sperm into a woman's vagina via a syringe.

asexual Without sexuality.

assertiveness When people feel comfortable enough with themselves to speak to others and make statements that represent their own feelings and thoughts; it is a balance between aggressive behavior and passive behavior.

assessing Determining personal strengths.

asthma A disease or allergic response characterized by bronchial spasms and difficulty in breathing.

atherosclerosis Hardening of the arteries; a degenerative cardiovascular disease that occurs when fat deposits build up in arteries.

attitude A feeling or emotion about a fact or behavior.

aversion therapy A type of treatment by which a specific behavior, in this case smoking, is made undesirable through negative reinforcement.

B

bacteria Microscopic organisms that cause disease.

bag A single dosage unit of heroin.

balanced adjustment Returning to the same level of functioning that existed before the life event.

barbiturate Sedative-hypnotic drug; depressant; as drug of abuse, commonly called "downer."

barriers to change Factors inhibiting a change of behavior.

basal body temperature (BBT) method Keeping track of temperature changes during menstrual cycle in an attempt to pinpoint ovulation.

basic metabolic rate The speed at which the body burns fuel.

benign tumor An uncontrolled growth of cells that is not malignant but can disturb the function of an organ.

benzodiazepines General classification of tranquilizers that include the most widely prescribed drugs, Valium and Librium.

bereavement The experience of loss that occurs when someone close to us dies.

bestiality (zoophilia) Sexual contact with animals.

beta cells The cells in the islets of Langerhans of the pancreas that produce insulin.

biological dimension of human sexuality Involves physiological responses, reproduction, puberty, pregnancy, and growth and development.

biopsy A surgical procedure in which a small section of tumor is removed and microscopically examined for possible cancer.

birthing center A medical facility with a homelike atmosphere that is used for delivering babies.

bisexuality Enjoyment of sexual relationships with both sexes. (Also called ambisexuality.)

blood alcohol concentration (BAC) Percentage of alcohol in the blood; used to determine drunken driving.

blood pressure The force the flowing blood exerts against the artery walls.

body composition The percentage of fat versus lean tissue.

brainstorm The process of listing all possible solutions and evaluating them only after the list is complete.

breathalyzer A machine used to determine the BAC of a person's blood; usually used with suspected drunk drivers.

breech birth A birth in which the buttocks of the fetus is positioned to be delivered first.

bronchitis Inflammation of the bronchial tubes in the lungs.

bulbourethral glands (Cowper's glands) Tiny pea-shaped organs located below the prostate that secrete a fluid during sexual arousal.

bulimia A disorder characterized by uncontrolled binge eating followed by forced vomiting because of the person's fear of getting fat.

bypass surgery A surgical technique where cardiologists take blood vessels from another part of the body and use them to replace obstructed coronary arteries. Single, double, triple, or quadruple bypasses may occur where one, two, three, or four of the coronary arteries might be replaced.

C

calcium Mineral needed for growth and maintenance of strong bones and teeth.

calendar method   Keeping track of number of days in the menstrual cycle in an attempt to pinpoint ovulation.

calorie   A unit for measuring the energy of food.

cancer   A group of diseases characterized by the uncontrolled growth and spread of abnormal cells.

cancer in situ   Localized cancer that has not spread.

carbohydrate   A compound consisting of carbon, hydrogen, and oxygen; one of the nutrients.

carbon monoxide   A deadly gas that is a by-product of burning tobacco.

carcinogen   Substance that stimulates the development of cancer.

cardiopulmonary resuscitation (CPR)   An emergency measure to maintain breathing and heartbeat artificially.

cardiovascular disease   Disease of the heart and blood vessels.

carotid endarterectomy   Surgery used to remove plaque buildup in the carotid arteries of the neck.

caveat emptor   "Let the buyer beware."

cerebral embolism   A clot that is carried to the brain, where it blocks a small artery.

cerebral hemorrhage   Bleeding from a diseased artery that damages surrounding brain tissue.

cerebral thrombosis   The formation of a blood clot that blocks the flow of blood to the brain.

cervical cap   Rubber, plastic, or metal contraceptive device that fits snugly around the cervix.

cervical mucus method   Checking cervical mucus in an attempt to pinpoint ovulation.

cesarean section   The delivery of a baby through the abdominal wall by making an incision in the lower abdomen and wall of the uterus.

chemotherapy   The use of specific drugs to treat a disease.

chicken pox   A disease caused by a virus and resulting in a rash, skin eruptions, and fever; itching may be severe but can be treated with antihistamines or taking warm baths with baking soda.

child language   Made up of terms that parents often use with children to refer to body parts or body functions.

chiropractic   A system of manipulative treatment; it teaches that all diseases are caused by impingement on spinal nerves and can be corrected by spinal adjustments.

chlamydia   A disease that symptomatically is similar to gonorrhea. It results in the infections of several pelvic areas and may result in some scarring and damage of some of the reproductive organs.

chloral hydrate   The oldest sleep-inducing drug.

chlorine residual   Chlorine that remains in water to decontaminate any additional bacteria in the water system.

chlorofluorocarbons   A chemical used in aerosols that destroys the ozone.

cholesterol   A fatlike substance found in animal tissue and manufactured by the body; one of the major risk factors of cardiovascular disease.

chorionic villi sampling (CVS)   The method of removing pieces of the villi (thin tissue) protruding from the chorion (outer layer of the amniotic sac) and analyzing it for birth defects.

chromosome   The part of the cell that contains the hereditary factors.

chronic bronchitis   Persistent inflammation of the mucous membrane of the bronchi, evidenced by continual coughing and mucoid discharges.

chronic disease   A long, drawn-out disease; a disease that cannot be cured.

cilia   Hairlike processes, as in the bronchi, that wave mucus, pus, and dust particles upward and out.

circumcision   Surgical removal of the foreskin of a male's penis.

cirrhosis   A disease of the liver manifested by scarring that may be a complication of excessive alcohol consumption.

class action suit   One person takes legal action on behalf of all who have had the same problem.

Clean Air Act (CAA)   Established air standards for six pollutants and emission standards.

Clean Water Act   Passed in 1977 to implement the provisions of the 1972 amendment to the Federal Water Pollution Control Act. A program that perhaps affected the most dramatic improvement in water quality in the history of the United States.

clinical psychologist   Person with a Ph.D. degree who specializes in emotional and psychological adjustment.

codeine   A narcotic drug used for the relief of moderate pain.

codependency   When people are in a relationship with a problem drinker or alcoholic and are so entrapped by love and concern for the person that they lose their own identities in the process of trying to help.

cohabiting   Living together without being legally married.

coitus interruptus   Withdrawal of the penis from the vagina before ejaculation.

coliform bacteria   A group of bacteria whose presence in drinking water is suggestive of fecal contamination.

collateral circulation   Circulation of the blood through smaller vessels when a major vessel has become blocked.

combination pill   Contains both progesterone and estrogen and works by suspending ovulation.

communicable disease   Disease that can be passed from one person to another.

communication skills   Interpersonal dialogue that is represented by honest expression of feelings, facts, and emotions and by the other party listening empathetically.

commuter marriage   A liaison in which spouses set up separate households and live apart for days to months at a time.

complementary factor   Characteristic that is different but relates to its opposite.

complete protein   Food that contains all eight amino acids.

complex carbohydrates   Carbohydrates that are composed of three or more simple sugars bonded together.

conception   Fertilization of a female egg by a male sperm resulting in pregnancy.

condom   Rubber sheath that covers the penis; a birth-control device for men.

condyloma   A sexually transmitted anal or genital wart caused by human papillomavirus, treated with Podophyllin.

confluence   The combining or linking of activities or behaviors for time efficiency.

congenital heart defect   Abnormality in the structure of the heart present at birth.

congestive heart failure   A condition in which the heart cannot pump its required amount of blood, causing fluid to collect in the abdomen, legs, and/or in the lungs.

contraceptive   Any birth-control method or device.

contractual marriage   Marital relationship in which the partners periodically agree to review their marriage contract.

coronary   Pertaining to the heart.

coronary circulation   Circulation of the blood through the coronary arteries.

Cowper's glands   *See* bulbourethral glands.

crabs   Insect parasites that can be passed from one person to another during close bodily contact; another name for pubic lice.

crack   The free-based version of cocaine that is extremely potent, quick addicting, and extremely dangerous.

crank   A stimulant; nickname for methamphetamine or speed.

cremation   The process of burning a corpse in a furnace, which reduces the remains to ashes.

criteria air pollutants   A group of chemicals identified under the Clean Air Act for which outside air standards are set. The chemicals included are carbon monoxide, lead, nitrogen, dioxide, ozone, particulate, sulphur dioxide.

cross tolerance   The interaction of two different drugs on a person's system.

cunnilingus   Oral contact with the female genitalia.

D

decibel (db)   A numerical expression of the relative loudness of a sound.

decision tree   A diagram of the possible choices and steps in decision making.

dehydration   The excessive loss of water from the body's tissues.

delirium tremens (DTs)   Hallucinations and convulsive seizures that occur during withdrawal from alcohol.

delta-9-tetrahydrocannabinol (THC)   The major psychoactive drug found in marijuana.

delusions   False beliefs that may occur in users of hallucinogens.

dementia   Loss of mental functions including memory loss, loss of language functions, inability to think abstractly, personality change, or inability to care for oneself.

depressant   Drug used to decrease nervous or muscular activity; as drug of abuse, commonly called "downer."

designer drug   Drugs that use the chief ingredient fentanyl or a derivative of fentanyl, which produces a drug that is one hundred times as strong as morphine and twenty to forty times as strong as heroin. Designer drugs may imitate the narcotics, cocaine, or hallucinogens.

detoxification   The process of eliminating a drug from the user's system.

diabetes mellitus   A chronic disorder affecting the natural metabolism of carbohydrates, fats, and protein due to defective or deficient insulin production.

diaphragm   A round, latex, dome-shaped birth-control device for women that blocks the entrance to the uterus.

diastolic pressure   Lowest blood pressure measured when the heart relaxes.

diethylstilbestrol (DES)   A synthetic estrogen used as a "morning-after" pill.

dilation and curettage (D and C)   An abortion procedure that must be carried out during the first twelve weeks of pregnancy; also a procedure used to relieve excessive menstrual bleeding.

Dilaudid   A synthetic drug of abuse.

direct involuntary euthanasia   When a lethal injection or other form of causing death is administered to relieve a patient from pain or suffering with inevitable death. This occurs by medical professionals or family out of mercy. Mercy death.

direct voluntary euthanasia   When a lethal injection or other form of causing death is administered to relieve a patient from pain or suffering with inevitable death. This occurs usually by request from the person who has their life taken rather than deal with living.

disaccharide   A simple carbohydrate formed from two monosaccharides.

disorganization   A temporary state when one or more of the basic components of health become disrupted.

disruption   Being out of balance in one or more of the six basic health components. In the face of adversity, life events, challenges, or stressors, it is the process of being temporarily taken back, upset, discouraged, or unsure before coping and adjustment takes place.

dissociative disorders   Also called hysterical neurosis; disturbances in an individual's identity, memory, or consciousness, such as multiple personality disorder.

distress   Negative stress.

diuretics   A type of medication that causes the body to eliminate water through urination.

DNA   Deoxyribonucleic acid; a nucleic acid found in all living cells; it carries the organism's genetic information.

drug interaction   The effect that occurs when two different drugs are used at the same time.

E

ecstasy   Also called MDMA, a hybrid cross between amphetamines and the hallucinogen, mescaline, that acts much like cocaine.

ectopic pregnancy   A pregnancy in which the fertilized egg implants somewhere other than the upper section of the uterus.

ego defense mechanism   Ways that people deal with perceived inadequacies or stressors.

ejaculation   The expulsion of semen from the penis, usually accompanying orgasm.

electrocardiogram (EKG)   Electrical impulses within the heart; a test used to determine malfunctioning of the heart.

embalming   The process of removing the blood from a dead person and replacing it with a preserving fluid.

embolus   A wandering blood clot.

embryo   Unborn young in its early stage of development.

emotional health   The ability to control emotions and express them comfortably and appropriately.

emphysema   A chronic disease of the lungs that affects the air sacs and causes breathlessness; it can lead to death.

empty calories   A term given to items that contain few or no nutrients.

enabling   A constellation of ideas, feelings, attitudes, and behaviors that unwittingly allow and/or encourage alcohol problems to continue or worsen by preventing the alcohol abuser from experiencing the consequences of his or her condition.

endometrium   The lining of the uterus.

Environmental Protection Agency (EPA)   A branch of the national government agency responsible for the protection of clean air, clean water, and other environmental concerns.

epididymis   A coiled tube between the seminiferous tubules and the vas deferens, where sperm mature.

episiotomy   Incision in vaginal tissue before birth to prevent its tearing.

erotic phone calling   A form of erotic distancing where a person receives erotic gratification by making gross remarks over the phone.

essential amino acids   Chemical compounds that are the building blocks of protein; must be obtained through food each day since they cannot be made or synthesized in the body.

essential fat   The amount of fat necessary to stay alive and needed to maintain normal body functioning.

essential hypertension   High blood pressure in which the cause is unknown.

estrogen   A female hormone.

ethyl alcohol   A colorless liquid that is the intoxicating ingredient in alcoholic beverages formed in the fermentation of grains and fruits; C_2H_5OH.

euphemism   Expression used to avoid explicit term (such as "making love" or "sleeping together").

euphoric   Pertaining to a feeling of extreme well-being.

eustress   Positive stress.

euthanasia   Putting a person to death painlessly; mercy death.

excitement phase   The initial phase of human sexual response.

exhaustion stage   Third stage of the general adaptation syndrome characterized by the fatiguing of organs and depressed immune system with resultant disorders of the organs.

exhibitionism   Achievement of sexual gratification by showing genitals to observers.

exposure   One of the two factors that determine toxicity, with the other being the amount of the dose.

Exposure can occur through direct contact, touching, or breathing.

extended family   Parents, children, and other relatives living together under the same roof.

F

faith healing   A theory based on the belief that the mind, which controls the body, can cure disease through divine help.

fallopian tubes   A pair of tubes in the female providing passage from the ovaries to the uterus; also called oviducts.

family therapy   The process by which a mental-health professional works with a family as a unit to help one or more members cope with a mental-health problem; the focus is on relationships within the family.

fat cell hyperplasia   The process of increasing adipose tissue by increasing the total number of fat cells.

fat cell hypertrophy   The process of increasing adipose tissue by filling existing fat cells with fat.

fat-soluble vitamins   Organic substances that are transported and stored by the fat cells of the body. Include vitamins A, D, E, and K.

faulty adjustment   When the person has fewer protective mechanisms or skills than before the life event.

Federal Trade Commission (FTC)   An agency of the federal government that has the power to halt what it deems deceptive or unfair advertising.

Federal Water Pollution Control Act   Enacted in 1948, a law that for the first time announced the national goals for water quality.

fellatio   Oral contact with the male genitals.

fentanyl   A psychoactive substance that is the basis for some designer drugs.

fertility awareness   *See* rhythm method.

fetal alcohol effect (FAE)   A group of subtle abnormalities such as mental retardation or moderate behavioral problems caused by the mother's use of alcohol during pregnancy.

fetal alcohol syndrome (FAS) Irreversible damage to the fetus caused by the mother's heavy use of alcohol during pregnancy.

fetishism Sexual fixation on an object other than a human being.

fetoscopy Insertion of a viewing instrument into the womb to observe the fetus.

fetus The unborn young from the third month after conception.

fiber A complex carbohydrate that is found in the walls of plant cells and in the tough, structural parts of plants.

fight or flight response The alarm stage of the stress response or involuntary physiological response to sudden danger characterized by quick action.

flashback Recurrence of effects such as the intensification of color, the apparent motion of a fixed object, or the mistaking of one object for another.

follicle Saclike structure in the ovaries that contains a developing egg cell.

follicle-stimulating hormone (FSH) A hormone secreted by the pituitary gland that stimulates the egg follicle.

freeing Achieving freedom from disabling habits.

frigidity Female sexual dysfunction.

frottage The act of obtaining sexual pleasure from rubbing against another person.

frustration The thwarting of a desired goal.

fungi Parasitic organisms of simple structure that live in soil, rotting vegetation, and bird excreta.

G

gas chromatography/mass spectrometry (GC/MS) An accurate drug testing technique that breaks down each drug and spreads each substance on a printout for easy identification.

general adaptation syndrome (GAS) Describes the three stages through which our body responds to stress: alarm, resistance, and exhaustion stages.

generic drug Similar compound that is not necessarily produced under the same brand name.

genetic counseling Looking at one's hereditary characteristics with a trained counselor before deciding to have children.

gerontology The study of aging.

global warming The warming of the earth's atmosphere as a result of the greenhouse effect.

glomeruli A small cluster of capillaries located at the beginning of each uriniferous tubule in the kidney. Its function is to filter and remove wastes from the blood.

glucose Energy source for cells.

glycogen Extra glucose that is stored in the body for future use.

gonorrhea One of the sexually transmitted diseases; the most frequently reported communicable disease.

gout A form of arthritis that commonly affects the joints of the feet, especially the big toe.

grand mal convulsions Serious involuntary and violent muscle contractions.

greenhouse effect The effect that the accumulation of carbon dioxide and other gases in the earth's atmosphere has on the balance between the energy the earth receives from solar radiation and the energy it loses by radiation from its surface back to space.

grief Intense emotional suffering that is normal reaction to bereavement (loss); its physical symptoms include a tight throat, shortness of breath, the need to sigh, and feelings of emptiness.

H

habit A routine act done without thought.

hallucination Visions or imaginary perceptions.

hazardous air pollutants Substances in the air that are generally considered carcinogenic. The EPA has identified six, including asbestos, benzene, beryllium, mercury, radio nuclide, vinyl chloride.

health The word comes from an Old English root meaning "wholeness."

health maintenance organization (HMO) A prepayment plan for medical care.

hemodialysis The artificial kidney machine that purifies a person's blood when the kidneys cannot.

hemoglobin An iron-containing compound in red blood cells that transports oxygen to the cells.

hepatic failure Failure of the liver to function properly.

herbal medicine The use of naturally occurring plants, roots, and seeds to fight disease.

heroin A synthetic narcotic drug of abuse.

herpes genitalis An incurable sexually transmitted disease characterized by cold sore-like blisters caused by the herpes simplex virus type 2.

herpes simplex virus type 2 The virus that causes herpes and is closely related to the one that causes cold sores, fever blisters, and shingles. Blisters appear on the genitalia, and symptoms may last from one to three weeks. The recurrence of herpes is probable, and the disease is incurable.

hertz (Hz) A measure of how irritating and damaging sound is. A Hertz is the pitch as indicated by the speed of the vibrations of sound.

hierarchy of needs A progression of growth by the attainment of needs ranging from basic needs to more complex higher needs. The progression includes physiological, safety, love, self-esteem, and self-actualization.

high-density lipoprotein (HDL) Considered good cholesterol because it removes cholesterol from the walls of the arteries and transports it to the liver, where it is processed and excreted.

HIV (human immunodeficiency virus)
Present when the patient tests positive for the AIDS virus, but symptoms are less severe.

homophobia A fear of homosexual feelings in oneself or a fear of homosexuals.

homosexuality Sexual attraction and/or relations between persons of the same sex.

hormone A chemical glandular secretion that regulates or stimulates body processes.

hospice A comfortable, homey place where terminally ill persons can go to die, or a home service allowing people to die at home.

human chorionic gonadotropin (HCG) A hormone produced by the placenta once implantation has occurred.

human growth hormone (HGH) The natural hormone that exists in the body that promotes growth; is sometimes abused and can result in giantism and other problems.

hydroponics The technological growing of plants (marijuana) in nutrient solutions with or without dirt as a medium or support.

hydrostatic weighing A method of determining the proportion of fat to lean tissue by weighing a person by normal methods and then weighing the person under water.

hypertension High blood pressure.

hypertrophy Larger and stronger muscle fibers.

hypnosis A physically-induced sleeplike condition in which the person is in an altered state of consciousness and can respond, within limitations, to suggestions.

hypoglycemia Low blood sugar.

hypothalamus Directs the pituitary gland in the control of the stress response.

hysterectomy Surgical removal of the uterus.

hysterotomy A method of abortion in which an incision is made in the abdominal wall and the fetus is removed.

I

ice The crystalline rock form of methamphetamine (speed) that is more powerful and more addicting than the original methamphetamine.

imagery The ability to see, hear, smell, taste, and feel through the mind's eye; simply the ability to fantasize or daydream in meaningful ways.

immunization The administration of a vaccine that prevents a person from getting a particular disease.

immunoassay Less reliable drug testing technique using antibodies that bond to drugs.

immunosuppressive drugs Drugs that suppress an individual's immune system so that a transplanted heart will not be rejected or attacked.

impotence Male sexual dysfunction.

incest Sexual behavior between closely related persons.

incubation stage The disease stage between the time of infection and the appearance of symptoms.

indirect involuntary euthanasia When life-support systems are taken away from an individual so that he or she can die naturally. This occurs when family or physicians pursue and receive a court order to remove the life-support systems.

indirect voluntary euthanasia When life-support systems are taken away from an individual so that he or she can die naturally. This occurs usually by legal request from the person who has the life support taken away.

infertility The inability to reproduce.

injectable Long-acting injectable contraceptive.

insulin A hormone produced by the pancreas.

interdependence When positive interactions occur with people and positive relationships are established, mutual support occurs, ideas are created, and energy is produced.

interferon A chemical within our bodies that gives us natural immunity to specific diseases.

internal medicine A medical specialty in which the physician deals with the functions of the internal systems of the body.

intoxication The result of alcohol acting as a depressant on the central nervous system; drunkenness.

intrauterine device (IUD) A small plastic or stainless steel contraceptive device that is placed inside a woman's uterus by a physician.

involuntary smoking When a person is around or near a person who is smoking, it is the act of inhaling the smoke that is in the air.

isokinetic contraction A muscular contraction where the speed of the contraction is kept constant against a variable resistance.

isometric activities Activities that involve muscular force against an immovable object to cause muscular contraction.

isotonic activities Activities that involve exerting muscular force throughout the range of motion of a joint to cause muscular contraction.

J

Jarvik 7, Jarvik 7-70 An artificial heart that temporarily replaces a real heart until a donor heart can be found. The revised versions of the Jarvik 7 include the Jarvik 7-70 and the Utah Artificial Heart.

jellies, creams, and foams Nonprescription contraceptives.

K

Kaplan's triphasic model Conceptualized human sexual response as consisting of a desire phase, an excitement phase, and a resolution phase.

ketosis In unmanaged diabetes, an excess of ketone buildup bodies in the blood, which can cause coma or death.

kidney transplant   When a kidney fails, a donor kidney can be successfully implanted in the individual, and survival rates are vastly and steadily improving. It is important that the kidney tissue of the donor and the recipient be matched.

L

labor   The process of childbirth.

lactation   Breast-feeding.

lactogenesis   The initiation of milk production after delivery of a baby.

Lamaze method   A type of natural childbirth.

law of reversibility   When training is stopped, a significant loss of working capacity quickly begins.

lean tIssue   TIssue that is composed of muscle, cartilage, skin, bone, connective tissue, or nerves.

lesion   An abnormal change in an organ due to injury or disease.

Librium   A minor tranquilizer used to treat anxiety.

licensed clinical social worker   Person with academic training in social work who specializes in emotional or psychological adjustment.

life event   Something occurring in life that has an influence on health. Examples include stressors, experiences, risks, peer pressure, and many others.

life-style contracting   A systematic approach to making a commitment to life-style change.

limbic system   The seat of emotions and behaviors, which influences both the cortex (thinking center) and hypothalamus (controls stress response).

limerence   The quality of sexual attraction based on chemistry and sexual desire.

lipoprotein   Fatty proteins that transport cholesterol through the bloodstream.

living will   A statement that requests removal from life-support systems if conditions warrant.

low-density lipoprotein (LDL)   Considered bad types of cholesterol because they allow the cholesterol to circulate in the bloodstream.

luteinizing hormone (LH)   A female hormone.

lysergic acid diethylamide (LSD)   A hallucinogenic drug of abuse.

M

macrominerals   Inorganic compounds that are required in relatively large amounts by the body and include calcium, magnesium, sodium, potassium, phosphorus, sulfur, and chlorine.

malignant tumors   Cancerous growths.

masochism   Sexual gratification from experiencing pain.

masturbation   Self-stimulation for sexual pleasure.

maximal aerobic power   The point at which the heart and circulatory system cannot deliver more oxygen to the tissues without approaching exhaustion.

medical-scientific language   Concrete and technical words.

Medicare   Federally administered medical assistance plan for persons over the age of sixty-five.

meditation   The skill of focusing on a "mantra" to achieve a state of relaxation.

megadoses   Amounts of vitamins that are many times higher than the Recommended Dietary Allowances.

menarche   The onset of menstruation.

menopause   The cessation of menstruation.

menstrual cycle   Series of biological events in females that facilitate reproduction.

menstruation   Periodic discharge of blood from the uterus through the vagina.

mental disorders   A general term used to describe the entire range of disorders where the individual does not mentally function in a rational manner.

mental health   The capacity to cope with life situations, grow emotionally through them, develop to full potentials, and grow in awareness and consciousness.

mescaline   A hallucinogenic drug of abuse, derived from the peyote cactus.

metastasis   Detached cancer cells that are carried to other parts of the body.

methadone   A synthetic narcotic drug of abuse; used as a treatment for heroin addiction.

mifepristone (RU486)   Chemical that blocks hormonal action needed to begin or sustain pregnancy.

minerals   Inorganic elements essential for bodily functioning.

minipIll   Progestin-only pill. The progestin inhibits implantation and causes the cervical mucus to become thicker, making it more difficult for the sperm to get through.

miscarriage (spontaneous abortion)   A naturally occurring abortion.

monilia or candidiasis   A common vaginal infection (yeast infection) caused by flourishing candida albicans due to an upset in a woman's internal balance.

monosaccharide   A simple carbohydrate consisting of one molecule of sugar (glucose, fructose, or galactose) that is the basic structural unit of simple carbohydrates.

monounsaturated   A type of unsaturated fat that has little effect on the amount of cholesterol in the blood.

moral dimension of human sexuality   Involves questions of right and wrong.

morphine   A narcotic drug used to relieve pain; it can also be abused.

motivation   Reason for changing behavior.

mourning   The social response to the state of bereavement such as wearing black and having funerals.

multiphasic pill   Varies the amount of estrogen and progesterone throughout the menstrual cycle to more closely match the amounts of these hormones naturally occurring within the female.

mumps A childhood disease characterized by infected salivary glands and swollen parotid glands (floor of the mouth).

mutations When a gene makes a permanent change during the process of cell division.

myocardial infarction Heart attack.

N

narcotics Drugs of abuse containing opium and opium derivatives.

National Advertising Division (NAD) A division of the Council of Better Business Bureaus to promote standards and handle complaints.

natural childbirth Drug-free childbirth.

nicotine An alkaloid poison; the addictive drug that is in tobacco.

nicotine gum Sold under the name of nicorette, a gum that contains about two milligrams of nicotine designed to substitute for smoking cigarettes.

nicotine skin or arm patch Nicotine-containing patch placed on the arm that delivers about one milligram of nicotine per hour as a substitute for smoking.

nongonococcal urethritis (NGU) or nonspecific urethritis (NSU) Several diseases including chlamydia are included among the nongonococcal urethritis or nonspecific urethritis diseases because they cause the inflammation of the urethra but not by gonococcus bacteria.

nuclear family Parents and children living together under the same roof; also called conjugal family.

nurse practitioner Registered nurse with advanced training in a particular medical specialty.

nurturing Giving care and attention to the strength-producing dimension of life.

nutrients The elements in food that are useful to the body.

nymphomania An extremely high sex drive that dominates the lives of certain women.

O

obstetrics and gynecology One of the medical specialties; the scientific management of women during pregnancy, childbirth, and after birth.

occupational health Feelings of comfort and accomplishment related to one's daily tasks.

oligospermia Low sperm count.

ophthalmologist Medical doctor who treats and performs surgery for eye disorders.

optimizing Striving to reach high levels of health in one health dimension at a time.

optometrist Nonmedical trained person who specializes in measuring visual acuity and in vision correction.

oral contraceptive The birth-control pill; the pill.

orgasm The peak of pleasure in sexual excitement; usually accompanied in the male by ejaculation; one of the four phases of human sexual response.

osteoarthritis A type of arthritis characterized by degeneration of the joint cartilage.

osteopathic physician A physician who has been trained in a college of osteopathic medicine.

osteoporosis Loss of bone material, which may result in loss of bone mass.

ovary A gland in the female that provides ova and certain hormones.

Over the counter (OTC) Proprietary drugs that can be purchased without a doctor's signature.

overload principle A principle of exercise; it states that one must place stress on the relevant part of the body to improve physical capacity.

overstimulation When demands placed on an individual exceed the capability to respond.

oviduct Another name for the fallopian tube.

ovulation The release of an egg from the ovary.

ovum The female egg.

oxygen debt The amount of oxygen used during recovery from physical activity over and above the amount that usually would have been used during that time at rest.

ozone layer Part of the stratosphere that acts as a shield protecting against the sun's ultraviolet light.

P

pairing The process of anchoring in your brain desired emotions and then finding some trigger to access and assume the desired emotional state.

paranoid disorders Also called delusional disorder; characterized by the presence of persistent delusions (conditions that are not true).

paraphilia Various sexual opinions; means love *(philia)* beyond the usual *(para)*.

paraquat A defoliant (plant killer).

particulate matter Minute, harmful substances in cigarette smoke.

pediatrics Medical specialty dealing with the treatment of children.

pedophilia The use of children as sexual objects.

pelvic inflammatory disease (PID) Inflammation of the female genital tract; a complication of sexually transmitted disease.

peptic ulcer An ulcer in the stomach area.

perinatal death When an infant dies within hours or days after birth.

personality The mental mechanisms, traits, experiences, and complex intricacies of the individual that determine how they behave, feel, and think.

peyote A form of cactus; mescaline is derived from its buttons.

phencyclidine (PCP) A hallucinogenic drug of abuse; also called angel dust.

photochemical smog   The primary air pollutant; the product of sunlight and auto and industrial exhausts.

physical fitness   Cardiorespiratory capacity, flexibility, muscular endurance, and strength are possessed at levels that are optimal for health and functioning of the body.

physical health   Efficient bodily functioning, resistance to disease, and the physical capacity to respond to varied events.

physically dependent   A condition in which a person has a biochemical need to continue using a particular drug to prevent withdrawal symptoms.

physician assistant (P.A.)   Under a physician's supervision, a P.A. does many basic tasks of a physician.

physiological dependence   Heavy alcohol consumption from three to fifteen years that results in a dependency on alcohol evidenced by withdrawal symptoms when drinking is stopped or decreased.

pituitary gland   Small oval endocrine gland that receives stimuli from the hypothalamus to trigger the stress response by stimulating the adrenal glands (releasing adrenocorticotropic hormone) and the thyroid glands (releasing thyrotropic hormone).

placebo effect   Subjects show improvement just because there are expectations for improvement (e.g., taking a sugar pill).

placenta   The organ connecting the fetus to the uterus via the umbilical cord.

plateau phase   The second phase of human sexual response.

polyunsaturated   A fat or vegetable oil that is usually liquid at room temperature.

pornography   Pictures or words related to sexuality.

positive addiction   Activity that an individual participates in on a regular basis that provides strength, comfort, and support. If the activity is not done, it is upsetting.

positive reinforcement   A technique in which the positive aspects of a person's endeavor to break a habit, in this case smoking, are rewarded.

preeclampsia   A mild form of hypertension in women.

pregnancy   The condition of being with child.

prenuptial agreement   Arrangements made prior to marriage by those planning to be married regarding assets, conditions of the marriage, situations that may arise, possible breakup, and other personal aspects of the relationship.

primary prevention   Prevention of a disease before symptoms appear.

principle of specificity   In fitness training, the concept of training for the component the individual wants to improve.

problem drinking   Repetitive use of alcohol that causes physical, psychological, or social harm to the drinker and/or others.

problematic adjustment   The person has not adjusted and therapy is probably needed. Evident behaviors might include use of chemical substances to adjust, violence, and difficulty controlling behavior.

progesterone   A female hormone that works with estrogen to prepare the uterine lining for pregnancy.

proof   The measure of a beverage's alcohol content; it represents roughly twice the value of the percentage of alcohol.

prostaglandins   Fatty acid substances found naturally in the body; can possibly be used for inducing labor during an abortion (still in research stage).

prostate gland   A male organ located below the bladder; it secretes the fluid that is part of semen.

prostitution   Refers to any situation in which one person pays another for sexual gratification.

protective skill   Skill used to prepare people to deal with life's problems while promoting higher levels of health.

protein   A compound consisting of carbon, oxygen, hydrogen, and nitrogen; one of the nutrients.

psychiatry   Medical specialty dealing with the diagnosis, treatment, and prevention of mental illness.

psychoanalysis   A type of psychotherapy in which the patient reflects on his or her life to find solutions to problems.

psychogenic psychosomatic disorder   Structural or functional disorders such as migraine headaches, ulcers, and asthma, that are worsened or caused by mental or emotional distress.

psychological dependence   A state in which the user's craving for a particular drug may be so intense as to alter behavior.

psychological dimension of human sexuality   Reflects attitudes and feelings toward ourselves and others.

psychological hardiness   Psychological characteristics that seem to protect an individual against the effects of type A behavior, including personal control, commitment, and challenge.

psychosis   Mental illness.

psychosomatic disease   Physical symptoms that have an emotional or mental origin.

Q

quackery   Methods and/or devices used to deceive the public about health/medical care.

R

radioactive pollution   Addition of enough radioactive matter to a natural body of water that the aquatic ecosystem is damaged.

rape   Forced sexual intercourse.

RDA (Recommended Dietary Allowances)   The levels of nutrient intake that are necessary for the maintenance of good nutrition of practically all healthy people.

recycle   The reusing of specific elements, such as aluminum cans.

reflective listening   Paraphrasing a speaker's words to be sure that the message was communicated.

refractory period   The period following sexual intercourse in which the male is unable to have another erection.

rehabilitation   The process of restoring a person's bodily or psychological functioning for a healthier life-style.

resilient adjustment   The optimal type of adaptation resulting from learning new skills, developing more self-understanding, and better comprehending personal, social, and environment influences. There are more protective factors and skills to use in the future. The process of coping with disruptive, stressful, or challenging life events in a way that provides the individual with additional protective and coping skills than prior to the disruption.

resistance stage   The second stage of the general adaptation syndrome characterized by the body attempting to return to homeostasis by building energy stores and hormones.

resolution phase   One of the four phases of human sexual response; a time when the body tends to return to its preexcitement stage.

responsible drinking   Making provision to be taken home if planning to drink, understanding limits through the calculation of blood alcohol concentration, and recognizing when enough alcohol has been consumed.

Rh incompatibility   Refers to a situation in which a mother's blood is Rh negative and her child's is Rh positive, which can create complications in future pregnancies because the mother develops antibodies in response to the child's positive Rh factor.

rheumatic heart disease   An inflammatory disease centered in the valves of the heart.

rheumatoid arthritis   The most crippling form of arthritis characterized by inflammation of the joints, stiffness, swelling, and pain.

rhythm method (fertility awareness)   A method of birth control based on abstinence from intercourse during the woman's fertile period.

rickettsiae   Minute bacteria-like organisms just visible with a light microscope; they demand the presence of living tissue and cannot be grown in a laboratory. They grow in the intestinal tract of insects called vectors. They are considered to be borderline between bacteria and viruses. They may cause diseases such as typhus and Rocky Mountain spotted fever.

risk assessment   Applies to the study of environmental health. It is a scientific estimation of likelihood of health problems occurring as a result of exposure to chemicals.

RU 486   See mifepristone.

rubella, or German measles   A childhood disease caused by a virus that results in a rash and perhaps a fever and swollen lymph glands.

rubeola, or red measles   A severe form of measles with rash, fever, coughing, and runny nose.

S

sadism   Sexual gratification from inflicting pain on another.

saline induction   A type of abortion in which a saline solution is injected into the amniotic sac; it is used during the second trimester of pregnancy.

sanitary landfill   Area where solid waste is buried.

satiety center   The area of the brain that signals fullness after eating.

saturated   A fat derived mainly from animal sources. It is usually solid at room temperature.

satyriasis   Excessive sexual drive in a male.

schizophrenic disorders   Presence of deteriorating psychotic symptoms such as hallucinations, delusions, and disturbances in emotions and thinking.

scopophilia   See voyeurism.

secondary prevention   Treatment of a disease at an early stage that attempts to keep it from worsening.

self-actualization   Fulfilling human potential along with the fulfilling of basic needs (physiological, safety, love, self-esteem).

self-counseling   The process of asking yourself key questions, allowing time to let your brain process, sort through emotions and facts, and ultimately arrive at acceptable solutions or resolutions.

self-esteem   Perceived sense of self-worth, self-confidence, and satisfaction with oneself.

seminal vesicles   A pair of glands in the male; they provide a portion of the ejaculate that contributes to the activation of the sperm.

seminiferous tubules   Coiled tubes in the male testes in which the sperm are produced.

sexual abuse   Forcing one's will upon another in sexual behavior.

sexual dysfunction   Chronic inability to respond sexually in a way that one finds satisfying.

sexual harassment   Sexual abuse, including verbal abuse, sexist remarks, unwanted physical contact, leering or ogling, demand for sexual favors in return for some favorable treatment, and actual physical assault.

sexuality   A four-dimensional (social, psychological, moral, biological) aspect of each person's personality that influences total well-being.

sexually transmitted diseases (STDs)   Diseases spread by sexual contact (venereal diseases) such as gonorrhea, syphilis, and herpes genitalis.

sidestream smoke   Smoke that comes directly from the source, such as cigarette, cigar, or pipe, or exhalation from a smoker that still contains the negative elements of tobacco smoke.

similarity factors Characteristics that are alike.

simple carbohydrates The building blocks of carbohydrates, which consist of fructose, glucose, and galactose.

single-parent family Family with only one parent.

sinsemilla Marijuana that is grown with hi-tech hydroponics, which produces THC levels much higher than when grown in natural mediums.

sinusitis Inflammation of the sinuses.

smokeless tobacco Tobacco that is used orally in three forms—snuff, looseleaf, and plug forms.

snuff A type of tobacco that is inhaled through the nostrils, chewed or placed against the gums.

social dimension of human sexuality Sum of cultural factors that influence thoughts and actions.

social health Good relations with others, a supportive culture, and successful adaptation to the environment.

social pressure The desire to (or the belief that we need to) go along with or rebel against others.

sodium A macromineral that is involved in the regulation of acid-base balance, the maintenance of osmotic pressure of body fluid, and the preservation of muscle irritability and the permeability of cells.

sodomy Technically applies to anal intercourse; however, the term is commonly used to refer to any sexual activity the speaker considers unnatural.

somatoform disorder A disorder that occurs when the brain, subconsciously, determines that the person is sick and the body develops physical symptoms.

somatogenic psychosomatic disorder Disorder that occurs when the body's resistance (immune system) is weakened as a result of stress.

sperm The male reproductive cell.

spermicide Sperm-killing chemical.

sphygmomanometer The instrument used to measure blood pressure.

spiritual health The ability to discover and articulate a personal purpose in life, to learn how to experience love, joy, peace, and fulfillment, and to help yourself and others achieve full potential.

sponge Contraceptive method that absorbs and kills sperm and serves as a barrier.

spontaneous abortion *See* miscarriage.

spontaneous remission When a disease reverses or cures itself without medical intervention.

spot reduction The attempt to remove fat from a certain part of the body.

stages of alcoholism The gradual decline from social drinking to alcoholism, including the early stage (increased drinking and tolerance), middle stage (conceals drinking, drinks alone, normal functioning affected, feels bad), and final stage (lives to drink, extreme personality changes).

stages of dying Five predictable but not universally applicable psychological stages through which a person passes during the course of a chronic terminal disease. The stages generally include denial, anger, bargaining, depression, and acceptance.

starch A complex carbohydrate from a plant source.

stepfamily When one or both parents have children from a previous marriage.

stereotyping Shared conventional expectations of how people in a certain group should behave; falsely assuming that all members of a group have common characteristics.

sterilization A surgical procedure that renders the individual incapable of reproduction.

stillborn When an infant is born dead.

storage fat The extra fat maintained by the body in the fat cells.

street language The language of graffiti—learned from peers.

strength intervention Includes four stages: assessing, nurturing, freeing, and optimizing.

stress The nonspecific response of the body to any demand made on it.

stress response The physiological arousal that occurs as a result of stressors.

stressor People, situations, or thoughts that trigger the stress response.

stroke A cardiovascular disease in which the blood supply is cut off to a portion of the brain, causing paralysis, aphasia, and/or death.

subcutaneous fat Fat beneath the skin.

substitution Substituting positive behaviors for negative behaviors or for nonproductive time.

sucrose Sugar.

suction curettage A type of abortion in which the uterine contents are sucked out through a narrow tube; it is the most widely used method of abortion performed up until the twelfth week of pregnancy.

sudden infant death syndrome (SIDS) The death of babies between one and three months of age; they die suddenly without warning, generally while sleeping.

suicide The intentional killing of oneself.

support group Group of people who can aid behavior change.

surgery Medical specialty dealing with operative procedures for correction of disease or deformity.

surgicenter A facility capable of providing minor, low risk, outpatient surgery.

susceptible host An organism that is vulnerable to harboring and nourishing a parasite.

swinging A mutual agreement in which a couple opens up their relationship to include sexual encounters with others.

symptothermal method Combination of BBT and cervical mucus methods.

synergistic Describes the effects of two different drugs that in combination are greater than the sum of their individual effects—a multiplying of effects.

syphilis   An infectious sexually transmitted disease caused by a bacterium *(Treponema pallidum)* with an incubation period of twelve to twenty days.

systematic enhancement   An approach to using a strength to deal with a weakness.

systolic pressure   The highest point of the blood pressure, measured when the heart contracts.

T

target zone   Sixty to 80 percent of maximal aerobic power.

teetotaler   Person who does not drink alcoholic beverages; abstainer.

teratogen   Substances that may cause birth defects or diseases in infants.

tertiary prevention   Rehabilitation; the lessening or eliminating of the serious effects of a disease.

testes   Two oval glands in the scrotum of the male that produce sperm and testosterone.

testosterone   The male hormone that affects the development of male sex characteristics and sex drive.

thanatologist   A person who studies death and dying.

thermal pollution   Addition of enough heat to a natural body of water that the aquatic ecosystem is damaged.

thrombus   A blood clot, usually one located at the point of its formation, in a blood vessel or a chamber of the heart.

thyroid gland   An endocrine gland that is stimulated by the pituitary gland to secrete thyroxine, which increases metabolic functions.

tolerance   A condition in which it takes increasingly larger amounts of alcohol to produce the same effects previously felt at lower levels of alcohol intake.

toxicity   When a chemical becomes poisonous; it depends upon the exposure and dose of chemicals and negative effects.

trace minerals   Inorganic compounds that are required in small amounts.

tranquilizer   A depressant drug used medically to relieve tension and anxiety; a drug of abuse as a "downer."

transsexual   A person who feels trapped in the body of the wrong sex.

transvestite   A person who gets sexual gratification from wearing clothes of the opposite sex.

trichomoniasis   Inflammation of the vagina and urethra caused by infection with trichomonas vaginalis (a protozoan parasite).

trigger response   Reminder that can help support behavior change, such as music, a poster, or a future reward.

triglyceride   The main type of lipid (fatty substance) in food. It is composed of three fatty acids that are bonded to glycerol. It is associated with an increased risk of cardiovascular disease.

troilism   Having sexual relations with a person while a third person watches.

tubal ligation   A female sterilization procedure in which the fallopian tubes are severed.

tumors   A mass of tissue.

type A behavior pattern   A person who is competitive, impatient, a polyphasic thinker (thinks of two or more things at once), has a sense of time urgency, and is openly or inwardly hostile.

type B behavior pattern   A person who lacks the characteristics of the type A behavior pattern, that is, who takes one thing at a time, concentrates effectively, is flexible, and does not get upset if daily tasks are not completed.

type I diabetes   Also called insulin-dependent diabetes mellitus, formerly called juvenile onset diabetes; the more severe form of diabetic cases, characterized by the absolute lack of insulin.

type II diabetes   Also called noninsulin-dependent diabetes mellitus, accounts for 85 percent to 90 percent of all diabetic cases. This form of diabetes is not as severe and generally occurs later in life (generally after forty). Insulin is produced by the beta cells but is insufficient to deal with glucose load.

U

ultrasound   The use of sound waves for medical detection and treatment purposes.

umbilical cord   The cord that provides nourishment from the mother to the fetus.

unsaturated   A fat derived mainly from vegetable sources; it is usually liquid at room temperature.

uremia   The accumulation of waste products in the body's tissues.

urethra   The tube through which urine passes from the bladder out of the body.

urgent care center   A facility that provides treatment without an appointment for minor problems such as sprained ankles, sore throats, and cuts needing stitches.

USRDA (U.S. Recommended Daily Allowances) Standards used to assess nutritional status and evaluate food supply.

uterus   The stretchable, pear-shaped organ in the female in which a baby develops; the womb.

V

vaccine   A preparation of dead or live attenuated (weakened) viruses or bacteria used to prevent infectious diseases by inducing active immunity.

vagina   The female organ that receives the penis during coitus and provides passage for the infant during birth.

vaginal douche   A stream of water or other liquid directed into the vagina for sanitary or medical reasons.

Valium   A widely prescribed tranquilizer that causes drowsiness and respiratory depression.

value   Something one believes and cherishes.

value-behavioral congruence   The harmony between what someone believes to be right and behaving or acting in accordance with that belief. Value-behavioral congruence results in inner peace and incongruence results in guilt.

vas deferens   A pair of tubes in the male extending from the epididymis to the prostate; they serve as the passageways for the sperm.

vasectomy   A male sterilization procedure in which the vas deferens are severed.

vasoconstrictor   A drug that narrows the blood vessels and reduces the oxygen supply.

vasodilators   Drugs or nerves that cause a widening of the opening of blood vessels.

vectors   Organisms that transmit disease from one host (person) to another.

vegetarian   Someone who consumes the majority of nutrients from plant sources.

very low-density lipoprotein (VLDL)   Considered bad types of cholesterol because they allow the cholesterol to circulate in the bloodstream.

virus   The smallest intracellular infectious parasite that is capable of living and reproducing only in living cells. Viruses cause numerous diseases such as measles, mumps, AIDS, hepatitis, herpes, rabies, and many others. Viruses are most difficult to control.

vitamins   Complex organic substances found in food or chemically made; they are essential in small amounts for body processes.

voyeurism   Refers generally to obtaining pleasure from watching people who are undressing or engaging in sexual behavior (same as scopophilia).

W

water-soluble vitamins   Organic substances that are not stored in the body and need to be replaced every day. Include the eight B vitamins and vitamin C.

withdrawal   Symptoms that occur because of physical dependence on a drug when use of the drug is stopped. Also, symptoms that occur because of physical dependence on alcohol when use of alcohol is stopped, ranging from a hangover to the delirium tremens.

Y

yoga   A system of flexibility exercises used to obtain mental and bodily control.

Z

Zilbergeld and Ellison's model   A five-component model of sexual response.

zoophilia   *See* bestiality.

zygote   A single cell resulting from the union of a sperm and an egg.

Credits

Illustrations

Chapter 1

Figure 1.4: This figure is reprinted with permission from the Journal of Health Education 21(6):33–39, 1990. Journal of Health Education is a publication of the American Alliance for Health, Physical Education, Recreation and Dance, 1900 Association Drive, Reston, Va 22091.

Chapter 3

Figure 3.2: "The Cholesterol Maze." Copyright 1991 by Consumers Union of U.S., Inc., Yonkers, NY 10703-1057. Reprinted by permission from *Consumer Reports On Health,* November 1991. **Figure 3.4:** From Nanci Hellmich, "Consumer Guide to Reading the New Food Label" in *USA Today,* December 3, 1992. Copyright 1992, USA TODAY. Reprinted with permission.

Chapter 4

Figure 4.2: From L. Zohman, M.D., *Beyond Diet: Exercise Your Way to Fitness & Heart Health,* CPC International, Englewood Cliffs, New Jersey.

Chapter 5

Figure 5.1: From *USA Today,* January 22, 1992. Data from Bruskin/Goldring Research poll of 1,002 for Ultra Slim-Fast. Copyright 1992, USA TODAY. Reprinted with permission. **Figure 5.3:** Reprinted by permission. In Eating Disorders Information Packet, The National Anorexic Aid Society of Harding Hospital, Columbus, Ohio, 1990.

Chapter 7

Figure 7.5: From William H. Masters and Virginia E. Johnson, *Human Sexual Response,* p. 5. Little, Brown, Boston, 1966.
Figure 7.6: From William H. Masters and Virginia E. Johnson, *Human Sexual Response,* p. 5. Little, Brown, Boston, 1966.

Chapter 8

Figure 8.1: From John W. Hole., Jr., *Human Anatomy and Physiology,* 5th edition. Copyright © 1990 Wm. C. Brown Communications, Inc., Dubuque, Iowa. All Rights Reserved. Reprinted by permission. **Figure 8.2:** From John W. Hole., Jr., *Human Anatomy and Physiology,* 5th edition. Copyright © 1990 Wm. C. Brown Communications, Inc., Dubuque, Iowa. All Rights Reserved. Reprinted by permission. **Figure 8.5:** From John W. Hole., Jr., *Human Anatomy and Physiology,* 5th edition. Copyright © 1990 Wm. C. Brown Communications, Inc., Dubuque, Iowa. All Rights Reserved. Reprinted by permission. **Figure 8.6:** From Stuart Ira Fox, *Human Physiology,* 4th edition. Copyright © 1993 Wm. C. Brown Communications, Inc., Dubuque, Iowa. All Rights Reserved. Reprinted by permission. **Figure 8.8:** From Kent M. Van De Graaff and Stuart Ira Fox, *Concepts of Human Anatomy and Physiology,* 3d edition. Copyright © 1992 Wm. C. Brown Communications, Inc., Dubuque, Iowa. All Rights Reserved. Reprinted by permission. **Figure 8.13:** Reproduced with the permission of The Alan Guttmacher Institute from Susan Harlap,

Kathryn Kost, and Jacqueline Darroch Forrest, *Preventing Pregnancy, Protecting Health: a New Look at Birth Control Choices in the United States,* 1991. **Figure 8.14:** From John W. Hole, Jr., *Human Anatomy and Physiology,* 5th edition. Copyright © 1990 Wm. C. Brown Communications, Inc., Dubuque, Iowa. All Rights Reserved. Reprinted by permission.

Chapter 13

Figure 13.7: Reproduced with permission. (c) "How Stroke Affects Behavior," 1992. Copyright American Heart Association.
Figure 13.8: Used by permission, American Cancer Society, Inc.

Chapter 15

Figure 15.3: From *World Population Prospects as Assessed in 1980* (United Nations publication, Sales. No. E.81.XIII.8). **Figure 15.4:** From *World Population Prospects as Assessed in 1980* (United Nations publication, Sales. No. E.81.XIII.8). **Figure 15.5:** From Anne Nadakavukaren, *Man and Environment: A Health Perspective,* 2d edition, p. 281. Copyright © 1986 Waveland Press, Prospect Heights, Ill. Reprinted by permission.

Computer Graphics by Publication Services, Champaign, IL: 3.2, 3.3, 3.4, 4.3, 5.1, 11.3, TA 14.4, TA 5.1
Computer Graphics by WCB Illustration, Dubuque, IA: 1.3, 4.1, 8.1, 8.14, 13.7

Index

Exhibitionism, 152
Expectorants, 264
Extended families, 135
External stressors, 33–34, 46–48
Extramarital sexual activity, 139–40
Exxon Valdez disaster, 346

F

Facial cleansers, advertising claims for, 353
Fackelmann, K. A., 245, 252
FAE (fetal alcohol effect), 232
Faith healing, 368–69
Fallopian tube (oviduct), 166
Fallout, radiation from, 348
Families, 9, 134–37
Family history, 281
Family relationships, homosexuality and, 153–54
Family therapy, 56
Family violence, alcohol and, 225
Farley, D., 360, 376
FAS (fetal alcohol syndrome), 171, 231–32
Fast foods, nutrition and, 81
Fat, 73–76
Fat cell hyperplasia, 115
Fat cell hypertrophy, 115
Fat cravings, 114–15
Fat-soluble vitamins, 73, 76
Fat tissue, 111
Fatty acids, 74
Federal Comprehensive Smoking Education Act, 241
Federal Trade Commission (FTC), 356, 359, 362
Federal Water Pollution Control Act of 1948, 340
Fein, J., 155, 160
Fellatio, 152
Felten, D. L., 25, 26
Feltman, J., 377
Female condom, 180, 274–75
Females, 97, 315. *See also* Gender eating disorders in, 120, 121
Fentanyl, 205–6
Fertility awareness (rhythm method), 181, 185
Fertility drugs, 169
Fetal alcohol effect (FAE), 232
Fetal alcohol syndrome (FAS), 171, 231–32
Fetishism, 152
Fetoscopy, 172, 302
Fetus, 167
Fiber, 69
Fight-or-flight response, 44
First aid kit, 386
Fischman, J., 37, 57
Fitness, 94–96
Fitness program, 101–5
"Five-Day Plan," for smoking cessation, 249–50
Flach, F. F., 14, 24
Flagyl, 274
Flannery, R. B., 38, 57
Flax, E., 133, 144, 156, 160

Fluid replacement, in diets of athletes, 85–86
Follicles, 164
Follicle-stimulating hormone (FSH), 163–64
Food additives, 81
Food and Drug Administration (FDA), 236, 356, 373, 383
    heart transplantation and, 289
    nutrition labeling and, 83
    product approval process of, 362
    regulation of serving sizes, 84
Food and Nutrition Board (National Research Council), 65
Food choices, 63, 79–81
Food endorsement program (AHA), 84
Food Guide Pyramid (USDA), 79–80
Food irradiation, 83
Food labeling, misinformation in, 84
Forced matrix, for problem solving, 49
Forrest, J. D., 185, 190
Fox, E., 131, 144
Fox, Stuart Ira, 173
Frantz, T. T., 327, 330
Free-basing, 208
Friedman, H., 253
Friedman, M., 37, 57
Frigidity, 151
Frottage, 153
Frustration, 33–34, 46
FSH (follicle-stimulating hormone), 163–64
FTC (Federal Trade Commission), 356, 359, 362
Fulton, G. B., 188, 190
Funerals, 324–25
Fungi, 263
Furey, E. M., 232, 234

G

Galizio, M., 229, 231, 234
Gallager, W., 205, 206, 216
Galli, N., 9, 24, 367–69, 376
Gangrene, diabetes mellitus and, 299
Gas chromatography/mass spectrometry (GC/MS), 212, 213
GAS (general adaptation syndrome), 44–45
Gauthier, M. M., 97, 106
Gavin, J., 102, 106
Gaylord, S. A., 311, 330
GC/MS (gas chromatography/mass spectrometry), 212, 213
Gender. *See also* Females; Males
    aging and, 314–15, 317
    cancer and, 290, 291
    eating disorders and, 120, 121
    pedophilia and, 156
    smoking and, 245
    stroke and, 287
General adaptation syndrome (GAS), 44–45
Generic drugs, 359
Genetic counseling, 172
Genetic disease, 302
Genetic influences, on pregnancy, 170–72
Genetic mutations, 290
Genital warts (condylomas), 274
Gerald, M., 205, 209, 210, 216

German measles (rubella), 266–67
Gerontology, 311
Getz, K. A., 267, 276
Gibbons, B., 222, 234
Gilbert, S., 119, 121, 123
Girdano, D. A., 45, 47, 51, 57, 203, 208, 209, 216, 220, 234, 243, 246, 252
Glasgow, R. E., 244, 252
Glasser, W., 39, 57
Global warming, 342–44
Glomeruli, 299
Glucose, 65
Glutethimide (Doriden), 209, 210
Glycogen, 69, 72
Godin, G., 103, 107
Goepp (cervical) cap, for birth control, 182
Gonorrhea, 271, 382
Goodloe, N. R., 5, 24
Gordon, S., 137, 138, 144
Gout, 302, 303
Grand mal convulsions, depressants and, 209
Green, D. E., 244, 252
Greenberg, J., 86, 88, 151, 160
Greenberg, J. S., 12, 24
Greenhouse effect, 342–43
Grieger, L., 289, 304
Grieving, 325–28
Grisham, J. W., 345, 351
Grocery Manufacturers Association, 84
Groves, M. M., 136, 144
Gruber, J. R., 157, 160
Guest, responsibilities of, 227–28
Gurin, J., 116, 123
Guthrie, H., 65, 88
Guthrie, O., 139, 144
Gwinnell, Donald, 226
Gynecology, 365

H

Hallfrisch, J., 311, 330
Hallucinogens, 210–11
Hamburger, M. I., 266, 276
Hamilton, K., 119, 123
Hamrick, M. H., 10, 24
Hansen, G. R., 264, 276
Hansen, J. C., 327, 330
Hanson, P. G., 44, 57
Hantula, R., 188, 190
Haraldsson, E., 322
Harvard Medical School definition of death, 320
Hastings Center Report on euthanasia, 321
Hatcher, R., 178, 190
Hawks, R. L., 213, 216
Hazardous air pollutants, 341
Hazardous waste incidents, 346
Hazard recognition, disaster preparedness and, 388
HCG (human chorionic gonadotropin), 170
HDL (high-density lipoprotein), 283
Health, 5–6, 8, 14–15
    weight control and, 109
Health actions, 10

Y

Z